CLINICAL NEUROSURGERY

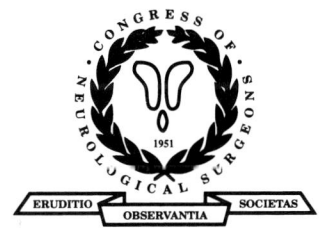

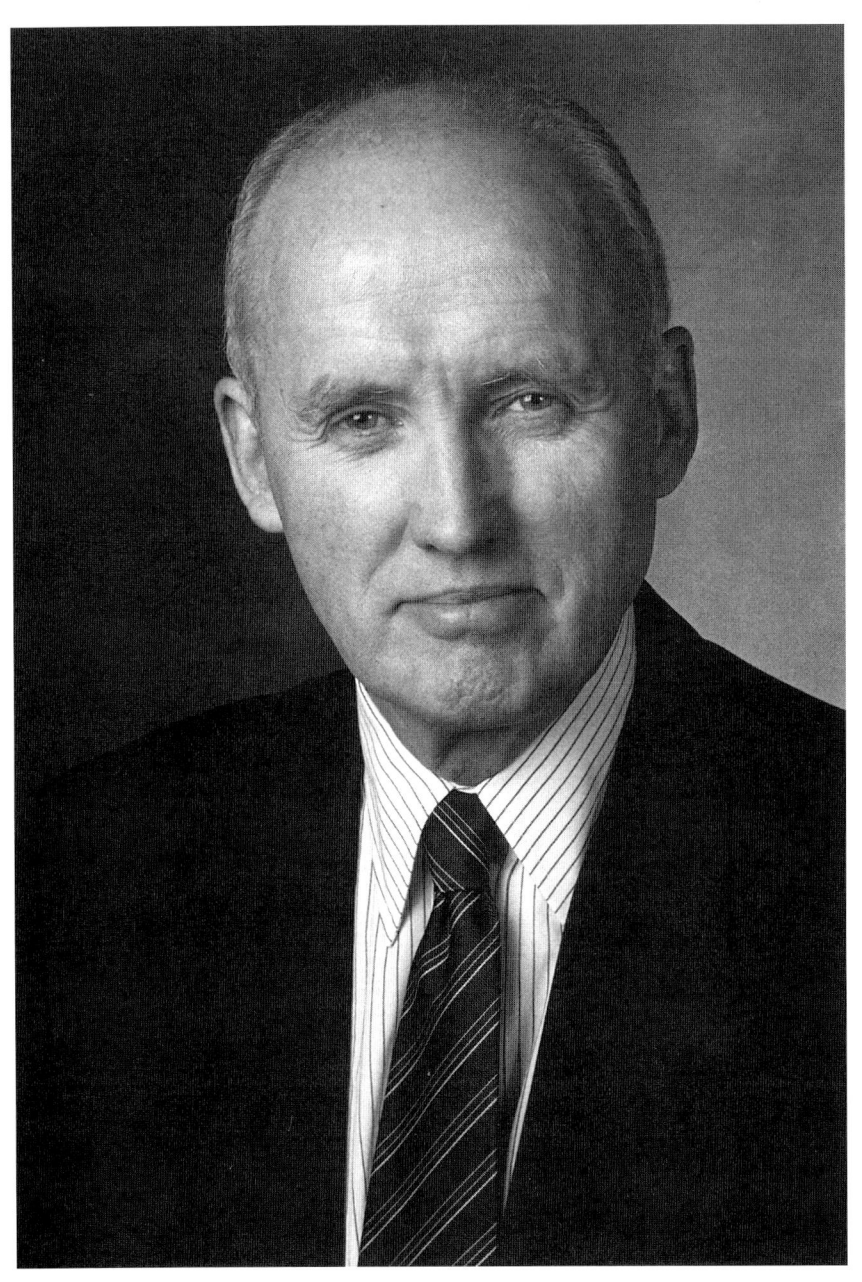

John M. Tew, Jr., M.D., FACS

CLINICAL NEUROSURGERY

Volume 46

Proceedings

OF THE
CONGRESS OF NEUROLOGICAL SURGEONS

Seattle, Washington
1998

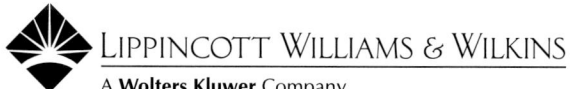

A **Wolters Kluwer** Company
Philadelphia • Baltimore • New York • London
Buenos Aires • Hong Kong • Sydney • Tokyo

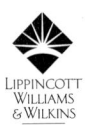

Copyright © 2000
THE CONGRESS OF NEUROLOGICAL SURGEONS

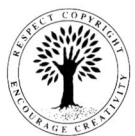

All rights reserved. This book is protected by copyright. No part of this book may be reproduced in any form or by any means, including photocopying, or utilized by any information storage and retrieval system without written permission from the copyright holder.

Accurate indications, adverse reactions, and dosage schedules for drugs are provided in this book, but it is possible that they may change. The reader is urged to review the package information data of the manufacturers of the medications mentioned.

Printed in the United States of America
(ISBN 0-7817-2533-X)

Preface

The 48th Annual Meeting of the Congress of Neurological Surgeons was held at the Washington State Convention and Trade Center in Seattle Washington for October 3–8, 1998. Volume 46 of Clinical Neurosurgery represents the official compendium of the platform presentations from that meeting.

The Annual Meeting Chairman, Dr. Mark N. Hadley, and the Scientific Program Chairman, Dr. Issam A. Awad, organized and led an outstanding meeting. The honored guest, Dr. John M. Tew, contributed to the high caliber of the meeting with his thoughtful and clear descriptions of skull base disorders and bringing technical innovations into neurosurgery. Dr. William A. Friedman, in his Presidential Address, challenged us to reflect on the meaning of life with his patient vignettes. As part of the long standing tradition of the Congress, the CNS Resident Award, given to Dr. Robert Friedlander, for his work on reduction of apoptotic cell loss after traumatic brain injury using caspase inhibitors is included in this volume.

The members and guests of the Congress enjoyed glorious sunny weather in a city renowned for rain (and as a resident of that city for 12 years, I can attest to the weather patterns!). All participants of the multiple meeting committees should be congratulated on their work. I would like to thank the contributors to Clinical Neurosurgery for their cooperation and timeliness in submitting their manuscripts and to my associate editors for their prompt and thorough editing of those manuscripts. I would also like to thank Vicki Vaughn at Lippincott Williams & Wilkins who has been extraordinarily patient in getting this volume together as I transitioned from the University of Washington to my present position at the University of Pennsylvania. Finally, I would like to acknowledge the efforts of my secretary at the University of Washington, Rosetta Marx, for her organizational skills in assembling this text. This is my last volume as editor and I wish my successor the best.

M. SEAN GRADY, M.D.
Editor

MATTHEW A. HOWARD III, M.D.
Associate Editor

MARYLOU HLAVIN, M.D.
Associate Editor

RICHARD OSENBACH, M.D.
Associate Editor

Honored Guests

1952—Professor Herbert Olivecrona, Stockholm, Sweden
1953—Sir Geoffrey Jefferson, Manchester, England
1954—Dr. Kenneth G. McKenzie, Toronto, Canada
1955—Dr. Carl W. Rand, Los Angeles, California
1956—Dr. Wilder G. Penfield, Montreal, Canada
1957—Dr. Francis C. Grant, Philadelphia, Pennsylvania
1958—Dr. A. Earl Walker, Baltimore, Maryland
1959—Dr. William J. German, New Haven, Connecticut
1960—Dr. Paul C. Bucy, Chicago, Illinois
1961—Professor Eduard A. V. Busch, Copenhagen, Denmark
1962—Dr. Bronson S. Ray, New York, New York
1963—Dr. James L. Poppen, Boston, Massachusetts
1964—Dr. Edgar A. Kahn, Ann Arbor, Michigan
1965—Dr. James C. White, Boston, Massachusetts
1966—Dr. Hugh A. Kravenbühl, Zurich, Switzerland
1967—Dr. W. James Gardner, Cleveland, Ohio
1968—Professor Normal M. Dott, Edinburgh, Scotland
1969—Dr. Wallace B. Hamby, Cleveland, Ohio
1970—Dr. Barnes Woodhall, Durham, North Carolina
1971—Dr. Elisha S. Gurdjian, Detroit, Michigan
1972—Dr. Francis Murphey, Memphis, Tennessee
1973—Dr. Henry G. Schwartz, St. Louis, Missouri
1974—Dr. Guy L. Odom, Durham, North Carolina
1975—Dr. William A. Sweet, Boston, Massachusetts
1976—Dr. Lyle A. French, Minneapolis, Minnesota
1977—Dr. Richard C. Schneider, Ann Arbor, Michigan
1978—Dr. Charles G. Drake, London, Ontario, Canada
1979—Dr. Frank H. Mayfield, Cincinnati, Ohio
1980—Dr. Eben Alexander, Jr., Winston-Salem, North Carolina
1981—Dr. J. Garber Galbraith, Birmingham, Alabama
1982—Dr. Keiji Sano, Tokyo, Japan
1983—Dr. C. Miller Fisher, Boston, Massachusetts
1984—Dr. Hugo V. Rizzoli, Washington, DC
    Dr. Walter E. Dandy (posthumously), Baltimore, Maryland
1985—Dr. Sidney Goldring, St. Louis, Missouri
1986—Dr. M. Gazi Yasargil, Zurich, Switzerland
1987—Dr. Thomas W. Langfitt, Philadelphia, Pennsylvania

1988—Professor Lindsay Symon, London, England
1989—Dr. Thoralf M. Sundt, Jr., Rochester, Minnesota
1990—Dr. Charles Byron Wilson, San Francisco, California
1991—Dr. Bennett M. Stein, New York, New York
1992—Dr. Robert G. Ojemann, Boston, Massachusetts
1993—Dr. Albert L. Rhoton, Jr., Gainesville, Florida
1994—Dr. Robert F. Spetzler, Phoenix, Arizona
1995—Dr. John A. Jane, Charlottesville, Virginia
1996—Dr. Peter J. Jannetta, Pittsburgh, Pennsylvania
1997—Dr. Nicholas T. Zervas, Boston, Massachusetts
1998—Dr. John M. Tew

Officers of the Congress of Neurological Surgeons
1998

WILLIAM A. FRIEDMAN, M.D.
President

H. HUNT BATJER, M.D.
President-Elect

MITCHELL S. BERGER   MARK N. HADLEY
Vice-President   *Secretary*

STEPHEN M. PAPADOPOULOS, M.D.
Treasurer

EXECUTIVE COMMITTEE

ISSAM A. AWAD, M.D.
DANIEL L. BARROW, M.D.
JAMES R. BEAN, M.D.
PAUL J. CAMARATA, M.D.
MARK H. CAMEL, M.D.
CURTIS A. DICKMAN, M.D.
EMILY DANE FRIEDMAN, M.D.

DOUGLAS S. KONDZIOLKA, M.D.
MICHAEL L. LEVY, M.D.
PAUL C. McCORMICK, M.D.
EVANDRO de OLIVEIRA, M.D.
GERALD E. RODTS, JR., M.D.
VINCENT TRAYNELIS, M.D.

Editors-in-Chief
Clinical Neurosurgery

Volume	Date	Editor-in-Chief
1	1953	Raymond K. Thompson, M.D.
2	1954	Raymond K. Thompson, M.D. & Ira J. Jackson, M.D.
3	1955	Raymond K. Thompson, M.D. & Ira J. Jackson, M.D.
4	1956	Ira J. Jackson, M.D.
5	1957	Robert G. Fisher, M.D.
6	1958	Robert G. Fisher, M.D.
7	1959	Robert G. Fisher, M.D.
8	1960	William H. Mosberg, Jr., M.D.
9	1961	William H. Mosberg, Jr., M.D.
10	1962	William H. Mosberg, Jr., M.D.
11	1963	John Shillito, Jr., M.D., & William H. Mosberg, Jr., M.D.
12	1964	John Shillito, Jr., M.D.
13	1965	John Shillito, Jr., M.D.
14	1966	Robert G. Ojemann, M.D. & John Shillito, Jr., M.D.
15	1967	Robert G. Ojemann, M.D.
16	1968	Robert G. Ojemann, M.D.
17	1969	Robert G. Ojemann, M.D.
18	1970	George T. Tindall, M.D.
19	1971	George T. Tindall, M.D.
20	1972	Robert H. Wilkins, M.D.
21	1973	Robert H. Wilkins, M.D.
22	1974	Robert H. Wilkins, M.D.
23	1975	Ellis B. Keener, M.D.
24	1976	Ellis B. Keener, M.D.
25	1977	Ellis B. Keener, M.D.
26	1978	Peter W. Carmel, M.D.
27	1979	Peter W. Carmel, M.D.
28	1980	Peter W. Carmel, M.D.
29	1981	Martin H. Weiss, M.D.
30	1982	Martin H. Weiss, M.D.
31	1983	Martin H. Weiss, M.D.
32	1984	John R. Little, M.D.
33	1985	John R. Little, M.D.
34	1986	John R. Little, M.D.
35	1987	Peter McL. Black, M.D., Ph.D.
36	1988	Peter McL. Black, M.D., Ph.D.
37	1989	Peter McL. Black, M.D., Ph.D.
38	1990	Warren R. Selman, M.D.
39	1991	Warren R. Selman, M.D.

40	1992	Warren R. Selman, M.D.
41	1993	Christopher M. Loftus, M.D.
42	1994	Christopher M. Loftus, M.D.
43	1995	Christopher M. Loftus, M.D.
44	1996	M. Sean Grady, M.D.
45	1997	M. Sean Grady, M.D.
46	1998	M. Sean Grady, M.D.

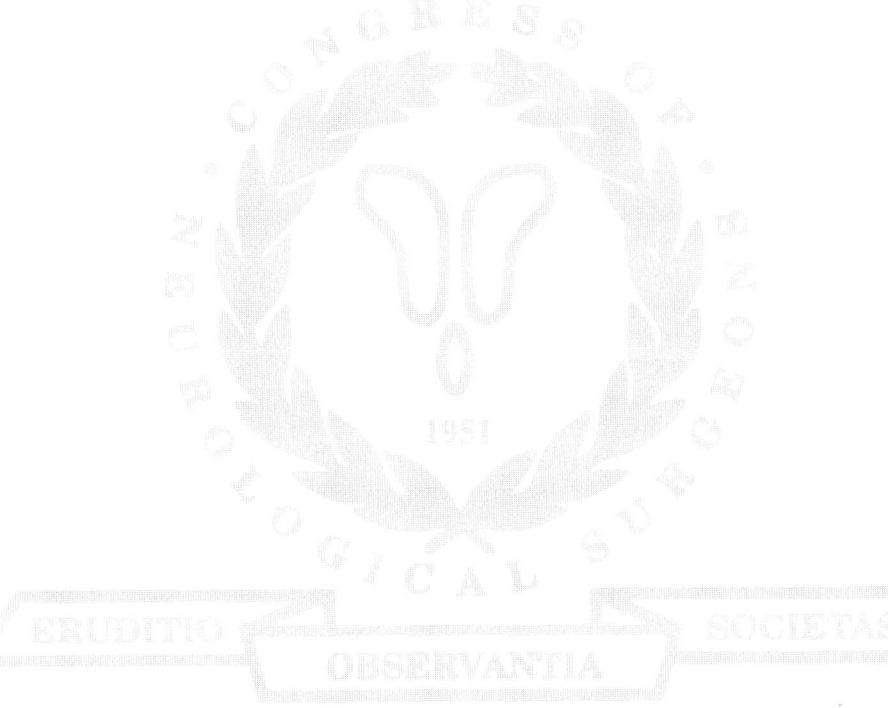

Contributors

CARGILL H. ALLEYNE, JR., M.D., Assistant Professor, Chief, Division of Stroke and Cerebrovascular Surgery, Department of Neurosurgery, University of Rochester, Rochester, New York (Chapter 25)

BRIAN T. ANDREWS, M.D., F.A.C.S., Attending Neurosurgeon, Department of Neurosurgery, University of Califonria at San Francisco, San Francisco, California (Chapter 14)

L. JOHN ANDREWS, M.D., Department of Neurosurgery, Harvard Medical School, Boston, Massachusetts (Chapter 2)

RONALD I. APFELBAUM, M.D., Department of Neurosurgery, University of Utah Health Sciences Center, Salt Lake City, Utah (Chapter 33)

MICHAEL L. J. APUZZO, M.D., Professor of Neurological Surgery, University of California School of Medicine, Los Angeles, California (Chapter 4)

ROCCO A. ARMONDA, M.D., M.A.I., M.C., U.S.A., Director, Section of Cerebrovascular Surgery & Interventional Neuroradiology, Walter Reed Army Medical Center, Washington, DC (Chapter 18)

ISSAM A. AWAD, M.D., M.Sc., F.A.C.S., The Nixdorff-German Professor, Department of Neurosurgery, Yale University School of Medicine, New Haven, Connecticut (Chapter 27)

KHALED M. ABDEL AZIZ, M.D., Research Fellow, Department of Neurosurgery, University of Cincinnati College of Medicine, Cincinnati, Ohio (Chapter 38)

DANIEL L. BARROW, M.D., MBNA/Bowman Professor and Chairman, Department of Neurosurgery, Emory University School of Medicine, Atlanta, Georgia (Chapters 21, 28)

H. HUNT BATJER, M.D., Michael J. Marchese Professor and Chair, Department of Neurological Surgery, Northwestern University Medical Center, Chicago, Illinois (Chapter 23)

M. FLINT BEAL, M.D., Neurochemistry laboratory, Massachusetts General Hospital, Harvard Medical School, Boston, Massachusetts (Chapter 2)

JOHN BENTSON, M.D., Professor, Department of Radiology/Neuroradiology, UCLA, Los Angeles, California (Chapter 22)

MIKHAIL BOGDANOV, M.D., Neurochemistry Laboratory, Massachusetts General Hospital, Harvard Medical School, Boston, Massachusetts (Chapter 2)

JEFFREY A. BROWN, M.D., F.A.C.S., Professor and Chairman, Department of Neurological Surgery, Medical College of Ohio, Toledo, Ohio (Chapter 32)

KIM J. BURCHIEL, M.D., F.A.C.S., John Raaf Professor and Chairman, Department of Neurological Surgery, Oregon health Sciences University, Portland, Oregon (Chapter 30)

WILLIAM E. BUTLER, M.D., Neurosurgical Service, Department of Surgery, Massachusetts General Hospital, Harvard Medical School, Boston, Massachusetts (Chapter 2)

BOB S. CARTER, M.D., Ph.D., Neurosurgical Service, Massachusetts General Hospital, Boston, Massachusetts (Chapter 26)

C. MICHAEL CAWLEY, M.D., Assistant Professor, Department of Neurosurgery, Emory University School of Medicine, Atlanta, Georgia (Chapter 28)

JOSEPH C.T. CHEN, M.D., Ph.D., Department of Neurological Surgery, University of California School of Medicine, Los Angeles, California (Chapter 4)

RANDALL M. CHESNUT, M.D., F.A.C.C.M., Associate Professor Neurosurgery, Adjunct Associate Research Professor, Emergency Medicine and Director, Neurotrauma and Neurosurgical Critical Care, Department of Neurosurgery, Oregon Health Sciences University, Portland, Oregon (Chaper 13)

PAUL W. DETWILER, M.S., M.D., Chief Resident, Division of Neurological Surgery, Barrow Neurological Institute, Phoenix, Arizona (Chapter 37)

CURTIS A. DICKMAN, M.D., Director of Spinal Research, Associate Chief of Spinal Neurosurgery, Division of Neurological Surgery, Barrow Neurological Institute, Phoenix, Arizona (Chapter 37)

CURT DOBERSTEIN, M.D., Professor, Department of Neurosurgery, Brown University, Providence, Rhode Island (Chapter 22)

MATTHIAS ENDRES, M.D., Stroke and Neurovascular Regulation, Neurosurgical Service, Departments of Surgery and Neurology, Massachusetts General Hospital, Harvard Medical School, Charlestown, Massachusetts (Chapter 2)

KLAUS B. FINK, M.D., Stroke and Neurovascuolar Regulation, Neurosurgical Service, Departments of Surgery and Neurology, Massachusetts General Hospital, Harvard Medical School, Charlestown, Massachusetts (Chapter 2)

JEFFREY I. FRANK, M.D., Director, Neuromedical and Neurosurgical Intensive Care and Associate Professor, Neurology and Surgery (Neurosurgery), The University of Chicago, Chicago, Illinois (Chapter 19)

ROBERT M. FRIEDLANDER, M.D., Neurosurgical Service, department of Surgery, Brigham and Women's Hospital, Neurosurgical Service,

Department of Surgery, Massachusetts General Hospital, Harvard Medical School, Boston, Massachusetts (Chapter 2)

WILLIAM A. FRIEDMAN, M.D., Department of Neurosurgery, University of Florida, Gainesville, Florida (Chapter 1)

HARSHA GOPAL, M.D., Department of Otolaryngology, Beth Israel Deaconess Medical Center, Boston, Massachusetts (Chapter 35)

MARK N. HADLEY, M.D., Department of Neurological Surgery, University of Alabama, Birmingham, Alabama (Chapter 11)

M. PETER HEILBRUN, M.D., Department of Neurosurgery, University of Utah School of Medicine, Salt Lake City, Utah (Chapter 6)

CARL B. HEILMAN, M.D., Assistant Professor, Department of Neurosurgery, Tufts University School of Medicine, Boston, Massachusetts (Chapter 35, 38)

MARTIN HOLLAND, M.D., Department of Neurosrugery, University of California, San Francisco, California (Chapter 16)

IAIN H. KALFAS, M.D., F.A.C.S. Head, Section of Spinal Surgery, Department of Neurosurgery, Cleveland Clinic Foundation, Cleveland, Ohio (Chapter 5)

ANDREW H. KAYE, M.D., M.B.B.S., F.R.A.C.S., Head of Department of Surgery, Director of Neurosurgery, Director of The Melbourne Neuroscience Centre, The Royal Melbourne Hospital, The University of Melbourne, Melbourne, Australia (Chapter 34)

SOHAIL Q. KHAN, M.D., Neurosurgical Service, Department of Surgery, Brigham and Women's Hospital, Harvard Medical School, Boston, Massachusetts (Chapter 2)

ROHIT KHANNA, M.D., Neurosurgeon, Daytona Beach, Florida (Chapter 22)

MICHAEL P. B. KILBURN, M.D., Department of Neurological Surgery, University of Alabama, Birmingham, Alabama (Chapter 11)

ANDREW J. KOKKINO, M.D., Assistant Professor, Department of Neurosurgery, Loyola University Medical Center, Maywood, Illinois (Chapter 38)

SUNGHOON LEE, M.D., Assistant Resident, Department of Neurosurgery, Yale University School of Medicine, New Haven, Connecticut (Chapter 27)

ADAM I. LEWIS, M.D., Jackson Neurosurgery Clinic, Jackson, Mississippi (Chapter 20)

MINGWEI LI, M.D., Neurosurgical Service, Department of Surgery, Brigham and Women's Hospital, Harvard Medical School, Boston, Massachusetts (Chapter 2)

MICHAEL J. LINK, M.D., Department of Neurosurgery, Mayo Clinic, Rochester, Minnesota (Chapter 24)

THOMAS G. LUERSSEN, M.D., F.A.C.S., F.A.A.P., Professor of Neurological Surgery and Director, Pediatric Neurosurgery Service, James Whitcomb Riley Hospital for Children, Indiana University Medical Center, Indianapolis, Indiana (Chapter 12)

LAWRENCE F. MARSHALL, M.D., San Diego, California (Chapter 7)

NEIL A. MARTIN, M.D., Professor, Department of Surgery/Neurosurgery, UCLA School of Medicine, Los Angeles, California (Chapter 22)

MARC R. MAYBERG, M.D. Department of Neurosurgery, Cleveland Clinic, Cleveland, Ohio (Chapter 17)

JEFFREY D. MCDONALD, M.D., PH.D., University of Neurosurgery, University of Utah, Salt Lake City, Utah (Chapter 6)

RICHARD J. MEAGHER, M.D., Department of Neurosurgery, Temple University Hospital, Philadelphia, Pennsylvania (Chapter 9)

MICHAEL A. MOSKOWITZ, M.D., Stroke and Neurovascular Regulation, Neurosurgical Service, Department sof Surgery and Neurology, Massachusetts General Hospital, Harvard Medical School, Charlestown, Massachusetts (Chapter 2)

SHOBU NAMURA, M.D., Stroke and Neurovascular Regulation, Neurosurgical Service, Departments of Surgery and Neurology, Massachusetts General Hospital, Harvard Medical School, Charlestown, Massachusetts (Chapter 2)

RAJ K. NARAYAN, M.D., Department of Neurosurgery, Temple University Hospital, Philadelphia, Pennsylvania (Chapter 9)

CHRISTOPHER S. OGILVY, M.D., Associate Professor of Surgery and Director, Brain AVM/Aneurysm Center, Massachusetts General Hospital, Boston, Massachusetts (Chapter 26)

ROBERT G. OJEMANN, M.D., Professor of Surgery, Neurosurgical Service, Massachusetts General Hospital, Boston, Massachusetts (Chapter 26)

VICTOR O. ONA, M.D., Neurosurgical Service, Department of Surgery, Brigham and Women's Hospital, and Neurosurgical Service, Department of Surgery, Massachusetts General Hospital, Harvard Medical School, Boston, Massachusetts (Chapter 2)

LAWRENCE H. PITTS, M.D., UCSF/Neurosurgery, San Francisco, California (Chapter 16)

RANDALL W. PORTER, M.D., Chief Resident, Division of Neurological Surgery, Barrow Neurological Institute, Phoenix, Arizona (Chapter 37)

JOHN T. POVLISHOCK, Ph.D., Professor and Chair, Department of Anatomy, Medical College of Virginia, Virginia Commonwealth University, Richmond, Virginia (Chapter 8)

CHRISTOPHER PUTMAN, M.D., Director, Neuro-Interventional Service, Massachusetts General Hospital, Boston, Massachusetts (Chapter 26)

ELIE E. REBEIZ, M.D., Assistant Professor, Department of Otolaryngology, Tufts University School of Medicine, Boston, Massachusetts (Chapter 35)

ROBERT H. ROSENWASSER, M.D., F.A.C.S., Professor of Neurosurgery and Director, Division of Cerebrovascular Surgery and Interventional Neuroradiology, Thomas Jefferson University Hospital, Philadelphia, Pennsylvania (Chapter 18)

OREN SAGHER, M.D., Department of Surgery, Section of Neurosurgery, University of Michigan, Ann Arbor, Michigan (Chapter 31)

WILLIAM A. SHUCART, M.D., Professor and Chairman, Department of Neurosurgery, Tufts University School of Medicine, Boston, Massachusetts (Chapter 35)

ROBERT F. SPETZLER, M.D., Director, BNI; J.N. Harber Chairman of Neurological Surgery, Division of Neurological Surgery, Barrow Neurological Institute, Phoenix, Arizona (Chapter 25)

JAMAL M. TAHA, M.D., Assistant Professor, Department of Neurosurgery, University of Cincinnati College of Medicine, Cincinnati, Ohio (Chapter 29)

CHARLES TEO, M.B.B.S., F.R.A.C.S., Queen's Park, N.S.W. Australia (Chapter 36)

JOHN M. TEW, JR., M.D., Frank H. Mayfield Professor and Chair, Department of Neurosurgery, University of Cincinnati College of Medicine, Cincinnati, Ohio (Chapters 3,20,24,29,38)

THOMAS A. TOMSICK, M.D., Professor, Department of Neuroradiology, University of Cincinnati College of Medicine, Cincinnati, Ohio (Chapter 24)

A. GIANCARLO VISHTEH, M.D., Neurosurgeon, Quantum Neurological Surgeons, PC, Phoenix, Arizona (Chapter 25)

BEVERLY C. WALTERS, M.D., M.Sc., F.R.C.S.C., F.A.C.S., Chief of Neurosurgery, The Miriam Hospital and Associate Professor, Clinical Neurosciences (Neurosurgery), Brown University School of Medicine, Providence, Rhode Island (Chapter 15)

JACK E. WILBERGER, M.D., Professor and Chairman and Vice Dean of School of Medicine, Department of Neurosurgery, Allellgheny University Hospitals, Allegheny General Hospital, Pittsburgh, Pennsylvania (Chapter 10)

JUNYING YUAN, M.D., Department of Cell Biology, Harvard Medical School, Boston, Massachusetts (Chapter 2)

Biography of John M. Tew, Jr., M.D., F.A.C.S.

John M. Tew, Jr., M.D., FACS was born and raised on a farm in eastern North Carolina. He graduated from Campbell and Wake Forest Universities Cum Laude in 1957. He attended Bowman Gray School of Medicine of Wake Forest Univesity and graduated AOA in 1961.

Dr. Tew studied general surgery for two years at Cornell-New York Hospital and Peter Bent Brigham, where he worked with Dr. Francis Moore in transplantation research. He was a fellow in neuro-physiology with Dr. Cho Lu Li at the National Institutes of Health NINCDS where they development intracellular recordings in the human cerebral cortex and thalamus. This was also an important personal time because John met Susan Smyth and they were later married in Boston in 1966.

In 1965, Dr. Tew returned to Boston for a research fellowship and neurosurgical residency at the Massachusetts General Hospital. Working with Drs. Sweet, Kjelberg and Ballantine, Dr. Tew brought the technique for microelectrode recording to the stereotaxic operation room. In 1967, Dr. Tew spent a year at the Boston Children's Hospital with Dr. Donald Matson, where he learned pediatric neurological surgery. During the final years of residency with Dr. Robert Ojemann, micro-neurosurgery was being born. The second Van Wagenen Fellowship was awarded to Dr. Tew to study with Professor Gazi Yasargil in Zurich. The experience was career focusing and later led to the development of the Cincinnati and the Mayfield Clinic as a center for education and application of micro-neurosurgery.

In Cincinnati, Dr. Tew came under the wise mentorship of Dr. Frank Mayfield, who taught him humility, patience, and instilled a heightened sense of community service. With Drs. Mayfield, Dunsker and other associates, a community based neurosurgical program was developed. The program became outstanding and was merged with the University of Cincinnati in 1983 to integrate the best aspects of each institution into a top academic program. In 1992, Dr. Tew became the first Frank Mayfield Chairman of Neurological Surgery at the University of Cincinnati. The neurological services were later integrated into The Neurological Institute, which was inaugurated in 1998 with Dr. Tew as Medical Director. The Neuroscience Institute is a nationally recognized center for treatment, education and research in neurological disorders. It is the result of mutual respect, coordination and excellence in research, education and clinical care by the University of Cincinnati departments.

Dr. Tew is especially proud of the residents and fellows who have been educated in Cincinnati since 1969. More than 150 in number, today they are teaching and practicing neurological surgery in the major clinics and schools of medicine throughout the United States and many other countries.

Dr. Tew has served as President of the Congress of Neurological Surgeons and the Academy of Neurological Surgeons. He has received recognition from Campbell University (honorary Doctorate in Humane Letters, 1985) and from Wake Forest University (Distinguished Alumni Award, 1991). As a member of the Cincinnati Community, he has served the Board of Trustees of Xavier University for nine years and received the Xavier leadership medallion in 1998. He received the Papal Pro Ecclesia Et Pontifica Medical from Pope John Paul II, delivered by Archbishop Daniel Pilarczyki in 1990, and the Distinguished Service Citation from the National Conference of Christians and Jews in 1995.

Dr. Tew is indebted to the community of Cincinnati, which has nurtured his family, the College of Medicine and the Mayfield Clinic. He maintains a very active involvement in community affairs, business and religious organizations. He continues a very active practive, is interested in constant change, whether in technology, patient care or economics of medical practice. He is one of neurosurgery's leaders in search of new concepts of facial pain, cerebrovascular disease brain tumors and disorders of the spine. His bibliography includes more than 250 publications, including many in history and biography, which were written as a member of The Literary Club of Cincinnati.

Bibliography of John M. Tew, Jr., M.D., F.A.C.

PUBLICATIONS

LI CL, TEW JM JR: Reciprocal activation and inhibition of cortical neurones and voluntary movements in man: Cortical cell activity and muscle movement. **Nature 203**:264–265, 1964

LI C, FRIAUF W, COHEN G, TEW JM JR: A method of recording single cell discharges in the cerebral cortex of man. **EEG and Neurophys 18**:187–190, 1965

WESTLAKE RJ, TEW JM JR: Urinary amines in patients undergoing thalamotomy for Parkinson's disease. **Neurology 16**:619–620, 1966

LI C, TEW JM JR: The effect of cerebellar stimulation and neuronal activity in the motor cortex. **Exp Neurol 14**:317–327, 1966

KRAYENBUHL HA, YASARGIL MG, FLAMM ES, TEW JM JR: Microsurgical treatment of intracranial saccular aneurysms. **J Neurosurg 37**:678–686, 1972

MOORE D, TEW JM JR, MAYFIELD FH: Ocular manifestations of sphenoid mucoceles (Case Report and Discussion). **Ohio State Med J 68**:1100–1104, 1972

CROWELL RM, TEW JM JR, MARK VH: Aggressive dementia associated with normal pressure hydrocephalus. Report of two unusual cases. **Neurology 23**:461–464, 1973

TEW JM JR, MAYFIELD FH: Trigeminal neuralgia: A new surgical approach. Percutaneous electrocoagulation of the trigeminal nerve. **Laryngoscope 83**:1096–1101, 1973

TEW JM JR, WIET RJ, MAYFIELD FH: Early diagnosis and management of acoustic neuromas. **Ohio State Med J 70**:365–367, 1974

TEW JM JR: Percutaneous electrocoagulation of the trigeminal nerve in the treatment of trigeminal neuralgia. **Radionics Procedure Technique Series,** 1974

TEW JM JR: Nerve coagulation controls tic douloureux. **JAMA 230**:652, 1974

TEW JM JR: Reconstructive intracranial vascular surgery. **Med Col VA Q 10**:139–145, 1974

TEW JM JR, MAYFIELD FH: Proceedings: Anterior cervical discectomy—a microsurgical approach. **J Neurol Neurosurg Psychiatry 38**:413, 1975

TEW JM JR: A view of medical education and medical practice. **Cinti J Med 56:**291–292, 1975

TEW JM JR, LOCKWOOD P, MAYFIELD FH: Treatment of trigeminal neuralgia in the aged by a simplified surgical approach. (Percutaneous electrocoagulation). **J Am Geriatr Soc 23:**426–430, 1975

LUKIN RR, CHAMBERS AR, MCLAURIN RL, TEW JM JR: Thrombosed giant middle cerebral aneurysms. **Neuroradiology 10:**125–129, 1975

TEW JM JR: RECONSTRUCTIVE INTRACRANIAL VASCULAR SURGERY FOR PREVENTION OF STROKE. CLIN NEUROSURG 22:264–280, 1975

TEW JM JR, LOCKWOOD P, MAYFIELD FH: The treatment of trigeminal neuralgia in the aged patient by a simplified surgical approach. **Cinti J Med 57:**29–33, 1976

TEW JM JR: Medical liability crisis: Is there a solution? **Cinti J Med 57:**219–220, 1976

TEW JM JR, MAYFIELD FH: COMPLICATIONS OF SURGERY OF THE ANTERIOR CERVICAL SPINE. CLIN NEUROSURG 23:424–434, 1976

TEW JM JR: Intracranial reconstructive vascular surgery: Indications and operative results. **International Congress Series, Neurological Surgery 433:**249–251, 1977

RAYMOND LA, TEW JM JR, FOGELSON MH: Ophthalmoplegic migraine of early onset. **J Pediatr 90:**1035–1036, 1977, (Letter)

TEW JM JR, GREINER AL, BERGER TS, DUNSKER SB, BUDDE RB: Intracranial vascular bypass: Can it prevent stroke? **Modern Medicine 45:**58–61, 1977

TEW JM JR, KELLER JT: The treatment of trigeminal neuralgia by percutaneous radiofrequency technique. **Clin Neurosurg 24:**557–578, 1977

ALVIRA M, SHAHBABIAN S, LUKIN R, TEW JM JR: The pathology of surgically treated cryptic arteriovenous malformations. **Am J Clin Pathol 70:**329–330, 1978

YAMAMOTO I, KUROKAWA K, TEW JM JR, DUNSKER SB, MAYFIELD FH: Anterior cervical discectomy with and without fusion: Clinical and experimental study. **No Shinkei Geka (Japan) 6:**781–787, 1978

TEW JM JR, KELLER JT, WILLIAMS DS: Application of stereotactic principles to the treatment of trigeminal neuralgia. **Appl Neurophysiol 41:**146–156, 1978

RAYMOND LA, TEW JM JR: Large suprasellar aneurysms imitating pituitary tumor. **J Neurol Neurosurg Psychiatry 41:**83–87, 1978

TEW JM JR: Techniques of supratentorial cerebral revascularization. **Clin Neurosurg 26:**330–345, 1979

JANNETTA PM, TEW JM JR: Treatment of trigeminal neuralgia. **Neurosurgery 4:**93–94, 1979

ABRAHAMSON IA JR, BALUYOT ST, TEW JM JR, SCIOVILLE G: Frontal sinus mucocele. **Ann Ophthalmol 11:**173–178, 1979

TEW JM JR: Biography of Frank Henderson Mayfield, M.D. **Clin Neurosurg 27:**23–25, 1980

TEW JM JR: Management of carotid artery occlusive disease. **Contemp Neurosurg 3:**1–6, 1980

JAZY FK, SHEHATA WM, TEW JM JR, MEYER RL, BOSS HH: Primary intracranial lymphoma of the dura. **Arch Neurol 37:**528–529, 1980

HARLESS MA, LIWNICZ BH, KELLER JT, TEW JM JR: Adrenoleukodystrophy: White matter disease with adrenal changes in a 33-year-old man. **Neurosurgery 7:**174–178, 1980

HAFNER CD, TEW JM JR: Surgical management of the totally occluded internal carotid artery: A ten-year study. **Surgery 89:**710–717, 1981

FRANK EH, TEW JM JR, PAGANI L: The prolonged Q-T syndrome presenting as a focal neurological lesion. **Surg Neurol 16:**333–335, 1981

YEH H, TEW JM JR, RAMIREZ R: Microsurgical treatment of intractable hemifacial spasm. **Neurosurgery 9:**383–386, 1981

YAMAMOTO I, TEW JM JR, TOMSICK TA: The use of balloon catheters in the treatment of carotid cavernous sinus fistula. **No Shinkei Geka (Japan) 10:**1175–1181, 1982

TEW JM JR: Frank Henderson Mayfield. **Surg Neurol 17:**1–3, 1982

FRANK EH, BERGER TS, TEW JM JR: Basilar impression and platybasia in osteogenesis imperfecta tarda. **Surg Neurol 17:**116–119, 1982

FRANK EH, BERGER TS, TEW JM JR: Bilateral epidural hematomas. **Surg Neurol 17:**218–222, 1982

STEIGER HJ, TEW JM JR, KELLER JT: The sensory representation of the dura mater in the trigeminal ganglion of the cat. **Neurosci Lett 31:**231–236, 1982

VAN LOVEREN HR, TEW JM JR, KELLER JT, NURRE MA: A ten-year experience in the treatment of trigeminal neuralgia: A comparison of percutaneous stereotaxic rhizotomy and posterior fossa exploration. **J Neurosurg 57:**757–764, 1982

FRANK EH, TEW JM JR: Normal-pressure hydrocephalus: Clinical symptoms, diagnosis, pathophysiology, and treatment. **Heart Lung 11:**321–326, 1982

VASCIK JM, TEW JM JR: Foreign body embolization of the middle cerebral artery: Review of the literature and guidelines for management. **Neurosurgery 11:**532–536, 1982

GUP RS, SHEELER LR, MAEDER MC, TEW JM JR: Pituitary enlargement and primary hypothyroidism: A report of two cases with sharply contrasting outcomes. **Neurosurgery 11:**792–794, 1982

Shehata WM, Meyer RL, Jazy FK, Tew JM Jr, Hall JM, Ignatius J, Reed RL, Liwnicz BH: Management of glioblastoma multiforme by irradiation and chemotherapy. **Ill Med J 163:**30–34, 1983

Tew JM Jr, van Loveren HR, Keller JT: Trigeminal neuralgia. **Neurosurgeons (Japan) 2:**251–265, 1983

Welling RE, Taha A, Goel T, Cranley J, Krause R, Hafner C, Tew JM Jr: Extracranial carotid artery aneurysms. **Surgery 93:**319–323, 1983

Tew JM Jr, Yeh H, Miller GW, Shahbabian S: Intratemporal schwannoma of the facial nerve. **Neurosurgery 13:**186–188, 1983

Tobler WD, Tew JM Jr, Cosman E, Keller JT, Quallen BL: Improved outcome in the treatment of trigeminal neuralgia by percutaneous stereotactic rhizotomy with a new, curved tip electrode. **Neurosurgery 12:**313–317, 1983

Tew JM Jr, Yeh H: Hemifacial Spasm. **Neurosurgeons (Japan) 2:**267–278, 1983

Keller JT, Saunders MC, Ongkiko CM Jr, Johnson J, Frank EH, van Loveren HR, Tew JM Jr: Identification of motoneurons innervating the tensor tympani and tensor veli palatini muscles in the cat. **Brain Res 270:**209–215, 1983

Tew JM Jr: Presidential address: Medical competence—education and ethics. **Clin Neurosurg 31:**1–8, 1984

Tomsick TA, Tew JM Jr, Lukin RR, Johnson JK: Balloon catheters for aneurysms and fistulae. **Clin Neurosurg 31:**135–164, 1984

Tew JM Jr, Tobler WD: The laser: History, biophysics and neurosurgical applications. **Clin Neurosurg 31:**506–549, 1984

Yamamoto I, Sato O, Tew JM Jr, Tomsick TA: Use of detachable balloon catheters in the treatment of carotid cavernous fistula. **Neurol Med Chir (Tokyo) 24:**678–688, 1984

Liwnicz BH, Liwnicz RH, Huff JS, McBride BH, Tew JM Jr: Giant granular cell tumor of the suprasellar area: Immunocytochemical and electron microscopic studies. **Neurosurgery 15:**246–251, 1984

Yeh HS, Keller JT, Brackett KA, Frank EH, Tew JM Jr: Human umbilical artery for microvascular grafting: An experimental study in the rat. **J Neurosurg 61:**737–742, 1984

Ross DL, Tew JM Jr, Benton C, Eisentrout C: Trigeminal schwannoma in a child. **Neurosurgery 15:**108–110, 1984

Tew JM Jr: Medical competence—education and ethics. **Neurosurgery 15:**1–3, 1984

Tew JM Jr, Feibel JH, Sawaya R: Brain tumors: Clinical aspects. **Semin Roentgenol 19:**115–128, 1984

Yeh H, Tew JM Jr: Tic convulsif, the combination of geniculate neuralgia and hemifacial spasm relieved by vascular decompression. **Neurology 34:**682–683, 1984

STEIGER HJ, TEW JM JR: Hemorrhage and epilepsy in cryptic cerebrovascular malformations. **Arch Neurol 41:**722–724, 1984

YEH H, TEW JM JR: Anterior interhemispheric approach to aneurysms of the anterior communicating artery. **Surg Neurol 23:**98–100, 1985

TEW JM JR, VAN LOVEREN HR: Surgical treatment of trigeminal neuralgia. **Am Fam Physician 31:**143–150, 1985

KIM LYS, TEW JM JR: Saccular aneurysms, subarachnoid hemorrhage, and the timing of surgery. **Heart Lung 14:**68–74, 1985

TEW JM JR, TOBLER WD, NURRE-MILLER MA: Application of lasers in neurological surgery—a special emphasis on inaccessible tumors of the skull and spinal cord. **Neurosurgeons (Japan) 4:**415–445, 1985

TEW JM JR, TOMSICK TA, LUKIN RR: Applications of interventional neuroradiology in the treatment of arteriovenous malformation and other vascular disorders of the brain. **Neurosurgeons 4:**331–356, 1985

YEH H, TOMSICK TA, TEW JM JR: Intraventricular hemorrhage due to aneurysms of the distal posterior inferior cerebellar artery: Report of three cases. **J Neurosurg 62:**772–775, 1985

JABRE A, BALL JB JR, TEW JM JR: Anterior sacral meningocele: Current diagnosis. **Surg Neurol 23:**9–13, 1985

SAWAYA R, MANDYBUR T, ORMSBY I, TEW JM JR: Antifibrinolytic therapy of experimentally grown malignant brain tumors. **J Neurosurg 64:**263–268, 1986

SHEHATA WM, MEYER RL, PANKE TL, TEW JM JR, RATH RK, SAMMARCO GJ: Primary lymphocytic lymphoma of the dorsal spine apparently cured by radio-chemotherapy. **Spine 11:**1035–1036, 1986

TOBLER WD, SAWAYA R, TEW JM JR: Successful laser-assisted excision of a metastatic midbrain tumor. **Neurosurgery 18:**795–797, 1986

OLIVI A, WANER M, SAWAYA R, WESSELER T, CASSINI P, LIWNICZ BH, PENSAK M, TEW JM JR: Photodynamic therapy of brain tumors: Studies on the distribution of DHE (di-hematoporphyrin ether) in normal and experimental neoplastic brain tissue in rats. **Adv Biosci 58:**169–174, 1986

BULLITT E, TEW JM JR, BOYD J: Intracranial tumors in patients with facial pain. **J Neurosurg 64:**865–871, 1986

LIWNICZ RH, WU SZ, TEW JM JR: The relationship between the capillary structure and hemorrhage in gliomas. **J Neurosurg 66:**536–541, 1987

WEIL SM, VAN LOVEREN HR, TOMSICK TA, QUALLEN BL, TEW JM JR:

Management of inoperable cerebral aneurysms by the navigational balloon technique. **Neurosurgery 21:**296–302, 1987

YEH H, HEISS JD, TEW JM JR: Persistent hypoglossal artery associated with basilar artery aneurysm. **Neurochirurgia 30:**158–159, 1987

WELLING RE, SAUL TG, TEW JM JR, TOMSICK TA, KREMCHEK T, BELLAMY MJ: Management of blunt injury to the internal carotid artery. **J Trauma 27:**1221–1226, 1987

JACOBSON GP, TEW JM JR: Intraoperative Evoked Potential Monitoring. **J Clin Neurophysiol 4:**145–176, 1987

BUCKINGHAM MJ, CRONE KR, BALL WS, TOMSICK TA, BERGER TS, TEW JM JR: Traumatic intracranial aneurysms in childhood: Two cases and a review of the literature. **Neurosurgery 22:**398–408, 1988

JACOBSON GP, TEW JM JR: The origin of the scalp recorded P14 following electrical stimulation of the median nerve: Intraoperative observations. **Electroencephalogr Clin Neurophysiol 71:**73–76, 1988

HEISS JD, TEW JM JR: Diskogenic diseases of the spine: Clinical aspects. **Sem Roentgenol 23:**93–99, 1988

KASHIWAGI S, TEW JM JR, VAN LOVEREN HR, THOMAS G: Trapping of giant basilar trunk aneurysms. **J Neurosurg 69:**442–445, 1988

TSAI S, TEW JM JR, MCLEAN JH, SHIPLEY MT: Cerebral arterial innervation by nerve fibers containing calcitonin gene-related peptide (CGRP): I. Distribution and origin of CGRP perivascular innervation in the rat. **J Comp Neurol 271:**435–444, 1988

YEH HS, TEW JM JR: Management of arteriovenous malformations of the brain. **Contemp Neurosurg 9:**1–8, 1988

ZUCCARELLO M, YEH H, TEW JM JR: Morbidity and mortality of carotid endarterectomy under local anesthesia: A retrospective study. **Neurosurgery 23:**445–450, 1988

ZUCCARELLO M, MANDYBUR TI, TEW JM JR, TOBLER WD: Acute effect of the Nd:YAG Laser on the cerebral arteriovenous malformation: A histological study. **Neurosurgery 24:**328–333, 1989

FUKOKA S, YEH H, MANDYBUR TI, TEW JM JR: Effect of insulin on acute experimental cerebral ischemia on gerbils. **Stroke 20:**396–399, 1989

SANBERG PR, CALDERON SF, GIORDANA M, TEW JM JR, NORMAN AB: The quinolinic acid model of Huntington's disease: Locomotor Abnormalities. **Exp Neurol 105:**45–53, 1989

KELLER JT, WEIL SM, ONGKIKO CM, TEW JM JR, MAYFIELD FH, DUNSKER SB: Repair of spinal dural defects with Vicryl (Polyglactin 910) mesh. **J Spinal Disord 2:**87–92, 1989

PENSAK ML, VAN LOVEREN HR, TEW JM JR: The surgical anatomy and approaches to lesions of the lower basilar artery and vertebral artery union. **Am J Otol 10:**351–357, 1989

KASHIWAGI S, VAN LOVEREN HR, TEW JM JR, WIOT JG, WEIL SM, LUKIN RA: Diagnosis and treatment of vascular brain-stem malformations. **J Neurosurg 72**:27–34, 1990

YEH HS, KASHIWAGI S, TEW JM JR, BERGER T.S.: Surgical management of epilepsy associated with cerebral arteriovenous malformations. **J Neurosurg 72**:216–223, 1990

SCODARY DJ, TEW JM JR., THOMAS GM, TOMSICK TA, LIWNICZ BH: Radiation-induced cerebral aneurysms. **Acta Neurochir (Wien) 102**:141–144 Fasc.3–4, 1990

WEIL SM, TEW JM JR: Surgical management of brain stem vascular malformations. **Acta Neurochir (Wien) 105**:14–23, 1990

VAN LOVEREN HR, KELLER JT, EL-KALLINY M, SCODARY DJ, TEW JM JR: The Dolenc technique for cavernous sinus exploration (cadaveric prosection). **J Neurosurg 74**:837–844, 1990

EL-KALLINY M, TEW JM JR, VAN LOVEREN HR, DUNSKER SB: Surgical approaches to thoracic disc herniations. **Acta Neurochir (Wien) 111**:22–32,1991

PENSAK ML, TEW JM JR, KEITH RW, VAN LOVEREN HR: Management of the acoustic neuroma in an only hearing ear. **Skull Base Surgery 1**:93–96, 1991

TEW JM JR: Deep intracranial vascular malformations. **Neurosurg Consult 2**:1–8, 1991

TEW JM JR: The physician's role as a community leader: Being more than just good. **W V Med J,** 1991

FICK J, TEW JM JR: Percutaneous Radiofrequency Rhizolysis for Trigeminal Neuralgia. **The American Association of Neurological Surgeons 1**:405–416, 1991

TEW JM JR: FRANK H. MAYFIELD, M.D., 1908–1991. **J Neurosurg 75**:347–348, 1991

EL-KALLINY M, VAN LOVEREN HR, KELLER JT, TEW JM JR: Tumors of the lateral wall of the cavernous sinus. **J Neurosurg 77**:508–514, 1992

LARSON JJ, TEW JM JR, WIOT JG, DE COURTEN-MYERS GM: Association of meningiomas with dural "tails": surgical significance. **Acta Neurochir (Wien) 114**:59–63, 1992

TSAI SH, TEW JM JR, SHIPLEY MT: Development of cerebral innervation: synchronous development of neuropeptide Y (NPY) — and vasoactive intestinal polypeptide (VIP) — containing fibers and some observations on growth cones. **Dev Brain Res 69**:77–83, 1992

TEW JM JR, TAHA JM: Treatment of intramedullary spinal cord tumors (ependymomas). **Findings 1(1)**:4–6, 1992

YEH HS, TEW JM JR, GARTNER M: Seizure control after surgery on cerebral arteriovenous malformations. **J Neurosurg 78**:12–18, 1993

TASDEMIROGLU E, ZUCCARELLO M, TEW JM JR: Recovery of vision after transcranial decompression of pituitary apoplexy characterized by third ventricular hemorrhage. **Neurosurgery 32:**121–124, 1993

TEW JM JR: The operative theater and operative planning. **Neurosurgeons 12:**27–28, 1993

MILLER CG, VAN LOVEREN HR, KELLER JT, PENSAK M, EL-KALLINY M, TEW JM JR: Transpetrosal approach: Surgical anatomy and technique. **Neurosurgery 33:**461–469, 1993

TEW JM JR, SKIDMORE BA: Treatment of the adult Chiari malformation. **Findings 2(2):**4–5, 1993

TOMSICK TA, TEW JM JR: Guglielmi detachable coil for the treatment of intracranial aneurysms. **Findings 2(2):**1–3, 1993

TAHA JM, TEW JM JR: Surgical treatment of trigeminal neuralgia. **Crit Rev Neurosurg 4:**156–163, 1994

BOUTHILLIER A, VAN LOVEREN HR, TEW JM JR: Anterior approaches to the clivus: classification & indications. **Contemporary Neurosurg 16:**1–8, 1994

BRENEMAN JC, TEW JM JR: Stereotactic radiosurgery for arteriovenous malformations. **Findings 3(1):**1–2, 1994

LEWIS AI, TEW JM JR: Treatment of thalamic-striate arteriovenous malformations. **Findings 3(1):**2–4, 1994

LEWIS AI, TEW JM JR, PAYNER TD, YEH HS: Dural cavernous angiomas outside the middle cranial fossa: a report of two cases. **Neurosurgery 35:**498–504, 1994

LEWIS AI, TOMSICK TA, TEW JM JR: Management of tentorial dural arteriovenous malformations: transarterial embolization combined with stereotactic radiation or surgery. **J Neurosurg 81:**851–859, 1994

LEWIS AI, TOMSICK TA, TEW JM JR: Treatment of carotid-cavernous fistulas with electrodetachable platinum coils. **Findings 3(1):**4–5, 1994

LEWIS AI, CRONE KR, TAHA JM, VAN LOVEREN HR, YEH HS, TEW JM JR: Surgical resection of third ventricle colloid cysts. **J Neurosurg 81:**174–178, 1994

PENSAK ML, VAN LOVEREN HR, TEW JM JR, KEITH RW: Transpetrosal access to meningiomas juxtaposing the temporal bone. **Laryngoscope 104:**814–820, 1994

PERATA HJ, TOMSICK TA, TEW JM JR: Feeding artery pedicle aneurysms: association with parenchymal hemorrhage and arteriovenous malformation in the brain. **J Neurosurg 80:**631–634, 1994

SHEHATA WM, PLOYSONGSANG SS, ARON BS, GERSON JW, TEW JM JR, TOBLER WD: Interstitial brain brachytherapy. **Appl Radiol 23:**11–14, 1994

TAHA JM, TEW JM JR, KEITH RW, PAYNER TD: Intraoperative monitoring of the vagus nerve during intracranial glossopharyngeal and upper vagal rhizotomy: technical note. **Neurosurgery 35:**775–777, 1994

SHINOURA N, HEFFELFINGER SC, MILLER M, SHAMRAJ OI, MIURA NHC, LARSON, JJ, DE TRIBOLET N, WARNICK RE, TEW JM JR: RNA expression of complement regulatory proteins in human brain tumors. **Cancer Letters 86:**143–149, 1994

BINDAL AK, DUNSKER SB, TEW JM JR: Chiari I malformation: Classification and management. **Neurosurgery 37:**1069–1074, 1995

BINDAL AK, TEW JM JR: Surgical management of the Chiari I malformation. **Crit Rev Neurosurg 5:**1–6, 1995

LARSON JJ, TEW JM JR, SIMON M, MENON AG: Evidence for clonal spread in the development of multiple meningiomas. **J Neurosurg 83:**705–709, 1995

LARSON JJ, TEW JM JR, TOMSICK TA, VAN LOVEREN HR: Treatment of aneurysms of the internal carotid artery by intravascular balloon occlusion: long-term follow-up of 58 cases. **Neurosurgery 36:**23–30, 1995

LARSON JJ, VAN LOVEREN HR, BALKO MG, TEW JM JR: Evidence of meningioma infiltration into cranial nerves: Clinical implications for cavernous sinus meningiomas. **J Neurosurg 83:**596–599, 1995

LEWIS AI, TOMSICK TA, TEW JM JR: Management of 100 consecutive direct carotid-cavernous fistulas: results of treatment with detachable balloons. **Neurosurgery 36:**239–245, 1995

LEWIS AI, VAN LOVEREN HR, TEW JM JR: Management of brain-stem vascular malformations: Advances in surgical technique and long-term results. **Neurosurgery Quarterly 5:**217–228, 1995

SIMON M, VON DEIMLING A, LARSON JJ, WELLENREUTHER R, KASKEL P, WAHA A, WARNICK RE, TEW JM JR, MENON AG: Allelic losses on chromosomes 14, 10, and 1 in atypical and malignant meningiomas: a genetic model of meningioma progression. **Cancer Res 55:**4696–4701, 1995

TAHA JM, TEW JM JR: Long-term results of radiofrequency rhizotomy in the treatment of cluster headache. **Headache 35:**193–196, 1995

TAHA JM, TEW JM JR: Long-term results of surgical treatment of idiopathic neuralgias of the glossopharyngeal and vagal nerves. **Neurosurgery 36:**926–931, 1995

TAHA JM, TEW JM JR, BUNCHER CR: A prospective 15-year follow up of 154 consecutive patients with trigeminal neuralgia treated by percutaneous stereotactic radiofrequency thermal rhizotomy. **J Neurosurg 83:**989–993, 1995

Taha JM, Tew JM Jr, van Loveren HR, Keller JT, El-Kalliny M: Comparison of conventional and skull base surgical approaches for the excision of trigeminal neurinomas. **J Neurosurg 82:**719–725, 1995

Taha JM, Tew JM Jr, Keith RW: Proximal-to-distal facial amplitude ratios as predictors of facial nerve function after acoustic neuroma excision. **J Neurosurg 83:**994–998, 1995

Tew JM Jr, Taha JM: An outpatient surgery to heat the pain away. TNAlert 1–3, 1995

Tew JM Jr, Lewis AI, Reichert KW: Management strategies and surgical techniques for deep-seated supratentorial arteriovenous malformations. **Neurosurgery 36:**1065–1072, 1995

Timperman PE, Tomsick TA, Tew JM Jr, van Loveren HR: Aneurysm formation following carotid occlusion. **AJNR 16:**329–331, 1995

Tomsick TA, Ernst RJ, Tew JM Jr, Brott TG, Breneman JC: Adult choroidal vein of Galen malformation. **AJNR 16:**861–865, 1995

Lewis AI, Tomsick TA, Tew JM Jr, Lawless MA: Long-term results of direct carotid-cavernous fistulas after treatment with detachable balloons. **J Neurosurg 84:**400–404, 1996

Kawase T, van Loveren HR, Keller JT, Tew JM Jr: Meningeal architecture of the cavernous sinus: Clinical and surgical implications. **J Neurosurg 39:**527–536, 1996

Simon M, Kokkino AJ, Warnick RE, Tew JM Jr, von Diemling A, Menong A: Role of genomic instability in meningioma progression. **Genes, Chromosomes & Cancer 16:**265–269, 1996

Taha JM, Tew JM Jr: Comparison of surgical treatments for trigeminal neuralgia: reevaluation of radiofrequency rhizotomy. **Neurosurgery 38:**865–871, 1996

Tew JM Jr, Kokkino AJ: Magnetic resonance imaging and its application for acoustic neuroma. **ANA Notes 57:**1–8, 1996

van Loveren HR, Liu SS, Tew JM Jr: Transcondylar approach. Operative Techniques in **Otolaryngology 7:**151–158, 1996

Payner TD, Tew JM Jr: Recurrence of hemifacial spasm after microvascular decompression. **Neurosurgery 38:**686–691, 1996

Lewis AI, Rosenblatt SS, Tew JM Jr: Surgical management of deep-seated dural arteriovenous malformations. **J Neurosurg 87:**198–206, 1997

Rosenberg WS, Tew JM Jr: Tew Cranial/Spinal Retractor. **Neurosurgery 40:**1096–1098, 1997

Pensak ML, Boulos O, Keigh RW, Tew JM Jr, van Loveren HR: Combination of auditory and somatosensory evoked potential monitoring during skull base tumor removal. **Laryngoscope 108:**770–775, 1997

TOMSICK TA, TEW JM JR, VAN LOVEREN HR: Subarachnoid hemorrhage due to aneurysms of the anterior communicating artery region after balloon occlusion: report of two cases. **AJNR 157:**213–219, 1997

GHOBASHY A, TEW JM JR, VAN LOVEREN HR, PENSAK MK, KEITH RW. A Continuing Role for Retrosigmoid Suboccipital Approach for the Treatment of Acoustic Schwannoma. **Egypt J Neurol Psychiat Neurosurg 33:**235–243, 1997

JONES BV, ERNST RJ, TOMSICK TA, TEW JM JR. Spinal dural arteriovenous fistulas: recognizing the spectrum of magnetic resonance imaging findings. **J Spinal Cord Med 20:**43–48, 1997

MEYERS P, LEACH J, TOMSICK T, GOLNIK K, TEW JM JR. Reversible cortical blindness following endovascular coil occlusion of a basilar terminus artery aneurysm. **J Neurovasc Disease** January/February:35–38, 1997

O'SULLIVAN MG, VAN LOVEREN HR, TEW JM JR. The surgical resectability of meningiomas of the cavernous sinus. **Neurosurgery 40:**238–247, 1997

TOMSICK TA, AUFFREY C, VAN LOVEREN HR, TEW JM JR. Cost-effectiveness of treatment of unclippable extradural internal carotid artery aneurysm. **J Neurovasc Disease 2:**149–162, 1997

FRIEDMAN RA, PENSAK ML, TAUBER M, TEW JM JR., VAN LOVEREN HR. Anterior petrosectomy approach to infraclinoidal basilar artery aneurysms: the emerging role of the neuro-otologist in multidisciplinary management of basilar artery aneurysms. **Laryngoscope 107:**977–983, 1997

LARSON JJ, BALL WS, BOVE KE, CRONE KR, TEW JM JR. Formation of intracerebral cavernous malformations after radiation treatment for central nervous system neoplasia in children. **J Neurosurgery 88:**51–56, 1998

BOOKS AND CHAPTERS IN BOOKS

Books

SAWAYA R, TEW JM JR: ***Neurosurgery: State of the Art Reviews.*** Hanley & Belfus: Philadelphia, Vol 2, 1987

DOWNING EF, ASCHER PW, CERULLO LJ, NEBLETT CR, ROBERTSON JH, TEW JM JR: ***Lasers in Neurosurgery.*** Springer-Verlag: Wein and New York, 1988

TEW JM AND VAN LOVEREN HR: *Atlas of Operative Microneurosurgery, Volume I.* W.B. Saunders: Philadelphia, 1994

TEW JM AND VAN LOVEREN HR: *Atlas of Operative Microneurosurgery, Volume II.* In Press.

Chapters in Books

MAYFIELD FH, TEW JM JR: Neurosurgery. In: *Textbook of Otolaryngology,* Paparella MM, Shumrick DA (eds). W.B. Saunders: New York, pp. 833–872, 1973

TEW JM JR: Percutaneous rhizotomy in the treatment of intractable facial pain (trigeminal, glossopharyngeal, and vagal nerves). In: *Current Techniques In Operative Neurosurgery,* Schmidek HH, Sweet WH (eds). Grune & Stratton: New York, pp. 409–426, 1977

TEW JM JR, KELLER JT: Percutaneous rhizotomy in the treatment of intractable facial pain. In: *Pain Management,* Fletcher LJ (ed). Williams and Wilkins: Baltimore, pp.145–165, 1977

TEW JM JR: Trigeminal neuralgia (tic douloureux) method of John M. Tew, Jr., M.D. In: *Current Therapy,* Conn H (ed). W.B. Saunders: New York, pp. 145–165, 1979

TEW JM JR, KELLER JT, WILLIAMS DS: Functional surgery of the trigeminal nerve: Treatment of trigeminal neuralgia. In: *Functional Neurosurgery,* Rasmussen T, Marino R (eds). Raven Press: New York, pp. 129–141, 1979

TEW JM JR, SAUL TG, MAYFIELD FH: Neurosurgery. In: *Otolaryngology, Second Edition.* Paparella M, Shumrick D (eds). W.B. Saunders: Philadelphia, pp. 900–950, 1980

TEW JM JR: Painful neuralgias of the trigeminal, glossopharyngeal, vagus, and geniculate nerves. In: *Current Diagnosis,* Conn H (ed). W.B. Saunders: Philadelphia, pp. 907–909, 1980

TEW JM JR, MAYFIELD FH: Surgery of the anterior cervical spine: Prevention of Complications. In: *Cervical Spondylosis,* Dunsker SB (ed). Raven Press: New York, pp. 191–208, 1981

TEW JM JR: Guidelines for management and surgical treatment of intracranial aneurysms. In: *Controversies in Neurology,* Thompson RA, Green JR (eds). Raven Press: New York, pp. 139–154, 1982

TEW JM JR: Treatment of trigeminal neuralgia by percutaneous rhizotomy. In: *Neurological Surgery,* Youmans J (ed). W.B. Saunders: Philadelphia, pp. 3564–3579, 1982

TEW JM JR: Treatment of pain of glossopharyngeal and vagus nerves by percutaneous rhizotomy. In: *Neurological Surgery,* Youmans J (ed). W.B. Saunders: Philadelphia, pp. 3609–3612, 1982

TEW JM JR: Nonsurgical treatment of lumbar disc disease. In: *Lumbar*

Disc Disease, Hardy RW (ed). Raven Press: New York, pp. 111–118, 1982

TOMSICK TA, TEW JM JR, LUKIN RR, MCLENNAN J: Intracranial arteriovenous malformation with increased intracranial pressure: Response to embolization. In: ***Vascular Malformations and Fistulas of the Brain,*** Smith R, Haerer A, Russell W (eds). Raven Press: New York, pp. 119–127, 1982

TOMSICK TA, TEW JM JR, LUKIN RR, EGGERS FM: Detachable balloon closure of carotid cavernous fistula. In: ***Vascular Malformations and Fistulas of the Brain,*** Smith R, Haerer A, Russell W (eds). Raven Press: New York, pp. 241–250, 1982

TEW JM JR, TOBLER WD, VAN LOVEREN HR: Percutaneous rhizotomy in the treatment of intractable facial pain (trigeminal, glossopharyngeal, and vagal nerves). In: ***Operative Neurosurgical Techniques,*** Schmidek HH, Sweet WH (eds). Grune & Stratton: New York, pp. 1083–1100, 1982

TEW JM JR: Guidelines for management and surgical treatment of intracranial aneurysms. In: ***Controversies in Neurology,*** Thompson R, Green J (eds). Raven Press: New York, pp. 139–154, 1983

TEW JM JR, VAN LOVEREN HR, KELLER JT, NURRE MA: A 10-year experience in the treatment of trigeminal neuralgia: A comparison of percutaneous stereotaxic rhizotomy and posterior fossa exploration. In: ***Pain Therapy,*** Rissi R, Elsevier V (eds). Biomedical Press: New York, pp. 321–337, 1983

TEW JM JR, STEIGER HJ: ANEURYSM CLIPS. IN: ***Neurosurgery,*** Wilkins RH, Rengachary SS (eds). McGraw Hill: New York, pp. 1530–1534, 1983

TEW JM JR, STEIGER HJ: Instrumentation for microneurosurgery. In: ***Neurosurgery,*** Wilkins RH, Rengachary SS (eds). McGraw Hill: New York, pp. 1108–1123, 1984

TEW JM JR, JOHNSON JK, TOMSICK TA: TRAUMATIC LESIONS OF THE CAROTID ARTERY. IN: ***Stroke and the Extracranial Vessels,*** Smith RR (ed). Raven Press: New York, pp. 307–319, 1984

TEW JM JR, VAN LOVEREN HR: Painful neuralgias of the trigeminal, glossopharyngeal, vagus, and geniculate nerves. In: ***Current Diagnosis,*** Conn R (ed). W.B. Saunders: Philadelphia, pp. 890–891, 1985

TOMSICK TA, TEW JM JR, LUKIN RR: Vascular interventional neuroradiology. In: ***Practice of Surgery,*** Hoff J, Chandler W (eds). J.B. Lippincott: Philadelphia, pp. 1–26, 1985

TEW JM JR, TOBLER WD: Present status of lasers in neurosurgery. In: ***Advances in Technical Standards In Neurosurgery,*** Symon L (ed). Springer-Verlag: Wien and New York, Vol 13, pp. 3–36, 1986

TEW JM JR, TOBLER WD, PENSAK ML, JACOBSON GP: Use of the laser for resection of the cranial base tumors. In: *Tumors of the Cranial Base: Diagnosis and Treatment,* Sekhar LN, Schramm VL Jr (eds). Futura: Mount Kisco, pp. 135–148, 1987

TEW JM JR: Lasers in neurosurgery: Past, present, and future. In: *Neurosurgery: State of the Art Reviews,* Sawaya R, Tew JM Jr (eds). Hanley & Belfus: Philadelphia, Vol 2, No 2, pp. 351–355, 1987

HEISS JD, TEW JM JR: Transsphenoidal laser microsurgery. In: *Neurosurgery: State of the Art Reviews,* Sawaya R, Tew JM Jr (eds). Hanley & Belfus: Philadelphia, Vol 2, pp. 411–425, 1987

TOBLER WD, TEW JM JR: The role of the carbon dioxide laser in skull base tumors. In: *Neurosurgery: State of the Art Reviews,* Sawaya R, Tew JM Jr (eds). Hanley & Belfus: Philadelphia, Vol 2, pp. 397–409, 1987

VAN LOVEREN HR, WEIL SM, TEW JM JR: Complete excision of thalamic arteriovenous malformations with neodymium: YAG laser. In: *Neurosurgery: State of the Art Reviews,* Sawaya R, Tew JM Jr (eds). Hanley & Belfus: Philadelphia, Vol 2, pp. 1987

TEW JM JR, TOBLER WD: The history of lasers in neurosurgery. In: *Lasers in Neurosurgery, Volume 1,* Robertson JH, Clark WC (eds). Kluwer Academic Publishers: Norwell, pp. 3–7, 1988

TEW JM JR, VAN LOVEREN HR: Percutaneous rhizotomy in the treatment of intractable facial pain (trigeminal, glossopharyngeal, and vagal nerves). In: *Operative Neurosurgical Techniques, 2nd Edition,* Schmidek HH, Sweet WH (eds). Grune & Stratton: Orlando, 1988; pp. 1111–1123, 1988

TOBLER WD, TEW JM JR: Neurosurgical applications of laser technology: In: *Advances in Nd:YAG Laser Surgery, Volume 19,* Joffe SN, Oguro Y (eds). Springer-Verlag: New York, pp. 118–130, 1988

ZUCCARELLO M, LIWNICZ BH, KELLER JT, TEW JM JR, TIERNEY B: Intracisternal synthetic substance P increases vascular permeability. In: *Cerebral Vasospasm,* Wilkins RH (ed). Raven Press: New York, pp. 187–193, 1988

TEW JM JR, TOBLER WD, ZUCCARELLO M: The treatment of arteriovenous malformations of the brain with the neodymium:YAG laser. In: *Lasers in Neurosurgery,* Downing EF, Ascher PW, Cerullo LJ, Neblett CR, Robertson JH, Tew JM Jr (eds). Springer-Verlag: Wein and New York, pp. 19–48, 1988

CRONE KR, BERGER TS, TEW JM JR: Laser applications in pediatric neurosurgery. In: *Lasers in Neurosurgery,* Downing EF, Ascher PW, Cerullo LJ, Neblett CR, Robertson JH, Tew JM Jr (eds). Springer-Verlag: Wein and New York, pp. 105–118, 1988

VAN LOVEREN HR, TEW JM JR, THOMAS GM: Trigeminal neuralgia therapy and surgical treatment. In: *Current Therapy in Neurological Surgery.* B.C. Decker, pp. 307–310, 1989

OLIVI A, TEW JM JR, VAN LOVEREN HR: Fibromuscular dysplasia. In: *Neurosurgery: State of the Art Reviews,* Sawaya R, Tew JM Jr (eds). Hanley & Belfus: Philadelphia, pp. 193–200, 1989

TEW JM JR, ZUCCARELLO M: Laser surgery of tumors and arteriovenous malformations of the diencephalon. In: *Surgery of the Diencephalon,* Holtzman RNN, Stein BM (eds). Plenum Publishing, pp. 231–236, 1989

TEW JM JR, SAWAYA R, PENSAK ML: Neurosurgery of the head and neck. In: *Otolaryngology, 3rd Edition,* Parparella MM, Shumrick DA, Meyerhoff WL, Gluckman JL (eds). W.B. Saunders: Philadelphia, pp. 2983–3031, 1991

BUCKINGHAM MJ, TEW JM JR, WIOT JG: The diagnosis and surgical treatment of craniocervical junction tumors. In: *Cervical Tumors/Vascular Disorders;* pp. 497–506, 1992

VAN LOVEREN HR, EL-KALLINY M, KELLER JT, TEW JM JR: Surgery of the Cavernous Sinus. In: *Neurosurgical Operative Atlas,* Wilkins RH (ed). Williams & Wilkins: Baltimore, pp. 355–365, 1992

TEW JM JR, SCODARY DJ: Basic techniques and surgical positioning. In: *Brain Surgery: Complication, Avoidance and Management,* Apuzzo M (ed). Churchill Livingstone: New York, pp. 31–50, 1993

TEW JM JR, SCODARY DJ: Surgical Positioning. In: *Brain Surgery: Complication Avoidance and Management,* Apuzzo MLJ (ed). Churchill Livingstone: New York, pp. 1609–1620, 1993

REICHERT KW, TEW JM JR, TOMSICK T: Intraoperative temporary balloon occlusion as an aid in basilar artery aneurysm clipping. In: *The 3rd International Workshop on Cerebrovascular Surgery,* Takakura K, Sasaki T (eds). University of Tokyo Press: Tokyo, pp. 58–61, 1993

REICHERT KW, TEW JM JR: Management of thalamic-basal ganglia arteriovenous malformations. In: *The 3rd International Workshop on Cerebrovascular Surgery,* Takakura K, Sasaki T (eds). University of Tokyo Press: Tokyo, pp. 166–171, 1993

BUCKINGHAM MJ, TEW JM JR, WIOT JG: The diagnosis and surgical treatment of craniocervical junction tumors. In: *Disorders of the Cervical Spine,* Camins MB, O'Leary PF (eds). Williams & Wilkins: Philadelphia, pp. 497–506, 1993

TEW JM JR, VAN LOVEREN HR, FERNANDEZ P: Operative positioning and perioperative management. In: *Surgery for Cranial Nerves of the Posterior Fossa,* Barrow DL (ed). Neurosurgical Topics, Book 13, 1993

EL-KALLINY M, KELLER, JT, VAN LOVEREN HR, TEW JM JR: Anatomy of the anterior clinoid process: a surgical perspective. In: *Skull Base Surgery. First International Skull Base Congress,* Samii M (ed). Basel: Karger, pp. 75–77, 1994

KUMAR R, GUTHIKONDA M, TEW JM JR: Advances in the medical management of severe head injury. In: *Advances in Clinical Neurosciences,* Sinha KK, Chandra P (eds). Association of Neuroscientists of Eastern India: Ranchi, pp. 169–186, 1994

LEWIS AI, TEW JM JR: Management of thalamic-basal ganglia and brainstem vascular malformations. In: *Clinical Neurosurgery,* Loftus CM (ed). Williams & Wilkins: Baltimore, pp. 83–111, 1994

TEW JM JR, HEISS JD: Anterior cervical discectomy. In: *Anterior Cervical Spine Surgery,* Whitecloud TS III, Dunsker SB (eds). Raven Press: New York, 1994

VAN LOVEREN HR, FERNANDEZ PM, KELLER JT, TEW JM JR, SHUMRICK K: Neurosurgical applications of Le Fort I-type osteotomy. In: *Clinical Neurosurgery,* Loftus CM (ed). Williams & Wilkins: Baltimore, pp. 425–443, 1994

REICHERT KW III, LEWIS AI, TEW JM JR: Surgical management of thalamic-basal ganglia vascular malformations. In: *Operative Neurosurgical Techniques,* Schmidek HH, Sweet WH (eds). W.B. Saunders: Philadelphia, pp. 1501–1521, 1995

REICHERT KW III, TEW JM JR: Surgical management of brainstem vascular malformations. In: *Operative Neurosurgical Techniques,* Schmidek HH, Sweet WH (eds). W.B. Saunders: Philadelphia, pp. 1485–1499, 1995

TEW JM JR, TAHA JM: Percutaneous rhizotomy in the treatment of intractable facial pain (trigeminal, glossopharyngeal, and vagal nerves). In: *Operative Neurosurgical Techniques,* Schmidek HH, Sweet WH (eds). W.B. Saunders: Philadelphia, pp. 1469–1484, 1995

TEW JM JR, LEWIS AI: Surgical management of brainstem vascular malformations. In: *Operative Neurosurgical Techniques,* Schmidek HH, Sweet WH (eds). W.B. Saunders: Philadelphia, pp. 1485–1499, 1995

TEW JM JR, TAHA JM: Treatment of trigeminal and other facial neuralgias by percutaneous techniques. In: *Neurological Surgery,* Youmans JR (ed). Williams & Wilkins: Baltimore, pp. 3386–3403, 1995

LEWIS AI, TEW JM JR: Effects of venous hypertension on dural arteriovenous malformations. In: *Surgery of the Intracranial Venous System,* Hakuba A (ed). Springer-Verlag: Tokyo; 395–405, 1995

LEWIS AI, TOMSICK TA, TEW JM JR: Carotid-cavernous fistulas and intracavernous aneurysms. In: *Neurosurgery, 2nd edition,* Wilkins RH, Rengachary SS (eds). McGraw Hill: New York, pp. 2529–2539, 1996

PAYNER TD, TEW JM JR, STEIGER HJ: Aneurysm clips. In: *Neurosurgery, 2nd edition,* Wilkins RH, Rengachary SS (eds). McGraw Hill: New York, pp. 2271–2276, 1996

PAYNER TD, TEW JM JR, STEIGER HJ: Instrumentation for neurosurgery. In: *Neurosurgery, 2nd edition,* Wilkins RH, Rengachary SS (eds). McGraw Hill: New York, pp. 531–538, 1996

TAHA JM, TEW JM JR: Surgical management of vagoglossopharyngeal and other uncommon neuralgias. In: Tindall GT, Cooper PR, Barrow DL (eds) *The Practice of Neurosurgery.* Williams & Wilkins: Baltimore; pp 3065–3080, 1996

TEW JM JR, SATHI S: Cavernous malformations. In: *Primer on Cerebrovascular Diseases,* Welch KM, Caplan L, Reis D, Weir B, Seisjo B (eds). Academic Press: New York; 549–556, 1997

LEWIS AI, SATHI S, TEW JM JR. Intracranial vascular malformations. In: *Principles of Neurosurgery.* Grossman RS, Loftus CM (eds). Philadelphia: Lippincott-Raven, 1997

TAHA JM, TEW JM JR. Treatment of trigeminal neuralgia by percutaneous radiofrequency rhizotomy. In: *Neurosurgery Clinics of North America: Neurosurgical Perspectives on Trigeminal Neuralgia.* Brown JA (ed). Philadelphia: W.B. Saunders, pp. 31–39, 1997

VAN LOVEREN HR, TAUBER M, LEWIS AI, AND TEW JM JR. Direct surgical treatment of carotid cavernous fistulas. In: *Carotid Cavernous Fistulas,* Tomsick TA (ed). Cincinnati: MRI Foundation, pp. 83–93, 1997

TAHA JM, AND TEW JM JR. Radiofrequency rhizotomy for trigeminal and other cranial neuralgias. In: *Textbook of Stereotactic and Functional Neurosurgery,* Gildenberg PL and Tasker RR (eds). New York: McGraw-Hill, pp. 1687–1696, 1998

ROSENBLATT S, LEWIS AI, TEW JM JR. Combined interventional and surgical treatment of arteriovenous malformations. In: *Neurovascular Malformations: Diagnosis and Intervention,* Neuroimaging Clinics of North America, Russell EJ, Meyer JR (eds). Philadelphia: W.B. Saunders, pp. 469–482, 1998

ABSTRACTS

WILLIAMS DS, KELLER JT, TEW JM JR: Neuroanatomical interrelationships pertaining to the percutaneous coagulation procedure for the treatment of trigeminal neuralgia. **Clin Res 25:**636A, 1977

Tew JM Jr: The management of carotid artery occlusive disease. **Proc Inst Med Chic 33:**146–147, 1980

Tomsick TA, Tew JM Jr, Lukin R, Sprick W, McLennan J, Eisentraut C, Chambers A: Computerized tomography as a prognostic indicator in subarachnoid hemorrhage due to ruptured aneurysm. **Stroke 11:**2, 1980

Frank EH, Keller JT, Burge B, Tew JM Jr, Mayfield FH: Tissue cultured arachnoid cells: The response to chemical irritation. **Neurosurgery 9:**474, 1981

Keller JT, Saunders MC, Ongkiko CM Jr, Frank EH, Tew JM Jr: Identification of motoneurons innervating the tensor tympani and tensor veli palatini muscles in the cat. **Anat Rec 202:**94-A, 1982

Larson JJ, de Tribolet N, Tew JM Jr, van Loveren HR, Warnick RE, Menon AG: Evidence for the clonal origin of primary and recurrent meningiomas and their malignant transformation. **J Neurosurg 82:**346A, 1995

Larson JJ, van Loveren HR, Balko GM, Tew JM Jr: Evidence of meningioma invasion into cranial nerves: clinical implication for cavernous sinus meningiomas. **J Neurosurg 82:**360A, 1995

Lewis AI, Brockman DE, Kossenjans W, Myatt L, Zuccarello M, Tew JM Jr: Increased expression of constitutive nitric oxide synthase in response to cerebral vasospasm after experimental subarachnoid hemorrhage. **J Neurosurg 82:**372A, 1995

Lewis AI, Lawless M, Tomsick TA, Tew JM Jr: Long-term results of direct carotid-cavernous fistulas after treatment with detachable balloons. **J Neurosurg 82:**343A, 1995

Lewis AI, Tomsick TA, deCourten-Meyers G, Tew JM Jr: Effects of venous hypertension on dural arteriovenous malformations. **J Neurosurg 82:**352A, 1995

Taha JM, Tew JM Jr: A prospective 15-year follow-up of 100 patients with trigeminal neuralgia treated by percutaneous stereotactic radiofrequency rhizotomy. **J Neurosurg 82:**365A-366A, 1995

Lewis AI, Tomsick TA, Tew JM Jr, Lawless MA: Long-term results of direct carotid-cavernous fistulas after treatment with detachable balloons. **J Neurosurg 82:**343A, 1995

Sathi S, Mascott CR, Liu SS, et al: Recurrence of arteriovenous malformations in children. **J Neurosurg 84:**364A-365A, 1996

Larson JJ, Tew JM Jr, van Loveren HR, Tomsick TA. Delayed complications after permanent balloon occlusion of the internal carotid artery (ICA) for treatment of aneurysms of the ICA. **J Neurosurg 86:**364A, 1997

Lewis AI, Tew JM Jr., and Zimmerman GA. True sylvian fissure arteriovenous malformations: a report of eight cases. **J Neurosurg 88:**200A, 1998

REVIEWS

TEW JM JR, KELLER JT: Book Review on *Principles of Neurology* by JB Angevine Jr and CW Cotman. **J Neurosurg 57:**577, 1982

TEW JM JR, WARNICK RE: Neurosurgical procedures: personal approaches to classic operations (book review). **J Neurosurg 34:**763–764, 1994

Professional Societies and Activities

1969	Academy of Medicine of Cincinnati, *Member, Media Resource* (1992)
1969	American Medical Association
1969	Ohio State Medical Association
1969	Ohio State Neurosurgical Society, *President* (1979)
1969	Cincinnati Society of Neurology and Neurosurgery, *President* (1980)
1969	Congress of Neurological Surgeons, *Executive Committee* (1975–1986), *President* (1982–1983)
1971	American College of Surgeons, *Fellow*
1972	American Association of Neurological Surgeons, *Chairman, Education Committee* (1981–1982)
1973	International Neurosurgical Society, *Founder*
1974	Section of Cerebrovascular Surgery of the AANS-CNS, *Founder and Chairman* (1978–1979)
1974	American Academy of Neurological Surgery, *Chairman, Future Sites Committee* (1992–1994), *President* (1995–1996)
1974	American Trauma Society, *President, Ohio Division Board of Trustees* (1975)
1975	American Heart Association, *Fellow in Stroke Council*
1975	Neurosurgical Society of America
1979	World Federation of Neurological Surgery, *Delegate* (1986-Present)
1979	Society of Neurological Surgeons
1980	Foundation for International Education in Neurological Surgery, Inc., *Board of Trustees*
1983	LANSI (Laser Association of Neurological Surgeons International), Founder and Board of Trustees, *President* (1992)
1986	Society of Medical Consultants to the Armed Forces
1988–1989	Society for Neuroscience
1988	Southern Neurosurgical Society, *Chairman, Future Sites Committee* (1993–1997)
1988	International Society of Pituitary Surgeons
1988	North American Skull Base Society
1992	Trigeminal Neuralgia Association, *Medical Advisory*

	Board Member, Chairman of the Finance & Development Committee
1992	Acoustic Neuroma Association, *Medical Advisory Board Member*
1992	Ohio Surgical Panel, Inc., *Member*
1992	Ohio Medical Instrument Company, *Member, Board of Directors*
1992	International Federation of Biomedical Laser Research Centers, *Member*
1993	The Vanderbilt-Meacham Neurosurgical Society, *Member*

Editorial Board

1977	*Neurosurgery,* Chairman, Publication Committee, 1984
1978	*Microsurgery*
1984	*Lasers in Medicine and Surgery*
1984–1995	*Acta Neurochirurgica*
1990	*Professional Healthcare Marketing,* Editorial Advisory Board
1993–1998	*Critical Reviews in Neurosurgery*
1996	*Neurologica Medico-chirurgica,* Commentary Board

Book Review Contributor

Neurosurgery
Journal of Neurosurgery

NATIONAL INSTITUTES OF HEALTH

1. Clinical Associate, National Institute of Neurological Diseases and Blindness, Bethesda, MD, 1963–1965
2. National Advisory Council, National Institute of Neurological and Communicative Disorders and Stroke, 1982–1985

TEACHING AND RESEARCH APPOINTMENTS

Presiously Held

1970–1982	Instructor in Surgery (Neurosurgery), University of Cincinnati Medical Center
1975–1988	Chairman, Section of Neurosurgery, The Deaconess Hospital
1977–1991	Chairman, Section of Neurosurgery, Good Samaritan Hospital
1982–1985	National Advisory Council, National Institute of Neurological and Communicative Disorders and Stroke, National Institutes of Health

1984–1997	United States Army Reserve, Colonel, MC Consultant to Surgeon General
1985–1987	Member, Washington Committee for Neurosurgery
1986–1991	Executive Committee, University of Cincinnati Medical Center

Current

1978-Present	Associate Professor of Anatomy
1982-Present	Professor and Chairman, Department of Neurosurgery, University of Cincinnati Medical Center
1982-Present	Chief of Neurosurgery, Children's Hospital Medical Center
1982-Present	Director, Division of Cerebrovascular Surgery, Department of Neurosurgery, University of Cincinnati College of Medicine
1984-Present	Delegate, World Federation of Neurological Surgery
1985-Present	Trustee, Foundation for International Education in Neurological Surgery, Inc.
1986-Present	Consultant, Hipple Cancer Research Center
1992-Present	Mayfield Professor of Neurosurgery, University of Cincinnati Medical Center
1995-Present	Board of Directors, Mayfield Clinic
1995-Present	Professor of Radiology, University of Cincinnati College of Medicine
1998-Present	Medical Director, The Neuroscience Institute

NAMED LECTURES

April 30, 1997	University of Michigan, Ann Arbor, Michigan Fred Coller Lecturer for Michigan Chapter of the American College of Surgeons; "Principles of Microsurgery"
October 19–21, 1978	Krayenbuhl Lecture. Zurich, SWITZERLAND
April 24–25, 1980	182nd Annual Meeting of Medical and Chirurgical Faculty. University of Maryland, Baltimore, Maryland Ridgeway Memorial Lecture: "Diagnosis and Treatment of Cerebrovascular Disease—A Neurological Perspective"
March 1–6, 1983	*Southern Neurosurgical Society.* Sea Island, Georgia Eustace Semmes Lecturer: "Laser Applications in Neurosurgery"

September 13, 1984	University of Alabama, Birmingham, Alabama Galbraith Lecturer: "Current Diagnosis and Treatment of Pituitary Tumors"
April 1–4, 1986	*Handa Memorial Lecture.* Kyoto, JAPAN "Surgical Treatment of the Thalamic and Deep AVMs With Microsurgical Laser Technology"
October 10–12, 1986	*Bowman Gray School of Medicine Alumni Weekend.* Wake Forest University, Winston-Salem, North Carolina Distinguished Alumni Lecturer for Class of 1961 "Can Neurosurgery Keep Pace with the Revolution in Neuroscience?"
March 30-April 2, 1988	Southern Neurosurgical Society. The Homestead, Hot Springs, Virginia William Henry Hudson Lecture "Neural Transplantation: Challenge for the Neurosurgeon"
December 5, 1990	Georgetown University Medical Center, Washington, D.C. Fulcher Visiting Professor; "Treatment of Arteriovenous Malformations"
August 15, 1991	*West Virginia State Medical Association.* White Sulphur Springs, West Virginia The Thomas L. Harris Address: "The Physician as a Caring Citizen: Being More than Just Good"
March 15–16, 1994	*Gurdjian Lecture.* Wayne State University School of Medicine, Detroit, Michigan "Arteriovenous Malformation of Brain and Dural Sinuses" and "Trigeminal Neuralgia"
June 8–9, 1995	*George Cohn Lecture,* Buffalo General Hospital, Buffalo, New York "Skull Base Meningiomas"; "Deep Arteriovenous Malformations"; and "Trigeminal Neuralgia"
October 16–17, 1997	*Raaf Lecturer,* Oregon Health Science University, Portland, Oregon "Cerebrovascular Disease—A Model for Change"

January 10–12, 1998	Northwestern University Medical Center, Evanston/Chicago, Illinois Bennett-Tarkington Visiting Professorship "New Concepts in the Treatment of Deep Brain Vascular Malformations" "Surgical Treatment of Skull Base Meningiomas"
May 22–23, 1998	*Andy Neal Lecturer* Joint Neurosurgery Society of Louisiana, Mississippi and Arkansas University of Mississippi, Jackson, Mississippi "Treatment of Aneurysms, Coiling or Clipping: A 5-year Experience"

HONORS

1957	*Cum Laude,* Wake Forest University, Winston-Salem, North Carolina
1961	*Alpha Omega Alpha,* Bowman Gray School of Medicine, Winston-Salem, North Carolina
1970	*William P. Van Wagenen Fellowship,* Awarded by American Association of Neurological Surgeons
1974	*The Hull Award,* Given by the AMA for outstanding scientific exhibit entitled Trigeminal Neuralgia: A New Surgical Approach"
1975	*Outstanding Young Physician, The Cincinnati Post,* Cincinnati, Ohio
1975	*The Billings Award,* Given by the AMA at the annual meeting for the exhibit entitled: "Trigeminal Neuralgia: A New Surgical Approach"
1975	*Silver Plaque for Excellence in Teaching,* Awarded by the Ohio State Medical Association for the exhibit on Trigeminal Neuralgia
1980	*Gold Plaque for 1st Place Award in Teaching,* Awarded by the Ohio State Medical Association for exhibit on Reconstructive Cerebrovascular Surgery
1980	*Bronze Plaque,* For the Ridgeway Trimble Lecture: "Diagnosis and Treatment of Cerebrovascular Disease: A Neurosurgical Prospective," to the 182nd Annual Meeting of Medical and Chirurgical Faculty of the State of Maryland
1980	*Honorary Member,* Neurological Society of Colombia
1981	*Distinguished Alumni Award,* Campbell University, Buies Creek, North Carolina

1985	*Honorary Doctor of Human Letters,* Campbell University, Buies Creek, North Carolina
1986	*Distinguished Alumni Lecturer, Class of 1961,* Bowman Gray School of Medicine, Winston-Salem, North Carolina
1988	*Paul Harris Fellow Award,* Presented by the Rotary Club of Cincinnati, Cincinnati, Ohio
1989	*Pro ecclesia et pontifice medal,* Papal honor presented by Archbishop Daniel E. Pilarczyk
1991	Distinguished Alumni Award, Bowman Gray School of Medicine, Wake Forest University, Winston-Salem, North Carolina
1992–1998	Listed *Best Doctors In America*
1992	Appointed *Frank H. Mayfield Professor of Neurosurgery,* Chairman, Department of Neurosurgery, University of Cincinnati College of Medicine, Cincinnati, Ohio
1994	*1994 Hospital Hero,* University of Cincinnati Medical Center, Cincinnati, Ohio
1995	Distinguished Service Citation, National Conference of Christians and Jews
1996–1998	Recognized as One of the Country's Best Neurosurgeons, *Good Housekeeping,* March 1996
1997	*Distinguished Service Award,* University of Cincinnati Medical Center, Department of Otolaryngology—Head and Neck Surgery Cincinnati, Ohio
1997	The Japan Neurosurgical Society, *Honored Member*
1998	*Xavier University Leadership Medallion,* Xavier University, Cincinnati, Ohio
1998	*Honored Guest,* Congress of Neurological Surgeons Meeting, Seattle, Washington

NON PROFESSIONAL SOCIETIES AND ACTIVITIES

Rotary Club of Cincinnati (and International)
Cincinnati Country Club
Queen City Club
The Travel Club
Cincinnati Tennis Club
The Literary Club
Optimist Club
Commonwealth Club, *Vice President,* 1998
Bellarmine Chapel
Campbell University, *Presidential Board of Advisors*
The Commercial Club
Xavier University, *Board of Trustees,* 1986–1995

1977	Challenge Fund Drive, Class Agent, Bowman Gray School of Medicine, Winston-Salem, North Carolina
1979	Fund Drive, Trinity College, Washington, D.C.
1980	Fund Drive for Establishing an Ecumenical Chair, Xavier University, Cincinnati, Ohio
1980-Present	Member, Dinner Committee, National Conference of Christians and Jews, Cincinnati, Ohio
1981-Present	Men's Committee, Cincinnati Art Museum, Cincinnati, Ohio
1981	Sesquicentennial Fund Drive, Historical Society of Cincinnati, Cincinnati, Ohio
1984-Present	Fund Drive, Robert Taft II Finance Committee, Cincinnati, Ohio
1985-Present	Board of Trustees, Union Central Life Insurance Company, Cincinnati, Ohio
1985–1990	Chairman, Good Samaritan Hospital Division of United Appeal, Cincinnati, Ohio
1985–1995	Board of Trustees, Xavier University, Cincinnati, Ohio
1986	Fund Drive, United Fine Arts Fund, Cincinnati, Ohio
1989	Citizens Committee for the new Drake Hospital, Cincinnati, Ohio
1989–1992	Cornerstone Fund Drive, Xavier University, Cincinnati, Ohio
1990–1993	Alumnae Council, Wake Forest University, Winston-Salem, North Carolina
1991	Daniel Drake Society, United Way, Cincinnati, Ohio
1991	Co-Chairman, Tax Levy Committee, University Hospital, Cincinnati, Ohio
1992-Present	Board of Directors, Blue Chip Venture Capital Fund
1993	Medical Committee, Greater Cincinnati Convention Alliance, Cincinnati, Ohio
1995	Kids Helping Kids, Cincinnati, Ohio

Contents

Preface v
Honored Guests vii
Officers of the Congress of Neurological Surgeons ix
Editors-in-Chief xi
Contributors xiii
Biography of John M. Tew, Jr., M.D., F.A.C.S. xix
Bibliography of John M. Tew, Jr., M.D., F.A.C.S. xxi

CHAPTER 1
Presidential Address: "What is the Meaning of Life?"
William A. Friedman, M.D. 1

CHAPTER 2
CNS Resident Award: Role of Interleukin-1β Converting
Enzyme in Experimental Traumatic Brain Injury
Robert M. Friedlander, M.D., M.A., Klaus B. Fink, M.D.
L. John Andrews, B.A., William E. Butler, M.D.,
Victoria O. Ona, M.D., Mikhail Bogdanov, M.D.,
Matthias Endres, M.D., Mingwei Li, M.D.,
Sohail Q. Khan, B.A., Shobu Namura, M.D.,
M. Flint Beal, M.D., Michael A. Moskowitz, M.D.,
Junying Yuan, Ph.D. 12

I

GENERAL SCIENTIFIC SESSION I

CHAPTER 3
Honored Guest Presentation—Integrating Technical Innovations
in Everyday Practice
John M. Tew, Jr., M.D., F.A.C.S. 27

CHAPTER 4
Localizing the Point: Evolving Principles of Surgical Navigation
Joseph C.T. Chen, M.D. Ph.D., Michael L. J. Apuzzo, M.D. 44

CHAPTER 5
Image-guided Spinal Navigation
Iain H. Kalfas, M.D., F.A.C.S. 70

CHAPTER 6
The Future of Image-guided Surgery
M. Peter Heilbrun, M.D., Jeffery D. McDonald, M.D., Ph.D. 89

II

GENERAL SCIENTIFIC SESSION II

Chapter 7
Epidemiology and Cost of Central Nervous System Injury
Lawrence F. Marshall, M.D. 105

Chapter 8
Pathophysiology of Neural Injury: Therapeutic Opportunities and Challenges
John T. Povlishock, Ph.D. 113

Chapter 9
The Triage and Acute Management of Severe Head Injury
Richard J. Meagher, M.D., Raj K. Narayan, M.D. 127

Chapter 10
Contemporary Treatment Paradigms in Head Injury
Jack E. Wilberger, M.D. 143

Chapter 11
Contemporary Treatment Paradigms in Spinal Injury
Michael P. B. Kilburn, M.D., Mark N. Hadley, M.D. 153

Chapter 12
Neurological Injuries in Infants and Children: An Overview of Current Management Strategies
Thomas G. Luerssen, M.D., F.A.C.S., F.A.A.P. 170

Chapter 13
Evolving Models of Neurotrauma Critical Care: An Analysis and Call to Action
Randall M. Chestnut, M.D., F.A.C.C.M. 185

Chapter 14
Core Curriculum in Neurosurgical Critical Care
Brian T. Andrews, M.D., F.A.C.S. 196

Chapter 15
Outcomes Science and Neurotrauma: A National Database
Beverly C. Waters, M.D., M.Sc., F.R.C.S.C., F.A.C.S. 203

Chapter 16
Trauma: The Neurosurgeon's Domain
Lawrence H. Pitts, M.D., Martin Holland, M.D. 216

III

GENERAL SCIENTIFIC SESSION III

Chapter 17
Organizing Cerebrovascular Care Teams
Marc R. Mayberg, M.D. 231

CHAPTER 18
Diagnostic Imaging for Stroke
Robert H. Rosenwasser, M.D., F.A.C.S.,
 Rocco A. Armonda, M.D., M.A.I., M.C., U.S.A. 237

CHAPTER 19
Contemporary Acute Ischemic Stroke Therapy with Intravenous
 Recombinant Tissue Plasminogen Activator
Jeffrey I. Frank, M.D. 261

CHAPTER 20
Honored Guest Presentation: Management Strategies for the
 Treatment of Intracranial Arteriovenous Malformations
John M. Tew, Jr., M.D., F.A.C.S., Adam I. Lewis, M.D. 267

CHAPTER 21
Controversies in Neurosurgery: Microsurgery versus
 Radiosurgery for Arteriovenous Malformations—
 The Case for Microsurgery
Daniel L. Barrow, M.D. 285

CHAPTER 22
Therapeutic Embolization of Arteriovenous Malformations:
 The Case For and Against
Neil A. Martin, M.D., Rohit Khanna, M.D.,
 Curt Doberstein, M.D., John Benston, M.D. 295

CHAPTER 23
Treatment Decisions in Brain AVMs: The Case For and
 Against Surgery
H. Hunt Batjer, M.D. 319

CHAPTER 24
Honored Guest Presentation: Therapeutic Carotid Occlusion
Michael J. Link, M.D., Thomas A. Tomsick, M.D.,
 John M. Tew, Jr., M.D., F.A.C.S. 326

CHAPTER 25
Therapeutic Carotid Occlusion:
 The Case for Prophylactic Bypass
A. Giancarlo Vishteh, M.D., Cargill H. Alleyne, Jr., M.D.,
 Robert F. Spetzler, M.D. 339

CHAPTER 26
Selective Use of Extracranial-Intracranial Bypass as an Adjunct
 to Therapeutic Internal Carotid Artery Occlusion
Bob S. Carter, M.D., Ph.D., Christopher S. Ogilvy, M.D.,
 Christopher Putman, M.D., Robert G. Ojemann, M.D. 351

CHAPTER 27
Therapeutic Carotid Occlusion: Current Management Paradigms
Sunghoon Lee, M.D., Issam A. Awad, M.D., M.Sc., F.A.C.S. 363

CHAPTER 28
Therapeutic Carotid Occlusion: Indications and Potential Complications
Daniel L. Barrow, M.D., C. Michael Cawley, M.D. 392

CHAPTER 29
Honored Guest Presentation: Therapeutic Decisions in Facial Pain
Jamal M. Taha, M.D., John M. Tew, Jr., M.D., F.A.C.S. 410

———————————— IV ————————————

GENERAL SCIENTIFIC SESSION IV

CHAPTER 30
Facial Pain Syndromes: Practical Considerations
Kim J. Burchiel, M.D., F.A.C.S. 435

CHAPTER 31
Contemporary Medical Management of Facial Pain
Oren Sagher, M.D. 443

CHAPTER 32
Percutaneous Treatment of Trigeminal Neuralgia: Advances and Problems
Jeffrey A. Brown, M.D. 455

CHAPTER 33
Neurovascular Decompression: The Procedure of Choice?
Ronald I. Apfelbaum, M.D. 473

CHAPTER 34
Trigeminal Neuralgia: Vascular Compression Theory
Andrew H. Kaye, M.D., M.B.B.S., F.R.A.C.S. 499

CHAPTER 35
Endoscopic Pituitary Surgery
Carl B. Heilman, M.D., William A. Shucart, M.D.,
  Elie E. Rebeiz, M.D., and Harsha Gopal, M.D. 507

CHAPTER 36
Endoscopic-Assisted Tumor and Neurovascular Procedures
Charles Teo, M.B.B.S., F.R.A.C.S. 515

CHAPTER 37
Endoscopic Spine Surgery
Curtis A. Dickman, M.D., Paul W. Detweiler, M.S., M.D.,
Randall W. Porter, M.D. 526

Chapter 38
Honored Guest Presentation: Contemporary Treatment of Skull Base Meningiomas
Andrew J. Kokkino, M.D., Khaled M. Abdel Aziz, M.D., John M. Tew, Jr., M.D. 554

Author Index 575

Subject Index 577

CHAPTER

1

Presidential Address: "What is the Meaning of Life?"

WILLIAM A. FRIEDMAN, M.D.

Dr. Rhoton, thank you for that wonderful introduction—I'm certain that even my mother, who is here today, was embarrassed by your lavish praise! It was almost exactly twenty years ago that I, as a young resident, sat and watched you give your CNS Presidential Address. I never imagined at that moment that I would have the opportunity to stand in your shoes someday. Most of you know that Dr. Rhoton has been my teacher, colleague, and friend for 22 years. He has had more impact on my development as a neurosurgeon, and as an individual, than anyone other than my parents. Dr. Rhoton, thank you again for the privilege you have afforded me by your introduction today.

Although it is impossible in the time allotted to do justice to the many individuals in this audience to whom I owe thanks, I would like to mention just a few. I would like to acknowledge the incredible efforts of Annual Meeting Chairman, Mark Hadley, and Scientific Program Chairman, Issam Awad. They deserve the lion's share of the credit for any successes we've enjoyed this year. I'm very proud to have several of my closest colleagues and friends here in Seattle, including Bruce Woodham, Salvatore Goodwin, Frank Bova, and John Buatti. I'm delighted that my sisters, brothers-in-law, and father-in-law are here to share this moment with me. Mom and Dad, thank you for your constant love and guidance over these many years. Most of all, I would like to acknowledge my wife, Ransom, and my three children, Daniel, Abigail, and David. As much as I love my work, and as much time as it has demanded from all of us, never forget that you are the most important part of my life. Thank you for your patience, support, understanding, and love, without which none of this would have been possible or worthwhile for me.

Members and guests of the Congress of Neurological Surgeons, it has been a great pleasure to serve this past year as your President. It has also been the greatest honor of my professional career. There are many issues with which the CNS has dealt this year. They include our relationship with the AANS, new publications, changes in Medicare, fellowship requirements, recertification, physician manpower, AMAP, evaluation and management coding, etc. Any of these issues could serve as the basis of a Presidential Address. Yet, I have chosen to turn toward another issue, which I believe, ultimately, has a greater impact on our personal and professional lives than all of the aforementioned topics thrown together. For my Presidential Address, I have chosen to discuss a simple question: What is the Meaning of Life?

Now some of you are probably convinced that I have finally lost all contact with reality. How can I hope, in the space of 30 minutes, to answer a question which has occupied lifetimes of study and contemplation by some of our most brilliant philosophers, authors, playwrights, artists, and poets? Bear with me, I plead. I am going to present you with four stories, four vignettes which I have chosen from thousands of patient interactions. I hope that they will remind each of you of similar experiences in your own lives. I contend that by pausing to reflect upon these episodes, we will be able to gain important insight into the great question, What is the Meaning of Life?

C.M.

C.M. was a 50-year-old white female who presented in 1996 with a 12-year history of symptoms consistent with Parkinson's disease. She noted severe freezing spells, alternating with severe dyskinesia. She also had severe dysarthria. Our neurologists felt she had medically intractable Parkinson's disease and was a candidate for pallidotomy.

The procedure was uneventful. Immediately after lesion placement, the patient experienced dramatic improvement in her tone and speech. However, I was later called to the recovery room because the patient had become aphasic and hemiplegic. A CT revealed a small hemorrhage at the lesion site. Over the next few days she made substantial but incomplete improvement.

On rounds with my resident, we sat trying to talk with the nearly mute C.M. She was, however, able to use her good arm to spell out messages on an alphabet board. She made it clear that she had an important message to give me. I expected that she would express disappointment or anger. Imagine my reaction as she slowly, agonizingly, spelled out, letter by letter, "IT'S NOT YOUR FAULT."

It's not your fault! I was stunned by her gesture as consideration for my feelings. Who was this woman? In an instant I understood, and I lowered by gaze. As Richard Selzer (6), a Yale surgeon and author, wrote, "One is not bold in an encounter with a god." I remembered that the gods appeared in ancient Greece as mortals, and I held my breath, and let the wonder in.

A.K.

A.K. was a distinguished professor of Pathology at the University of Florida. One Wednesday noon, I sat and chatted with him over lunch in the faculty dining room. We talked of the usual things: the weather, medical center politics, a planned vacation. The next morning, I was summoned to the emergency room. A deranged graduate student, distraught over his failure to pass his written qualifying exams, had appeared at A.K.'s door early that morning. He wife answered. The student asked for A.K. When he appeared at the door, the student shot him in the head. He then sat down and waited for the police and ambulance to arrive.

When I examined A.K., he was brain dead. There was nothing that I or anyone else could do except to try to comfort the family.

Selzer (6), I wiped a piece of brain from his shoulder to make his smashed body more presentable to his son. Now I stood with his son by the stretcher. We were arm-in-arm, like brothers. All at once, there was that terrible silence of discovery. I glanced at his son, followed his gaze and saw that there was more brain upon A.K.'s shoulder, newly slipped form the cracked skull. His son bent forward a bit. He had to make certain. It was A.K.'s brain! I watched the knowledge expand upon his face, so like his father's. I, too, stared at the fragment flung wetly, now drying beneath the bright lights of the emergency room, its cargo of thoughts evaporating from it, mingling for this little time with his son's, with mine, before dispersing in the air.

A.B.

A.B. was an 18-month-old baby girl. She and her mother were out for a long drive early one Sunday morning. Mom was exhausted and fell asleep at the wheel. The car careened out of control and struck the median guard rail. In an instant the air bags deployed. Mom awakened and brought the car under control. But baby A.B., having been struck full-force by the air bag, was unresponsive.

In the pediatric intensive care unit, I examined this blond, blue-eyed, beautiful girl. She was unresponsive, with no brainstem reflexes or spontaneous respiration. A nuclear medicine bedside scan confirmed the absence of cerebral blood flow.

I walked with the pediatric intensivist to the waiting room. There, a large family, comprising perhaps 25 people, waited for us to speak. I slowly, gently relayed the inescapable truth: baby was gone. Eager, hopeful faces broke into sobs and tears. And upon Mom's face was a look, all too familiar to me, a look of absolute woe. "Why," she cried, had God taken her baby? "It's my fault—I fell asleep at the wheel!" "No, you must be wrong, it can't be true!" And, finally, when the words were gone, there was nothing left but to hold each other and pray for strength.

J.F.

J.F. was a 32-year-old ER nurse who presented with a seizure and was found to have a posteromedial right frontal mass. I performed a craniotomy and gross total resection of a low-grade mixed glioma. She underwent postoperative radiotherapy. Shortly thereafter she returned to work full-time. Subsequently, she quit her ER job, formed a brain tumor support group, and devoted most of her time to writing patient support literature and to helping other patients with brain tumors.

Three years later she was found to have a recurrence. On repeat craniotomy, she had a frank glioblastoma. She began chemotherapy but later succumbed.

J.F. was a physically beautiful woman. She was also vivacious, intelligent, and caring. She was unfailingly positive and optimistic, regardless of what her MRI scans seemed to show. She never, ever lost hope.

When I last saw her, her external beauty was marred by hair loss and Cushingoid symptoms from steroid therapy. She and I both knew that time was short and there was little more that medicine could offer. We talked, nonetheless, at length about her plans for the future. She thanked me for all of my efforts. I thanked her for allowing me to be her physician. When we hugged each other at the end of her visit, we knew we would not meet again in this world.

As Selzer (6) wrote, "Far away from the operating room, the surgeon is taught that some deaths are undeniable, but this does not deny their meaning. To *perceive* tragedy is to wring from it beauty and truth. It is a thing beyond mere competence and technique, or the handsomeness to precisely cut and stitch. Further, he learns that love can bloom in the stoniest desert."

Selzer writes further, "I do not know when it was that I understood that it is precisely his hell in which we wage our lives that offers us the energy, the possibility to care for each other. A surgeon does not slip from his mother's womb with compassion smeared upon him like the drippings of his birth. It is much later that it comes. No easy shaft of grace this, but the cumulative murmuring of the numberless wounds he has dressed, the incisions he has made, all the sores and ulcers and cavities he has touched in order to heal. In the beginning it is barely audible, a whisper, as from many mouths. Slowly it gathers, rises from the steaming flesh until, at last, it is a pure *calling*—an exclusive sound, like the cry of certain solitary birds—telling that out of the resonance between the sick man and the one who lends him there may spring that profound courtesy that the religious call Love."

So, you ask, what do these sad stories have to do with the question, "What is the meaning of life?" Rabbi Harold Kushner (4) explored this topic in his short but meaningful book, When Bad Things Happen to Good People. "Let me suggest," says Kushner, "that the bad things that happen to us in our lives do not have a meaning when they happen to us. They do not happen for any good reason which would cause us to accept them willingly. But we can give them a meaning. We can redeem these tragedies from senselessness by imposing meaning on them. . . . When a person is dying of cancer, I do not hold God responsible for the cancer or for the pain he feels. They have other causes. But I have seen God give such people the strength to take each day as it comes, to be grateful for a day full of sunshine or one in which they are relatively free of pain. . . . When people who were never particularly strong become strong in the face of adversity, when people who tended to think only of themselves become unselfish and heroic in an emergency, I have to ask myself where they got these qualities which they would freely admit they did not have before. . . . In the final analysis, the question of why bad things happen to good people translates itself into some very different questions, no longer asking why something happened, but asking how we will *respond,* what we intended to *do* now that it has happened."

John Gunther (3), a distinguished writer, published a book in the 1940s wherein he chronicled his son's struggle with a glioblastoma. That book, *Death Be Not Proud* should be read by every neurosurgeon. Listen to Gunther's words, as he finds meaning in Johnny Jr.'s tragedy: "All that goes into a brain—the goodness, the wit, the sum total of enchantment in a personality, the very will, indeed the ego itself—being killed inexorably, remorselessly, by an evil growth! Everything that makes a human being what he is, the inordinately subtle and exquisite combination of memory, desire, impulse, reflective capacity, power of association, even consciousness—to say nothing of sight and hearing, muscular movement and voice, and something so taken for granted as the ability to chew—is encased delicately in the skull, working there within the membranes by processes so marvelously interlocked as to be beyond belief. All this—volition, imagination, the ability to have even the simplest emotion, anticipation, understanding—is held poised and balanced in the normal brain with silent, exquisite efficiency. And all this was what was being destroyed. It was, we felt, as if reason itself were being ravaged away by unreason, as if the pattern of Johnny's illness were symbolic of so much of the conflict and torture of the external world. A primitive to-the-death struggle of reason against violence, reason against disruption, reason against brute unthinking force—this was what went on in Johnny's head. . . . For others, I would say that it was his spirit, and only his spirit, that kept him invincibly alive against such dreadful obstacles for so long, this is the central pith and substance of what I am trying to write, as a mournful tribute not only to Johnny but to the *power, the wealth, the unconquerable beauty of the human spirit, will, and soul."*

Viktor Frankel (2) was a young, brilliant Viennese psychiatrist when he and his wife were sent to Auschwitz. He never saw his 24-year-old wife again, for she perished there. He himself barely survived. He lived to write about his experiences in the concentration camp. He founded a new school of psychotherapy, called logotherapy, based on his conviction that man's most profound driving force is to find meaning.

One day, exhausted, frozen, and hungry, on a work detail far from the camp, Frankel's companion mentioned his wife. Frankel later wrote,

"That brought thoughts of my own wife to mind. And as we stumbled on for miles, slipping on icy spots, supporting each other time and again, dragging one another up and onward, nothing was said, but we both knew: each of us was thinking of his wife. Occasionally I looked at the sky, where the stars were fading and the pink light of the morning was beginning to spread behind a dark band of clouds. But my mind clung to my wife's image, imagining it with an uncanny acuteness. I heard her answering me, saw her smile, her frank and encouraging look. Real or not, her look was then more luminous than the sun which was beginning to rise. A thought transfixed me: for the first time in my life I saw the truth as it is set into song by so many poets, proclaimed as the final wisdom by so many thinkers. The truth—that *love* is the ultimate and highest goal to which man can aspire. Then I grasped the *meaning* of the greatest secret that human poetry and human thought and belief have to impart: *The salvation of man is through love and in love.* I understood how a man who has nothing left in this world still may know bliss, be it only for a brief moment, in the contemplation of his beloved. In a position of utter desolation, when man cannot express himself in positive action, when his only achievement may consist in enduring his sufferings in the right way—an honorable way—in such a position man can, through loving contemplation of the image he carries of his beloved, achieve fulfillment. For the first time in my life I was able to understand the meaning of the words, "The angels are lost in perpetual contemplation of an infinite glory. . . ."

Frankel notes, ". . . we can discover the *meaning of life* in three different ways: 1) by creating a work or doing a deed, 2) by experiencing something or encountering someone, and 3) by the attitude we take toward unavoidable suffering.

As Nietzche said, "Was mich nicht umbringt, macht mich starker."— That which does not kill us makes us stronger. In other words, what matters is to make the best of any given situation. "The best," Frankel wrote, is that which in Latin is called optimum—hence, the reason I speak of a tragic optimism, that is, an optimism in the face of tragedy and in view of the human potential which at its best always allows for: 1) turning suffering into a human achievement and accomplishment, 2) deriving from guilt the opportunity to change oneself for the better, and 3) deriving from life's transitoriness an incentive to take responsible action" (2).

Kushner, Gunther, and Frankel all tell us that each patient vignette which I have presented does provide a profound answer to our question, What is the Meaning of Life? Each patient or family, when faced with tragic illness, used the opportunity to "answer life's question to them, to redeem these tragedies from senselessness by imposing meaning on them, to turn suffering into a human achievement and accomplishment." I submit to you that as we care for our patients, truly care for them, we see, with amazing frequency, people who were never particularly strong become strong in the face of adversity, people who tended to think only of themselves become unselfish and heroic. Each time I see this happen, I "let the wonder in," for I believe that in such moments I am witnessing evidence of the divine spark which may exist deep within us all.

So, I have suggested a means by which we can see, and perhaps help our patients see, the meaning of their lives. But what of the physician? What is the meaning of life for the practicing neurosurgeon?

My colleague, Albert Rhoton, wrote about this topic in his CNS Presidential Address, "Neurosurgeons share a great professional gift; our lives have yielded an opportunity to help our fellow men in a unique and exciting way. For this presidential address, I want to share some of my sense of gratitude for and inner pride and joy in our specialty, although I know that for many of us the appreciation for this opportunity, this profession, this gift, is greater than the spoken word can convey."

And, our friend Frankel (2) has written, ". . . mental health is based on a certain degree of tension, the tension between what one has already achieved and what one still ought to accomplish, or the gap between what one is and what one should become." Such a tension is inherent in the human being and therefore is indispensable to mental well-being. We should not, then, be hesitant about challenging man with a potential meaning for him to fulfill. It is only thus that we evoke his will to meaning from its state of latency. I consider it a dangerous misconception of mental hygiene to assume that what man needs in the first place is equilibrium or, as it is called in biology, homeostasis—i.e., a tensionless state. What man actually needs is not a tensionless state but rather the striving and struggling for a worthwhile goal, a freely chosen task. What he needs is not the discharge of tension at any cost but the *call of a potential meaning waiting to be fulfilled by him.*

Frankel describes what he calls an "existenial vacuum," wherein we cannot find the meaning of our lives and, instead, pursue other directions. He says, "Moreover, there are various masks and guises under which the existential vacuum appears. Sometimes the frustrated will to meaning is vicariously compensated for by a will to power, including the most primitive form of the will to power, the *will to money.* In other cases, the place of the frustrated will to meaning is taken by the will to pleasure. How true his words should ring for us. As my colleague, Arthur Day stated in his CNS Presidential Address, "The HMOs, the federal government and its bureaucrats, the insurance companies, the lawyers, and the paperwork are not our enemies, although certainly they are major obstacles to our art. Our enemies are the malignant glioma, the ruptured aneurysm with vasospasm, spinal cord injuries, and their treatment with impersonal low-quality medicine. If we continually emphasize self-serving complaints—threats to our incomes, our lifestyles, and our freedom to practice only as we see fit—we will remain unheard, isolated, impotent, and unfulfilled. To greet these changes, we must return our focus to our primary responsibility, to serve as advocates for our patients' best interests. . . ." As Osler said, "Happiness lies in the absorption in some vocation which satisfies the soul . . . we are here to add what we can to, not to get what we can from, life."

I attended Ohio State Medical School from 1973–1976. There, a plaque is affixed to the wall, just inside the entrance of the main education building. It reads, "Dr. Isaac Burt Harris, 1873–1953, Master of the healing arts for half a century, philosopher and friend of man, chief of staff, St. Francis Hospital, Professor, Ohio State University, THOUSANDS LIVED BECAUSE HE LIVED. I have ever been profoundly impressed by these words. What an outstanding memorial to Dr. Harris, and what an outstanding statement regarding the meaning of life for a physician.

As the surgeon and author Richard Selzer (6) said, "But I believe that the truly great writing about doctors has not yet been done. I think it must be done by a doctor, one who is through with the love affair with his technique, who recognizes that he has played Narcissus, raining kisses on a mirror, and who now, out of the impacted masses of his guilt, has expanded into self-doubt, and finally into the high state of wonderment. . . . I must confess that the priestliness of my profession has ever been impressed on me. In the beginning there are vows, taken with all solemnity. Then there is the endless harsh novitiate of training, much fatigue, much sacrifice. At last one emerges as celebrant, standing close to the truth lying curtained in the Ark of the body. Not surplice and cassock but mask and gown are your regalia. You hold no chalice, but a knife. There is no wine, no wafer. There are only the facts of blood and flesh."

In the brilliant movie "Shindler's List," Steven Spielberg recounts the story of the Shindlerjuden—the hundreds of Jews saved by the actions of Oskar Shindler during World War II. In gratitude, they made, as a present for Shindler, a gold ring from extracted dental fillings. On it they inscribed the ancient Talmudic saying (referring to the instructions given to a jury in a capital case): HE WHOSE SAVES ONE LIFE SAVES THE WORLD ENTIRE (7). As physicians we are granted the amazing opportunity to save lives. The meaning of our lives is to save lives, to help thousands live because we live.

To quote Frankel (2) again "... we can discover the *meaning of life* in three different ways: 1) by creating a work or doing a deed, 2) by experiencing something or encountering someone; and 3) by the attitude we take toward unavoidable suffering." Neurosurgeons have the phenomenal opportunity to discover the meaning of their lives by "creating a work or doing a deed," that is, practicing the art and science of medicine. We are, daily, presented with situations where we can additionally find the meaning of lives by "experiencing something or encountering someone," because we are interjected into the lives of countless patients who need our skills and our compassion. And, finally, and most remarkably, the meaning of our lives constantly intersects with the meaning of our patients' lives, as they struggle "with the attitude they take toward unavoidable suffering."

Allow me, if you will, to tell you one more sad story. Chuck Shank (*Fig. 1.1*) was a resident in neurosurgery at the University of Florida until 1990. Prior to entering medical school, he was an army helicopter pilot in Vietnam. During his 13-month assignment there, his aircraft was shot down twice. He received 21 air medals, the Distinguished Flying Cross, two Bronze Stars, and the Vietnamese Cross of Gallantry. The tragedy he witnessed in Vietnam motivated him ultimately to attend medical school. He was the single most gifted surgeon I have had the opportunity to help train. We became close during his time in Gainesville. After finishing training he went into private practice in Ft. Worth. His practice grew and his young family prospered. In 1997 he developed some vague abdominal discomfort, then some back pain. An ultrasound exam was done, looking for gallstones. Instead a pancreatic tumor was identified. Chuck underwent a Whipple procedure at M.D. Anderson hospital, followed by many rounds of chemotherapy and some radiation.

During the last year of his life, Chuck remained unfailingly optimistic. He bore his illness with courage and strength. He spent much time with his loving wife and two young children. When I visited him in Ft. Worth, he was then weak and feverish. We talked for hours—he told me of his love for neurosurgery, his lack of interest in money, and his great joy in caring for and loving his patients. I believe he knew then, with certainty, that his life's meaning had been to save lives, to render compassionate care, and to help his patients deal with their own search for meaning. Chuck is gone, but hundreds of grateful patients live on with loving memories of his life. HE WHO SAVES ONE LIFE SAVES THE WORLD ENTIRE.

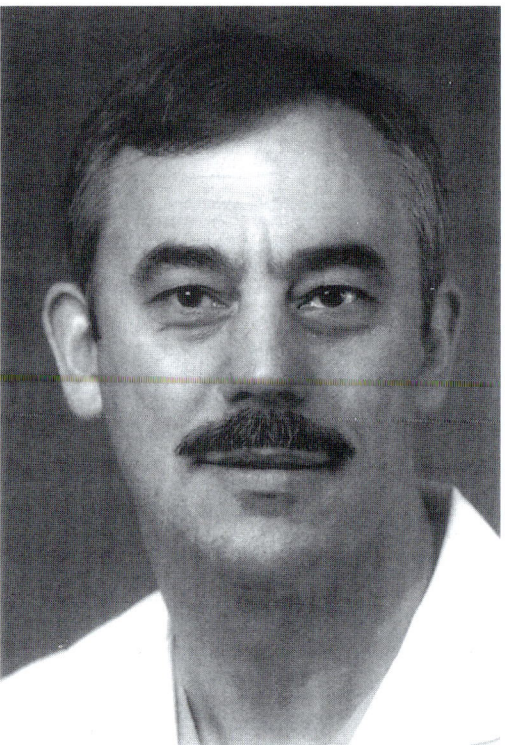

FIG. 1.1 Chuck Shank, 1948–1998.

So, what is the meaning of life? My answer, and that of Kushner, Frankel, and Selzer, is that life has a different meaning for each person. We neurosurgeons have been granted the incredible gift of finding the meaning of our lives as we do our daily work, while witnessing and helping our patients as they find theirs (1). In closing, I recall the words of Moses Maimonides. Moses Maimonides was the most important Jewish philosopher of the middle ages. He and his family fled to Cairo because of rising anti-Semitism in Spain. There, he worked as a physician, but he also became a scholar of Jewish law and a philosopher. In fact, he was asked by Richard the Lionhearted to become his Royal Physician, but he declined. He did become physician to the Sultan, Saladin. Among his many contributions is the following physician's oath, now know as the Oath of Maimonides:

> Thy eternal providence has appointed me to watch over the life and health of Thy creatures. May the love for my art actuate me at all

times: may neither avarice nor miserliness, nor thirst for glory or for a great reputation engage my mind; for the enemies of truth and philanthropy could easily deceive me and make me forgetful of my lofty aim of doing good to Thy children. *May I never see in the patient anything but a fellow creature in pain.*

Grant me the strength, time, and opportunity always to correct what I have acquired, always to extend its domain; for knowledge is immense and the spirit of man can extend indefinitely to enrich itself daily with new requirements.

Today he can discover his errors of yesterday, and tomorrow he can obtain a new light on what he thinks himself sure of today. Oh God, Thou has appointed me to watch over the life and death of Thy creatures; here am I ready for my vocation and I turn unto my calling.

REFERENCES

1. Day AL: Keeping neurosurgery special. **Neurosurgery** 34: 1052–1057, 1994.
2. Frankel VE: Man's search for meaning. New York, Simon & Schuster, 1959.
3. Gunther J: Death be not proud. New York, Harper & Row, 1965.
4. Kushner HS: When bad things happen to good people. New York, Avon Books, 1983.
5. Rhoton AL: Improving Ourselves and the specialty. **Clin Neurosurg** 26: 8–19, 1979.
6. Selzer R: Mortal lessons. New York, Simon & Schuster, 1975.
7. The Talmud, Mishnah Sanhedrin 4:5.

CHAPTER

2

CNS Resident Award: Role of Interleukin-1β Converting Enzyme in Experimental Traumatic Brain Injury*

ROBERT M. FRIEDLANDER, M.D., M.A., KLAUS B. FINK, M.D.,
L. JOHN ANDREWS, B.A., WILLIAM E. BUTLER, M.D., VICTORIA O. ONA, M.D.,
MIKHAIL BOGDANOV, M.D., MATTHIAS ENDRES, M.D., MINGWEI LI, M.D.,
SOHAIL Q. KHAN, B.A., SHOBU NAMURA, M.D., M. FLINT BEAL, M.D.,
MICHAEL A. MOSKOWITZ, M.D., AND JUNYING YUAN, PH.D.

Traumatic injury is the third leading cause of death in the western world, superseded only by cancer and heart disease. Half of traumatic deaths are directly attributed to brain injury (3). Despite the societal impact of traumatic brain injury (TBI), the basic mechanisms mediating cell death after TBI are not completely understood. Traditional notion attributes cell death to necrosis as the major mechanism following TBI (24). This view has been recently challenged with the detection of apoptotic cells in experimental brain injury models (2,22,28), as well as in humans following head trauma (26). Understanding the pathways mediating posttraumatic apoptosis might lead to novel approaches to rational pharmacotherapy of TBI.

Mechanistically, apoptotic cell death is mediated by a family of cysteine proteases known as caspases. Caspases are mammalian homologues of the *Caenorhabditis elegans* death gene product CED-3 (29,30), which executes, together with CED-4 apoptotic cell death in the nematode. Interleukin-1β converting enzyme (ICE; caspase-1), the first identified member of the caspase family, is a cysteine protease responsible for the activation of pro-Interleukin-1β (proIL-1β) (19,27). The involvement of caspase-1 in apoptosis has been demonstrated in a variety of experimental paradigms (18,19). Caspase-1 activation, as demonstrated by the detection of mature IL-1β, has been identified during apoptosis both in vitro as well as in vivo (14–16,18). We have shown previously that endogenously produced mature IL-1β, processed following caspase-1 activation, plays an important role in apoptosis (11). We have

---

*Reprinted with permission from Fink et al. Reduction of post-traumatic brain injury and free radical production by inhibition of the caspase-1 cascade. **Neuroscience** 94:1213–1215, 1999.

generated a transgenic mouse expressing a dominant negative inhibitor of caspase-1, which has the active site cysteine substituted for glycine (C285G), in neurons under the control of the neuron-specific enolase promoter (NSE-M17Z) (10). We demonstrated that caspase-1 is activated following cerebral ischemia and that expression of the M17Z transgene decreased ischemia-induced cerebral infarct as well as mature IL-1β production (10,14,15). Furthermore, synthetic peptide inhibitors of ICE-like caspases reduced infarct size following focal cerebral ischemia (15). Caspase-1 mediated cell death also plays a role in the progression of amyotrophic lateral sclerosis in its familiar transgenic mouse model (9). The above evidence implicates ICE-like caspases as important mediators of cell death in a variety of neurological conditions.

Although apoptosis has been detected in experimental brain injury models (2,22,28), our report is the first to specifically investigate the role of the caspase-1 cell death pathway in vivo following cerebral trauma. Inhibition of this apoptotic pathway might attenuate traumatic cerebral injury. We report that caspase-1 is activated in a traumatic brain injury model and that inhibition of the caspase-1 cell death cascade, both by genetic and pharmacological means, reduces traumatic brain injury. Because reactive oxygen species (ROS) are potent mediators of cell death, we also investigated whether ICE-like caspases played a role in the modulation of free radical production.

MATERIAL AND METHODS

Traumatic Brain Injury

Brain trauma experiments and lesion quantification were performed essentially as described (1). Spontaneously ventilating adult mice were initially anesthetized with halothane in 70% N_2O and 30% O_2 and fixed in a stereotactic frame. Before trauma, an atraumatic craniectomy was performed by removing the right parietal bone posterior to the coronal, lateral to the sagital, and anterior to the lambdoid suture. Laterally, the craniectomy was extended to the insertion of the temporalis muscle. A piston, which was 3 mm in diameter and had an excursion of 3 mm, was then placed over the craniectomy defect. A 20-g weight was dropped inside a cylinder from a height of 150 mm onto the piston. Twenty-four hours after trauma, brains were removed and sectioned into five coronal (2 mm) slices and stained with 2% 2,3,5-triphenyltetrazolium chloride (TTC) as described for a weight drop trauma model (1). Surgical procedure as well as quantification of lesion size was performed by an investigator naive to the animal identity. Lesion volume was calculated using an image analysis system (M4, Imaging Research, St. Catherines, Ontario, Canada) from the total lesion volume integrated from the volumes of each single section, after subtracting the volume of the deficient cortex as caused by piston penetration. The volume of the piston penetration was calculated as that of a cylinder ($\pi r^2 h = 3.14 \times 1.5^2 \times 3$ mm^3 = 21.2 mm^3), where r is the radius of the piston, and h the depth of penetration. The trauma protocol was approved by the IACUC. NSE-M17Z mice were genotyped as previously described (9). zVAD-fmk (480 ng) or AcYVAD-cmk (200 ng) or vehicle (0.4% dimethyl sulfoxide) was injected i.c.v. (2 μl; bregma: 0.9 mm lateral, 0.1 mm posterior, 3.1 mm deep) 1 hour before or, in one series of experiments with zVAD-fmk, 1 hour after trauma.

IL-1β Determination

Mature IL-1β quantification was performed as previously described using an enzyme-linked immunosorbent assay kit (Genzyme, Cambridge, MA) (15). Brains were removed 4 hours following trauma or sham operation, and each hemisphere without 2 mm from frontal and occipital poles was homogenized in lysis buffer. Sham-operated mice were craniectomized but not traumatized.

DNA Fragmentation Analysis

DNA was end-labeled with [^{32}P]ddATP, electrophoresed on a 2% agarose gel, and autoradiographed as described by Endres et al. (6). For analysis of DNA damage, tissue samples corresponding to the striatum in slice 3 were obtained 24 hours after trauma.

TUNEL Immunohistochemistry

In situ terminal deoxynucleotidyl transferase-mediated DNA nick-end labeling was performed as described by Namura et al. (20).

Hydroxyl Radical Detection

Hydroxyl radical production was determined in mice that underwent weight drop trauma as well as in sham-operated mice. Fifteen minutes prior to craniectomy, mice were intraperitoneally injected with 400 mg of 4-hydroxybenzoic acid (4-HBA)/kg body weight, and sacrificed 30 minutes after trauma/craniectomy. Brains were removed, and the hemispheres were separated minus 2 mm of the frontal and occipital lobes. Tissue was homogenized in 0.2 mol/L perchloric acid (1:5, w:v) at 4°C, vortexed, and centrifuged (12,000 rpm, 15 min, 4°C). Supernatant was analyzed using high-pressure liquid chromatography/EC. The high-pressure liquid chromotography system consisted of a dual piston pump (ESA Model 480 pump; ESA Inc., Chelmsford, MA), two pulse dampers in series, a refrigerated autosampler (CMA/200, CMA/microdialysis), and a Coulochem II (Model 5200A, ESA Inc.) electrochemical detector. Data collection was performed using an ESA501 data station. Analytes were separated on a SuperODS 5 cm × 4.6 mm, 2-μm column (TosoHaas; Montgomeryville, PA) kept at 29°C. The mobile phase delivered at 1 ml/min consisted of 100 mM NaH_2PO_4, pH 2.8, with phosphoric acid, 6.5% methanol (v/v). Analytes were detected using dual coulometric electrode analytical cell (Model 5011, ESA Inc.). The potentials applied to the first and the second electrodes were +150 mV and +700 mV, respectively. 3,4-Dihydroxybenzoic acid (3,4-DHBA) was detected on the first electrode and 4-HBA on the second. Potential of the guard cell (Model 5020, ESA Inc.), placed between the pump and the injection valve, was set at +200 mV. Under these conditions, the limit of detection for 3,4-DHBA was about 1 pg on the column, and the chromatogram was completed in less than 6 min.

RESULTS

DNA Fragmentation following TBI

To determine whether apoptotic cell death develops as a consequence of direct impact brain injury, we examined traumatized tissue for the presence of oligonucleosomal DNA fragmentation. In the lesioned hemisphere, we found extensive DNA fragmentation 24 hours following trauma. DNA damage was not detected in brain tissue from sham-operated mice, which had only been craniectomized but not traumatized (*Fig. 2.1*). DNA fragments appeared on agarose gels as a ladder reflecting oligonucleosomal DNA fragmentation superimposed upon a smear reflecting random DNA degradation. Random DNA degradation

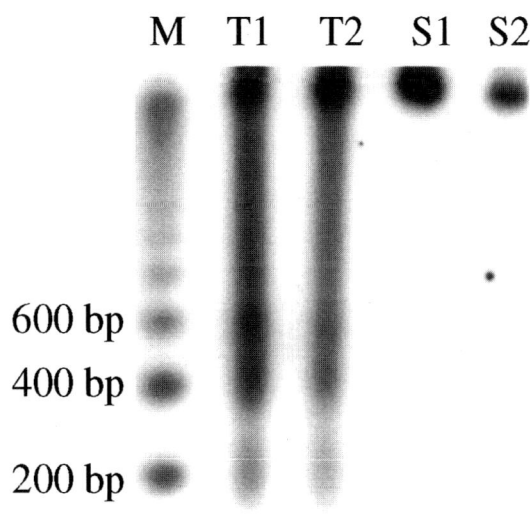

FIG. 2.1 DNA damage in the lesioned hemisphere of wild-type mice. *Lane 1* shows the DNA size marker (M), lanes 2 and 3 (T1 and T2) the DNA ladder, prepared from right coronal sections 6 mm from frontal pole 24 hours after weight drop trauma, and lanes 4 and 5 (S1 and S2) the DNA from the corresponding section of the right hemisphere of sham-operated animals. As characteristic for apoptosis, oligonucleosomal DNA fragmentation ("ladder") occurs at about 180-bp intervals. T1, T2, S1, and S2 were taken from different animals.

results from necrotic cell death, whereas oligonucleosomal DNA fragmentation occurs following apoptotic cell death. This result indicates that both necrotic as well as apoptotic cell death pathways are activated and likely play a role in experimental TBI. As previously reported by others, we also detected a marked increase number of cells showing TUNEL-positive nuclei 24 to 72 hours following TBI when compared with sham-operated mice (data not shown) (2).

Mature IL-1β in Traumatized Brain

ProIL-1β processing requires functional caspase-1 activity as demonstrated in caspase-1 knock-out mice following lipopolysaccharide challenge (17). Detection of mature IL-1β has been employed as direct evidence for caspase-1 activation (10,11,14,15,17,18). In traumatized mice, brain tissue mature IL-1β levels were significantly increased to 165.1 ± 40.3 pg/g brain tissue as compared with 19.1 ± 2.8 pg/g brain tissue in the ipsilateral hemisphere of sham-operated mice, indicating posttraumatic caspase-1 activation (*Fig. 2.2*). Mature IL-1β levels in the contralateral hemisphere (18.4 ± 2.8 pg/g tissue) did not signifi-

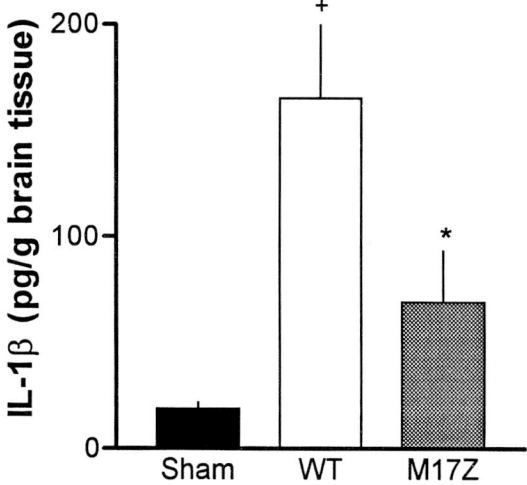

FIG. 2.2 Trauma-induced elevation of mature IL-1β levels in brain from transgenic NSE-M17Z mice expressing a dominant negative inhibitor of ICE (M17Z) or from wild-type littermates (WT). IL-1β levels were quantified 4 hours after trauma using an enzyme-linked immunosorbent assay specific for mature IL-1β detection. Sham-operated mice were craniectomized but not traumatized. Data are presented as mean +SEM (n = 6 in duplicate); $^+P < 0.005$ versus ipsilateral hemisphere in sham-operated wild-type mice (Sham); $^*P < 0.03$ versus ipsilateral hemisphere in traumatized wild-type mice (WT).

cantly differ from corresponding levels in sham-operated mice (14.9 ± 1.4 pg/g tissue). In NSE-M17Z trangenic mice, the increase in mature IL-1β level in the traumatized hemisphere was significantly lower than in wild type, indicating that the M17Z transgene is inhibiting caspase-1 (69.2 24.0 pg/g brain tissue; Fig. 2). There was no difference between mature IL-1β levels in sham wild type and sham NSE-M17Z mice. Elevated levels of mature IL-1β were not detected 24 hours following injury. Early elevation of caspase-1 activity is consistent with that previously reported during apoptosis (5,14,15).

Trauma-mediated Brain Damage

Because caspase-1 is activated following TBI, we evaluated whether caspase-1 inhibition might reduce trauma-mediated brain injury. We previously demonstrated that the M17Z transgene behaves as a dominant negative inhibitor of caspase-1 (9,15). To evaluate if caspase-1 inhibition might attenuate brain trauma-mediated damage, we compared lesion size in NSE-M17Z transgenic mice with that of wild-type littermates 24 hours post-impact. Total lesion volume in the NSE-M17Z mice, 24 hours following trauma, was significantly reduced by 42% when compared with wild-type mice (*Fig. 2.3A*). The M17Z mutant caspase-1 gene confers tissue protection following traumatic injury, implicating ICE-like caspases as mediators of traumatic-induced cell death.

Protection from cerebral ischemia-mediated injury in the NSE-M17Z transgenic mouse correlates with protection by synthetic peptide ICE family protease inhibitors (10,15). We evaluated whether zVAD-fmk (a nonselective ICE family protease inhibitor) or AcYVAD-cmk (a selective caspase-1 inhibitor) would diminish traumatic tissue damage as was demonstrated in the NSE-M17Z transgenic mouse. Wild-type mice were injected with zVAD-fmk (480 ng) or AcYVAD-cmk (200 ng) into the lateral cerebral ventricle 1 hour prior to impact. Total lesion volume 24 hours following trauma in the treated mice was significantly reduced in zVAD-fmk-treated mice by 53% when compared with the vehicle-injected mice (*Fig. 2.3C*). After AcYVAD-cmk injection, total lesion volume was reduced by 56% compared with controls (*Fig. 2.3B*). Treatment with the cathepsin B inhibitor, *N*-benzyloxycarbonyl-Phe-Ala-fluoromethylketone (zFA-fmk), as an inactive amino acid control sequence had no effect (data not shown). Moreover, lesion volume was reduced by 20% if zVAD-fmk was administered 1 hour following trauma (*Fig. 2.3D*). In the latter case, statistical significance was only reached in the anterior two out of five slices, suggesting that a therapeutic window exists for the treatment of TBI with caspase inhibitors. These results further confirm that the caspase family plays a role in traumatic

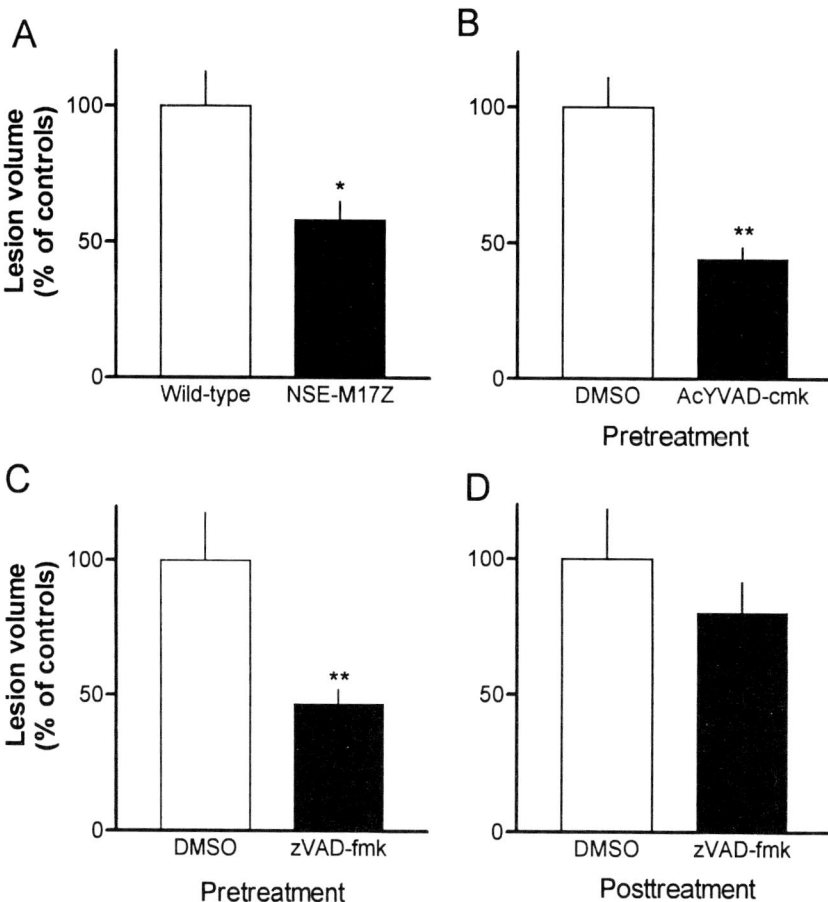

FIG. 2.3 Total lesion volume after traumatic brain injury in NSE-M17Z transgenic mice or corresponding wild-type littermates (A) or in C57BL/6 mice (B–D). Lesion size was assessed 24 hours following weight drop impact to the right hemisphere. AcYVAD-cmk (200 ng) was injected i.c.v. 1 hour before trauma (B). zVAD-fmk (480 ng) was injected i.c.v. either 1 hour before trauma (C) or 1 hour after trauma (D). Total lesion volume is calculated from lesion areas determined in each of five coronal sections (2 mm) from anterior (2 mm behind frontal pole) to posterior (10 mm). Total lesion volume was decreased in NSE-M17Z transgenic mice and after injection of zVAD-fmk or AcYVAD-cmk 1 hour before trauma. Although total lesion volume in animals injected with zVAD-fmk 1 hour after trauma was not significantly different, the size of lesion in the treated mice in the two most anterior sections (2–6 mm) was significantly reduced ($P < 0.05$; n = 5; data not shown), indicating a trend of a protective effect. Data are presented as mean + SEM (n = 5–6). *$P < 0.05$ or **$P < 0.01$ versus vehicle or, in case of transgenic mice, versus wild-type littermates.

brain injury-mediated apoptosis and suggest that strategies of ICE family inhibition may be useful to ameliorate the consequences of brain trauma.

Free Radical Formation after TBI

Little is known regarding the actual mechanisms by which caspase-1 activation mediates cell death. Caspase-1 can activate caspase-3, and caspase-3 has been recently shown to activate a DNase that mediates apoptotic cell death (4,25). Clearly, additional pathways must be recruited following caspase-1 activation that play a role in mediating cell death. Free radical production has been implicated as an important downstream mediator of cell death (13,23). Free radical production increases following traumatic brain injury (12). For this reason, we evaluated whether caspase-1 inhibition in vivo might attenuate free radical production. Elevation of free radical production following trauma was significantly decreased by 43% in NSE-M17Z transgenic mice compared with its wild-type littermates. No difference in baseline free radical production was detected between sham-operated wild-type and NSE-M17Z mice (*Fig. 2.4*).

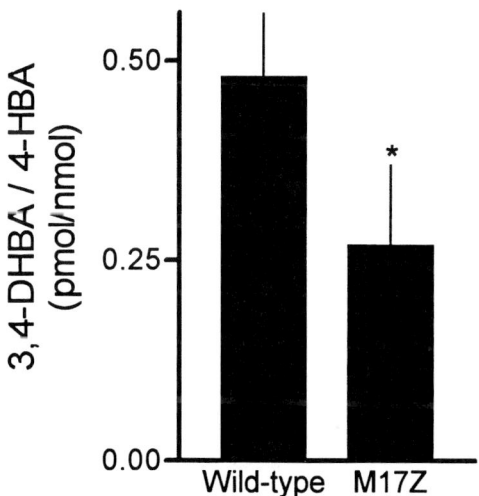

FIG. 2.4 Trauma-induced increase in free radical production in M17Z and wild-type mouse brain homogenates. Results are shown as 3,4-DHBA/4-HBA ratio and represent the change in free radical production when compared with ipsilateral hemispheres of sham-operated mice. Data are presented as mean + SEM (n = 7); *$P = 0.03$.

DISCUSSION

These results provide evidence that ICE-like caspase-family-induced apoptosis plays an important role in mediating posttraumatic cerebral damage. First, we demonstrate caspase-1 activation following traumatic injury. Apoptotic cell death was shown by DNA laddering and by TUNEL in situ. Second, we document reduced injury in a transgenic mouse expressing a dominant negative caspase-1 inhibitor following trauma. Third, we show that injection of a non-selective ICE-like caspase family inhibitor (zVAD-fmk), as well as a selective caspase-1 inhibitor (AcYVAD-cmk), reduced the volume of traumatic lesion in this brain injury model. Our results confirm reports by other groups indicating that apoptosis, as well as caspases, contribute to cellular injury following experimental TBI (28). The reported data extend previous findings by implicating ICE-like caspase activation in TBI and by demonstrating tissue protection from TBI by inhibiting the caspase cascade.

Caspases are involved in the induction and execution of programmed cell death in acute and chronic neurological disorders (8). Caspase-1 itself does not seem to play a significant role in developmental apoptotic cell death as demonstrated in caspase-1 knock-out mice (17) and in the NSE-M17Z transgenic mouse (18). However, in view of the prominent role that caspase-1 and ICE-like caspases play in ischemia, amyotrophic lateral sclerosis, and trauma, we propose that alternate apoptotic pathways might be preferentially activated during pathological and developmental apoptosis (9,10,14,15).

It might be argued that the time course of the apoptotic process in the TBI model as presented here is very fast. In fact, speed of the cell death process depends on the triggering event. We have previously demonstrated in transient focal ischemia that it just takes 6 hours following severe 2 hours of ischemia until oligonucleosomal DNA fragmentation is detected (14); however, it takes 1 to 3 days after mild 30 minutes of ischemia to find a similar degree of DNA fragmentation (16). Hence, the time course and sensitivity to detecting apoptotic cell death may also vary in different trauma models. Although slower development of apoptosis after TBI has been reported (2), the time 24 hours after TBI selected in this study is consistent with other reports (28).

There is substantial in vitro evidence implicating formation of ROS in certain forms of neuronal apoptosis (13). In some forms of apoptosis, generation of ROS initializes cell damage and thus is an early signal in the apoptotic cascade (13). Similarly, SOD depletion increased peroxynitrite formation, which finally lead to activation of ICE-like caspases and apoptotic cell death (21). Recently, it was shown in a BDNF deprivation model that increased peroxynitrite formation causes protein nitration, DNA fragmentation, and apoptotic cell death (7). In other forms of apoptosis, ROS generation is a downstream event, as caspase-1 inhibitors block their generation (23). In TBI-induced apoptosis, ROS generation also seems to be downstream from caspase-1 activation. This is the first report to demonstrate that caspase-1 is activated following traumatic brain injury and that in vivo inhibition of the caspase-1 cell death family reduces formation of ROS. Taken together, caspase-1 mediated free radical formation seems to be a downstream effector of caspase-induced apoptosis in vivo. Traumatic induced injury, as well as cell death in other disorders featuring apoptosis, may be treated with inhibitors aimed at modulating ICE family activity to reduce brain injury and preserve brain function.

SUMMARY

Necrotic and apoptotic cell death both play a role mediating tissue injury following brain trauma. The interleukin-1β converting enzyme (ICE; caspase-1) is activated, and oligonucleosomal DNA fragmentation is detected in traumatized brain tissue. Reduction of tissue injury and free radical production following brain trauma was achieved in a transgenic mouse expressing a dominant negative inhibitor of caspase-1 in the brain. Neuroprotection was also conferred by pharmacological inhibition of caspase-1 by intracerebroventricular administration of the selective inhibitor of caspase-1, acetyl-Tyr-Val-Ala-Asp-chloromethylketone (AcYVAD-cmk), or the nonselective caspase inhibitor N-benzyloxycarbonyl-Val-Ala-Asp-fluoromethylketone (zVAD-fmk). These results indicate that inhibition of caspase-1 like caspases reduces trauma-mediated brain tissue injury. In addition, we demonstrate an in vivo functional interaction between ICE-like caspases and free radical production pathways, implicating free radical production as a downstream mediator of the caspase cell death cascade.

REFERENCES

1. Chan PH, Epstein CJ, Himouchi H, et al.: SOD-1 transgenic mice as a model for studies of neuroprotection in stroke and brain trauma. **Ann NY Acad Sci** 738:93–103, 1994.
2. Conti AC, Raghupathi R, Trojanowski JQ, McIntosh TK: Experimental brain injury induces regionally distinct apoptosis during the acute and delayed post-traumatic period. **J Neurosci** 18:5663–5672, 1998.
3. Department of Health and Human Services: *Interagency Head Injury Task Force Report,* 1989.
4. Enari M, Sakahira H, Yokoyama K, et al.: A caspase-activated DNase that degrades DNA during apoptosis, and its inhibitor ICAD. **Nature** 391:43–50, 1998.

5. Enari M, Talanian RV, Wong WW, Nagata S: Sequential activation of ICE-like and CPP32-like proteases during Fas-mediated apoptosis. **Nature** 380:723–726, 1996.
6. Endres M, Namura S, Shimizu-Sasamata M, et al.: Attenuation of delayed neuronal death after mild focal ischemia by inhibition of the caspase family. **J Cereb Blood Flow Metab** 18:238–247, 1998.
7. Estévez AG, Spear N, Manuel SM, et al.: Nitric oxide and superoxide contribute to motor neuron apoptosis induced by trophic factor deprivation. **J Neurosci** 18:923–931, 1998.
8. Friedlander RM, Yuan J: ICE, neuronal apoptosis and neurodegeneration. **Cell Death Differ** 10:823–831, 1998.
9. Friedlander RM, Brown RH, Gagliardini V, et al.: Inhibition of ICE slows ALS in mice. **Nature** 388:31, 1997.
10. Friedlander RM, Gagliardini V, Hara H, et al.: Expression of a dominant negative mutant of ICE in transgenic mice prevents neuronal cell death induced by trophic factor withdrawal and ischemic brain injury. **J Exp Med** 185:933–940, 1997.
11. Friedlander RM, Gagliardini V, Rotello RJ, Yuan J: Functional role of interleukin-1β (IL-1β) in interleukin-1β converting enzyme-mediated apoptosis. **J Exp Med** 184:717–724, 1996.
12. Globus MY, Alonso O, Dietrich WD, et al.: Glutamate release and free radical production following brain injury: Effects of posttraumatic hypothermia. **J Neurochem** 65:1704–1711, 1995.
13. Greenlund LJS, Deckwerth TL, Johnson EM Jr: Superoxide dismutase delays neuronal apoptosis: A role for reactive oxygen species in programmed neuronal death. **Neuron** 14:303–315, 1995.
14. Hara H, Fink K, Endres M, et al.: Attenuation of transient focal cerebral ischemic injury in transgenic mice expressing a mutan ICE inhibitor protein. **J Cereb Blood Flow Metab** 17:370–375, 1997.
15. Hara H, Friedlander RM, Gagliardini V, et al.: Inhibition of interleukin-1β converting enzyme family proteases reduces ischemic and excitotoxic damage. **Proc Natl Acad Sci USA** 94:2007–2012, 1997.
16. Hogquist KA, Nett MA, Unanue ER. Chaplin DD: Interleukin 1 is processed and released during apoptosis. **Proc Natl Acad Sci USA** 88:8485–8489, 1991.
17. Li P, Allen H, Banerjee S, et al.: Mice deficient in IL-1β converting enzyme are defective in production of mature IL-1β and resistant to endotoxic shock. **Cell** 80:401–411, 1995.
18. Miura M, Friedlander RM, Yuan J: Tumor necrosis factor-induced apoptosis is mediated by a CrmA-sensitive cell death pathway. **Proc Natl Acad Sci USA** 92:8318–8322, 1995.
19. Miura M, Zhu H, Rotello R, et al.: Induction of apoptosis in fibroblasts by IL-1β converting enzyme, a mammalian homolog of the C. elegans cell death gene ced-3. **Cell** 75:653–660, 1993.
20. Namura S, Zhu J, Fink K, et al.: Activation and cleavage of caspase-3 in apoptosis induced by experimental cerebral ischemia. **J Neurosci** 18:3659–3668, 1998.
21. Park DS, Morris EJ, Troy CM, et al.: Multiple pathways of neuronal death induced by DNA-damaging agents, NGF deprivation, and oxidative stress. **J Neurosci** 18:830–840, 1998.
22. Rink A, Fung KM, Trojanowski JQ, et al.: Evidence of apoptotic cell death after experimental traumatic brain injury in the rat. **Am J Pathol** 147:1575–1583, 1995.
23. Schulz JB, Weller M, Klockgether T: Potassium deprviation-induced apoptosis of cerebellar granule neurons: A sequential requirement for new mRNA and protein

synthesis, ICE-like protease activity, reactive oxygen species. **J Neurosci** 16: 4696–4706, 1996.
24. Shapira Y, Shohami E, Sidi A, et al.: Experimental closed head injury in rats: Mechanical, pathophysiologic, and neurologic properties. **Crit Care Med** 16: 258–265, 1998.
25. Tewari M, Quan LT, O'Rourke K, et al.: Yama/CPP32β, a mammalian homolog of CED-3, is a crmA-inhibitable protease that cleaves the death substrate poly(ADP ribose) polymerase. **Cell** 81:801–809, 1995.
26. Thomas LB, Gates DJ, Richfield EK, et al.: DNA end labeling (TUNEL) in Huntington's disease and other neuropathological conditions. **Exp Neurol** 133:265–272, 1995.
27. Thornberry NA, Bull HG, Calay JR, et al.: A novel heterodimeric cysteine protease is required for interleukin-1β processing in monocytes. **Nature** 356:768–774, 1992.
28. Yakovlev AG, Knoblach SM, Fan L, et al.: Activation of CPP32-like caspases contributes to neuronal apoptosis and neurological dysfunction after traumatic brain injury. **J Neurosci** 17:7415–7424, 1997.
29. Yuan J, Horvitz HR: The Caenorhabditis elegans genes ced-3 and ced-4 act cell autonomously to cause programmed cell death. **Dev Biol** 138:33–41, 1990.
30. Yuan J, Shaham S, Ledoux S, Ellis HM, Horvitz HR: The C. elegans cell death gene ced-3 encodes a protein similar to mammalian interleukin-1β-converting enzyme. **Cell** 75:641–652, 1993.

I

General Scientific Session I

CHAPTER

3

Integrating Technical Innovations in Everyday Practice

JOHN M. TEW, JR., M.D.

Man's nature is such that he has always been fascinated by technology. Throughout the ages, humans have sought to overcome the unpredictability of nature by reformatting existing knowledge in the search of new principles. By a slow but orderly process, science—both basic and clinical—has given birth to new concepts. Practicing physicians then determine whether the concepts have practical application to human disease. Some concepts are miracles for a day and then become routine; others quickly become relics of the past.

You, or your progeny, will one day look back on the proceedings of this Congress with amused tolerance as new technological advances exceed our current imagination. Lack of vision should not deter us because technical achievement is not our principal mission. The skillful application of advanced technologies is essential for the care of each patient. However, our society does not afford neurosurgeons their high position of respect because of our limited technical achievements alone. Some of our members do become renowned or win high recognition by the public for a day because of their technical achievements. But such praise does not accord a high place in the fraternity of humans unless the individual also deserves respect based on a philosophy that is centered on the needs of others. We will be judged on the basis of our response to the needs of society and the strict application of standards of moral excellence, competence, and honest conduct. We must be ever mindful of the value of human life expressed in individual terms. Our most important commitment remains compassion for our patient. With the goal in mind to refine knowledge and technology for application to our patients, I direct this discussion toward integrating technical innovations into everyday practice. Medicine, one of the youngest sciences, can credit many of its advances as a result of superior technology and science. These are advances that our patients greatly appreciate.

HISTORY

Neurosurgeons have always been quick to recognize the value of new technology and to devote great energy and creativity toward bringing their discoveries to practical application. The creative capacity of neurological surgeons is remarkably demonstrated by the example provided by their contributions to stereotactic and image-guided surgery. In 1908, Horsley and Clarke (2) developed the stereotactic frame and the concept for stereotactic surgery (*Fig. 3.1*). They developed an atlas based on cranial landmarks for functional exploration of the cerebellum in small animals, but they never applied the technology in clinical practice. Spiegel and Wycis (4) in 1947 performed the first operation on humans using the stereoencephalotome (*Fig. 3.2*). Spiegel and Wycis understood that the development of stereotactic operation was dependent on the use of a precise frame attached to the skull and the ability to reliably target three-dimensional space within the frame using the internal coordinates of the pineal gland and foramen of Monro. Early stereotactic guidance for functional neurosurgery used brain atlases reconstituted from cross sections. Radiographic images demonstrated brain anatomy following introduction of air or contrast material into

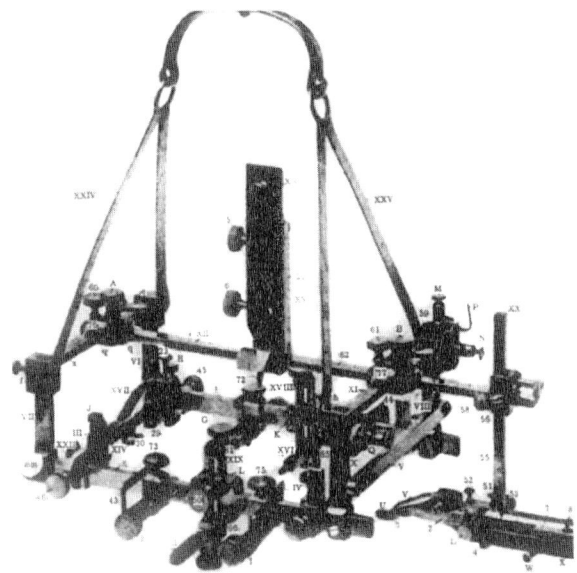

FIG. 3.1 First stereotactic frame developed by Horsley and Clarke in 1908 (reprinted with permission: Oxford University Press, New York).

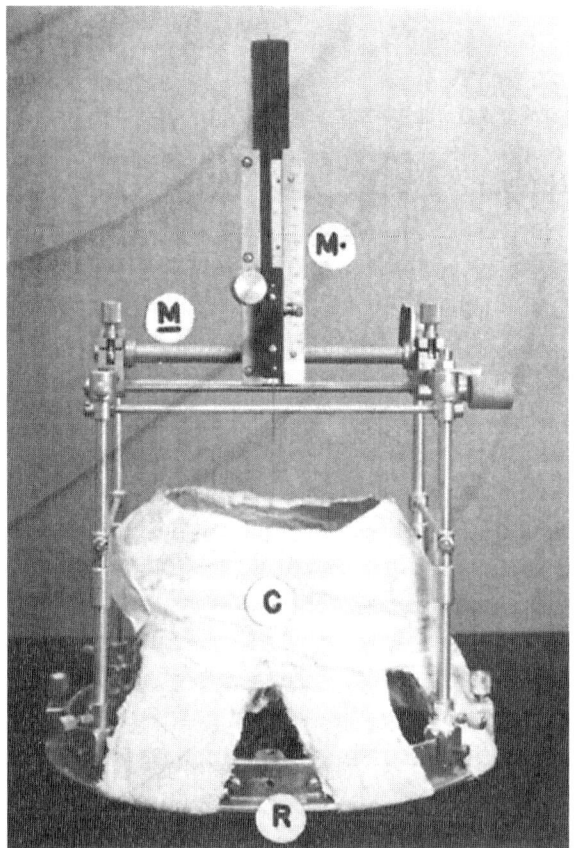

FIG. 3.2 Stereoencephalotome developed by Spiegel and Wycis (reprinted with permission: Spiegel EA, Wycis HT: Methods and stereotaxic atlas of the human brain, part I, in Spiegel EA (ed): *Stereoencephalotomy (Thalamotomy and Related Procedures)*. New York, Grune & Stratton, 1952).

the ventricular cavities. The introduction of computed tomography (CT) by Hounsfield (3) in 1973 stimulated Brown (1) in 1979 to unify brain imaging and stereotactic guidance for safe, precise documentation of minute brain targets.

Magnetic resonance imaging (MRI) provided exquisite images of surface and deep brain anatomy. CT and MRI images offer complementary features. For example, bone and calcification are best seen on CT images, whereas MRI provides better resolution of soft-tissue structures. Clinical diagnosis and surgical planning are increasingly based on complementary use of this information. CT and MRI provide little functional data, whereas positron emission tomography and single-photon emission computed tomography scans display aspects of brain function and provide metabolic measurements. Modern frame systems can incorporate CT, MR, and positron emission tomography images and coregister multimodal image volumes acquired with the patient in the frame.

Stereotactic frame systems have acquired a wide variety of applications for functional surgery, brain biopsy, and neurosurgery. Frame-based systems, although accurate, are subject to inaccuracies associated with image resolution. Frame-based technology is difficult to manage and cumbersome to apply for open surgical procedures because of the bulk and configuration of the equipment. Simplified systems that use a single site for skull attachment became attractive for biopsy and localization techniques. The Pelorus is an example of a simplified system (*Fig. 3.3*), allowing the surgeon to localize deep-seated lesions, pinpoint the lesion with a guide, and contour the craniotomy without the

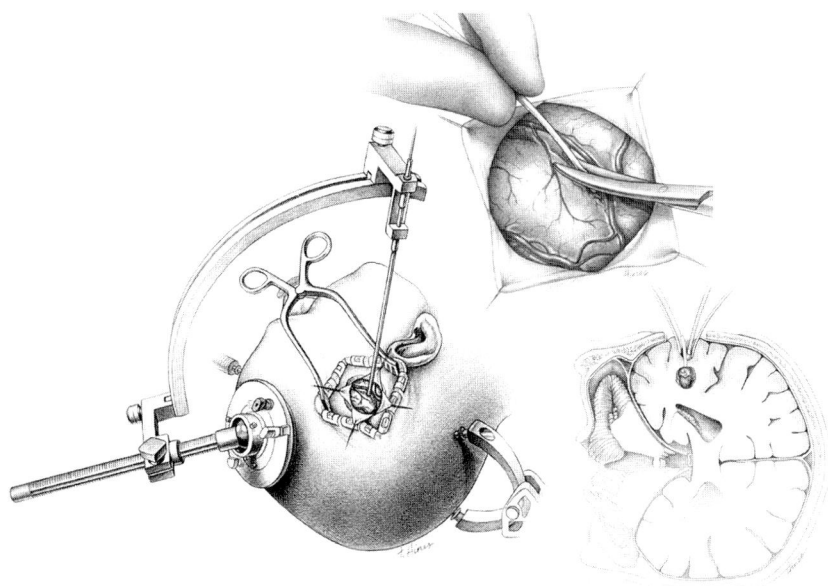

FIG. 3.3 Mark III Pelorus Stereotactic System (Ohio Medical Instrument Company, Cincinnati, OH) is used to pinpoint a small temporal lobe lesion. A silastic cannula is inserted through the probe to the edge of the lesion and serves as a guide for the cortical dissection to the lesion (reprinted with permission: Tew JM Jr, van Loveren HR: *Atlas of Operative Microneurosurgery,* Vol. I. Philadelphia, WB Saunders, 1994).

encumbrance of a frame system. Despite the accuracy and precision provided by a frame-based technology, stereotactic methods were performed in a majority of intracranial procedures other than biopsy. Neurosurgeons sought the advantages of imaging adjuncts, cineradiography, ultrasonography, and intraoperative angiography. Although these techniques were valuable, the requirements for effective image-guided surgery were not met. It was recognized that the surgeon needed a three-dimensional registration of the image matched to the anatomy of the patient's head. The surgeon needed to be able to view the images and create a road map to effectively plan the trajectory and outline the lesion. The surgeon needed to be able to document in real time his relationship to the target in three-dimensional planes. The accuracy of the system should allow comparison of preoperative, intraoperative, and postoperative images and minimize the need for other intraoperative localizing techniques.

No frame-based image-guided system can meet these demands. In 1987, Watanabe et al. (5) presented the new concept of frameless computer-directed surgery. This innovative concept and subsequent refinements have demonstrated the great interest and brilliant future for technological developments related to the application of the computer in neurosurgery.

INTEGRATING TECHNICAL INNOVATIONS INTO EVERYDAY PRACTICE

In this article, I discuss a paradigm or model for integrating technology into everyday practice. Hopefully, this model and the associated six principles will be of value as an example of our responsibility to build relationships among team members, our institutions, and business colleagues in a manner that is scientifically based, fiscally sound, humane, and sensitive to the individual needs of each patient. The saying is attributed to Harvey Cushing that "Neurosurgery is 20% science, 75% artistry, and 5% community service." Recent applications of computers in neurosurgery creatively document the marked increase in science and artistic technology in our profession. Cushing is also alleged to have dreamed of the day when a neurosurgeon with no hands could be successful. That vision is now possible; virtual reality and voice-activated computer navigation of the brain are visionary projects. Today's dream can be tomorrow's common practice.

By elucidating six principles, I want to share with you our team's approach to combining science, technology, and service in a model that: (1) seeks to focus attention on the individual patient, (2) seeks a creative environment in which technology is evaluated for its effectiveness according to established practices, and (3) seeks to develop and nurture a team

Model for Integrating Technology

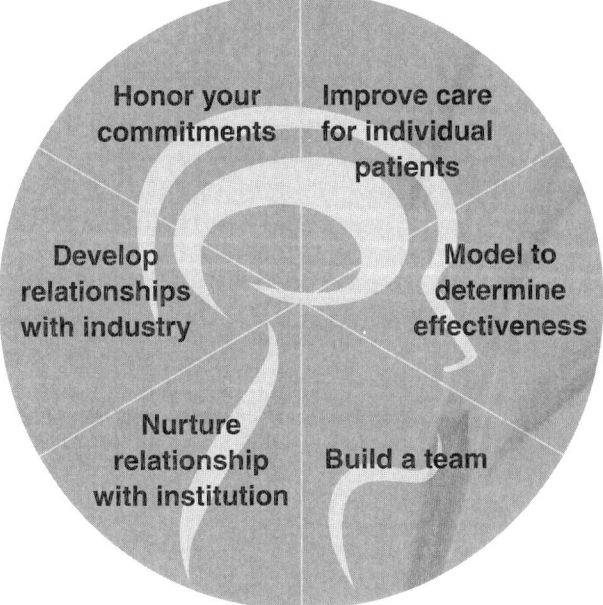

FIG. 3.4 Six-part model for integrating technology by combining science, technology, and service to focus attention on the individual patient.

of interdependent people who work together in a secure creative environment. In this model, the team includes institutions, which in our profession are hospitals, medical centers, and universities that join together into partnerships with industrial providers of technology. Our model consists of the following six principles (*Fig. 3.4*): (1) improve the care for individual patients; (2) establish a model or process to determine the effectiveness of the new technology; (3) build a multidisciplinary team; (4) nurture the relationship with your institution; (5) develop a relationship with industry based on value, respect, and collaboration; and (6) nurture and honor your commitment with industrial partners.

The functional success of this model is not limited to the large clinic or university practice. The model can be equally successful if applied by an individual or by a small group of professionals in community practice. I would like to discuss the six principles and illustrate how we have applied them in the use of computer technology for everyday practice in our institutions.

Improve the Care for Individual Patients

The first guiding principle of technical innovation is to explore and develop technology that will heighten our art, skills, and competence in a manner that improves the care of individual patients. Outcome analysis should provide a systematic method to answer the questions we ask of each patient: How do you feel? How are you?

EXAMPLE AT CINCINNATI

Frame-based stereotactic surgery has been applied since 1947, when Spiegel and Wycis documented their application of the stereoencephalotome (4). A new dimension of neurosurgery was created. Subsequently, generations of patients with functional neurological disorders, parkinsonism, dystonia, pain, epilepsy, multiple sclerosis, and affected disorders have benefited. A constant state of evolution in technology has resulted in increased precision such that stereotactic-guided surgery has gained renewed application in the treatment of movement disorder, such as tremors and akinesia. Precise localization of the globus pallidum by image-guided frame-based surgery when augmented by microelectrode recording of tremor cells and the optic track provides micrometer accuracy necessary for lesioning and placement of depth electrodes for stimulation (*Fig. 3.5*). The computer-generated atlas of the target and postoperative MRI image documents the exact location and size of the lesion in the globus pallidus interna.

Establish a Model or Process to Determine the Effectiveness of New Technology

Does the technology achieve a desired result? Is the tumor completely removed? Is survival and quality of life improved? Is patient satisfaction increased? Is the technology cost-effective? Is the length of hospital stay decreased? These are the types of questions that our model for outcomes must analyze to document effectiveness.

EXAMPLE AT CINCINNATI

Frame-based image-guided surgery reached a pinnacle of effectiveness when applied to individual patients with functional disorders (5) and for biopsy and radiosurgery. Yet, the transition of this technology to the broad spectrum of neurosurgical procedures required the adaptation of imaging, three-dimensional registration of images for the creation of a safe trajectory to the lesion, and a map of the boundaries of the target. To accomplish the critical transition from frame-based to frameless image-guided surgical procedures, CT and MRI imaging provide spacial information that replaces the point-to-point system inher-

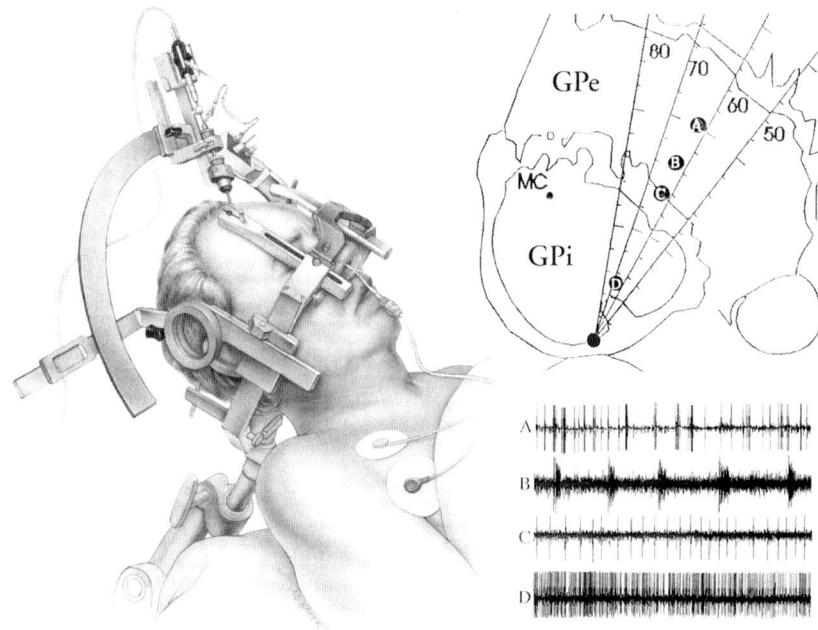

FIG. 3.5 Leksell stereotactic frame (Elekta Instruments, Inc., Atlanta, GA) used for microelectrode recordings of tremor cells in the globus pallidus interna and optic track. Once the target is appropriately localized, a thermal lesion is created (reprinted with permission by Mayfield Clinic, Cincinnati, OH).

ent in frame-based systems with the three-dimensional location of each pixel in the image set. This new concept of tracking the surgical position in physical space while displaying the position in image space eliminated the necessity for a frame-based point-to-point process. The new procedure, called frameless or image-guided surgery, has three main components: (1) a three-dimensional spatial localizer, (2) a registration technique, and (3) a display of the anatomy in image space. The majority of three-dimensional surgical localizers are of two basic types: articulated mechanical arms and triangulated emitters. Each has an advantage; therefore, we have participated actively in the process of developing both systems.

Bill Tobler, M.D., working with the Ohio Medical Instrument Company of Cincinnati, OH, developed the Mayfield ACCISS system (*Fig. 3.6*), an operating arm involving mechanical link sections and electrically encoded moveable joints that connect the three sections of the arm to enable a wide range of angular and positional freedom of motion. This small, lightweight mechanical arm is mounted directly onto the halo retractor device in a fixed relationship to the operative field.

A ball-and-socket assembly can be attached to the mechanical arm and used to generate stereotactic trajectories to a target. The computer workstation calculates the distance to the target and provides a view of trajectory to the lesion.

Simultaneously, Ron Warnick, M.D., led another team that collaborated with Radionics, Inc. (Burlington, MA) in the development and application of an operating arm system (*Fig. 3.7*) and an optical tracking system.

We were able to compare the advantages and disadvantages of both concepts simultaneously. Both systems have certain technical and practical advantages. The operating arm system offers high precision, simplicity, stability, and convenience of a self-contained unit. Disadvantages of the mechanical arm system include (1) inconvenience of hardware that is attached directly to the head frame and (2) limitations of maneuverability of the apparatus about the surgical field.

The optical tracking system involves a lightweight set of light-emitting diodes, lights that can be attached to a probe and surgical instruments (5). The light-emitting diodes are tracked by triangulated cameras that view the operative field. This freehand system provides an advantage of freedom of movement that is unencumbered, lightweight, and unobtrusive. The light-emitting diodes may be attached to a mi-

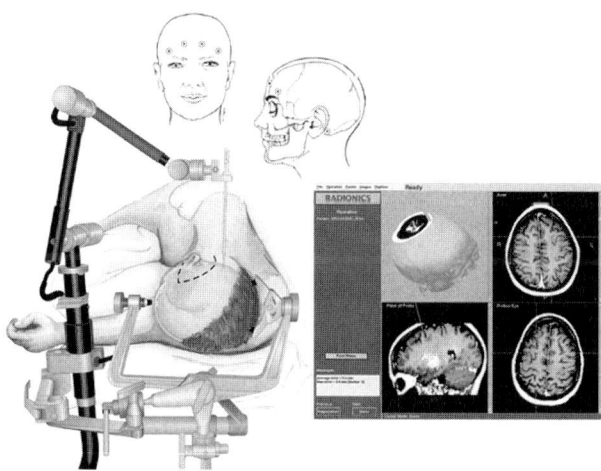

FIG. 3.6 Mayfield ACCISS system featuring the AccuPoint targeting sphere attached to the Budde Halo retractor system (Ohio Medical Instruments, Inc., Cincinnati, OH).

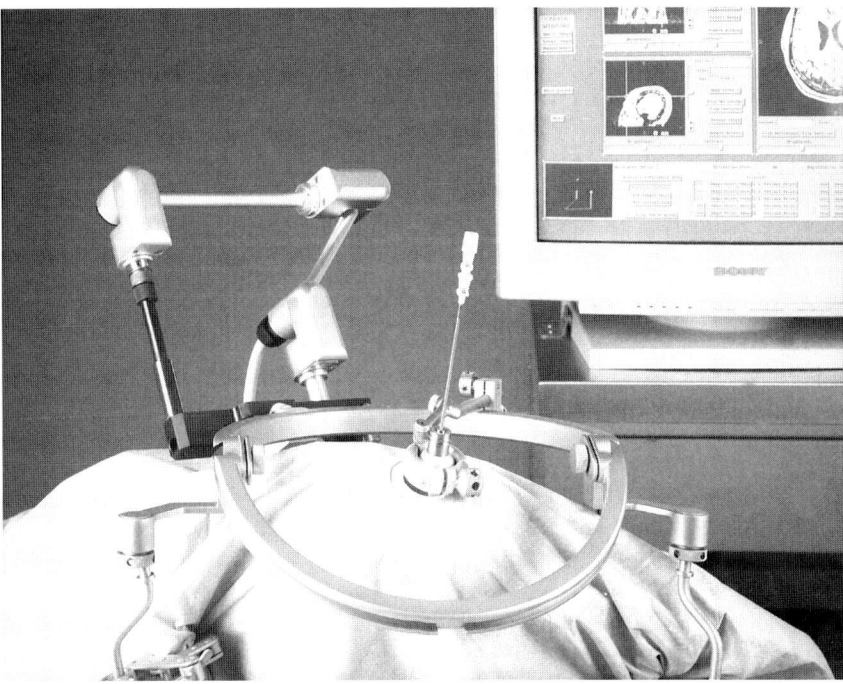

FIG. 3.7 Illustration of the Operating Arm System (Radionics, Burlington, MA) showing correct attachment to the Mayfield headholder. Four fiducials across the forehead and one fiducial at the mastoid register the patient with three-dimensional image space (reprinted with permission by Mayfield Clinic, Cincinnati, OH).

croscope or spinal instruments to enhance applications of the technology. A disadvantage is that the camera requires an unobstructed view of the operative field and the instruments.

The two systems can be complementary if software and graphics packages are compatible. Frameless, or image-guided, surgery has gained broad application in tumor, vascular, functional, and spinal neurosurgery. In the investigation of each technology, a process has been followed.

A clinical trials team conducts a thorough review for each system aided by the Institutional Review Board. Safety and clinical effectiveness of each device has been documented. FDA approval has been acquired for clinical application after rigid evaluation of case studies from multiple centers.

The results of application have been presented in peer-reviewed journals and at meetings. Finally, the evaluation of cost-effectiveness of the technology has been completed. Ron Warnick and his neuro-oncology team documented that although the operating room (OR) time was prolonged, attributed to the introduction of new technology, the hospital stay was significantly reduced. The costs of learning a new technology were therefore offset. Gross total resection of tumors was achieved, and analysis of neurologic outcomes indicates that the introduction of new technology was not harmful to the study patients.

Build a Multidisciplinary Team

Team building requires synergetic behavior based on trust and trustworthiness. Interdependence is preferred to independence. Cross-functional cooperation, communication, and respect must replace competition, turfism, and barriers to effectiveness. Basically, a sense of internal security must be built so that the organization can be flexible in changing its culture. Hospitals and medical practices have long been top-down cultures characterized by limited opportunity for creative change. Bureaucracy causes organizations to fossilize and become incapable of quick adaptation to change. People who possess a sense of purpose and feel secure can become transformers in any organization. Our challenge is to find and nurture courageous leaders who can, through their initiative, persistence, patience, and desire for excellence, inspire others. This alignment of purpose enables the maximum use of human resources and potential.

The team approach embraces the entire institution, including its community and academic components, crosses departmental barriers, and expresses concern for interrelated contributions of all members. Building a successful clinical team can be the basis for effective collaboration in many projects and activities that ultimately will serve good patient care.

EXAMPLE AT CINCINNATI

Team building does not come naturally to most neurosurgeons. We spend so much of our effort in early professional development creating our intellectual and technical expertise. Yet, our profession requires an extraordinary level of cooperation to build an effective organizational unit. I believe that team building is one of our most important challenges. We can view with pride the example provided by our neurosurgical leaders, Drs. Roberto Heros and Julian Hoff, who have been instrumental in establishing the Brain Attack Coalition. By their efforts, we have been encouraged to build and nurture our local team to combat stroke, the leading cause of death and disability in our society.

Now, I would like to call your attention to one specific example of cross-departmental team building that has provided synergistic benefit for our patients, colleagues, and institutions.

I refer to the radiosurgery program. Initially, some of us imagined that radiosurgery conceived by neurosurgeons as a surgical procedure should be controlled by surgeons. Of course, radiotherapists with access to linear accelerators were concerned. As a result of previous good collaboration, we elected to build this program with our radiation colleagues. Following the leadership of Bill Friedman, Peter Black, and others, we established an alignment with our Radiology Department's division of radiotherapy, thus creating an atmosphere of collaboration and dedication to creativity. The effort has diminished competition in our own institution such that there is only one radiosurgery center in the region. The center is growing. Community practitioners have privileges to bring their cases to the center, where education and patient care are co-mingled.

Nurture the Relationship with Your Institution

First, a cooperative relationship between the hospital and physician should be based on respect, joint commitment, and shared responsibility.

Second, the joint project must share the goal of improving patient care.

Third, The project must be fiscally sound and based on resource allocation. A jointly developed and approved business plan is advisable. A story about my first project at the University Hospital in Cincinnati may illustrate how relationships can be built. The story also illustrates how business plans have changed over the last two decades. The year was 1982, and the hospital was called Cincinnati General. The neurosurgery service was on a general surgery floor, where we had no intensive care unit for neurologic patients. At that time, the General was largely a hospital for the care of indigent patients. The administration was becoming interested in improving service and making it more attractive for customers. I inquired, "How can we get an integrated unit and an ICU for neurology and neurosurgical patients?" The Director of the hospital, undoubtedly anticipating the opportunity, replied that "we could make a deal if the physicians would keep four beds occupied with private patients." This was an early lesson in building partnerships that might not be appreciated today because the goal is more directed to keeping the beds unoccupied. Many years later when the University Hospital was privatized and became a member of the Health Alliance of Cincinnati, our team was prepared with a carefully developed strategic plan to create a neuroscience institute. After multiple revisions and presentations of the plan to the Alliance directors and community leaders without success, we finally recognized that a critical ingredient might be missing. Whereupon, I asked a friend who chaired the board to tell me what was wrong with our proposal. He replied, "Your concept is great, but you have no business plan." He continued, "In today's market, we can't invest in good ideas. We need market analysis to document that your plan will return 10% on investment. We need answers to these questions: How much equity do you need? How will you invest the resources and how much return will you get on our investment?" After 6 months and a six-figure investment for market consultants, we had a business plan that would please Proctor & Gamble. We rolled out The Neuroscience Institute in partnership with six other departments and the Health Alliance into a new era of meeting the expectations of a business partnership.

Fourth, the partnership must commit the resources to develop and support clinical studies to track outcomes. Outcome analysis must be built into the business plan.

EXAMPLE AT CINCINNATI

In an earlier story, I recalled the value of building a strong relationship with your institution. A partnership based on joint responsibility and respect is needed. If that sense of partnership is shared, worthy projects that contain high risk can be considered.

The implementation of an MRI-surgery program is such a high-risk project. Our surgeons felt that this project was justified on the basis of our perceived need for advances in image-guided surgery. In constructing a plan, we sought to maximize the functional operation of the unit, control costs, and minimize the risk of failure.

Functional operation was enhanced by collaboration with Hitachi to build an open MRI system into a complete OR suite (*Fig. 3.8*). To control costs, the magnet was built on the foundation of the ground floor rather than on the suspended floor of the hospital OR. An adjacent state-of-the-art neurosurgical OR and support space was designed to provide capacity for major or minor image-guided procedures. Functional capacity of the MRI was ensured by building the unit near the Emergency Center so that it would serve diagnostic purposes as well as emergency procedures, such as evacuation of intracerebral hematomas.

Collaboration with the Departments of Radiology and Surgery made the project more acceptable to our hospital administrators and ensured the commitment of Hitachi for a long-term relationship.

The deal was a win–win arrangement for the hospital, for Hitachi, and for our team of neuroscientists. Mary Gaskill, of the Department

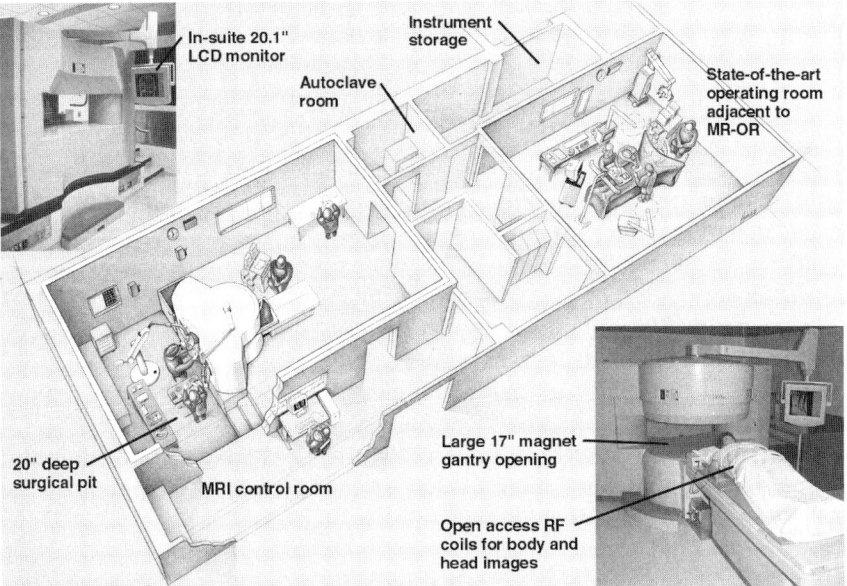

FIG. 3.8 Magnetic resonance operating room featuring the ARIS II Open MRI (Hitachi Medical Systems America, Twinsburg, OH). The magnetic resonance operating room is designed to accommodate diagnostic, minimally invasive, and open surgical procedures. If required, procedures can begin in the adjacent OR and then be transferred to the MRI without breaking the sterile field.

of Neuroradiology, has performed a clinical outcomes study similar to that done for intraoperative angiography. The study demonstrates that MRI-guided transsphenoidal surgery results in more complete resections of extrasellar lesions. Some concern has been raised that intraoperative imaging may induce the surgeon to exceed the limits of ordinary caution associated with standard operating procedures. For this reason, real-time assisted surgery is becoming increasingly attractive.

Develop a Relationship with Industry Based on Value, Respect, and Collaboration

Development of innovative and improved technology is the goal of all industrial collaborations. Meaningful contact occurs at meetings like the Congress, and follow-up continues on returning home. Industrial leaders are truly interested in communication with young creative, innovative neurosurgeons who are accessible and are motivated to collaborate on projects. These interactions are not limited to surgeons in academic practice or large clinics. In fact, we began many of our programs in an industry that is increasingly building consortiums and partnerships with surgeons who are in small groups, are in clinical practice, and who can demonstrate ability to conduct effective clinical trials with less cost and resources. Access to an institutional review board and ample volume of clinical material can provide the elements for building a partnership with industry and be the beginning of a valued relationship.

EXAMPLE AT CINCINNATI

Technical advances in my early career were largely related to the transition from macroscopic to microscopic surgery. Surgical anatomy, surgical planning, and execution was macroscopic. The three-dimensional road map was in our head. Loupes were used to magnify objects, and headlights had changed little since Cushing's time. We purchased our first OPMI I microscope in 1968 and transported it to the autopsy room to perform dissections of all the operations that we could imagine. A generation of neurosurgeons were mentored by Professor Yasargil. When we returned home, we built a microsurgical lab at the Christ Hospital and started courses to teach ourselves and our colleagues the new method to perform surgery. The Carl Zeiss Company became our first partner in this new venture. Tabletop dissection microscopes were used first for practicing extracranial-to-intracranial bypass procedures. We collaborated closely with Zeiss for the development of a series of innovative changes in microscopes that included ceiling mounts, mobile track-mounted scopes, laser-assisted microsurgery, variable focus for variable working distance, as well as advanced illumination and optical resolution. Movement focus adjustment and magnification controlled by foot, hand, and mouth electromagnetic clutches allowed the microscope to be integrated with head motion and with free-flowing action. Continuous improvement has led to the marriage of image-guided technology to the microscope (*Fig. 3.9*).

Over 30 years of association, our team and institutions have been continuously supported by the Zeiss staff. We have collaborated in the development and testing of new technology. Our courses in Cincinnati, and at national and international meetings, have been supported by many industrial partners who are equally committed to innovation, education, and continuous improvement of patient care.

Nurture and Honor Your Commitment with Your Industrial Partners

Having an early understanding of each partner's primary mission is the basis for a longstanding relationship. All partners must share a mission to place the concerns of our patients first, followed by the

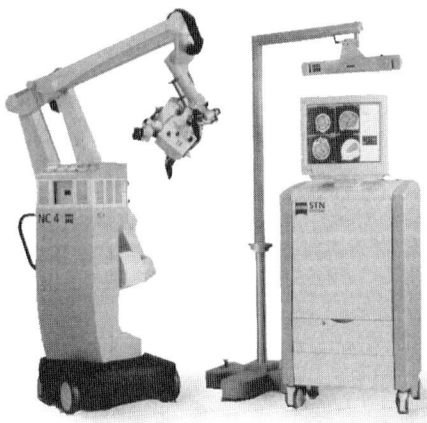

FIG. 3.9 OPMI NEURO/NC4 (Carl Zeiss, Inc., Thornwood, NY) for image-guided surgery represents the marriage of frameless stereotaxy with the operative microscope.

concerns of the team, the institutions, and the partnership. Rarely is there a subsequent disagreement when the goals and missions have been mutually accepted.

In time, surgeons, who are valued collaborators, become advisors for new designs, inventors of new products, and holders of patents. In some circumstances, a novel concept may lead to the incubation of a start-up company, acquisition of venture capital, and major opportunities for expression of creativity. The synergy of the collaboration requires objectivity by the surgeons and anticipates the publication of results and outcomes even when the results do not support the effectiveness of the product.

Association with a business partner provides another valuable opportunity. Knowledge-based training is intensely sought by most young businessmen. The relationship can be a very effective win–win exchange of scientific information and education in return for technical support, product consideration, or contributions to the education funds of the department or practice group.

EXAMPLE AT CINCINNATI

Throughout the long and productive relationship with industry, a mission characterized by mutual respect and primary concern for the needs of the patient has prevailed. These relationships have spanned generations. Our work with Bernie Cosman of Radionics Corp. began when I was a resident. Bernie developed one of the early radio frequency generators, and we coagulated many eggs and brain specimens to analyze lesion dynamics and thermal injury.

Subsequently, his son, Eric Cosman, Ph.D., then a professor at the Massachusetts Institute of Technology, and I developed a flexible electrode for radio frequency lesioning of the trigeminal nerve root. The partnership continued with development of image-guided surgery and stereotactic radiosurgery.

The depth of partnerships with our industrial colleagues has grown through the association with Jeff Keller, who heads our Goodyear Laboratory, where a continuous variety of educational courses have been conducted to instruct surgeons, nurses, and industrial personnel. Zeiss, Codman, Radionics, Midas Rex, Ohio Medical Instruments, US Medical, Hitachi, OMNI Medical, and many others have studied in Cincinnati and supported our courses at the Congress, AANS, and the Goodyear Laboratory and other sites where participation has been requested.

Today, and through the years, our goal is to meet the needs of each of our patients in the community. We are confident that we can best accomplish that goal by integrating technical innovations into our everyday practice in a scientifically measured, multidisciplinary team approach within our institutions and with our industrial partners, ensuring that the individual patient is always at the center of our collective focus.

REFERENCES

1. Brown RA: A computerized tomography-computer graphics approach to stereotactic localization. **J Neurosurg** 50:715–720, 1979.
2. Horsley V, Clarke RH: The structure and function of the cerebellum examined by a new method. **Brain** 31:45–124, 1908.
3. Hounsfield GN: Computerized transverse axial scanning (tomography): Description of the system. **Br J Radiol** 46:1016–1022, 1973.
4. Spiegel EA, Wycis HT, Marks M, Lee AS: Stereotactic apparatus for operation on the human brain. 106:349–350, 1947.
5. Watanabe E, Watanabe T, Manaka S, et al.: Three-dimensional digitizer (neuronavigator): New equipment for computed tomography-guided stereotactic surgery. **Surg Neurol** 27:543–547, 1987.

CHAPTER

4

Localizing the Point: Evolving Principles of Surgical Navigation

JOSEPH C. T. CHEN, M.D., PH.D., AND MICHAEL L. J. APUZZO, M.D.

HISTORY OF NAVIGATION

Surgical navigation has often been compared with its geographical equivalent. Although differing in detail, this comparison is apt, as they have similar conceptual histories. Both are concerned with "localizing the point," and the methods used are similar. Navigation charts and instrumentation in many senses provide a similar substrate for operation as imaging collages and stereotactic tools. They share developmental parallels in the evolution and increasing sophistication of fundamental instrumentation and conceptual components.

Dead Reckoning: Primordial Navigation

The advent of sea travel posed significant hurdles to the ancients. Lacking navigational tools, the ancients largely confined their sea travels to within visual range of the coast. Gradually, as navigational experience grew, a system of navigation using determinations of speed and heading lead to the development of dead reckoning methods of navigation. Dead reckoning (DR) comes from the term *deduced reckoning,* as it involves careful continuous assessment of speed and direction to determine location relative to a starting point. Navigators measured speed by tossing a buoy off the bow of the boat while singing a chant. As the buoy passed a marked point along the side of the boat, the navigator would stop his chant. The syllable upon which the chant was stopped correlated to the speed of the boat.

Directional heading was kept by knowledge of the direction of prevailing winds or position of the sun and moon. Keeping a steady directional heading, therefore, was very much a matter of the skill of the navigator. Changing weather conditions or cloud cover could result in significant difficulties in establishing a heading. The introduction of the compass to navigation therefore represents a significant milestone in the maritime arts.

It is likely that the earliest compasses were made of naturally occurring magnetic iron ore. Such lodestones, although rare commodities, could be found in natural deposits in Scandinavia, the Urals, and along the Chinese coast. These lodestones, by virtue of their ability to attract metal filings, were considered to be more valuable than gold. There is evidence that man-made magnets were being produced by the Chinese as early as the first century AD. It is likely that the magnet was used as a navigational tool by the Chinese as early as AD 1100. Over the next 200 to 300 years, the use of the magnet as a direction-finding device began to appear in Arab, Indian, and European navigation. Although the true origins of the compass are quite obscure, there are certain historical markers of note in its early history. In 1269, Pierre de Maricourt, a military engineer traveling with the crusades, wrote the first known manuscript on the action of the magnet and its use in navigation. He also described the construction of a box compass. It is said that the mariner's compass was invented in 1302 by an unknown navigator of Amalfi. This invention constituted the mounting of a 32-point compass rose onto a magnetized pin (18).

Regardless of its origin, the introduction of the compass allowed for reliable determinations of directional heading in foul or cloudy weather. The significance of the introduction of the compass is reflected in nautical charts of the age, where compass roses started to appear.

In Europe, DR methods were developed by Mediterranean sailors, where distances to be traveled were relatively short, and sea currents were not of a velocity that would confound the method (23). With navigators experienced in dead reckoning, long sea-faring trade routes throughout the Mediterranean were established.

The principles of celestial navigation, although known at least since Ptolemy's age in the first century AD, were not in general use for navigation as the techniques were difficult to employ on small sea-faring vessels. Furthermore, little was to be gained by celestial navigation in the waters of the Mediterranean as it has a narrow latitudinal dimension. In such waters, DR could serve more than adequately.

Although it is likely that earlier explorers had journeyed from Europe to the New World, it is Christopher Columbus among this group who has left the greatest amount of surviving evidence. Columbus, a Genoan, used the DR methods that he was familiar with to estimate his position in the Atlantic. Although he attempted celestial methods to estimate his position, these measurements were wildly inaccurate. Inspection of his navigational logs by modern historians revealed that the DR methods that he used lead to significant errors in estimation of his position (30).

Celestial Navigation

The development of celestial navigation was pioneered by the Portuguese under the patronage of Prince Henry the Navigator in the 15th century, contemporaneously with the voyages of Columbus. Celestial navigation enabled the Portuguese over a period of approximately 50 years to map the western coast of the African continent, opening up trade routes that would enrich the coffers and broaden the political influence of this small country.

The success of the principles of celestial navigation to precisely determine latitude spurred the development of a series of navigational instruments designed to measure accurately and precisely the altitude of celestial bodies above the horizon. These instruments included the quadrant, the astrolabe, and the sextant (*Fig. 1*).

Whereas latitude could be routinely determined in the 16th century, longitude could not. The only method available to calculate longitude in Columbus' day was by the observation of lunar eclipses, a relatively imprecise and unreliable method. It would not be until the 18th cen-

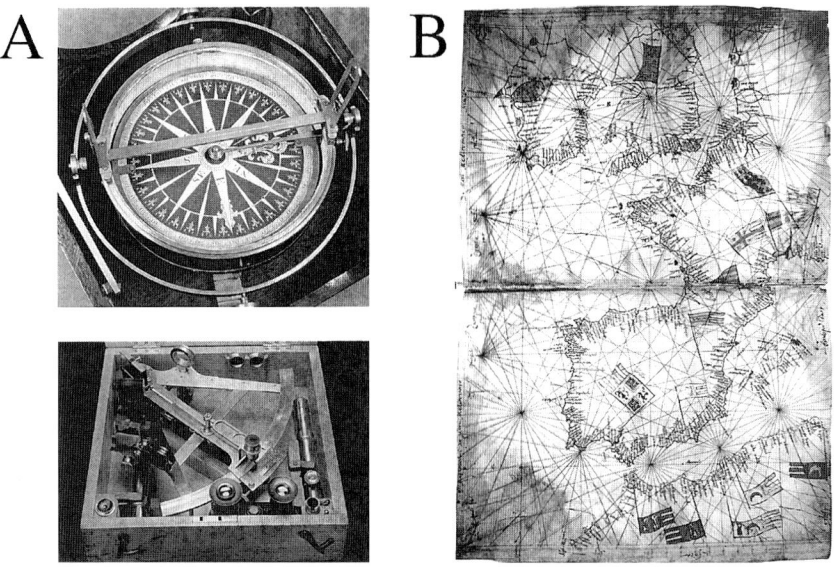

FIG. 4.1 Reliable nautical navigation involves the use of multiple instrumentation and techniques. *A*, navigational instrumentation including compass and sextant enabled long-distance navigation. *B*, ancient nautical chart c. 1350 constructed from dead reckoning techniques. Note numerous compass roses.

tury, when John Harrison would develop the first practical sea-going chronometers, that longitude could be reliably determined (61). Longitude could then be determined with the use of a celestial almanac in conjunction with accurate time keeping and a sextant. With this, the principal development of celestial navigation was complete (79). Navigation would in principle not change until the advent of the Global Positioning System, allowing instant determinations of absolute position independent of celestial observation.

HETEROGENEOUS NATURE OF BRAIN FUNCTION AND THE NEURON THEORY

Modern stereotactic neurosurgery is borne out of the knowledge that existent within the brain are distinct centers that subserve different aspects of neural function. As a concept, the localized nature of brain function is relatively new. The realization and subsequent development of this concept formed the primordial kernel for the initiation of "brain charts."

Although it had been known from at least as early as Hippocratic times that injuries to the brain produce weakness on the side opposite the lesion, concepts of localized brain function would remain murky until the 19th century, despite the rapidly accruing neuroanatomic discoveries in the 17th and 18th centuries.

An early important figure in the conceptual development of the localized nature of brain function was Thomas Willis, who in 1664 published a landmark monograph on brain anatomy notable for its physiological orientation. Willis, for the first time, divided the brain into functional parts, placing higher reasoning and emotion in the cerebrum and vegetative functions in the brainstem (80). This general division of brain function along anatomic lines would not go unchallenged, most notably by Albrect von Haller, who advocated a radically equipotential school of brain function (35). To Haller, it was uncertain if there was any division of neural function with the exception of the function of the peripheral nerves.

The debate between equipotential and localized function would continue at various levels with eminent proponents of both sides. The 19th century would herald an intensification of the debate, first catalyzed by the phrenologists Gall and Spurzheim. Phrenology stated that higher cortical function is localized and, further, that distinct personal qualities may be elucidated through the study of the shape of a person's head (68). These ideas would be popular with the general public but would remain controversial in scientific circles.

The birth of modern neuroanatomy and neurophysiology would be heralded by the work of a succession of physiologists, anatomists, and clinicians. These included Bell and Magendie, who independently discovered the directional nature of the ventral and dorsal spinal roots; Flourens who pioneered the cortical lesioning experiment; Broca, whose stunning observations of the patient "Tan" set the stage for a new school of cortical localization; and Cajal, who—with the development of the neuron theory coupled with his acute observations of the microscopic anatomy of the brain—developed a set of basic tenets to which all modern neuroscientific research can be traced.

The advent of a new school of neurological localization resulted in the advent of neurologically guided brain surgeries. It was Macewen who, in 1879, using David Ferrier's cortical map, performed the first neurologically directed removal of a brain tumor, heralding the modern age of neurological surgery (29, 48).

CRANIOMETRIC LOCALIZATION: NEUROSURGICAL DEAD RECKONING

Work had been made to geometrically describe important features of the brain at least since the time of Leonardo's efforts to localize the precise location of the seat of the soul in the third ventricle. Accurate descriptions of the anatomy of the brain were being produced during the Renaissance, and information on new anatomic discoveries were rapidly disseminated throughout Europe. These descriptions served as maps of the central nervous system. The advent of modern surgical technique turned the scientific study of anatomy into a practical matter.

Like early sailors navigating between Mediterranean ports, most neurosurgical procedures depend on standard landmarks and relative position. Such techniques are the most expedient methods for reaching points on the surface of the brain, especially in instances where there is not excessive distortion of brain anatomy.

Features of the skull serving as external landmarks have therefore been studied to determine their correlation with underlying brain structures. An example is the Taylor-Haughton line, described in 1900. These craniometrically based landmarks were developed to provide accurate localization of the Sylvian fissure and central sulcus on plainfilm x-rays. These lines have been demonstrated to be of surprisingly good accuracy in the localization of these features (73).

One of the major goals of neurosurgical training is the development of deduced reckoning skills in regard to operative procedures. The ability to make eidetic constructs on the basis of neurological and radiographic findings is the hallmark of a competent neurosurgeon.

Yet, dead reckoning has limitations. Whereas these methods have proven adequate for addressing lesions situated close to easily reachable landmarks, small deep-seated targets within brain parenchyma remained out of the reliable reach of surgeons. Until the advent of the computed tomography (CT) scanner, such lesions were uncommonly operated on, however, as imaging methods were until recently not of sufficient sophistication to resolve such lesions.

MODERN STEREOTAXY: NEUROSURGICAL CELESTIAL NAVIGATION—A NEXUS OF DISCIPLINES

It was the need to develop new tools for neuroanatomic investigations that would lead to the development of what is generally accepted to be the first stereotactic system. Horsely and Clarke introduced their stereotaxic device in 1908 for the purpose of reproducibly inserting electrodes into the dentate nucleus of the monkey (37). Although Mussen developed a version of this device for human use, it has never been used on humans (39, 54).

Despite what we now recognize as being the obvious practicality of the device for use in humans, the development of stereotactic methods for use in humans would languish until the late 1940s, when modern clinical stereotaxy would be introduced by Spiegel and Wycis (67).

Spiegel and Wycis for the first time integrated the use of a stereotactic frame with radiographic imaging, electrophysiological monitoring, and an anatomic atlas. This powerful melding of techniques was used to address a wide variety of surgical targets, treating patients with movement disorders (62, 64), epilepsy (66), pain (65), and psychiatric disease, thereby giving birth to a broad new discipline.

Evolving Stereotactic Techniques

As in nautical navigation, establishing a chart or map as a frame of reference for cerebral navigation was a fundamental imperative. Although advancements in stereotactic systems would change the details of stereotactic localization, the basic paradigm of a measurement device, radiographic localization, and anatomic atlas would remain key features. Therefore, the key technology that has driven the development of modern stereotactic systems is radiographic imaging. The strengths and limitations of each method have influenced the implementation of stereotactic instrumentation as well as the basic indications for stereotactic technique.

X-RAY

X-ray imaging of the ventricular system by pneumoencephalography and later contrast ventriculography for the first time allowed visualization of the ventricles and cisterns. The ventricular chamber then became a natural landmark or reference point by which lesions would be placed. These ventriculographic features would then be indexed relative to fixed points on the stereotactic apparatus.

ATLASES

Spiegel and Wycis understood that the inability to directly visualize brain structures by then-available radiographic techniques required an interpolative method to localize structures. They therefore studied a number of normal human brains in cross section to develop a stereotactic atlas. In 1952, Spiegel and Wycis published *Stereoencephalotomy,* the first of the modern stereotactic atlases (*Fig. 2*) (63). Recognizing that craniometric points were unreliable reference points for intracranial targets, Spigel and Wycis introduced the concept of using radiographically visible intracranial landmarks. Their initial landmarks included the center of the pineal gland, the habenular calcification, and the posterior commissure-pontomedullary line.

Although the radiographic landmarks of Spiegel and Wycis would later be supplanted by other landmarks, such as the anterior commissure–posterior commissure line (69) and the foramen of Monro–posterior commissure line (3), the principles of stereotactic atlas construction and use would remain the same to the present time and would be applied to all regions of the brain.

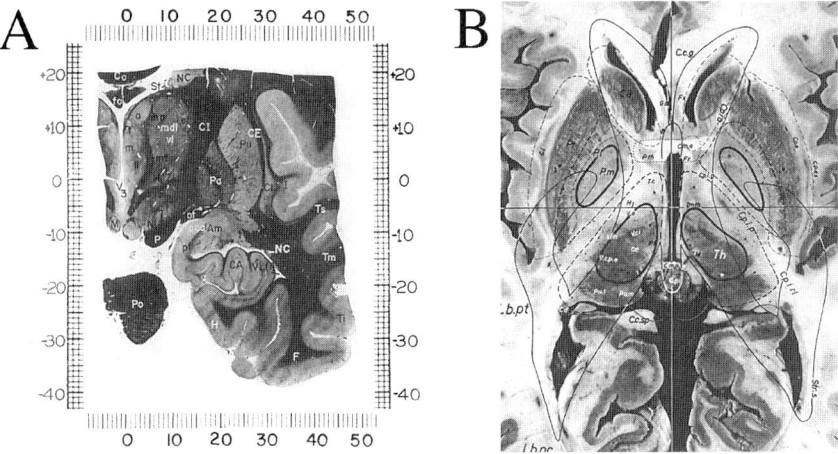

FIG. 4.2 Stereotaxic atlases have developed as interpolative devices to localize specific brain structures not visualized by radiographic imaging. *A,* The first anatomic atlas, Stereoencephalotomy (c. 1957). *B,* axial slice from Schaltenbrand and Wahren (c. 1977) demonstrating the plane of the AC-PC line 58.

Although analogous to nautical charts, the stereotactic atlas differs fundamentally in principle. The nautical chart describes unambiguously the position of geographic points of interest in reference to direction, distance, and celestial relations. By contrast, the use of an atlas in stereotactic procedures depends on the assumption that the relative position of brain structures across individuals may be described on a statistically accurate level to allow functional procedures.

As interpolative devices, stereotactic atlases cannot be relied upon to yield precise and accurate stereotactic coordinates for all patients. This variability of the relative location of brain structures has been recognized since Spiegel and Wycis's work and has been echoed by many subsequent investigators (3, 16, 76). What is evident from these studies is that significant variability may exist from one brain to the next. The stereotactic atlas can therefore only be used as a guide, and other methods should be used to obtain fine accuracy.

INSTRUMENTATION

The decade of the 1950s saw an exponential growth in stereotactic surgical procedures for functional disorders. In the age before the advent of modern neuropharmacology and psychopharmacology, attempts to surgically correct imbalances in various brain circuits were attempted for a number of diseases for which there was no other treatment. As the success of such procedures was growing, a number of eminent neurosurgeons were to develop their own instrumentation in a desire to improve upon the stereotactic methodology. Each instrument design reflects the biases and philosophical approach of its developers.

Two basic approaches have been used in the development of stereotactic instrumentation. In the first, a simple adjustable guide was used. This was exemplified by the devices developed independently by Austen and Lee (7), Cooper (24), and Todd, McCaul (49), Rand and others. With these devices, a burr-hole trephination was made, and the guide was then rigidly attached to the rim of the burr hole (*Fig. 3*). A probe was gradually introduced through this guide, and serial intraoperative ventriculograms were obtained as the probe was advanced toward its intended target. Corrections to the trajectory could be made during the passage to reach the target. This method, although intuitively simple, demanded a certain amount of manual skill from its users and could result in mistargeting. Yet, very good results were obtained by experienced surgeons (74). However, because of the experience needed to develop adequate facility with this method, and the potentially high complication rate in inexperienced hands, this method has been largely abandoned.

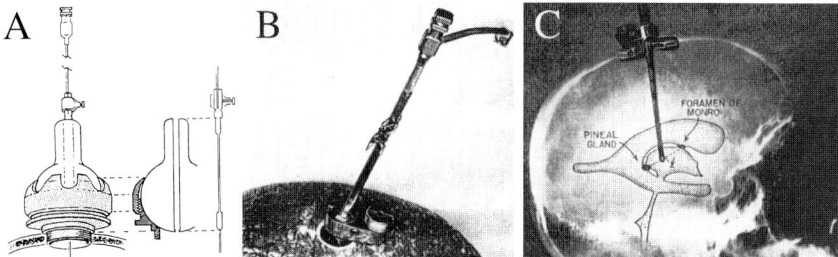

FIG. 4.3 Early stereotactic devices included burr hole-mounted devices to be used in conjunction with intraoperative plain-film radiography. Course corrections were made on the basis of plain-film radiographs obtained between successive small advancements of the stereotactic probe. Burr hole-mounted devices by Austin (*A*) and Todd (*B*) (c.1958). Technique of thalamotomy as illustrated by Todd using method espoused by Cooper (*C*).

In the second approach, a stereotactic frame is affixed to the patient's head, and localization of the target is made by centering the intended lesioning point within a targeting reticule as determined by fiducial markers. This approach has the advantage of eliminating the need to make continual adjustments to the trajectory of the lesioning probe, resulting in far more reproducible results and greater safety margins. Virtually all modern stereotactic devices are variations of this second type.

The prototypical frame-based device is the Horsely-Clark apparatus. This apparatus is a rectilinear one, with a probe mounted to sliders moveable in the anterior-posterior and lateral planes. Spiegel and Wycis, over a period of 20 years, developed a number of stereotactic apparatuses, each an improvement on the previous one. All of these were rectilinear devices, similar in conception to the original Horsely-Clark apparatus. Initial methods of fixation to the skull used plaster casts of the head affixed to the stereotactic instrumentation. Because of difficulties with this technique, especially in patients with mental illness, rubber-capped bolts were eventually used (*Fig. 4*).

Alterations in trajectory from normal angles to the frame required that trigonometric calculations be made to find the target (63). This particular difficulty was solved by Lars Leksell, who introduced the first of the arc-centered frame systems in 1949 (44). By placing the target at the center of a moveable arc, trajectories could be changed easily without requiring further calculations. Leksell was also the first to use skull fixation pins. Most of the later stereotactic frames take advantage of the arc-centered radius system (*Fig. 5*).

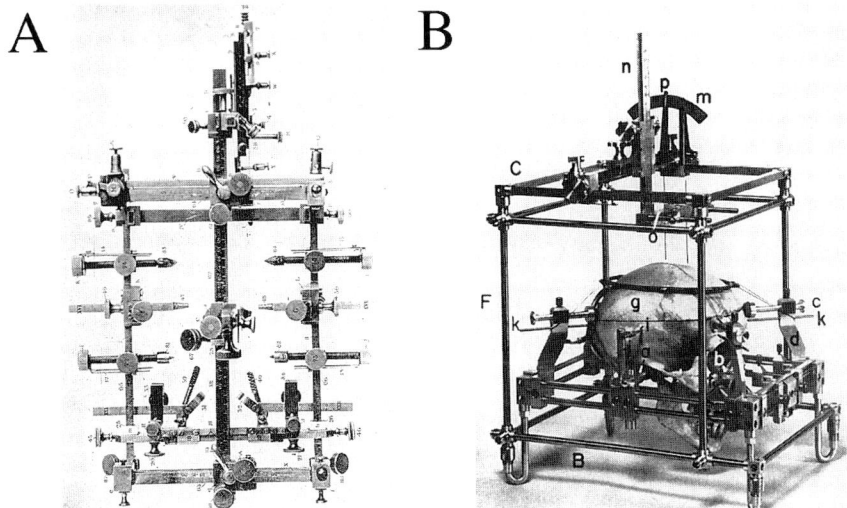

FIG. 4.4 Initial efforts at frame-based stereotactic instruments used rectilinear geometries. Such devices required trigonometric calculations to obtain angled trajectories to a target. *A*, Horsely and Clarke instrument, c. 1905, designed for use in macaque. *B*, Spiegel and Wycis' model III, c. 1952.

FIG. 4.5 The introduction of arc-centered devices by Leksell simplified the process of using angled trajectories by eliminating the need for trigonometric calculations. Arc-centered devices: *A*, Leksell frame, c.1949; *B*, Todd-Wells device, c. 1964.

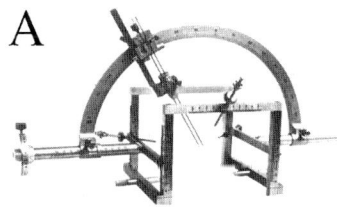

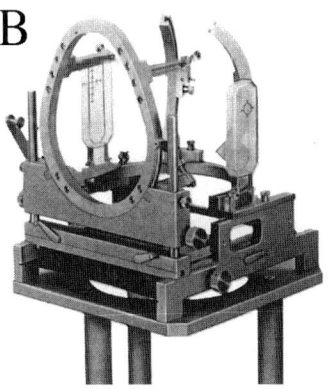

Specialized applications in one instance led to a close co-evolution of imaging and frame technology. The design of the Talairach apparatus was driven by the goal to eliminate the distorting magnifying effects of standard radiographic techniques. By using teleradiographic techniques in combination with angiographic studies and a rectilinear stereotactic apparatus, a comprehensive system was designed. In addition to its utility in diencephalic procedures, the Talairach apparatus is uniquely suited for stereoelectroencephalography depth electrode placement (70).

ELECTROPHYSIOLOGICAL LOCALIZATION

As experience accrued from functional procedures guided by plain-film radiography and atlas coordinates, it became clear that significant errors in target localization could occur, sometimes resulting in treatment failure or operative complications (26).

Because of the limits of then existent anatomic techniques, electrophysiological methods were introduced in an effort to more precisely localize functional targets. Three basic methods of neurophysiological localization have been used in human clinical subjects: electrical stimulation, impedance measurements, and microelectrode recording. Electrical stimulation is a provocative test, relying on the local stimulation of brain tissue to provoke responses (1). Impedance measurements rely on measurements of electrical impedance between the tip of a macro recording electrode and a distant ground. This method has proven to be an effective means of localization when applied to regions of the brain that have distinctive impedance profiles (43).

Electrical stimulation and impedance measurements are the most widespread used methods of electrophysiological localization, as they are the easiest to employ and have adequate spatial accuracy. Electrophysiological features discerned during the recording may serve as a clue to the location of the electrode, thereby serving as a guide to the direction in which the electrode must be moved if necessary.

Microelectrode recording methods are the most technically demanding yet precise and information-rich means of electrophysiological localization. The methods for human microelectrode recording are a direct translation of the in vivo microelectrode recording methods pioneered by neurophysiologists. Wetzel and Snider are likely the first to have used the technique in humans (78). This was quickly followed by the pioneering work of Guiot (34), Bertrand (13), and others.

Microelectrode recording can be difficult. The observer must be able to discern the characteristic firing patterns of neurons. Recording conditions may vary from day to day and from patient to patient, resulting in poor reliability. Single unit recordings may suffer from movements

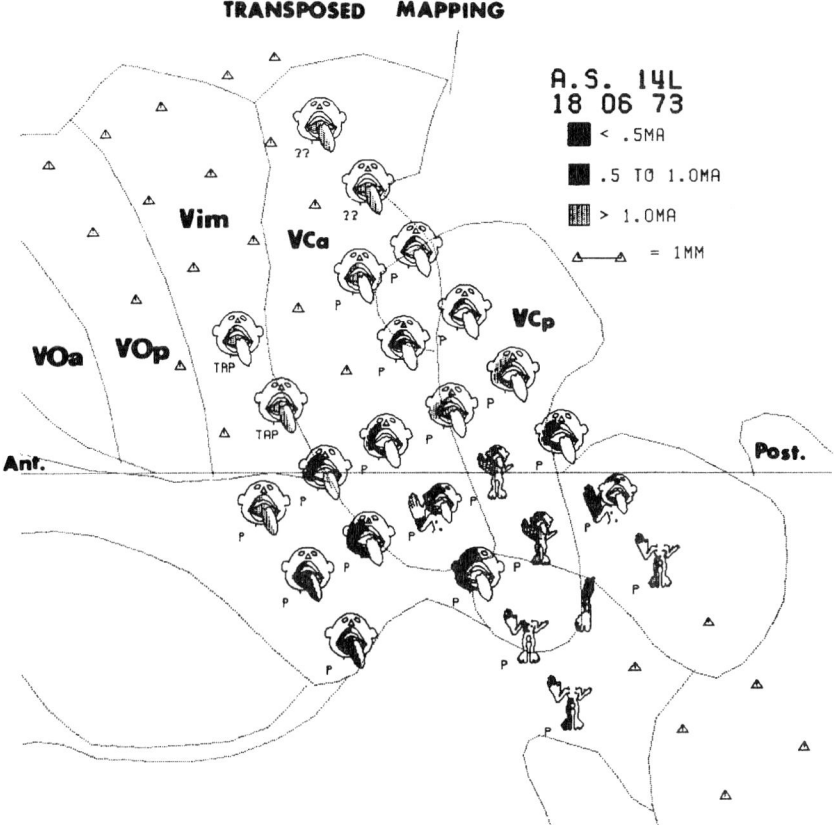

FIG. 4.6 Electrophysiological recording currently is the standard for localization of functional targets. Such recordings may provide detailed neurophysiological maps of both clinical and basic science interest. Pictured is a somatotopic map derived from electrophysiological recordings by Tasker et al. (c. 1981).

of the brain secondary to patient tremor, cardiac pulsations, and respiratory movement. The recording equipment can be very delicate, leading to intraoperative failures. The complexity of the method may significantly increase operative times. Further, multiple passes with a sharp electrode may increase the risk of hemorrhage.

Yet, despite these disadvantages, microelectrode recording is currently the gold standard for localization in functional procedures. In experienced hands, microelectrode recordings can generate detailed somatotopic maps of targeted structures, a level of resolution not likely to be approached by noninvasive radiographic techniques (*Fig. 6*) (72).

Presently, in the majority of major centers, electrophysiological recording is standard technique. However, the debate concerning the utility of microelectrode recording in functional procedures continues.

ADVANCES IN IMAGING: CT AND PLANAR IMAGING

Clinical stereotaxy, from its inception by Spiegel and Wycis, did not change in technical principle for approximately 30 years. This stasis nearly led to its demise as a discipline with the introduction of L-Dopa. Yet outside of the operating room, developments were occurring that would result in the rebirth of stereotaxy. This period of time, from the 1950s to early 1970s, coincides with the nascent period of computer technology and transistorized electronics. In the world of navigation, the military-industrial complex fueled the introduction of multiple computerized systems using cybernetic principles to provide high precision navigational and guidance abilities (*Fig. 7*). The computing devices initially developed for the defense sector would find eventual application in the medical field. In 1972, the first computed tomographic scanner was introduced (38). This device had a metric of 80 by 80 pixels, suitable for low resolution imaging of the brain and ventricular system.

The introduction of computed tomography allowed for the first time to directly visualize the internal anatomy of the brain in a noninvasive fashion. As the resolution of successive generations of CT scanners improved, its use in stereotactic surgery eventually became practical. The CT scanner's ability to discriminate pathological anatomy extended the scope of stereotactic surgery into the diagnosis and treatment of neoplasms and other intracranial mass lesions (6, 8, 36, 71). Neoplasms would supplant functional disorders as the principal indication of stereotactic methodology.

Because the method reliably produces a spatially accurate image, its use in stereotaxy has been rapidly accepted. Initial efforts were made to adapt CT methods to already existent stereotactic systems (12, 31), but it became clear that the new imaging modality would require the development of a new class of instrumentation to take advantage of the unique features and requirements of planar imaging.

CT-OPTIMIZED INSTRUMENTATION

One of the first devices specifically developed for use in conjunction with CT scanning was the Brown-Roberts-Wells (BRW) apparatus (19–22). Russell Brown, under the guidance of Theodore Roberts, developed a means of using external reference points to unambiguously describe points within stereotactic space. The device he developed in conjunction with the engineer Trent Wells introduced a localizing frame

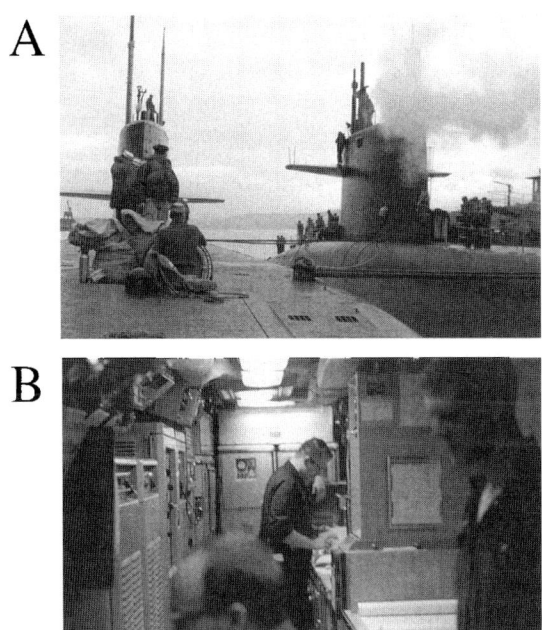

FIG. 4.7 National security-driven demands on the military-industrial complex led to the application of computerized devices using cybernetic principles to provide high precision navigation and guidance. A, masts on Polaris-class nuclear missile submarine (SSBN-601), c. 1970, contain automated celestial sextants, satellite tracking systems, as well as periscopes. These instruments, along with ship's inertial navigational guidance systems, long wave radio triangulation, and bottom contour mapping, served as a precise amalgam for point orientation on the global surface. B, navigational center on Polaris submarine using early mainframe computers as well as standard navigational charts.

with three sets of bars arranged in an N-shaped configuration. A CT-image slice through any plane containing the nine fiducial points could be used to localize a target within the scanned plane as well as define the relation of the scanned plane to the base ring (*Fig. 8*). Targeting was accomplished through the use of a computer program that, when provided with the coordinates of the localizing bars and the target point, would provide the settings to be made on a phantom base. The trajectory would be determined by the arrangement of interlocking rings. The BRW apparatus was used in the first large studies of the CT-guided stereotactic methodology as applied to intracranial lesions (6, 36). The elegance and simplicity of the N-bar and CT method led to its wide acceptance and adaptation to a number of stereotactic systems.

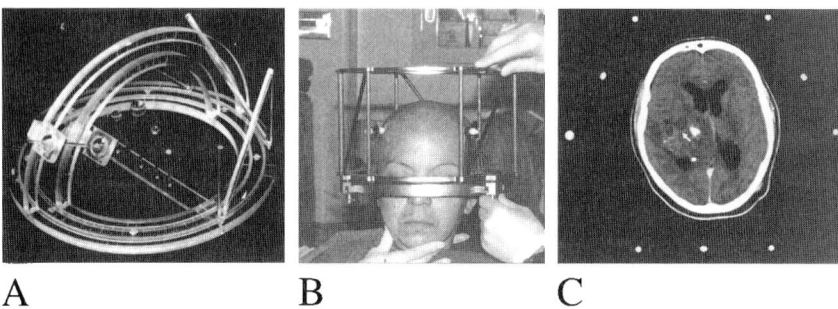

FIG. 4.8 Planar imaging extended the indications of stereotactic localization to neoplastic processes. *A,* prototype of BRW localizing system built by Russell Brown demonstrating the N-bar concept. *B,* production of the N-bar localizer on BRW head ring. *C,* CT scan demonstrating constellation of localizing bars serving as reference points for computerized targeting.

Other stereotactic systems have been similarly adapted to use with computed tomography with similar results (14, 33, 45).

ADVANCES IN IMAGING: MAGNETIC RESONANCE IMAGING (MRI)

MRI techniques represent a fundamental advance over previously available imaging techniques. In addition to its ability to generate high-resolution planar images of brain structures, MRI can generate information regarding vascular flow characteristics, tissue chemical composition, and regional functional characteristics. Most instrumentation systems designed for CT-guided techniques have been easily adapted for MR use.

The versatility of MRI, however, can come at the price of accuracy. Unlike the x-ray beams of CT, the magnetic fields used in MRI can be spatially distorted, resulting in inaccurate targeting. Conditions leading to magnetic susceptibility artifact are often not obvious and may vary from patient to patient (52, 57). Use of MRI-acquired images therefore requires the strictest quality control and rejection of the technique when there is suspicion of conditions leading to geometric distortion.

Despite these limitations, the high resolution and fine-tissue discrimination of MRI has resulted in its rapid acceptance by stereotactic surgeons (42). In part, this is due to the ability of the technique—for the first time—to directly visualize anatomic targets. In particular, with current techniques, it is not difficult to visualize the component structures of the basal ganglia. For the first time, the anatomic targets of functional procedures have become directly visible through these scanning methods. This essentially obviates the need for standard stereotactic atlases in certain procedures. For other targets, it is likely that new atlas coordinate systems based on MRI-observable landmarks may be introduced for the planning of functional procedures (32, 81).

MRI instrumentation is still evolving. Higher strength magnets in combination with evolving gradient coil and sequence architecture are resulting in ultra-high resolution imaging remarkable for precise anatomic detail (53) (*Fig. 9*). It is therefore likely that additional functional targets will become directly resolvable by MRI.

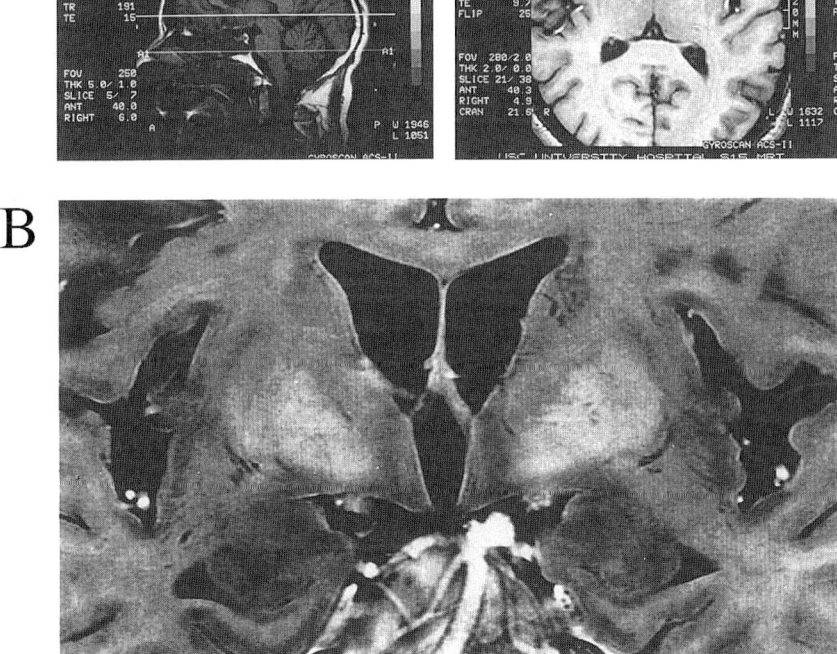

FIG. 4.9 Advanced radiographic techniques may alter the paradigm of localizing functional targets, providing individualized maps for each patient. *A,* stereotactic MRI at 1.5 tesla, demonstrating target of lesioning procedure. *B,* 3 tesla images created on research scanner demonstrating high-resolution images.

Current State Of The Art
MECHANICAL COUPLED POINT STEREOTAXY

The common thread of all stereotactic frame-based systems is the integration of a mechanical measuring device and instrument holder. A number of frame-based stereotactic devices have been developed by committed visionary neurosurgeons and engineers over the years (*Fig. 10*). Of the many devices that have been developed, three devices account for the vast majority of stereotactic procedures that have been executed in the short history of this discipline. These are the Leksell, the Todd-Wells, and the Brown-Roberts-Wells and Cosman-Roberts-Wells series of devices.

Following a visit to Philadelphia to observe the work of Spiegel and Wycis, Lars Leksell returned to Sweden and proceeded to develop his own stereotactic instrumentation (*Fig. 11*). The Leksell series of stereotactic devices has been continuously modified over the years and enjoys popular use in functional and radiosurgical procedures. The current Leksell G-frame is an integral part of the Gamma-Knife radiosurgical system. Approximately 1200 Leksell frames have been produced and are used in over 850 centers worldwide (28).

Edwin M. Todd trained under Gardner in Cleveland, Ohio and subsequently pursued fellowships first at Yale and then at the Royal Infirmary in Edinburgh under John Gillingham. Having gained experience

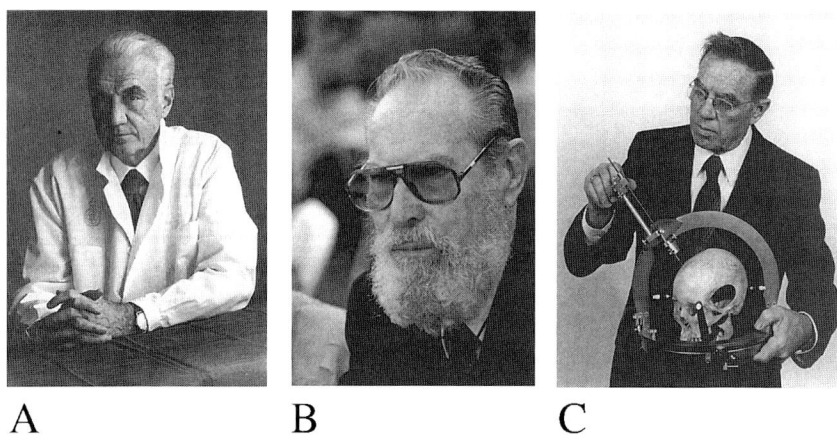

FIG. 4.10 Numerous stereotactic instruments have been created over the years by visionary neurosurgeons and engineers. Leaders in the development of stereotactic instrumentation. *A*, Lars Leksell; *B*, Edwin M. Todd; *C*, Trent H. Wells, Jr. with BRW frame.

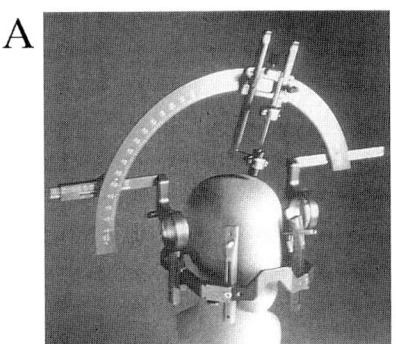 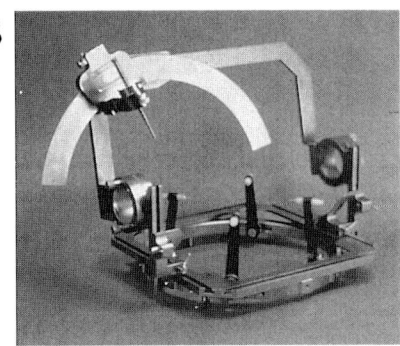

FIG. 4.11 Modern stereotactic instrumentation optimized for planar imaging techniques. *A*, Leksell G-frame; *B*, CRW frame.

in stereotactic surgery, he was to avidly pursue this in practice. In 1964, he joined the clinical staff at the University of Southern California. He, in collaboration with Trent H. Wells, Jr., developed the Todd-Wells stereotactic frame, which was introduced in 1964. It is characterized by robust construction and remarkable flexibility in application. Produced for approximately 20 years, it served as the de facto standard for stereotactic devices in North America. In all, approximately 2000 Todd-Wells devices were produced (77).

The youngest series of stereotactic devices are the BRW and CRW frames. This is a modular system with functionally interchangeable componentry. The CRW differs from the BRW by replacing the intersecting semicircle system with a more conventional arc-centered system (25). Presently, over 2000 BRW and 1500 CRW frames have been produced (55).

The high level of acceptance of these devices and other devices is a testament to the ease of use and sound principle of their operation as well as the ability to extend the scope of neurosurgical practice. Frame-based stereotaxy has been used in wide-ranging indications including movement disorders, pain, epilepsy (10), psychosurgery (9), cerebrovascular disease (2, 60), neoplasms, and cranial and spine trauma (50, 51). The success of frame-based stereotaxy is based on the ability to define a point in space and unambiguously reach that point with high margins of safety (5). The technique is by nature minimally invasive, being accomplished through small twist drill-sized burr holes.

FRAMELESS AND VOLUMETRIC STEREOTAXY

Soon after the introduction of planar computed tomographic and magnetic resonance imaging, it was recognized that serial scans could be reformatted into three-dimensional rendered images. This advance, coupled with the increasing availability of desktop computing power and advanced software, made possible the development of volumetric stereotactic methods, first adapted to rigid frame-based systems (41). Volumetric techniques are particularly suited for surgery of deep-seated intrinsic brain tumors, where they may increase the likelihood of gross total resections with minimal involvement of adjacent neurologically critical structures.

The volumetric paradigm was to give birth to a new form of stereotactic instrumentation, free of rigid constraints and specifically tailored as an aid for open neurosurgical procedures. This new class of instrumentation has spawned the field of image-guided or frameless stereotactic surgery. Initially described by Roberts et al., frameless devices use optical, acoustic, or magnetic sensors to measure relative positioning of a lesion or probe relative to arbitrarily defined fiducials (*Fig. 12*) (56, 59).

By nature, the method is volumetric in orientation, although it can be adapted to point stereotaxy. The frameless method creates a new

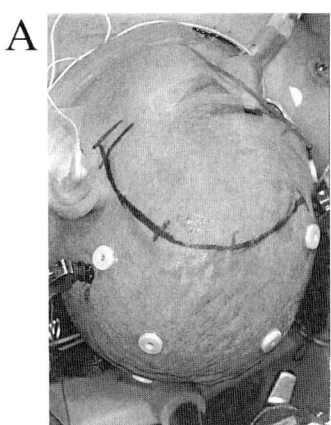
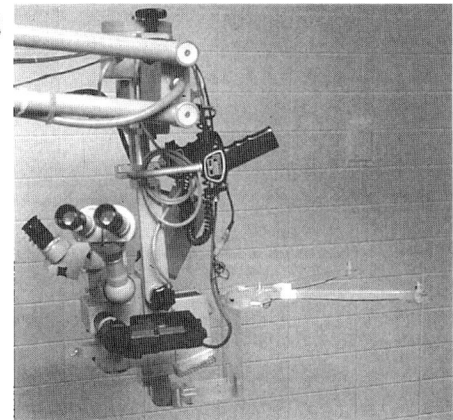

FIG. 4.12 Frameless stereotaxy is a relatively new paradigm in surgical navigation initially conceived as an aid to open cranial surgeries. *A*, device of Roberts et al., which tracks movement of microscope relative to lesion using a planar array of spark gaps with sonar disposition in ceiling of operating room. *B*, fiducial placement on scalp at arbitrary positions.

philosophical approach to the stereotactic methodology. Rather than being concerned with minimally invasive approaches directed toward getting to an unambiguous point, the technique supplements open procedures by reporting where a point is within the three-dimensional operative space.

Frameless-stereotactic systems are generally not suited for use in twist-drill approach biopsy and functional procedures but have become viable aids in traditional open procedures and neuroendoscopic procedures.

Despite widespread implementation of these devices, the advantages of such image-guided techniques are unclear, at least in the realm of open intracranial surgeries. Brain shift, registration errors, increased time of set-up, and requirement for additional skilled personnel all potentially may complicate its utility and acceptance. Dead reckoning methods, when implemented by properly trained and experienced surgeons, have proven effective, and the advantages of frameless systems in the majority of intracranial neurosurgical procedures are uncertain in regard to patient outcome, safety, and cost.

Frameless methods, however, may prove helpful in applications outside of intracranial neurosurgery, particularly in spinal surgery. Procedures difficult to execute with conventional flouroscopic imaging techniques, such as spinal screw instrumentation placement, may disproportionately benefit from image-guided techniques (17, 40).

FUTURE DIRECTIONS IN STEREOTAXY

One may look into the near future to speculate how stereotactic systems may change to take advantage of emerging developments in neuroscience and electronic technologies. It is certain that new technologies in radiographic imaging, robotics, and neuroscience will fundamentally alter the manner in which surgeries are carried out.

Imaging Techniques

Medical imaging science has and will continue to be a primary driving factor in the evolution of stereotactic surgery. Whereas it is impossible to foresee the introduction of fundamentally new imaging technologies, evolutionary improvements in present technologies will likely result in widespread changes in stereotactic methodology.

In contrast to the use of intraoperative plain-film radiographs, current planar imaging techniques largely force the temporal separation of the imaging session from the operative procedure. This "real time problem" gives rise to difficulties in stereotactic methodology, such as brain shift, rendering planning coordinates useless. The use of CT and

MRI technologies to the operating room promises an elimination of this problem and further will likely redefine the concept of image-guided surgery (15, 47, 75).

Although current devices are of limited utility as they suffer from poor ergonomics, high cost, and mediocre image quality, improvements in design and production processes will likely overcome these limitations in the near future. The intra-operative imaging device of the future, with rapid image acquisition and superimposition of real-time radiographic images onto the operative field, may result in improved operative safety and outcome.

Robotics

The capability of robots to precisely measure their movements makes them by nature stereotactic instruments. Robotic-assisted open and stereotactic procedures have already been introduced by neurosurgical researchers (11, 27). Current commercially available robotic technology consists of "dumb" robots, subject purely to the command of the surgeon. Such robots are currently in development to provide surgical services remote to the location of the surgeon. "Remote surgery" will also depend on new information display technologies, exemplified by the introduction of the surgical head-mounted display (46).

Continued refinements to frameless stereotactic systems have included the integration of robotic technology to image-guided surgery (e.g., the Zeiss MKM). Robotic stereotactic methods may allow accurate placement of functional lesions, spinal instrumentation, and biopsy probes on a purely automated basis.

Concurrent with improvements in the user-friendliness of robotic technology, robots will become "smarter." Pattern-recognition software will be able to interpret higher level commands and execute simple multistep movements in response. Later robots, in the roll of an intelligent surgical assistant, may suggest surgical stratagems to the surgeon user and will be able to carry out complex multistep procedures under direction.

Advances in Neuroscience

Localizing the point is but one aspect of stereotaxis that has undergone seismic changes over the last 20 years. Whereas functional stereotaxy has had its birth with ablative procedures, a new age of augmentative procedures is dawning. The lessons learned from early attempts at adrenal transplantation are now being applied to fetal transplants and the genetically engineered cells of the near future.

Targets of augmentative or ablation procedures will become more refined as the limitations of current stereotactic targets are appreciated and further research into the pathophysiology of movement and other disorders elucidates basic mechanisms of brain function.

Advances in neuroscience will likely change the manner in which functional disorders of the brain are addressed. Rather than seeking to retune a damaged system by placing destructive lesions in the brain, augmentative procedures have recently become a near reality. Such augmentation may occur through advances in biotechnology with implantation of specially developed cells to replace damaged neurotransmitter systems, or through the introduction of genetic material to induce repair of damaged systems. Alternatively, advances in microelectronics may allow biological interfaces to allow the development of direct brain-machine interfaces.

Factors Controlling Acceptance of Stereotactic Techniques

Our current social and economic revolution based on semiconductor technology has profoundly changed our daily lives. Methods of stereotactic localization have been similarly influenced and will continue to be refined and altered as new technologies are introduced. Significant developments have been made in every aspect of this discipline in the last 10 years. The technology dependence of stereotaxis promises advancements in stereotactic methodology and instrumentation far into the future (4).

Gordon Moore, a seminal figure in semiconductor technology, stated in 1965 that the number of transistors integrated onto a single chip would double every 18 to 24 months. This statement has surprisingly held true over 30 years and now is popularly known as "Moore's Law." With this tidal wave of computing power has come a bewildering array of new surgical navigation technologies and products. The plethora of new devices, coupled with the competitive medical marketplace, has encouraged many centers to purchase these technologies—sometimes before the technologies have been suitably tested, refined, and understood. With many of these systems, use makes painfully evident how short the reality falls short of the promise. Yet, before many of these devices and concepts have a chance to mature, they become obsolete as newer technologies enter the marketplace with ever more grandiose claims.

New technologies in stereotaxy will only be accepted in the long run if they significantly improve outcome and safety of surgery, if they enable the execution of procedures otherwise not performable, or if their use can result in significant cost savings. Stereotacticians, familiar with technological advances harnessed to "localize the point," should continue to be on the forefront of introducing advanced technologies to the neurosurgical discipline while recognizing the limitations of these technologies in the surgical theater.

REFERENCES

1. Alberts WW, Wright EW, Levin G, et al.: Threshold stimulation of the lateral thalamus and globus pallidus. **Electroencephalogr Clin Neurophysiol** 13:68–74, 1961.
2. Alksne J: Stereotaxic thrombosis of intracranial aneurysms. **N Engl J Med** 284:171, 1971.
3. Andrew J, Watkins ES: *A Stereotaxic Atlas of the Human Thalamus and Adjacent Structures: A Variability Study.* Baltimore, Williams & Wilkins, 1969.
4. Apuzzo ML: The Richard C. Schneider Lecture. New dimensions of neurosurgery in the realm of high technology—Possibilities, practicalities, realities. **Neurosurgery 38:**625–637; Discussion 637–639, 1996.
5. Apuzzo ML, Chandrasoma PT, Cohen D, Zee CS, Zelman V: Computed imaging stereotaxy: Experience and perspective related to 500 procedures applied to brain masses. **Neurosurgery** 20:930–937, 1987.
6. Apuzzo ML, Sabshin JK: Computed tomographic guidance stereotaxis in the management of intracranial mass lesions. **Neurosurgery** 12:277–285, 1983.
7. Austin G, Lee A: A plastic ball and socket type stereotaxic director. **J Neurosurg** 15:264–268, 1958.
8. Backlund EO, Von Holst H: Controlled subtotal evacuation of intracerebral hematoma by stereotactic technique. **Surg Neurol** 9:99–101, 1978.
9. Ballantine HT Jr, Cassidy WL, Flanagan NB, Marino R Jr: Stereotaxic anterior cingulotomy for neuropsychiatric illness and intractable pain. **J Neurosurg** 26:488–495, 1967.
10. Bancaud J, Angelergues R, Bernouilli C, et al.: Functional stereotaxic exploration (SEEG) of epilepsy. **Electroencephalogr Clin Neurophysiol** 28:85–86, 1970.
11. Benabid AL, Cinquin P, Lavalle S, Le Bas JF, Demongeot J, de Rougemont J: Computer-driven robot for stereotactic surgery connected to CT scan and magnetic resonance imaging. Technological design and preliminary results. **Appl Neurophysiol** 50:153–154, 1987.
12. Bergstrom M, Greitz J: Stereotaxic computed tomography. **Am J Roentgenol** 127:167–170, 1976.
13. Bertrand G, Jasper H: Microelectrode recording of unit activity in the human thalamus. **Conf Neurol** 26:205–208, 1965.
14. Birg W, Mundinger F, Klar M: A computer programme system for stereotactic neurosurgery. **Acta Neurochir (Wien)** 24[Suppl]:99–108, 1977.
15. Black PM, Moriarty T, Alexander E III, et al.: Development and implementation of intraoperative magnetic resonance imaging and its neurosurgical applications. **Neurosurgery** 41:831–842; Discussion 842–845, 1997.
16. Brierly JB, Beck E: The significance in human stereotactic brain surgery of individual variation in the diencephalon and globus pallidus. **J Neurol Neurosurg Psychiatry** 22:287–298, 1959.
17. Brodwater BK, Roberts DW, Nakajima T, Friets EM, Strohbehn JW: Extracranial application of the frameless stereotactic operating microscope: Experience with lumbar spine. **Neurosurgery** 32:209–213; Discussion 213, 1993.
18. Brown LA: *The Story of Maps.* New York, Little, Brown, 1969.

19. Brown RA: A computerized tomography-computer graphics approach to stereotaxic localization. **J Neurosurg** 50:715–720, 1979.
20. Brown RA: A stereotactic head frame for use with CT body scanners. **Invest Radiol** 14:300–304, 1979.
21. Brown RA, Roberts T, Osborn AG: Simplified CT-guided stereotaxic biopsy. **Am J Neuroradiol** 2:181–184, 1981.
22. Brown RA, Roberts TS, Osborn AG: Stereotaxic frame and computer software for CT-directed neurosurgical localization. **Invest Radiol** 15:308–312, 1980.
23. Castleman B: Navigators in the 1490's. **Proc U S Naval Inst** 118:39–43, 1992.
24. Cooper I: Chemopallidectomy: An investigative technique in geriatric parkinsonism. **Science** 121:217–218, 1955.
25. Couldwell WT, Apuzzo ML: Initial experience related to the use of the Cosman-Roberts-Wells stereotactic instrument: Technical note. **J Neurosurg** 72:145–148, 1990.
26. Dierssen G, Bergmann LL, Gioino G, et al.: Hemiballism following surgery for Parkinson's disease. **Arch Neurol** 5:627–637, 1961.
27. Drake JM, Joy M, Goldenberg A, Kreindler D: Computer- and robot-assisted resection of thalamic astrocytomas in children. **Neurosurgery** 29:27–33, 1991.
28. Elekta, personal communication.
29. Ferrier, D: *The Functions of the Brain.* London, Smith, Elder and Company, 1876.
30. Fuson RH: *The Log of Christopher Columbus.* Camden, Maine, International Marine Publishing, 1987.
31. Gildenberg PL, Kaufman HH, Murthy KS: Calculation of stereotactic coordinates from the computed tomographic scan. **Neurosurgery** 10:580–586, 1982.
32. Giller CA, Dewey RB, Ginsburg MI, Mendelsohn DB, Berk AM: Stereotactic pallidotomy and thalamotomy using individual variations of anatomic landmarks for localization. **Neurosurgery 42:**56–62; Discussion 62–65, 1998.
33. Gouda K, Freidberg S, Larsen C: Modification of the Gouda frame to allow stereotactic biopsy of the brain using the GE 8800 computer tomographic scanner. **Neurosurgery** 13:176–181, 1983.
34. Guiot G, Hardy J, Albe-Fessard D: Delimitation precise des structures sous-corticales et identification de noyaux thalamiques chez l'homme par electrophysiologie stereotaxique. **Neurochirurgie** 5:1–18, 1962.
35. Haller AV; *Elementa Physiologie.* Lausanne, Marci-Michael, Bosquet et Sociorum 1766.
36. Heilbrun MP, Roberts TS, Apuzzo ML, Wells TH Jr, Sabshin JK: Preliminary experience with Brown-Roberts-Wells (BRW) computerized tomography stereotaxic guidance system. **J Neurosurg** 59:217–222, 1983.
37. Horsley V, Clarke RH: The structure and function of the cerebellum examined by a new method. **Brain** 31:45–124, 1908.
38. Hounsfield GN: Computerized transverse axial scanning (tomography): I. Description of the system. **Br J Radiol** 46:1016–1022, 1973.
39. Jensen RL, Stone JL, Hayne, RA: Introduction of the human Horsley-Clarke stereotactic frame. **Neurosurgery** 38:563–567; Discussion 567, 1996.
40. Kalfas IH, Kormos DW, Murphy MA, et al.: Application of frameless stereotaxy to pedicle screw fixation of the spine. **J Neurosurg** 83:641–647, 1995.
41. Kelly P: Volumentric stereotactic surgical resection of intra-axial brain mass lesions. **Mayo Clin Proc** 63:1186–1198, 1988.
42. Kondziolka D, Flickinger JC: Use of magnetic resonance imaging in stereotactic surgery: A survey of members of the American Society of Stereotactic and Functional Neurosurgery. **Stereotact Funct Neurosurg** 66:193–197, 1996.

43. Laitinen L, Johansson GG, Sipponen P: Impedence and phase angle as locating method in human stereotaxic surgery. **J Neurosurg** 25:XXX–XXX, 1966.
44. Leksell L: A stereotaxic apparatus for intracerebral surgery. **Acta Chir Scand** 99:229–233, 1949.
45. Leksell L, Jernberg B: Stereotaxis and tomography: A technical note. **Acta Neurochir** 52:1–7, 1980.
46. Levy M, Chen J, Moffitt K, Corber Z, McComb J: Stereoscopic head-mounted display incorporated into microsurgical procedures: Technical note. **Neurosurgery** 43: 392–396, 1998.
47. Lunsford LD, Rosenbaum AE, Perry J: Stereotactic surgery using the "therapeutic" CT scanner. **Surg Neurol** 18:116–122, 1982.
48. Macewan W: Tumor of the dura mater removed during life in a person affected with epilepsy. **Glasgow Med J** 12:210–213, 1879.
49. McCaul I: A method for the localization and production of discrete destructive lesions in brain. **J Neurol Neurosurg Psychiatry** 22:109–112, 1959.
50. McFadden JT: Stereotaxic realignment of the dislocated cervical spine. **Surg Gynecol Obstet** 133:262–264, 1971.
51. McFadden JT, Horton CE: Stereotaxic localization of extracranial foreign bodies in the head. **Am Surg** 37:353–356, 1971.
52. Michiels J, Bosmans H, Pelgrims P, et al.: On the problem of geometric distortion in magnetic resonance images for stereotactic neurosurgery. **Magn Reson Imaging** 12:749–765, 1994.
53. Nakayama N, Nakada T: High-resolution T2-reversed magnetic resonance imaging on a high magnetic field system: Technical note. **J Neurosurg** 89:492–495, 1998.
54. Picard C, Olivier A, Bertrand G: The first human stereotaxic apparatus: The contribution of Aubrey Mussen to the field of stereotaxis. **J Neurosurg** 59:673–676, 1983.
55. Radionics, 1998.
56. Roberts DW, Strohbehn JW, Hatch JF, Murray W, Kettenberger H: A frameless stereotaxic integration of computerized tomographic imaging and the operating microscope. **J Neurosurg** 65:545–549, 1986.
57. Schad L, Lott S, Schmitt F, Sturm V, Lorenz WJ: Correction of spatial distortion in MR imaging: A prerequisite for accurate stereotaxy. **J Comput Assist Tomogr** 11:499–505, 1987.
58. Schaltenbrand G, Wahren W: *Atlas for Stereotaxy of the Human Brain.* 2nd ed. Stuttgart, Georg Thieme, 1977.
59. Smith KR, Frank KJ, Bucholz RD: The NeuroStation: A highly accurate, minimally invasive solution to frameless stereotactic neurosurgery. **Comput Med Imaging Graph** 18:247–256, 1994.
60. Smith RW, Alksne JF: Stereotaxic thrombosis of inaccessible intracranial aneurysms. **J Neurosurg** 47:833–839, 1977.
61. Sobel D: *Longitude: The True Story of a Lone Genius Who Solved the Greatest Scientific Problem of His Time.* New York, Walker & Co., 1995.
62. Spiegel EA, Wycis HT: Pallido-thalamotomy in chorea. **Arch Neurol** 64:495–496, 1950.
63. Spiegel EA, Wycis HT: *Stereoencephalotomy. Part 1.* New York, Grune & Stratton, 1952.
64. Spiegel EA, Wycis HT: Ansotomy in paralysis agitans. **Trans Am Neurol Assoc** 78:178–198, 1953.
65. Spiegel EA, Wycis HT: Mesencephalotomy in the treatment of "intractable" facial pain. **Arch Neurol** 69:1–13, 1953.

66. Spiegel EA, Wycis HT, Baird HW: Pallidotomy and pallidoamygdalotomy in certain types of convulsive disorders. **Arch Neurol** 80:714–728, 1958.
67. Spiegel EA, Wycis HT, Marks M, et al.: Stereotaxic apparatus for operations on the human brain. **Science** 106:349–350, 1947.
68. Spurzheim G: *The Anatomy of the Brain.* London, S Highley, 1826.
69. Talairach J, David M, Tournoux P, et al.: *Atlas d'Anatomie Stereotaxique.* Paris, Masson, 1957.
70. Talaraich J, Szikla G: *Atlas of Stereotaxic Anatomy of the Telencephalon.* Paris, Masson & Cie, 1967.
71. Tanikawa T, Amano K, Kawamura H, et al.: CT-guided stereotactic surgery for evacuation of hypertensive intracerebral hematoma. **Appl Neurophysiol** 48:431–439, 1985.
72. Tasker RR, Organ LW, Hawrylyshyn PA: *The Thalamus and Midbrain of Man: A Physiological Atlas Using Electrical Stimulation.* Springfield, IL, Charles C. Thomas, 1982.
73. Taylor AJ, Haughton VM, Syvertsen A, Ho KC: Taylor-Haughton line revisited. **Am J Neuroradiol** 1:55–56, 1980.
74. Todd E, Shelden C, Pudenz R, Crue B: Surgical management of dyskinesia. **Am J Surg** 102:265, 1961.
75. Tronnier VM, Wirtz CR, Knauth M, et al.: Intraoperative diagnostic and interventional magnetic resonance imaging in neurosurgery [see comments]. **Neurosurgery** 40:891–900; Discussion 900–902, 1997.
76. Van Buren JM, Bourke RC: *Variations of the Human Diencephalon,* Vol. II. Berlin, Springer-Verlag, 1972.
77. Wells T, personal communication.
78. Wetzel N, Snider R: Neurophysiological correlates in human stereotaxis. **Q Bull Northwest Univ Med School** 32:XXX–XXX, 1958.
79. Williams JED: *From Sails to Satellites: The Origin and Development of Navigational Science.* New York, Oxford University Press, 1992.
80. Willis T: *Cerebri Anatome: Cui Accessit Nervorum Descriptio et Usus.* London, J Martyn and J Allestry, 1664.
81. Young RF, Shumway-Cook A, Vermeulen SS, et al.: Gamma knife radiosurgery as a lesioning technique in movement disorder surgery. **J Neurosurg** 89:183–193, 1998.

CHAPTER

5

Image-guided Spinal Navigation

IAIN H. KALFAS, M.D., F.A.C.S.

Interactive image-guided navigation using surface reference fiducials in place of a stereotactic frame has been successfully applied to intracranial surgery (1, 2, 5, 9, 12, 13, 15, 16, 19). It provides an accurate and reliable means of *localizing* lesions within the brain and identifying underlying anatomic structures. This serves to minimize surgical morbidity and limit the length and expense of the procedure.

However, for most spinal procedures, localization is not a significant problem. An intraoperative lateral radiograph is sufficient in most cases to localize the appropriate spinal level. Image-guided spinal navigation is not needed to identify a lumbar disc herniation, a vertebral body fracture, or an extramedullary spinal neoplasm. For those cases in which an intramedullary neoplasm or syrinx is difficult to precisely localize, intraoperative ultrasonography has proved useful (6).

The purpose of applying stereotactic principles to spinal surgery is to improve the surgeon's orientation to the unexposed spinal anatomy. The three-dimensional anatomy of the spinal column can present difficulties for even the most experienced surgeon. Standard posterior surgical approaches expose only a portion of the spinal column at a given level. Although this partial exposure is not problematic for most laminectomy or discectomy procedures, it can be limiting in the setting of complex spinal column disorders, such as fractures, neoplasms, or deformities.

The ability to conceptualize the three-dimensional anatomy of the spinal column from any single surgical approach varies among surgeons. It is dependent not only on the surgeon's knowledge of the spinal anatomy but also on the correct interpretation of both preoperative and intraoperative imaging. Image-guided spinal navigation facilitates this image interpretation process by providing digitized images through multiple points and planes in the spinal column. This greatly enhances the surgeon's ability to "visualize" the unexposed spinal anatomy.

The evolution of spinal instrumentation devices, as well as the development of more involved surgical approaches to the spine, have expanded the options for managing complex spinal disorders. These procedures all require the surgeon to be oriented to the unexposed spinal anatomy. In particular, the variety of spinal fixation techniques involving the placement of bone screws into the pedicles of the thoracic, lumbar, and sacral spine; into the lateral masses and across joints of the cervical spine; and across the vertebrae of the thoracic and lumbar spine requires a thorough understanding of the spatial relationships of the unexposed spinal anatomy.

Although intraoperative fluoroscopy and serial radiography have proved useful as intraoperative imaging tools, they are limited to providing only two-dimensional imaging of a complex three-dimensional structure. Consequently, the surgeon is required to estimate the position of unexposed spinal structures based on an interpretation of these images and a knowledge of the pertinent anatomy. Such inference can result in varying degrees of inaccuracy when placing screws in the spinal column.

Several studies have shown the unreliability of routine radiography in assessing pedicle screw placement in the lumbrosacral spine. The rate of penetration of the pedicle cortex by an inserted screw ranges from 21 to 31% in these studies (7, 8, 17). However, Steinmann et al., using an image-based technique for pedicle screw placement that combined computed tomography (CT) axial images of cadaver spine specimens with fluoroscopy, were able to demonstrate a reduction of this screw insertion error rate to 5.5% (14).

The initial difficulty in adapting stereotactic principles to spinal surgery was identifying a frame of reference in which digitized images could be more directly applied to intraoperative anatomy. Unlike intracranial surgery, an external frame system is not practical for spinal surgery. Furthermore, the use of surface landmarks or fiducials creates problems of spatial accuracy because of skin movement with respect to bony landmarks (3, 4). This is less of a problem with intracranial applications because of the relatively fixed position of the overlying scalp to the attached fiducials.

The application of stereotactic technology to spinal surgery involves using the rigid spinal anatomy itself as a frame of reference. By selecting a series of corresponding points in a CT image set and in the exposed spinal anatomy, a point-to-point mapping of the image data onto the spinal anatomy can be performed. The image data can then be reformatted and presented to the surgeon in multiple planes to optimally demonstrate the unexposed spinal column (10).

However, unlike intraoperative ultrasonography or fluoroscopy, image-guided spinal navigation does not provide true real-time imaging. It does not show changes in the spinal anatomy as they occur. Instead, the role of this technology is to function as a confirmatory tool to assist the surgeon in identifying unexposed anatomic structures and relating their position and orientation to the exposed spinal anatomy. It is not intended to function as a substitute for a thorough understanding of the appropriate spinal anatomy and the correct surgical indications and techniques. It is an alternative method to the more conventional means of interpreting two-dimensional images of the spine provided by intraoperative fluoroscopy.

TECHNIQUE

Intraoperative localization for intracranial lesions using an armless, frameless stereotactic wand system has been previously described (1, 2). The primary components of the system used for spinal navigation include an image processing computer workstation (Picker International, Highland Heights, OH) interfaced with a two-camera optical localizer (Northern Digital, Waterloo, Ontario, Canada (*Fig. 5.1*). The op-

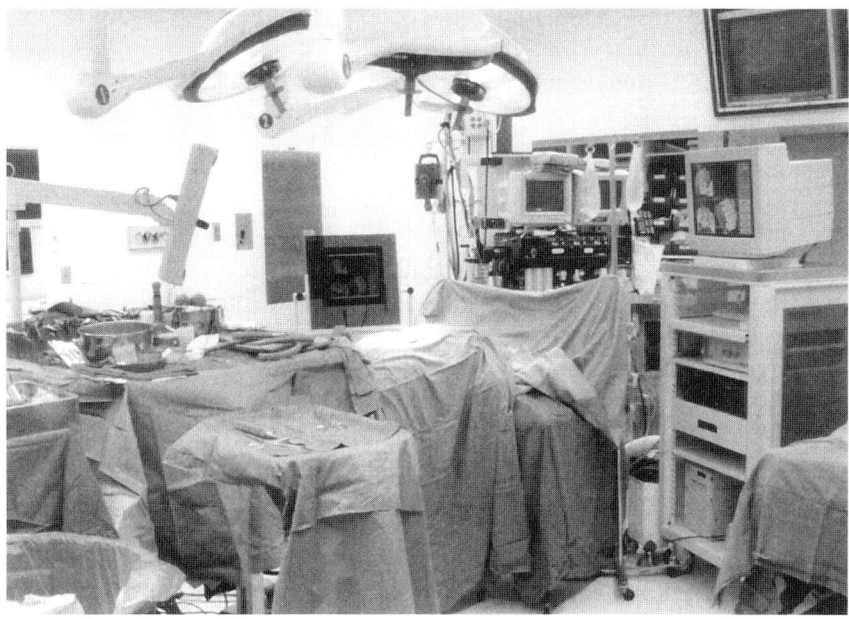

FIG. 5.1 Operating room arrangement for image-guided spinal navigation. For lumbosacral procedures, the infrared camera detector is positioned near the foot of the table and aimed rostrally. For cervical procedures, it is positioned at the head of the table and aimed caudally. The image processing workstation is positioned across the table from the surgeon. A separate flat panel display screen connected to the workstation is positioned across the table from the assistant.

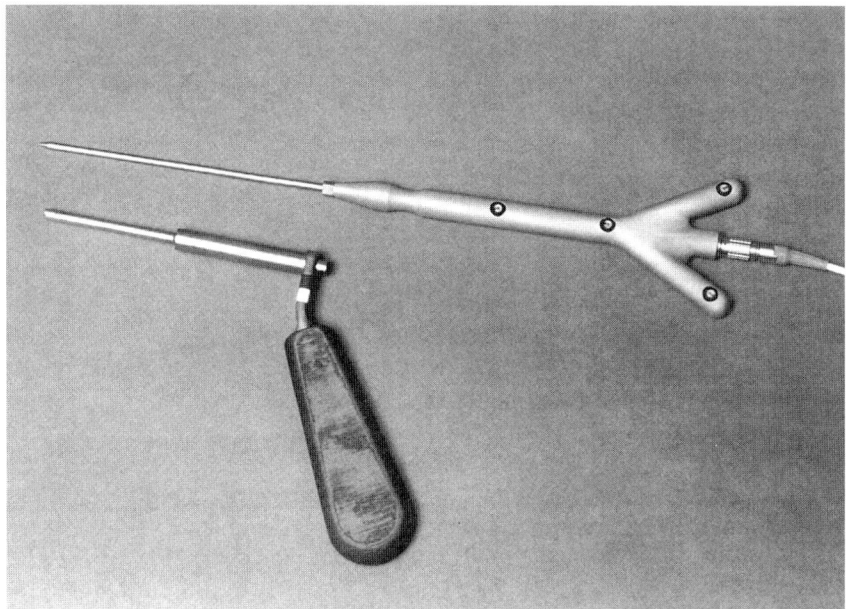

Fig. 5.2 Handheld wand and drill guide. The same wand is used for both registration and navigation. The drill guide is used during navigation to preserve the location of the entry point and the angle trajectory acquired during navigation. The wand can then be removed and a drill inserted through the drill guide.

tical localizer tracks infrared light emitted by a series of light-emitting diodes mounted on a customized handheld wand or selected surgical instruments (*Fig. 5.2*). The position of the wand or customized surgical instruments can then be tracked in space using mathematical principles of localization by triangulation. These instruments serve as the interface between the surgeon and the computer workstation.

The surface anatomy of the exposed spinal column provides the frame of reference necessary for image-guided navigation. Specifically, any bony landmark that can be identified intraoperatively as well as in the preoperative image data set can be used as a reference point. The spatial position of each point selected can be defined by its specific x, y, and z cartesian coordinates. The coordinates of a selected point in the image data set can be mapped onto its corresponding point in the surgical anatomy data set through a process termed *registration*.

Registration involves placing the cursor on the workstation screen on a preselected anatomic landmark in the CT magnetic resonance imaging data set while positioning the wand on the corresponding point in the surgical field. The position of the wand tip is precisely tracked by the camera localizer system. When the wand is placed on a specific reference point, the spatial location of that point is relayed to the computer workstation and linked to its corresponding image data point. Three to five reference points at a single exposed spinal level (e.g., tips of a spinous process and the two transverse processes) are required for the registration process.

Alternatively, the registration process can be performed by creating a contour map of the exposed spinal anatomy. With this technique, the localizing instrument is placed on numerous (30–40) arbitrarily selected points on the exposed and debrided surface of the spinal anatomy. These points are transmitted to the workstation, which then creates a topographical map of the selected anatomy and "matches" it to the stored CT data set of the same spinal anatomy.

The registration process represents the step during image-guided navigation that can contribute the greatest degree of inaccuracy to the procedure. It is dependent on the surgeon carefully selecting the correct registration points or performing the contour mapping process. However, if the registration process is properly performed, reformatted, mutliplanar CT or magnetic resonance images can be generated in near real time to precisely navigate through the unexposed spinal column and orient the surgeon to selected screw entry points and trajectories.

When applying image-guided technology to anterior spinal surgery, the registration process is less precise and more difficult to perform because of the lack of prominent bony landmarks on the anterior surface of the spinal column. For anterior thoracic fixation procedures, acceptable reference points include the junction of the head of a rib with the adjacent disc or pedicle, the disc spaces themselves, and selected points on the lateral surface of the vertebral body. Although these reference points may not provide the same degree of millimetric accuracy as that provided by the selection of more distinct posterior bony landmarks, the degree of accuracy required for screw placement across a thoracic vertebra is not as great as that required for screw insertion through a lumbar or thoracic pedicle or across the C1–2 facet joint. Regardless of the registration accuracy issue with anterior spinal surgery, image-guided navigation still provides intraoperative image data that exceed that provided by any other conventional localizing technique (e.g., fluoroscopy).

After each registration step, the navigational system compares the spatial relationship of the registration points selected in the surgical field with preselected registration points in the image data set. The degree of error in the registration process is conveyed to the surgeon. The accuracy requirements for each specific surgical procedure will dictate the degree of registration error that may be tolerated. Lumbosacral pedicle fixation, for example, will generally tolerate a registration error of 2.0 mm, whereas C1–2 transarticular screw fixation will generally not tolerate an error greater than 1.0 mm.

Although the navigational systems can illustrate the amount of registration error in millimeters incurred by the user, this figure represents only a relative indicator of accuracy. A more definitive accuracy verification step is performed immediately before beginning spinal navigation. This involves placing the wand or trackable instrument on several visible structures in the field. If the registration process has been properly performed, the computer cursor on the workstation screen will localize to the same selected points. If there is not a good correlation in this verification step, the registration process must be more carefully repeated.

Once the registration process is completed, the images are automatically reformatted and presented to the surgeon in multiple planes through any selected surface point. Typically, three different orthogonal planes oriented to the long axis of the wand are generated. As the axis of the wand changes with respect to the spinal column, the orientation of each plane will change. In most applications to spinal surgery, the three planes commonly displayed will represent a near-sagittal, a near-coronal, and a near-axial view. A cursor and a trajectory line with a diameter and width that can be adjusted in proportion to the selected screw diameter are presented on the workstation screen. These indicate the proposed location and trajectory path through the selected point in the operative field. The length of the trajectory line relative to the imaged spine is displayed in millimeters, providing for accurate screw length selection (*Fig. 5.3*).

The images can be manipulated intraoperatively to show corresponding spinal anatomy in multiple planes and at a range of depths. By adjusting the length of the trajectory line, a near-coronal reconstructed image corresponding to the end of the trajectory line can be generated. When the correct entry point and trajectory for a pedicle screw are selected, the near-coronal view will show a cursor lying within the boundaries of the pedicle on cross section at the selected trajectory depth. As the trajectory line is extended through the image set, the near-coronal plane will adjust accordingly to indicate the final position of a screw tip placed along that trajectory. Significant errors in sagittal angulation of the drill guide-wand assembly will place the cursor in either disc space adjacent to that pedicle. Errors in axial angulation of the drill guide-wand assembly or selected entry point in the

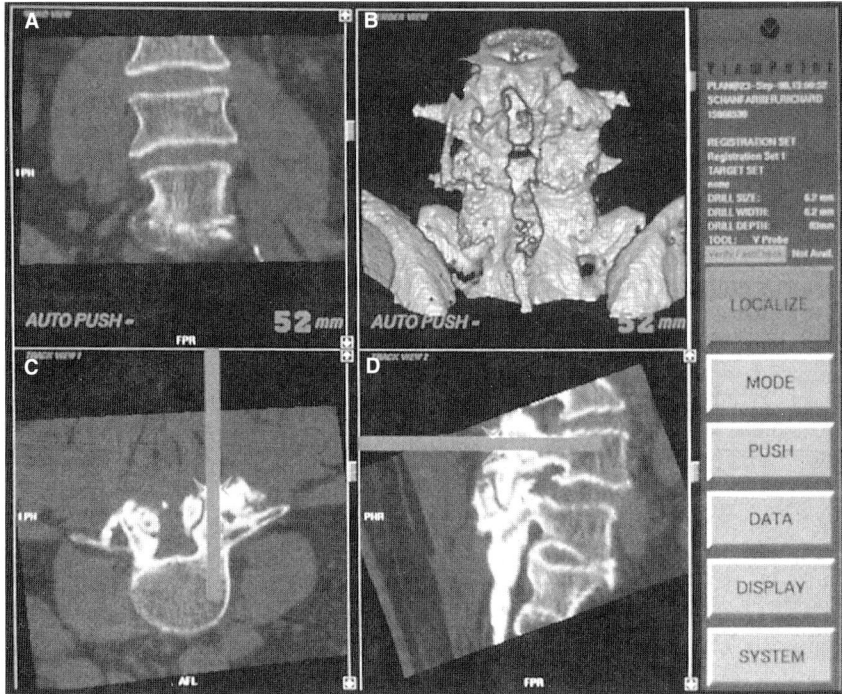

FIG. 5.3 Workstation screen demonstrating navigation through the right L4 pedicle in a patient who has previously undergone an L4–5 laminectomy with bilateral transverse process fusion. The depth of the trajectory line is 52 mm and measures the distance from the indicator on the trajectory line at the level of the fusion mass to the distal extent of the trajectory line. The cursor in the near-coronal view (A) indicates the distal endpoint of the trajectory line. The near-axial and near-sagittal views are shown in *panels* C and D, respectively. *Panel B* screen shows the surface rendered view of the lumbar spine with an incomplete fusion evident on the left side.

coronal plane will place the cursor outside the boundaries of the vertebral body or pedicle wall (*Fig. 5.4*).

CLINICAL APPLICATIONS

Image-guided spinal navigation was initially tested in the insertion of pedicle screws in the thoracic and lumbosacral spines of cadaver specimens. The accuracy of screw insertion was documented by plain-film radiography and thin-section CT imaging of the instrumented levels. All inserted pedicle screws was satisfactorily placed (11).

The clinical application of image-guided spinal navigation began in 1993 with its use in lumbosacral pedicle fixation (10). Other spinal applications gradually evolved, including cervical screw fixation, thoracic pedicle fixation, and anterior spinal decompression and fixation procedures. The application of image-guided navigation to spinal surgery is directed by the complexity of the procedure and, specifically, by the need to visualize the unexposed component of a spinal segment. Image-guided navigation can be used with or without standard intraoperative imaging techniques (e.g., fluoroscopy). In either case, image-guided navigation provides the surgeon with an improved orientation to the pertinent spinal anatomy, which subsequently facilitates the accuracy and effectiveness of the procedure.

Pedicle Fixation

Pedicle fixation has gained acceptance as an effective and reliable method of spinal stabilization (18). However, because of the variations

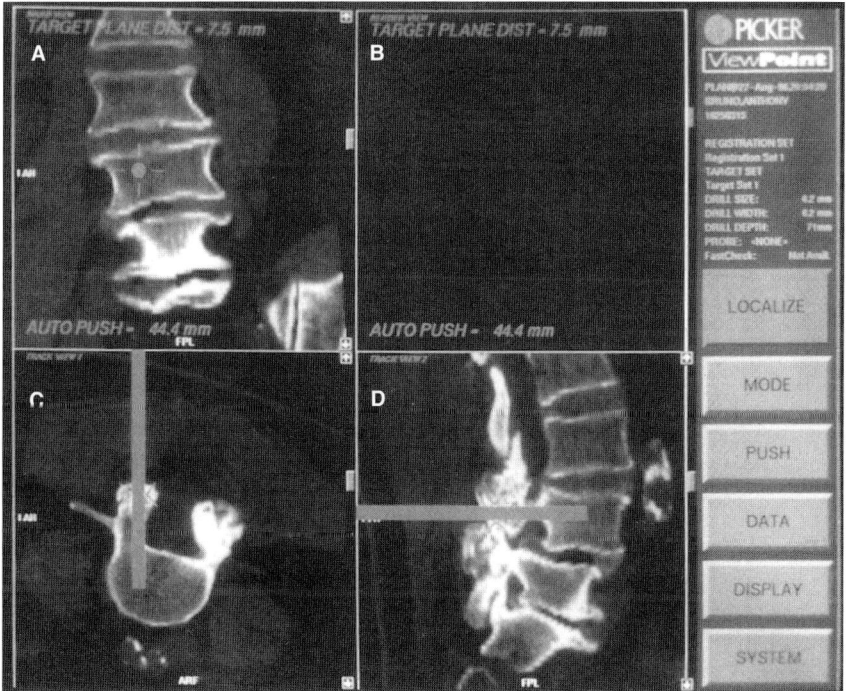

FIG. 5.4 Workstation screen indicating an error in positioning of the handheld wand. The near-axial view demonstrates that the trajectory selected through the L4 pedicle is too medial. A lateral fluoroscopic view would show only the sagittal trajectory seen in *Panels C* and *D* and could result in incorrect screw placement. Movement of the wand medially would result in a redirection of the trajectory line into a more appropriate position.

of pedicle anatomy within each patient, the safe and precise placement of pedicle screws can be difficult to achieve. Suboptimal screw placement can result in varying incidences of neural injury and fixation failure. These complications can be minimized if the surgeon is provided with a greater degree of spatial orientation to each pedicle to be instrumented before screw insertion.

During screw insertion, the pedicle is generally not visualized by the surgeon. Instead, posterior bony landmarks (transverse process, facet joint) are used to approximate the location of each pedicle. The diameter and axial angulation of each pedicle can be estimated from an analysis of radiographic studies and from a general understanding of the orientation of pedicles at each spinal level. Intraoperative imaging can then be used to help confirm screw positioning.

Two methods of intraoperative imaging are used to obtain anatomic orientation before pedicle screw placement. C-arm fluoroscopy provides real-time imaging of the pertinent spinal anatomy. However, the fluoroscopic views generated represent only two-dimensional images of a complex three-dimensional structure and can be easily misinterpreted. With manipulation of the fluoroscopic unit, the three dimensions can be visualized in a series of images, but these maneuvers can be cumbersome and time-consuming. Other disadvantages include the radiation exposure and the need to wear lead aprons during the procedure.

The second method of obtaining anatomic orientation in the spine is serial, intraoperative radiography. Before screw insertion, metal pins are positioned in each pedicle and a lateral radiograph is obtained to confirm the pins' relationship to the surrounding spinal column structures. If the position of the pins is not satisfactory, their trajectory is readjusted and a second radiograph is obtained. Once the pins are satisfactorily positioned, they are removed, and the pedicle screws are inserted along the same trajectory. This technique can be time-consuming and misleading in that only lateral radiographs are obtained. Oblique and anteroposterior views are difficult to acquire, and without these views, screws may be improperly positioned. Furthermore, the screw trajectory can change when the pins are removed and the screws are inserted unless a cannulated screw system is used.

Although both of these intraoperative imaging techniques provide the surgeon with information regarding the parameters of pedicle screw insertion, neither technique demonstrates the relationship of a proposed screw trajectory to an axial image of the spine. It is this view provided by image-guided navigation that makes it superior to the two standard methods of intraoperative imaging.

Preoperatively, a CT scan through the appropriate spinal segments is obtained. The images consist of a three-dimensional volume data set of contiguous axial CT images. Alternatively, magnetic resonance imaging data may also be used. The image data are then transferred to the computer workstation via optical disk or a high-speed data link (e.g., Ethernet). Three to five reference points for each spinal segment to be instrumented are selected and stored in the image data set.

Intraoperatively, a standard exposure of the spinal levels to be instrumented is performed. A lateral radiograph is obtained to confirm the appropriate level. The computer workstation and camera localizer are then positioned. The infrared camera detector is mounted at the foot of the table and aimed rostrally for thoracic and lumbosacral procedures. The camera is positioned at the head of the table and aimed caudally for cervical procedures.

The reference points previously selected for each spinal level are identified in the operative field and registered. The registration error is calculated by the system and displayed. If the computed error is significant (i.e., greater than 2.0 mm), the registration process is more carefully repeated. When a satisfactory registration error has been obtained, the accuracy verification step is performed immediately before proceeding with navigation.

Following registration, standard bony landmarks for pedicle localization are used to approximate the screw entry point. A drill guide is placed on this entry point and the wand is passed through the guide. The wand is activated and the multiplanar CT images through the localized point are generated. The near-axial and near-sagittal views can be manipulated via mouse or foot pedal control to show the "extension" of the wand through the selected entry point. This involves a lengthening of the trajectory line through each of the two views. The near-coronal view will adjust accordingly to show a cursor in the CT image set at the distal extent of the trajectory line.

The orientation of each pedicle to be instrumented can be assessed rapidly and accurately. Image manipulation occurs in near real time with the location of the trajectory line and screen cursor changing as the surgeon moves the wand through the surgical field. Any errors in trajectory or entry point selection can be determined and corrected by adjusting the position of the wand–drill guide assembly.

When a satisfactory screw entry point and trajectory has been selected, the wand is removed and a drill (3.2-mm diameter) is positioned through the guide. The drill guide preserves the navigational information when the wand is removed. A pilot hole is drilled through the pedicle into the vertebral body. A pedicle sound instrument is placed in the hole to confirm satisfactory hole placement. The hole is tapped, and the appropriate length screw is inserted. The process is repeated for each pedicle to be instrumented. C-arm fluoroscopy or serial radiographs are not required.

When screws are placed at a second spinal level, a new set of registration points are selected at that level. This method, termed *segmental registration,* eliminates any discrepancy in anatomic orientation that may be related to a change in patient position between the preoperative CT scan and surgery. The spatial relationship of anatomic points at a single vertebral level is not affected by changes in body position.

In addition to screw placement in the large pedicles of the lumbosacral spine, image-guided navigation can also facilitate screw placement into the smaller pedicles of the thoracic spine (*Fig. 5.5*). This fixation option is attractive when extending lumbar fixation rostrally

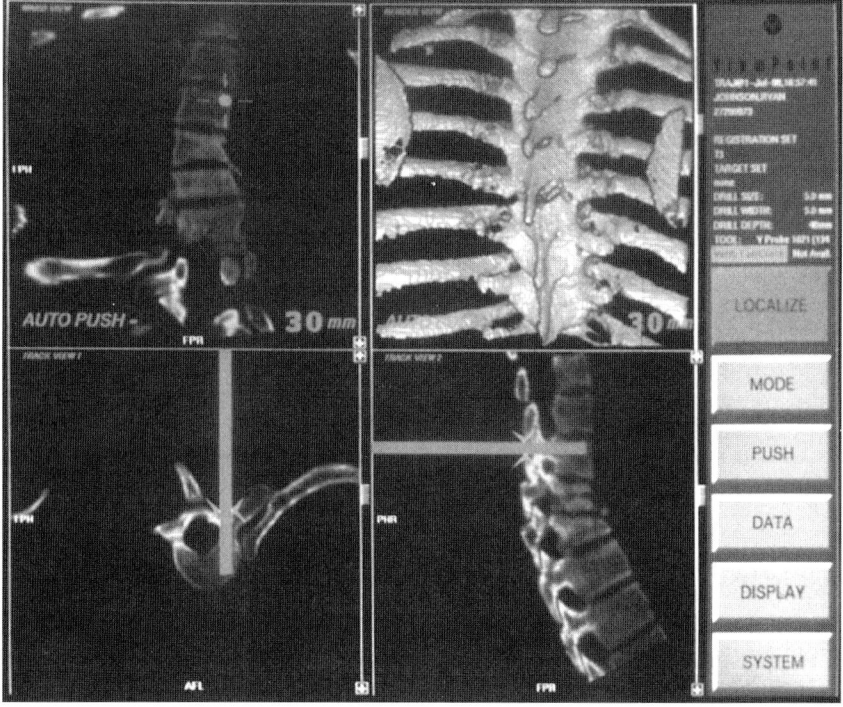

FIG. 5.5 Workstation screen demonstrating the selected trajectory for a T3 pedicle screw in a patient with a T4–5 wedge compression fracture. The width of the trajectory can be adjusted to correspond to the diameter of the pedicle screw. In this case, the width is set at 5.0 mm.

across the thoracolumbar junction or cervical fixation caudally across the cervicothoracic junction.

Posterior C1-2 Transarticular Screw Fixation

The placement of screws across the C1–2 facet joints has gained acceptance as a reliable method of supplementing a standard wire and bone graft fixation of the atlanto–axial complex. By providing rigid internal fixation, the transarticular screws reduce or eliminate the postoperative need for halo brace immobilization.

The procedure involves inserting a 3.5-mm or 4.0-mm-diameter screw into the C2 articular pillar and directing it rostrally and ventrally, through the pars interarticularis of C2, across the C1–2 facet joint, and into the lateral mass of C1. The procedure is usually performed bilaterally in conjunction with a C1–2 wire or cable and bone fixation.

The risks of inserting a screw into this region of the cervical spine include: 1) injury to the vertebral artery if the screw trajectory is too lateral or ventral, 2) injury to the spinal cord if the screw trajectory is too medial, and 3) failure to engage the lateral mass of C1 if the screw trajectory is too ventral. The insertion of a screw on either side may be contraindicated if the transverse foramina of C2 is in an abnormally posterior and medial position (e.g., narrow pars interarticularis of C2).

The selection of the appropriate screw entry site and trajectory requires a thorough understanding of the atlanto–axial anatomy. Although fluoroscopic guidance can be helpful, it may not consistently offer the millimetric precision necessary for this technique.

The technique for applying image-guided navigation to posterior C1–2 screw fixation involves obtaining a preoperative CT scan that extends from the lower occipital region to C3. The image data are then transferred to the computer workstation and can be used to create a preoperative screw trajectory plan. A proposed entry point and target can be selected at the C2 and C1 levels, respectively. These two points are then connected by a trajectory line with a width proportional to a 4.0-mm-diameter screw. The image data set can then be manipulated in multiple planes to demonstrate the position of a screw placed through the C2 pars interarticularis and its relationship to the corresponding transverse foramina. This information can be used preoperatively to determine the feasibility of safe screw placement. It allows the surgeon to plan for an alternative approach if the proposed screw trajectories intersect the path of the vertebral artery.

At the time of surgery, positioning of the patient and exposure of the posterior C1–2 complex is performed. A wire (cable) and bone graft stabilization procedure at the C1–2 level is performed before navigation and screw insertion. This helps minimize any independent motion between C1 and C2 during navigation. Three to five registration points are then selected from the image data at the C2 level. These points typically include the lateral margins of the C2–3 facet joints and the spinous process of C2. It is not necessary to register at the C1 level.

Although the technique involves the passage of a screw across two spinal segments, the primary difficulty of the procedure is the safe positioning of the screw within the narrow C2 pars interarticularis. The proximity of the vertebral artery to a transarticular screw is closest at the level of the narrow pars interarticularis of C2. The target (the lateral mass of C1) is relatively large and easily accessed provided the screw has been accurately passed through the appropriate C2 anatomy. Consequently, the procedure is more of an intrasegmental, rather than intersegmental, technique. The specific role of image-guided navigation is to facilitate safe screw placement across C2. Although the relative position of C1 and C2 in both the preoperative image set and the surgical field is important, it is not critical enough to interfere with the process of image-guided navigation.

If there is a minor discrepancy in the position of C1 and C2, it is typically related to translation in the sagittal plane. This discrepancy will only affect the position of the screw tip in the lateral mass of C1. If there is an anterior translation of C1 intraoperatively (compared with the preoperative images), the screw tip will be located more posteriorly in the lateral mass. If the translation of C1 is more posterior, the screw tip will have a more anterior location in the lateral mass. In either case, the screw tip will reach the lateral mass of C1, provided that accurate navigation through C2 has been achieved.

Following exposure and arthrodesis of the posterior C1–2 complex, two separate stab incisions are made on either side of the midline at the C7–T1 level. A drill guide is placed through one of the stab incisions, passed through the paravertebral musculature, and brought out into the operative field. The registration points are selected and the wand is then passed through the drill guide so that its tip lies close to the proposed screw entry points. Intraoperative navigation and orientation of the C1–2 complex is performed, and the precise screw entry point and trajectory are confirmed (*Fig. 5.6*). The length of screws required will also be displayed by the system. The wand is then removed from the drill guide and a drill is inserted. A hole is drilled along the selected trajectory, tapped, and the appropriate length screw is inserted. The same procedure is performed on the opposite side.

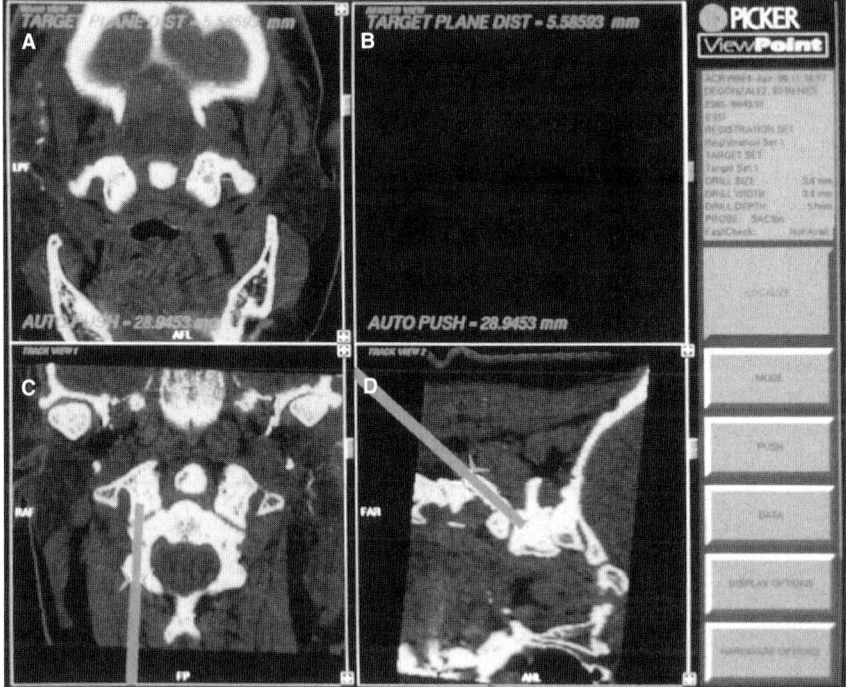

FIG. 5.6 Workstation screen demonstrating a trajectory for insertion of a C1–2 transarticular screw. *Panel D* shows the trajectory in the sagittal plane. *Panel C* represents an orthogonal plane lying between the true axial and true coronal planes. It demonstrates the medial–lateral direction of the selected trajectory. *Panel A* represents a plane that is perpendicular to the two other images. It demonstrates the location of the screw tip inserted along the selected trajectory at the indicated depth.

Cervical Lateral Mass Plate Fixation

Lateral mass plate fixation involves the insertion of screws into the lateral articular pillars of the cervical spine. The screws are directed rostrally and laterally to avoid injury to the exiting nerve root and the vertebral artery. Image-guided spinal navigation can be applied to this procedure to help identify the optimal entry point and trajectory for each screw.

After segmental registration, an approximate entry point over a lateral mass is selected. The optimal entry point and the trajectory in the sagittal and axial planes can then be obtained during the navigational process. When the C2 or C7 levels are included in the lateral mass plate construct, it may be difficult to pass a screw into the lateral masses because of the obliquity or absence of a suitable lateral mass at these two levels. At these levels, screws can be directed medially into the pars interarticularis of C2 or into the pedicle of C7.

Application to Anterior Thoracolumbar Surgery

Image-guided spinal navigation can be applied to anterior thoracolumbar surgery to monitor the orientation and extent of decompression and to facilitate the precise placement of fixation screws. Although the selection of reference points for anterior spinal surgery is limited by the relative lack of prominent bony landmarks on the anterior aspect of the spinal column, the degree of accuracy required is less than that needed for most posterior screw fixation procedures.

Potential registration points for the use of image-guided navigation in anterior thoracolumbar surgery include selected landmarks on the vertebral endplates, pedicles, head of the rib, and prominent ventral osteophytes. Registration errors of 3.0 mm or less are usually sufficient to obtain clinically relevant accuracy with image-guided navigation in most anterior thoracolumbar procedures. The verification step can further confirm the degree of registration accuracy achieved before proceeding.

Image-guided navigation can be used to monitor the extent of decompression during a thoracolumbar corpectomy (*Fig. 5.7*). The surgeon can verify the position of the epidural space as well as the contralateral margin of the spinal column (*Fig. 5.7*). After decompression, the system can be used to guide anterior fixation screws across the vertebrae adjacent to the corpectomy site.

Application to Spinal Neoplasms

Neoplasms involving the spinal column can produce varying degrees of spinal instability and/or neural compression. The surgical management of these lesions involves tumor excision and, frequently, spinal reconstruction. However, with larger neoplasms, the distant margins may be difficult to determine, and blind decompression may put adjacent neural and other soft tissue structures at risk. Image-guided navigation can be used to monitor the extent of tumor decompression and to identify the nonvisualized distant margins.

The procedure is similar to that of other applications of image-guided spinal navigation. Discrete bony landmarks on the exposed spinal column at the level of the neoplasm are selected and registered. As tumor removal proceeds, the wand can be placed within the cavity of the tumor or its exposed margin. The actual extent of tumor removal can be determined by noting the position of the wand tip relative to the non-

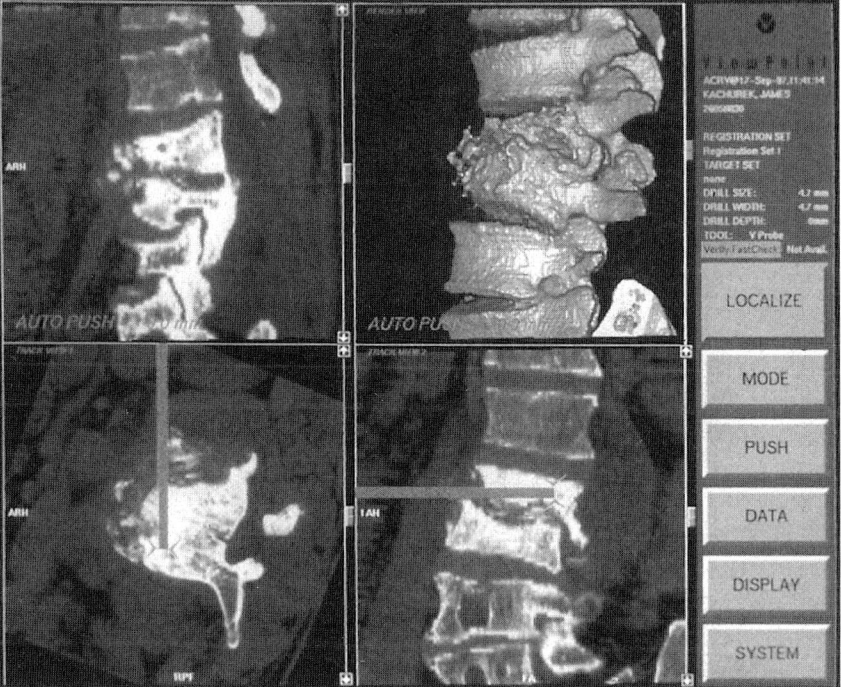

Fig. 5.7 Workstation screen demonstrating the use of image-guided spinal navigation during an L2–3 corpectomy for osteomyelitis. At various stages of the corpectomy, the wand can be placed into the partially decompressed site to orient the surgeon to the contralateral side of the spinal column as well as to the epidural space. The system can then be used to precisely direct anterior fixation screws into the adjacent L1 and L4 vertebrae.

visualized tumor margins on the workstation screen (*Fig. 5.8*). After tumor removal, image-guided navigation can facilitate any necessary screw fixation procedure for spinal stabilization.

CONCLUSION

Interactive frameless stereotactic technology has been successfully applied to spinal surgery. By linking digitized image data to spinal surface anatomy, image-guided spinal navigation facilitates the surgeon's orientation to unexposed spinal structures improving the precision and accruacy of the surgery. It is typically used to optimize the placement of spinal fixation screws and to monitor the extent of complex decompression procedures. It can also be used as a preoperative planning tool.

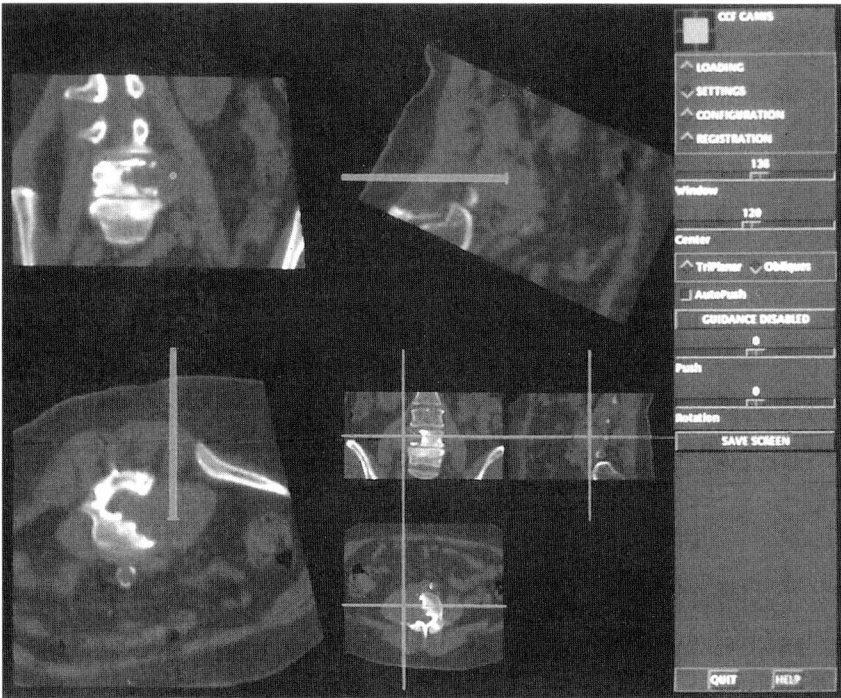

FIG. 5.8 Workstation screen during removal of an L4 neurofibroma. Following partial removal of the neoplasm, the wand is placed into the tumor bed. The relative location of the tumor's anterior and lateral margins can be readily determined.

Although image-guided spinal navigation is a versatile and effective technology, it is not a replacement for the surgeon having a thorough knowledge of the pertinent spinal anatomy as well as correct surgical techniques. It merely serves as an additional source of information used by the surgeon to make selected intraoperative decisions. In this way, it is similar to more conventional intraoperative imaging techniques (e.g., fluoroscopy), except that it provides a much greater degree of information to the surgeon.

Despite the advantages of image guidance, the surgeon must ultimately assess the information provided by this system and determine if it correlates with his or her estimation of the unexposed anatomy and the proposed surgical plan. If there is a good correlation between the two, the surgical step can be performed. However, if a correlation is not present, the surgeon must reassess both the spinal anatomy and the image-guided registration accuracy before proceeding.

Ideally, the clinical application of this technology to spinal surgery should facilitate a reduction in operative time, morbidity, and costs. It should be capable of minimizing or eliminating the need for conventional intraoperative imaging. It should be fast, easy to use, reliable, and capable of being used briefly to provide accurate intraoperative information while minimizing any disruption to the standard routine of each surgical procedure. Ultimately, beyond each individual surgical application, image-guided navigation technology must be clinically versatile. It is the routine use of this technology by multiple surgical specialties that will drive its continued evolution and development as well as establish it as a cost-effective surgical tool.

REFERENCES

1. Barnett GH, Kormos DW, Steiner CP, Weisenberger J: Intraoperative localization using an armless, frameless stereotactic wand: Technical note. **J Neurosurg** 78: 510–514, 1993.
2. Barnett GH, Kormos DW, Steiner CP, Weisenberger J: Use of a frameless, armless stereotactic wand for brain tumor localization with two-dimensional and three-dimensional neuroimaging. **Neurosurgery** 33:674–678, 1993.
3. Brodwater BK, Roberts DW, Nakajima T, Friets EM, Strohbehn JW: Extracranial application of the frameless stereotactic operating microscope: Experience with lumbar spine. **Neurosurgery** 32:209–213, 1993.
4. Bryant JT, Reid JG, Smith BL, Stevenson JM: A method of determining vertebral body positions in the sagittal plane using skin markers. **Spine** 14:258–265, 1989.
5. Bucholz RD, Heilbrun MP, McDurmont L: Use of an intraoperative optical digitizer in a system for free-hand stereotactic surgery. Presented at the 60th Annual Meeting of the American Association of Neurological Surgeons, San Francisco, CA, April 11–16, 1992.
6. Dohrmann GJ, Rubin JM: Intraoperative ultrasonic imaging of the spinal cord: Syringomyelia, cysts, and tumors—A preliminary report. **Surg Neurol** 18:395–399, 1982.
7. George DC, Krag MH, Johnson CC, Van Hal ME, Haugh LD, Grobler LJ: Hole preparation technique for transpedicle screws: Effect on pull-out strength from human cadaveric vertebrae. **Spine** 16:181–184, 1991.
8. Gertzbein SD, Robbins SE: Accuracy of pedicle screw placement in vivo. **Spine** 15:11–14, 1990.
9. Guthrie BL, Adler JR: Computer assisted pre-operative planning, interactive surgery and frameless stereotaxy. **Clin Neurosurg** 38:112–131, 1992
10. Kalfas IH, Kormos DW, Murphy MA, McKenzie RL, Barnett GH, Bell GR, Steiner CP, Trimble MB, Weisenberger JP: Application of frameless stereotaxy to pedicle screw fixation of the spine. **J Neurosurg** 83:641–647, 1995.
11. Murphy MA, McKenzie RL, Kormos DW, Kalfas IH: Frameless stereotaxis for the insertion of lumbar pedicle screws. **J Clin Neurosc** 1:257–260, 1994.
12. Reinhardt HF, Horstmann GA, Gratzl O: Sonic stereometry in microsurgical procedures for deep-seated brain tumors and vascular malformations. **Neurosurgery** 32:1–57, 1993.
13. Roberts DW, Strohbehn JW, Hatch JF, Murray W, Kettenberger H: A frameless

stereotaxic integration of computerized tomographic imaging and the operating microscope. **J Neurosurg** 65:545–549, 1986.
14. Steinmann JC, Herkowitz HO, El-Kommos H, Wesolowski DP: Spinal pedicle fixation: Confirmation of an image-based technique for screw placement **Spine** 18:1856–1861, 1993.
15. Tan KK, Grzeeszczuk R, Levin DN, Pelizzari CA, Chen GT, Erickson RK, Johnson D, Dohrmann GJ: A frameless stereotactic approach to neurosurgical planning based on retrospective patient-image registration: Technical note. **J Neurosurg** 79:296–303, 1993.
16. Watanabe E, Mayanagi Y, Kosugi Y, Manaka S, Takakura K: Open surgery assisted by the neuronavigator, a stereotactic articulated sensitive arm. **Neurosurgery** 28:792–800, 1991.
17. Weinstein JN, Spratt KF, Spengler D, Brick C, Reid S: Spinal pedicle fixation: Reliability and validity of roentgenogram-based assessment and surgical factors on successful screw placement. **Spine** 13:1012–1018, 1988.
18. Wiltse LL: History of pedicle screw fixation of the spine. **Spine** 6:1–10, 1992.
19. Zamorano L, Kadi AM, Dong A: Computer-assisted neurosurgery: Stimulation and automation. **Stereotact Funct Neurosurg** 59:115–122, 1992.

CHAPTER

6

The Future of Image-guided Surgery

M. PETER HEILBRUN, M.D.,
JEFFREY D. MCDONALD, M.D., PH.D.

As we approach the millennium and the end of this Decade of the Brain, the transition from frame-based stereotactic surgery to the broad world of surgical image guidance is clearly impressive. The advancements in this field have paralleled the explosion in computer and information technology that now impact every moment of our daily lives. Although we may yearn for times past, our daily lives, including the practice of neurosurgery, proceed at a rapid pace. Whether or not we embrace Moore's law, which links computer power to decreasing cost, the result stimulates us as neurosurgeons to pursue new challenges, opportunities, and horizons.

The objective of future modes of image guidance is to achieve improved neurosurgical capabilities in disease diagnosis, management, and outcome. This objective can be met if neurosurgeons bring into their daily practice the improved precision and safety that comes with well designed image guidance surgical systems. There are at least five evolving areas of image-guided surgery that will improve the safety, the precision, and the ease of use of these technologies: 1) methods of compensating for shift of intracranial structures after brain exposure, 2) the use of active robots as surgical assistants; 3) the use of coregistration of functional images to anatomic stereotactic templates to enhance resection, 4) the use of reprogramable stimulation techniques as a substrate for ablative lesioning methods in the management of movement disorders, and 5) the ability to shape radiation beams for both radiosurgery and fractionated radiation therapy.

BACKGROUND

Before looking at the future, a review of some of the pioneering steps and events that were taken in the mid 1980s and early 1990s to couple computed tomographic (CT) and magnetic resonance imaging (MRI) advancements to concepts of navigation in physical space is necessary. Substituting industrial grade three-dimensional digitizers and robots for stereotactic frames led to more flexible target access within the human body, particularly the nervous system. Neurosurgeons involved with the evolution of image guidance associating with radiation oncologists and physicists in the development of radiosurgery led to experimentation with digitizers and robots. These colleagues introduced us to the robotic techniques inherent in the design of linear accelerators to deliver precision radiation to the human body.

Although our radiation colleagues have their own heroes, as neurosurgeons we must look to Lars Leksell, who, in his broad range of stereotactic experiments in the 1960s, adapted a linear accelerator to his stereotactic frame (16, 17). This initial experiment by Leksell resulted in the design and construction of the first gamma knife. My own personal heroes in this field are my colleagues Ted Roberts, Russell Brown, and Trent Wells, who in the mid 1970s designed a new stereotactic frame compatible with the recently introduced CT scanner technology (6). Trent Wells is an engineer and World War II pilot who introduced many stereotactic neurosurgeons to his concepts of navigation and instrument design, concepts that are the foundation of the transition from frame-based to frameless image guidance.

The younger pioneers of the 1980s include Patrick Kelly, who developed a wide range of new techniques to take us from image-guided point biopsy to tumor volumetric resection and robotics; Dade Lunsford, who introduced gamma knife technology from Sweden to the rest of the world and the use of a dedicated CT scanner to the operating room for real-time stereotactic imaging; and Ken Winston, who adapted the Brown-Roberts-Wells stereotactic system so that cost-effective linac radiosurgery could become a mainstream part of neurosurgical disease management. Bill Friedman designed a new linac hardware and radiation planning hardware and software that would improve the accuracy and ease of use of the linac as a neurosurgical tool. (9, 12, 13, 20, 21, 29). However, two important neurosurgeons in establishing the foundation for the transition to frameless stereotaxy were David Roberts, who designed the first operating microscope that could be used as a surgical navigation tool by coupling a standard Zeiss Contraves microscope to a sonic three-dimensional digitizer, and Eli Watanabe, who coupled a linked industrial digitizer to software for image guidance (24, 25, 28). With these advancements in the late 1980s, the step from bench-top and operating room experiments required that neurosurgery's commercial partners recognize that these technologies would be attractive to the neurosurgical mind. At the 1990 fall CNS meeting, ISG Technologies, a Toronto company, introduced the Allegra passively linked arm as a frameless surgical guidance tool. At the 1991 spring

American Association of Neurological Surgeons (AANS) meeting, a group of neurosurgeons met with the vendors interested in these frameless systems and discussed whether this technology was ready for widespread use by the neurosurgical community. That summer, a small group of interested neurosurgeons, radiation oncologists, physicists, and imaging and stereotactic industry representatives surveyed the field. Phil Gildenberg summarized that meeting well with this statement that "The future is now. We must now build a bridge to bring the elegant imaging of the radiologist to the advanced navigation technology of the operating room." At the 1992 Congress of Neurological Surgeons meeting, the first practical workshop was organized to introduce several frameless guidance systems to our colleagues.

In the fall of 1998, the catalog of rapidly exploding applications of this technology into all areas of neurosurgical practice is huge. Today, it is possible to move large image data sets across the internet to our offices and operating rooms. As a result, in the past 2 years there has been a rapid consolidation of the systems available from imaging and neurosurgical instrument companies, all of whom have had significant input from neurosurgeons. This consolidation has resulted in the introduction of easily managed image guidance systems in large numbers to academic and community neurosurgical practices throughout this country and other parts of the world. The applications, which were initially limited to the intracranial vault for point biopsy and then extended to volumetric resection, now encompass all aspects of intracranial surgery from skull base surgical applications for monitoring proximity to critical vascular and cranial nerve structures to functional neurosurgical procedures, including ablative lesions and stimulation systems for Parkinson's disease, stereotactic placement of depth electrodes and grids, and selective image-guided selective amygdala-hippocampectomy for epilepsy of mesial temporal origin, as well as transpial transections for extratemporal epilepsy and some eplieptic type of autism. Modalities for limiting radiation to normal brain tissue surrounding lesions include static and dynamic conformal beam shaping for both single fraction and fractionated focused radiation. An expansion from intracranial to spinal applications provide precision guidance of spine stabilization instrumentation and now focused spinal column radiation.

FUTURE APPLICATIONS

Brain Shift

Throughout the era of both frame-based and now frameless image guidance, critics of this technology have been concerned with the inaccuracies due to the linkage of retrospective preoperative image data sets with brain structures, which shift after the opening of the skull and dura. Kelly demonstrated that these shifts minimally impact guided surgery as long as one takes precautions in minimizing skull openings, controlling intracranial pressure, avoiding cerebrospinal fluid loss, and positioning the patient's head to the trajectory from entry into the head to the target is vertically oriented (11).

The clear solution to this potential accuracy problem is to perform surgical approaches using concurrent real-time imaging. Neurosurgeons have a long history of using this methodology with the combination of intraoperative x-ray, using air or other radioopaque contrast materials to indirectly identify brain shifts, and the position of instruments in relation to bony structures in the cranial vault and spine. Another indirect measure was the use of ultrasound to identify midline shifts. In the 1980s, several stereotactic systems were designed that could be used for biopsy procedures in the CT scanner. However, to take advantage of the capability of direct visualization of structures with MRI, several imaging companies have produced open MRI systems that allow real acquisition of MR images during surgery. To date, these open MRI systems are expensive and cumbersome, and it is only recently that a wide range of nonmagnetic surgical instruments have been developed to allow the surgeon reasonable selection of operating tools (5). In the future, multiuse open MRI systems will become a standard neurosurgical tool. At the same time, less costly portably CT scanners are being introduced into the operating and critical care environment, which could serve the purpose of real serial monitoring of brain shift. There is the concern of radiation exposure with this application. Two reasonable applications that have demonstrated usefulness are linking ultrasound data and fluoroscopic x-ray data to the patient physical space with LEDs attached to ultrasound probes and portable C-arm fluoroscopes. The ultrasound data set can be reformatted in the stereotactic planning computer and manipulated so that the ultrasound image is oriented in the same plane as both anatomic and navigation MRI and CT views. With these data overlaid onto a preoperative CT or MR image, the shift can be serially or continuously monitored. Adaptation of these techniques is presently under evaluation (7, 27).

Operating Room Robotics

Another theme for the future, which will evolve further, will be the transition from computer-assisted to computer-directed surgery by coupling the robots to image guidance systems. The first widely used computer-directed systems, which are in place today, are both floor and ceiling-mounted robots that serve as platforms for operating microscopes to be used as stereotactic navigational pointing devices. Standard industrial robots adapted to hold surgical instruments within the brain were designed and tested in the 1980s. However, in the last 2 years, a mechanical robot designed specifically to guide instruments accurately along in oblique trajectories into the head are being introduced commercially, which will have important applications, particularly for biopsy and placement of probes and electrodes during awake functional procedures. This use of robots can assist the neurosurgeon in participating functional testing (2, 3, 30) (*Figs. 6.1 and 6.2*).

Magnetic image guidance of objects from surfaces to the subcortical regions of the brain is being tested in several centers. This technology, like robotics, will improve the surgeon's capability for safe hands-free delivery of devices and other therapeutic modalities to specific brain regions (10).

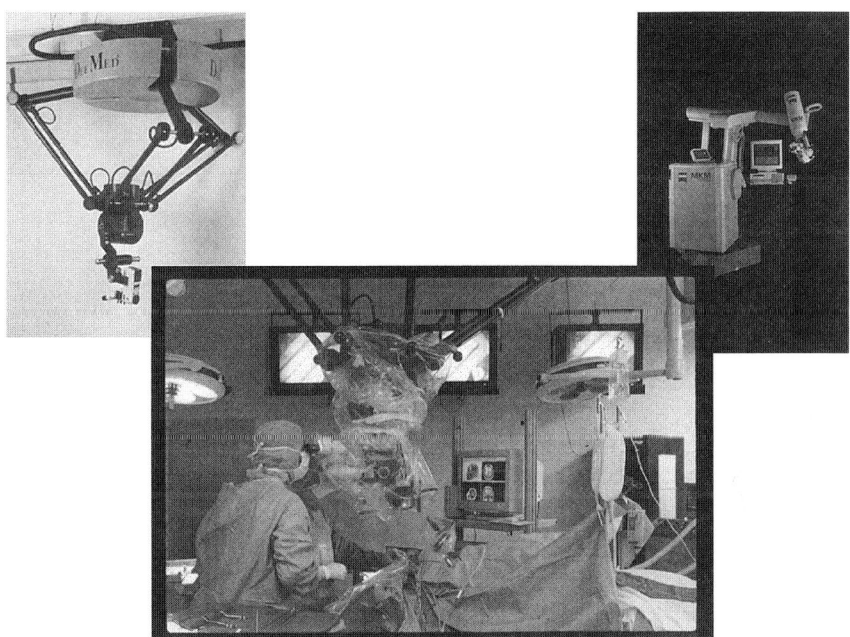

FIG. 6.1 Images of ceiling and floor stand-mounted robotic microscopes used for guidance with image of surgeon at place planning and resecting tumor seen in Figure 6.2.

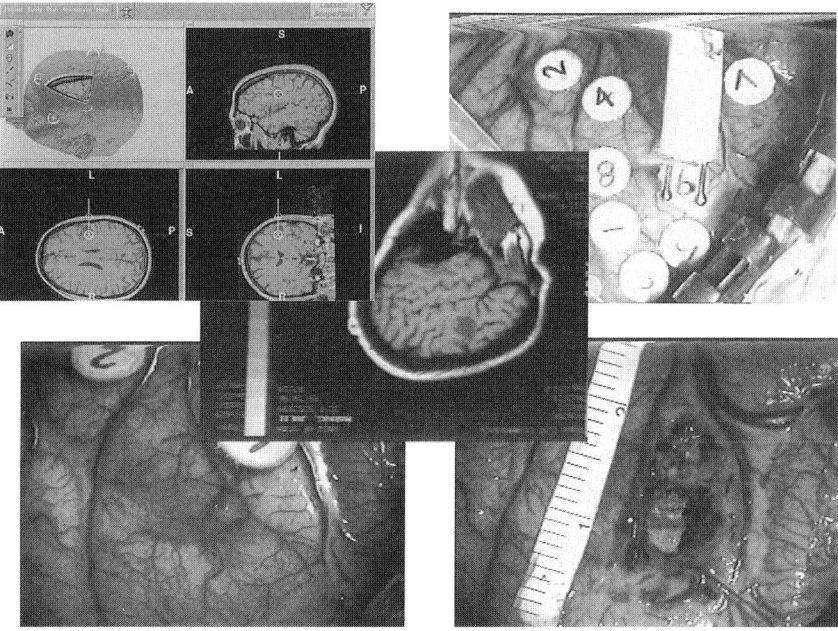

FIG. 6.2 Interactive image guidance demonstrating steps in awake, craniotomy, identification of subcortical tumor and cortical stimulation to identify facial and tongue motor function, and postresection view after microsurgical tumor resection.

Functional Imaging

The capability of obtaining functional data from the brain and the practical usefulness of such data in protecting normal brain and allowing safer, yet more complete lesion resections will occur as we develop the software for our surgical planning computers that will allow us to merge both anatomic and functional data sets within a single coordinate system, which can be easily linked to physical space. These systems will also be capable of storing individual data sets in massive databases for comparison of responses to both invasive and noninvasive provocative tests. Standard provocative tests that can be performed both preoperatively and intraoperatively during both awake and asleep craniotomies will allow us to identify sensory, motor, visual, auditory, and speech regions of the cortex. The sophisticated testing paradigms developed for positron emission tomography identification of both cortical and subcortical functional regions will be applied to the new technologies of functional MRI and magnetic source imaging (MSI). Functional MRI measures small regional changes in oxygen reduction states accompanying cortical activation and has the temporal resolution of analyzing epochs occurring in one- to several-second intervals MSI looks at activation and inactivation of neuronal signals in the millisecond range. Whereas the time course of MSI or magnetoencephalography (MEG) is similar to the measurement of neuronal electrical signals and electroencephalography (EEG), the artifact associated with volume conduction through the skull and scalp is eliminated. In addition, the combination of simultaneous MEG and EEG recordings with appropriate analysis has the potential of improving source analysis of the three-dimensional position of these signals.

MEG systems are presently in place in several institutions that have 120 sensors. Presently several centers are installing MEG machines with over 300 sensors. At this time, we can only imagine the possibilities of understanding brain function when we have the capability of measuring simultaneous millisecond epochs in over 300 cortical regions. Presently, most MSI is based on spherical models of the skull. However, with the ability to cross-register MEG sensor location to magnetic resonance anatomic surface templates of the brain, and with the decreasing cost of supercomputers, magnetic signal localization will be modeled more realistically. It is often asked why EEG, which is less expensive, cannot be used for these measurements. As stated, there are many constraints in measuring over 300 EEG signals, including the time and discomfort involved in attaching more than 20 disc or needle electrodes to the scalp. I would predict that the combination of looking at 1- to 2-second redox epochs in voxel volumes with functional MRI and millisecond MEG/MSI magnetic epochs in over 300 cortical regions will result in a new era of analysis of brain function. With MRI technology, we also have the capability of analyzing chemical events in the brain with standard spectroscopy. Spectroscopic data can now be mapped directly to anatomic MR images in relatively small regional clusters of voxels.

Another newly introduced MRI technology is diffusion scanning. This method of MR scanning allows identification of subcortical white matter tracks. Depending of their vertical or horizontal orientation, the relationship of these tracts with identifiable cortical functional areas such as speech, cortical sensory, and motor function can be assessed. These images can determine the integrity of myelin-containing fiber tracts. Thus, lesions such as tumors or cortical dysplasia that can cause disruption of myelin tracts can be identified with diffusion imaging (18, 23). This information, combined with analysis of cortical function, adds another level of sophistication to functional imaging. The continued confirmation of the validity of noninvasive functional imaging with direct cortical and subcortical electrical stimulation in both awake and asleep craniotomies will impact the necessity of awake craniotomies.

At the University of Utah, a neurosurgeon has access to a spectrum of functional imaging tools including high resolution single-photon emission computed tomography, functional MRI, MSI/MEG, MR diffusion, and MR spectroscopy. At this time, the majority of these data sets can be mapped stereotactically to an anatomically correct MRI or CT scan (22). In addition, these anatomic MRI templates can be configured in a range of sequences and slice thickness to accentuate tissue with varying concentrations of fat and water. With this wide range of anatomic and functional data sets, it becomes clear that we must initiate a process to determine which data sets are most useful for a suspected clinical diagnosis. Every sequence cannot be performed on every patient. For example, different sets of sequences may be necessary for problems such as hydrocephalus, epilepsy, ischemic strokes, tumors, and neurodegenerative disorders. To register accurately the functional sets of data to anatomically correct MRI/CT data also requires establishing common reference points, both deep in the brain and on the surfaces of the brain, on the skull, and on the head, including the face. For many linkages, identification of the anteroposterior commissures as well as midline points allows for accurate cross-registration of data sets and for correcting potential yaw, roll, and pitch deviations from standard axial, coronal, sagittal views along fixed anteroposterior and vertical planes. Eventually, anatomically correct matching of face, forehead, and ear surface features will accomplish accurate automatic cross-registration of data sets. The use of this stereotactic combination of functional image data sets with anatomic MRI/CT data sets is demonstrated in a patient with recurrent tumor located adjacent to functional cortex and white matter tracts.

CASE REPORT

Patient AW A 42-year-old right-handed woman had two prior craniotomies in 1982 and 1990 for resection of a right frontal oligo-astrocytoma located anterior to primary motor cortex. She underwent external beam radiation therapy, and multiple cycles of PCV chemotherapy were completed in 1992. In 1998, an MRI scan documented progression once again of her residual/recurrent tumor. The patient underwent preoperative noninvasive functional analysis by functional MRI and MSI, and the data were imported into the frameless stereotactic workstation before surgery. This allowed direct correlation with functional points mapped during surgery by cortical stimulation. This analysis confirmed highly concordant localization of function across testing modalities. The mapping data, combined with standard use of the stereotactic surgical anatomic information, facilitated a near-total resection of the lesion. A transient postoperative supplemental motor area deficit producing moderate contralateral arm and leg weakness resolved by 4 weeks postoperatively.

This case demonstrates that with the distortion of exquisite brain structures, particularly in the setting of recurrent tumor in which there can be a mixture of tumor glial and functional brain regions, it is appropriate to use a spectrum of functional tools including functional MRI, MSI, and diffusion imaging to identify on images functional brain regions related to sensation, motor function, and speech. In this case, both functional MRI and MSI were concordant with cortical stimulation in mapping wrist and hand function. However, leg motor function, which was identified with MSI and not with functional MRI, was confirmed with cortical stimulation of convexity cortex just adajcent to the midline. Deep white matter tracts, noted to be displaced posteriorly by the tumor mass on diffusion imaging, were identified by direct electrical stimulation of the descending internal capsule motor tracts. The limit of resection posteriorly was decided by the confirmation of the hand and leg motor areas by combining awake craniotomy and safe cortical stimulation levels, which were monitored with EEG after discharge (*Fig. 6.3*).

This patient, like many with slowly progressive oligodendrogliomas, can have a significant prolongation of survival coupled with satisfactory life quality if aggressive resections are guided by precision mapping of cortical and white matter tract function. The use of these techniques as an adjunct to anatomic image-guided resection will allow neurosurgeons to maximize the potential reduction of tumor burden in lengthening and improving the quality of survival time in patients with progressive disease. As we gain more experience with these techniques and confirm their accuracy and reliability, we will be able to discard in many instances awake craniotomy and cortical stimulation. At the present time, we are analyzing predominantly those cortical functions of which we have some understanding. Through the development of new neuropsychometric paradigms for testing associative cortical functions and using diffusion scans to identify connecting white matter tracts, the optimization and safety of intracranial resection will continue to improve.

Stimulation for Functional Disorders

With the recent resurgence of ablative pallidal and thalamic lesions for the surgical management of Parkinson's disease, new information about the impact of ablation and stimulation of excitatory and inhibitory circuits in the brain in the presence of patients receiving re-

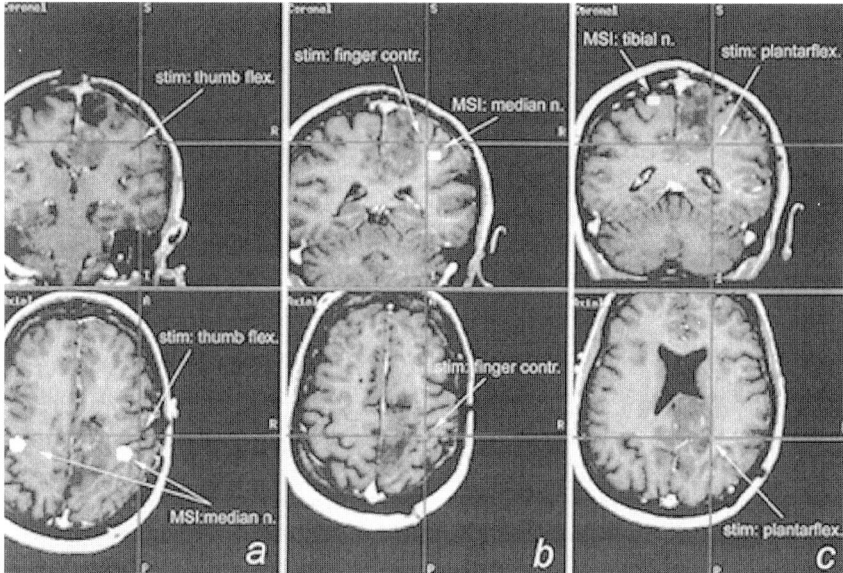

Fig. 6.3 Interactive image guidance using a combination of functional MRI, MSI, MR diffusion imaging, and cortical stimulation to resect recurrent tumor adjacent to eloquent cortex and white matter tracks. Images demonstrate correlation of MSI and cortical stimulation for finger and foot function.

placement medication to normalize brain dopamine levels is available (19, 26). This ablative lesion in the pallidum, in part, can modify the adverse effects of levodopa administration. The ablative lesion in the pallidum releases the inhibition of the pallidum and subthalamic nucleus and improves spontaneous activation of thalamocortical circuits. Appropriately placed thalamic and pallidal lesions also reduce tremor by eliminating the increased activation and synchronization of uninhibited thalamocortical circuits. Benebid's group has demonstrated that chronic thalamic stimulation improves tremor more effectively than thalamotomy in a high percentage of patients (4). The most disabling condition for the Parkinson's patient is the complex of gait impairments with freezing, festination, and falling. Gait problems are not significantly improved with pallidotomy. Benebid has also reported that bilateral chronic stimulation of the subthalamic nuclei at a rate to inhibit outflow to the pallidum and thalamocortical circuits does improve gait problems (14). Ablative lesions are permanent, whereas temporary lesions with stimulation systems allow the assessment of a range of stimulation parameters that can both inhibit and activate brain structures.

Conformal Radiation Delivery

Delivery of a lethal dose of radiation to lesions in the brain either as a single or fractionated doses requires dose design that kills the abnormal tissue while protecting surrounding normal tissue. The use of multiple isocenters to a lesion has been the best means to date of delivering high radiation doses to irregularly shaped lesions. However, the use of multiple isocenters results in the delivery of a heterogeneous dose to the lesion. This could result in "cold areas" that do not receive enough radiation to be effective. Demonstration of the feasibility of attaching a mechanical multivane collimator to a linear accelerator with the capability of shaping the radiation beam based on its changing "view" of the lesion has been demonstrated experimentally to provide for a more homogeneous dose while protecting surrounding tissue (8, 15). Multileaf collimators adjusted through computer servomotor control have been used for radiation delivery to extracranial lesions. Commercially available mini-multileaf collimators for standard linear accelerators, coupled with sophisticated computer dosimetry programs, are now avail-

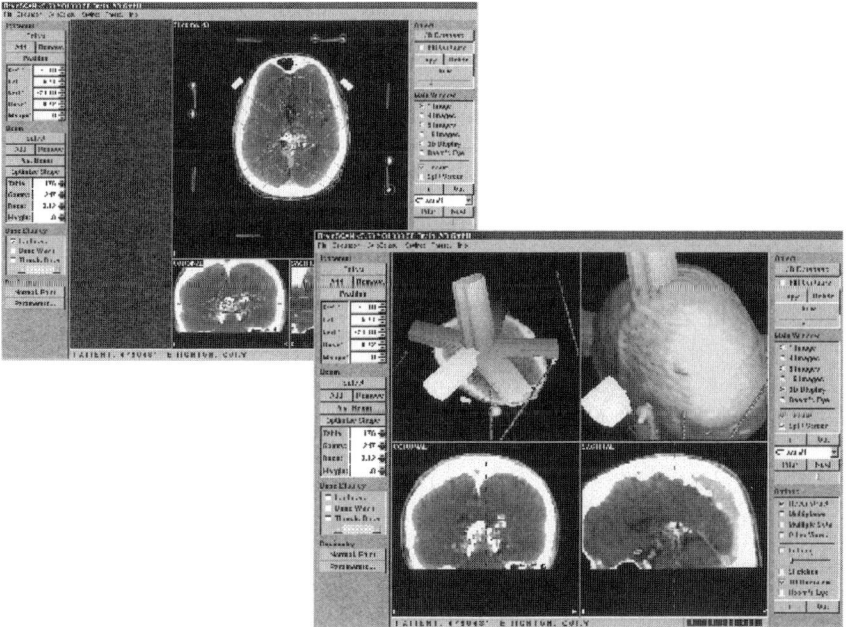

FIG. 6.4 Conformal radiosurgery planning software demonstrating dosimetry plan for treatment of a large bithalamic arteriovenous malformation with six static ports shaped using a cerrobend to shape collimator.

able and have the capability of providing both static and dynamic beam shaping. *Figure 6.4* demonstrates graphically the planning to use a shaped beam to provide a relatively homogeneous dose to the nidus of a large bithalamic arteriovenous malformation. This large lesion was treated with six noncoplanar static shaped fields. Adler and his group have demonstrated the feasibility of delivering radiation with three-dimensional homogeneity using the multiple axis capability of a miniature linear accelerator coupled to and guided by a large industrial robot (1). These beam-shaping advances will significantly improve the safety and effectiveness of radiation therapy.

In summary, this chapter reviews the status of five areas in which enhancement of image guidance techniques can improve the safety and precision of intracranial surgery. The combination of these advances will usher in an era in which neurosurgeons can accurately map brain function in physical stereotactic space, make real-time adjustments of shifts in brain structure related to maximized surgical resection, use robotics for assistance in defining and adjusting pathways to brain targets, both study and alter brain function with accurately placed electrode systems, and deliver with precision homogeneous radiation to brain targets.

REFERENCES

1. Adler JR, Jr., Chang SD, Murphy MJ, et al.: The Cyberknife: a frameless robotic system for radiosurgery. **Stereotact Funct Neurosurg** 69:124–128, 1997.
2. Benabid AL, Cinquin P, Lavalle S, et al.: Computer-driven robot for stereotactic surgery connected to CT scan and magnetic resonance imaging. Technological design and preliminary results. **Appl Neurophysiol** 50:153–54, 1987.
3. Benabid AL, Hoffmann D, Ashraf A, et al.: The robotization of neurosurgery: state of the art and future outlook]. **Bull Acad Natl Med** 181:1625–1635, 1997; Discussion 1635–1636.
4. Benabid AL, Pollak P, Gao D, et al.: Chronic electrical stimulation of the ventralis intermedius nucleus of the thalamus as a treatment of movement disorders [see comments]. **J Neurosurg,** 84:203–214, 1996.
5. Black PM, Moriarty T, Alexander E. 3rd, et al.: Developmental and implementation of intraoperative magnetic resonance imaging and its neurosurgical applications. **Neurosurgery** 41:831–842, 1997. Discussion 842–845.
6. Brown RA, Roberts TS, Osborn AG: Stereotaxis frame and computer software for CT-directed neurosurgical localization. **Invest Radiol** 15:308–312, 1980.
7. Bucholz RD, Greco DJ: Image-guided surgical techniques for infections and trauma of the central nervous system. **Neurosurg Clin North Am** 7:187–200, 1996.
8. Carol M, Grant WH, 3rd, Pavord D, et al.: Initial clinical experience with the Peacock intensity modulation of a 3-D conformal radiation therapy system. **Stereotact Funct Neurosurg** 66:30–34, 1996.
9. Friedman WA, Bova FJ: Mendenhall WM, Linear accelerator radiosurgerpy for arteriovenous malformations: the relationship of size to outcome [see comments]. **J Neurosurg** 82:180–189, 1995.

10. Howard MA 3rd, Henegar MM, Dacey RG, Jr., et al.: Magnetic neurosurgery: image-guided, remote-controlled movements of neurosurgical implants. **Clin Neurosurg** 43:382–391, 1996.
11. Kelly PJ: Computer assisted volumetric stereotactic resection of superficial and deep seated intra-axial brain mass lesions. **Acta Neurochir Suppl** 52:26–29, 1991.
12. Kelly PJ, Alker GJ Jr: A stereotactic approach to deep-seated central nervous system neoplasms using the carbon dioxide laser. **Surg Neurol** 15:331–334, 1981.
13. Kelly PJ, Kall B, Goerss S: Stereotactic CT scanning for the biopsy of intracranial lesions and functional neurosurgery. **Appl Neurophysiol** 46:193–199, 1983.
14. Krack P, Pollak P, Limousin P, et al.: Subthalamic nucleus or internal pallidal stimulation in young onset Parkinson's disease. **Brain** 121 (Pt. 3): 451–457, 1998.
15. Leavitt DD, Gibbs FA, Jr., Heilbrun MP, Moeller JH, Takach GA Jr.: Dynamic field shaping to optimize stereotactic radiosurgery. **Int J Radiat Oncol Biol Phys** 21:1247–1255, 1991.
16. Leksell L: Stereotactic radiosurgery. **J Neurol Neurosurg Psychiatry** 46:797–803, 1983.
17. Leksell L, Jernberg B: Stereotaxis and tomography. A technical note. **Acta Neurochir** 52:1–7, 1980.
18. Lewine JD, Orrison WW Jr.: Magnetic source imaging: basic principles and applications in neuroradiology. **Acad Radiol** 2:436–440, 1995.
19. Lozano AM, Lang AE, Hutchison WD, Dostrovsky JO: Microelectrode recording-guided posteroventral pallidotomy in patients with Parkinson's disease. **Adv Neurol** 74:167–174, 1997.
20. Lunsford LD, Rosenbaum AE, Perry J: Stereotactic surgery using the "therapeutic" CT scanner. **Surg Neurol** 18:116–122, 1982.
21. Lutz W, Winston KR, Maleki N: A system for stereotactic radiosurgery with a linear accelerator. **Int J Radiat Oncol Biol Phys** 14:373–381, 1988.
22. McDonald JD, Chong BW, Lewine JD, et al: Integration of preoperative and intraoperative functional brain mapping in a frameless stereotactic environment for lesions near eloquent cortex. Technical note. **J Neurosurg** 90:591–598, 1999.
23. Rezai AR, Mogilner AY, Cappell J, et al.: Integration of functional brain mapping in image-guided neurosurgery. **Acta Neurochir Suppl** 68:85–89, 1997.
24. Roberts DW, Nakajima T, Brodwater B et al.: Further development and clinical application of the stereotactic operating microscope. **Stereotact Funct Neurosurg** 58:114–117, 1992.
25. Roberts DW, Strohbehn JW, Friets EM, Kettenberger J, Hartor A: The stereotactic operating microscope: accuracy refinement and clinical experience. **Acta Neurochir Suppl** 46:112–114, 1989.
26. Tasker RR, Munz M, Junn FS, et al.: Deep brain stimulation and thalamotomy for tremor compared. **Acta Neuochir Suppl** 68:49–53, 1997.
27. Trobaugh JW, Richard WD, Smith KR, Bucholz RD: Frameless stereotactic ultrasonography: method and applications. **Comput Med Imaging Graph** 18:235–246, 1994.
28. Watanabe E, Mayanagi Y, Kosugi Y, Manaka S, Takakura K: Open surgery assisted by the neuronavigator, a stereotactic, articulated, sensitive arm. **Neurosurgery** 28:792–799, 1991; Discussion 799–800.
29. Winston KR, Lutz W: Linear accelerator as a neurosurgical tool for stereotactic radiosurgery. **Neurosurgery** 22:454–464, 1988.
30. Young RF: Application of robotics to stereotactic neurosurgery. **Neurol Res** 9:123–128, 1987.

II

General Scientific Session II

CHAPTER

7

Epidemiology and Cost of Central Nervous System Injury

LAWRENCE F. MARSHALL, M.D.

Head and spinal cord injuries, because of their prevalence in the young, take a particular toll in both human suffering and cost in all societies. In some Latin American countries and in Asia, head injury is, in fact, the leading cause of death. Many patients who suffer what are considered to be minor head injuries are left with long-term disabilities. A percentage called the "miserable minority" sees the loss of jobs and of family as the final outcome from a nonhospitalized minor head injury that results in personality changes and cognitive dysfunction. In a recent study from New Zealand (6), 5% of patients with a minor head injury sought medical attention for cognitive and behavioral problems more than 1 year after the incident.

The misery of spinal cord injury is even more obvious to the lay public. Although spinal cord injury is a much less frequent event than severe head injury, improved initial care coupled with a much better understanding of the sequelae of spinal cord injury has yielded hundreds of thousands of long-term survivors who suffer from lifelong impairments and face enormous obstacles, even in relatively sophisticated societies. It is encouraging to note, however, that policies designed to make vehicular travel safer, and preventive programs such as the "Feet First" program started by the neurosurgical community, seem to have impacted the incidence, if not the severity, of such injuries in some communities.

San Diego County is a particularly fertile region to study the incidence of such injuries because it has been characterized in previous work through the studies of Klauber (2) and Kraus (3–5). Because the region is limited on the West by the Pacific Ocean, to the South by the Mexican border, to the East by a formidable desert, and to the North by a large marine training base and almost uninhabitable mountains, it is quite well defined and lends itself to incidence studies. Moreover, because San Diego has almost exactly 1% of the American population within its county, with a large urban core surrounded by moderately populated suburbs, it mimics many of the characteristics of more traditional urban America. Although absolute conclusions cannot be made simply by multiplying the observations in San Diego County by 100, such statistical manipulations will give a relatively accurate picture of the epidemiology and cost of head and spinal cord injuries.

MATERIALS AND METHODS

The rubric used to capture the incidence of head and spinal cord injury in previous studies in San Diego County was applied to the period of 1992 to 1997. Data were collected from the San Diego County Trauma Registry for those years using the same ICD9 codes for the discharge diagnosis. San Diego County has mandatory reporting for these ICD9 codes. The definitions used for moderate and severe head injury were identical to those employed by Kraus: severe brain injury, Glasgow Coma Scale score of 8 or less at the time of admission; moderate brain injury, Glasgow Coma Scale score of 9 to 12 with an abnormal computed tomographic scan or the need for brain surgery. To calculate incidence data, we used population data published with the 1990 census and data available from the County of San Diego to calculate data for 1992 and 1997, the two index periods used.

Data were analyzed and compared with that collected in the two large epidemiology studies of head injury in San Diego County (2, 4).

Cost calculations for the acute care costs of minor head injury were taken from three trauma centers in San Diego County and averaged for those patients who were admitted for less than 48 hours. Cost data for the lifelong costs of severe head injury, using the definition provided in the text, were calculated based on data provided in 1984 by the Brain Foundation of Australia and corrected for inflation. The report here is in United States dollars, and the rate of conversion is appropriate for 1984.

The frequency of spinal cord injury was determined by a study of all trauma centers in San Diego County, including the Children's Hospital. Because transfer of patients with detectable spinal cord injury to a trauma center is mandated in our region, failure to capture significant spinal cord injury is unlikely, although surveys were not carried out in non-trauma center institutions. In the case of the ascertainment method used here, gunshot wounds were captured for both head and spinal cord injury. The results were compared with the report of DeVivo et al. (1).

RESULTS AND DISCUSSION

Table 7.1 compares the incidence of all head injuries, including moderate and severe head injuries, in San Diego County over a period of almost 20 years. As can be seen from the table, the rather dramatic reduction that occurred between 1978 and 1981 is coincident with the introduction of CT scanning and a regional plan for trauma management in San Diego. The trend toward reduced incidence slowed fairly dramatically by 1992, but a rather dramatic reduction in the frequency of moderate and severe injuries still occurred during the previous 11-year interval. Whereas a small further reduction in all head injuries admitted to the hospital was observed between 1992 and 1997, the frequency of moderate and severe injuries seems to have stabilized at approximately 34 per 100,000.

There has been no substantive decline in mortality when comparing the 30 per 100,000 noted in the report of Kraus et al. (4) and the most recent data of 29.2 per 100,000. However, because there was a rather substantial increase in the number of deaths caused by firearms in the most recent period, mortality from non-gunshot wounds seems to have fallen. A detailed analysis, however, has not been completed,.

Spinal Cord Injury

The frequency of spinal cord injury, defined as injuries to the cervical, thoracic, or upper lumbar spinal cord and excluding the cauda equina, seems to have remained remarkably stable over the last 5 years (*Table 7.2*). In an initial unpublished study carried out in 1980, the incidence of spinal cord injury patients reaching the hospital alive in San Diego County was approximately 51 per 1,000,000. Our most recent data suggest that there has been approximately a 20% decline in spinal cord injury and that the figure has stabilized at this level. Thus, in 1992, the incidence was approximately 40 per 1,000,000 and has remained at that level since.

TABLE 7.1
Incidence in a Defined Population of Head Injury

	All Head Injuries	Moderate and Severe Head Injuries
1978	295/100,000	40/100,000
1981 (Kraus)	180/100,000	44/100,000
1992	150/100,000	33/100,000
1997	144/100,000	34/100,000

TABLE 7.2
Spinal Cord Injury in San Diego County

Year	Number	Incidence per 10^6	Site	
1992	103	42	Cervical	55
			Thoracic	27
			Lumbar	21
1997	106	40	Cervical	58
			Thoracic	27
			Lumbar	21

TABLE 7.3
Spinal Cord Injury

	Average Length of Stay	
Year	Acute	Rehabilitation
1992	14	48
1997	9	32

The distribution of spinal cord injuries by location is also shown in *Table 7.2*. Here too, the distribution of the location of injury seems almost identical when a 5-year epic is compared. However, some changes have occurred in the region. The average length of stay for acute spinal cord injury, shown in *Table 7.3,* has declined between 1992 and 1997 from 14 days to 9 days, and rehabilitation days have declined to 32. This obviously reflects cost-containment pressures in the region, but whether there has been a compromise of rehabilitation care cannot be determined.

The Cost of Head Injury

The actual overall cost of head injury in the United States is difficult to determine. It is easier to calculate the charges for care, and they are truly enormous. Much more difficult, however, is the determination of the actual costs. Even more difficult than that to calculate is the cost of lost work, spousal abuse, child abuse, and the loss in quality of life for these patients and their families.

In San Diego County, the cost for a 36-hour stay for an uncomplicated minor head injury with a loss of consciousness is approximately $13,500. The basis for those costs, taken from a survey of the trauma centers, is shown in *Table 7.4*. As can be seen from the table, the activation of the trauma system within the hospital requiring the presence of a number of providers, including general surgeons, trauma surgeons, neurosurgeons, respiratory therapists, and radiologists, is very substantial. Mechanisms to determine the severity of injury in a more accurate manner from the field have reduced the number of trauma team activations, but there is still substantial overtriage. However, undertriage is quite dangerous, and the need for better scoring systems and better identification of patients at particular risk is needed.

If one extrapolates from the San Diego experience and separates simple minor head injury from cases where there are additional orthopedic or abdominal injuries, an estimate of approximately 180,000 admissions, or approximately 40% of all patients, are admitted with simple uncomplicated head injury. The cost of those patients, again using the San Diego charge figures, is almost 3 billion dollars, indicating that even a 15 or 20% reduction in the frequency with which the trauma system is activated, or, even better, preventing such injuries, would result in substantial dollar savings.

The average length of stay within intensive care units for patients with severe head injury is approximately 9 days. If one adds the charges for all services provided to such patients and includes only the acute care stay, the average charges approximate $100,000. This does not include the rehabilitation phase of care or the subsequent long-term costs for the care of such patients.

The lifelong costs for a profoundly disabled survivor are even more forbidding. In 1984, the Brain Foundation of Australia estimated lifelong care for head-injured males in Australia. The costs with corrections for inflation using a 4% per year figure since 1984 are shown in *Table 7.5*. In the example shown, it is assumed that the patient is awake and nonvegetative, but unable to walk or feed himself, and is incontinent of urine. It is further assumed that this patient's life span will be foreshortened by approximately one-third because of inability to participate in any meaningful activities.

In looking at these costs, a striking finding is the relatively limited cost of lost work years when compared with the overall total cost. Al-

TABLE 7.4
Costs of Head Injury

Uncomplicated Brief LOC	
Trauma team	$8,200.00
Radiology	$1,500.00
Hospital	$2,400.00
Pharmacy	$700.00
Ambulance	$700.00
Total	$13,500.00

TABLE 7.5
A 28-Year-Old Severely Head-Injured Patient[a]

Incontinent	$1,000,000.00
Not ambulatory	$1,200,000.00
Cannot feed himself	$1,200,000.00
Unemployed	$600,000.00
Total	$4,000,000.00

[a]Based on 1984 data corrected to 1998; 4% rate of inflation; death at age 60.

though the assumptions underlying these projected figures can be challenged, they do indicate that the focus in the care of the severely head injured, particularly those with survivable injuries but with extensive structural brain damage, should be restoration to a semi-independent state, rather than the patient's returning to work or school. It is unlikely, for many of the more seriously injured, that it is realistic to expect them to return to work or school.

Cost of Spinal Cord Injury

More rapid mobilization of spinal cord injury patients because of surgical stabilization and the introduction of a number of new assistive devices, including motorized wheelchairs, has reduced the initial costs of the care in the spinal cord injured. However, little is known as to the long-term effects of such changes, given the fact that motorized wheelchairs, for example, are much more expensive than manual devices and seem to need replacement as frequently. The passage of the Americans with Disabilities Act has added considerable societal cost because of the need to retrofit buildings and to incorporate changes into new structures. Of course, improvements in the quality of life because of those changes (e.g., building access) are more difficult to measure in dollar terms as an offset to increased expenses.

There is no question that the most effective means of reducing the cost of spinal cord injury lies in the continuing efforts to prevent such injuries. The fact that the frequency seems to have stabilized in our region suggests that alternative efforts beyond those presently employed to educate young people, particularly young males, is going to be necessary if further reductions in the frequency of such injuries is to occur.

CONCLUSION

The present comparative analysis seems to demonstrate a continuing decline, although one that is moderating, in the frequency of hospitalized head injury in San Diego County. Unfortunately, there has not been a coincident significant decline in the incidence of moderate and severe head injury, suggesting that further modifications, perhaps in vehicular design and certainly in education, are required if this is to be impacted. Data for the last 5 years in San Diego County paint a similar picture for spinal cord injury, where the incidence remains remarkably stable and the severity of injury at 6 months remains unchanged. It seems that the impact of mandatory seatbelt legislation and mandatory helmet legislation in California, along with improvements in vehicular design, were responsible for the changes seen in the frequency of moderate and severe head injury between 1981 and 1992. However, given the stable incidence of such injuries since 1992, it seems that there is a further need for modifications in vehicular design to, for example, protect pedestrians if one is going to make further progress in reducing the most significant injuries and those with the most dramatic long-term sequelae.

The snapshot offered here of spinal cord injury provides information requiring further analysis. Clearly, the lack of any change in the frequency of complete versus incomplete injuries and no further decline in the incidence of these injuries is disappointing. This would suggest that educational efforts, such as the "Feet First" program, have not had as dramatic an impact as one would have hoped, at least in San Diego County. More work is needed to better define the causes and potential public health interventions that could reduce the frequency and severity of spinal cord injury. It is possible that the trends demonstrated here are not an accurate reflection of the United States as a whole. However, until there is some demonstration that the present programs in prevention and education are effective, there is sobering news here that should lead to a critical examination of our present preventative efforts.

The present report continues to demonstrate a high frequency of admission for head injury. Extrapolating from the San Diego experience, one would expect approximately 400,000 patients to have been hospitalized in the United States during 1997. Given the region's sophisticated trauma system and well-defined protocols for patient discharge from emergency rooms or trauma centers without admission, it is probable that the frequency of admission elsewhere in the United States, at least in many instances, is somewhat higher. San Diego County's EMS system has served as a model for other regions, and reductions in admissions in cities and counties where similar policies have been adopted have also been observed. Even if the number of approximately 400,000 admissions is an accurate reflection and not an underestimate, it still represents the most frequent cause of admission in the United States for nervous system disease. Although the cost of such admissions overall is difficult to determine, the human cost is substantial. Death as a health care cost, if it occurs early, is inexpensive, but the cost to families, businesses, and communities is tremendous, particularly given the relative youth in many instances of fatal head injury. Moreover, the toll of minor head injury on children and spouses, where personality change and cognitive dysfunction is quite common, is substantial. The recent report by Wrightson and Gronwall (6) indicates that persistent symptoms are common in a substantial percentage of patients with minor head injuries and are disruptive to life function for more than a year in many. Thus, further improvements in vehicular safety and recreational education are necessary if the frequency of head and spinal cord injury are to be reduced.

REFERENCES

1. DeVivo MJ, Fine PR, Maetz HM, Stover SL: Prevalence of spinal cord injury: A reestimation employing life table techniques. **Arch Neurol** 37:707–708, 1980.
2. Klauber MR, Barrett-Connor E, Marshall LF, Bowers A: The epidemiology of head injury: Prospective study of an entire community—San Diego County, California, 1978. **Am J Epidemiol** 113:500–509, 1981.
3. Kraus JF, Nourjah P: The epidemiology of mild, uncomplicated brain injury. **J Trauma** 28(12):1637–1643, 1988.
4. Kraus JF, Black MA, Hessol N, et al.: The incidence of acute brain injury and serious impairment in a defined population. **Am J Epidemiol** 119:186–201, 1984.
5. Kraus JF, Fife D, Ramstein K, Conroy C, Cox P: The relationship of family income to the incidence, external causes, and outcomes of serious brain injury, San Diego, California. **Am J Public Health** 76(11):1345–1347, 1986.
6. Wrightson P, Gronwall D: Mild head injury in New Zealand: Incidence of injury and persisting symptoms. **N Z Med J** 27:99–101, 1998.

CHAPTER

8

Pathophysiology of Neural Injury: Therapeutic Opportunities and Challenges

JOHN T. POVLISHOCK, PH.D.

In this review, I will attempt to provide a brief, yet concise, overview of current thoughts on the pathophysiology of traumatic brain injury while suggesting potential new directions for the field to move in relation to pharmacological invention. This review will be framed by a sense of urgency and, to a point, frustration, in that despite the exponential advances in our understanding of the pathophysiology of traumatic brain injury over the past 20 years, these advances have not translated into the generation of new and better therapeutic strategies for the improved outcome of patients sustaining traumatic brain injury. What follows is a frank discussion of where we are in the field, where we have failed, and where we should be going.

BASIC PATHOPHYSIOLOGY OF TRAUMATIC BRAIN INJURY

As is well known to the neurosurgical community, the pathobiology of traumatic brain injury can be divided into focal and diffuse change (for a review, see Reference 8). Focal injuries entail contusion and/or hematoma formation and generally exert significant local destructive effects that impact mortality based on their location and overall progression. Diffuse injuries, on the other hand, are not confined to discrete anatomic foci but rather are distributed widely throughout the brain and brain stem. Typically, such diffuse injuries are characterized as either diffuse axonal injury or diffuse microvascular damage. In addition to these focal and diffuse changes, there is now significant evidence that widespread or generalized changes also occur in concert with the above described pathologies. In this context, it is well recognized that the traumatic episode can be associated with generalized neuroexcitation, involving the release of multiple neurotransmitter systems in which the neuroexcitatory amino acids have received the most consideration (for review, see Reference 33). In addition to this neuroexcitatory surge, there is also evidence of generalized brain oxygen free radical production that, in part, also may be linked to the above described neuroexcitatory storm as well as some of the other sequelae of traumatic brain injury (for a review, see Reference 9). Lastly, in concert with the above described events, there is generalized metabolic and microvascular alteration, with the changes in brain metabolism most likely reflecting a neuroexcitation-mediated response (for review, see Reference 12), whereas the vascular abnormalities may, in large part, have their genesis in the damaging consequences of the oxygen free radical generation (17). In the following passages, I will discuss the basic pathophysiology of each of these of these diffuse and generalized changes in an effort to provide a contemporary overview of the pathophysiology of traumatic brain injury, while providing the intellectual framework on which modern clinical trials for the treatment of traumatic brain injury have been based.

DIFFUSE AXONAL INJURY

Diffuse axonal injury is associated early in the traumatic course with the presence of swollen axons forming terminal clubs. These are replaced over time by a gliotic response, followed by delayed Wallerian degeneration. Importantly, in this process of diffuse axonal injury, diffuse deafferentation of brain target sites is the natural consequence (for a review, see Reference 30). It is well recognized that axons are not torn at the moment of injury but rather undergo sequential, focal changes that lead to swelling and disconnection over a multiple hour postinjury course (for a review, see References 19 and 29). In the case of severe traumatic brain injury, recent experimental evidence has demonstrated that the initiating event in the sequence of axonal swelling and disconnection is a traumatically induced focal alteration to the axolemma, which allows for the influx of substances normally confined to the extracellular front. In this scenario, it is envisioned that calcium passes through the impaired axolemma. Experimental evidence supports this assumption by the demonstration, within the first minutes postinjury, of the activation of calpain-mediated spectrin proteolysis in the subaxolemmal network (3). This calcium-mediated change in the subaxolemmal compartment further modifies the axolemma to lead to continuing posttraumatic axolemmal leakage. Concomitant with the above described subaxolemmal change, the related underlying cytoskeleton demonstrates a consistent triad of change reflected in neurofilament compaction, microtubular loss, and mitochondrial swelling. These intra-axonal changes remain stable for the first 30 to 60 minutes postinjury, but then, over time show continued progressive alterations associated with further cytoskeletal change and modification. It is this local cytoskeletal modification that leads to an impairment of axoplasmic transport, local swelling of the axon, and its disconnection (26). As the consequence of this delayed disconnection, the downstream, disconnected fibers degenerate, as do their terminal fields, leading to diffuse deafferentation of target sites. In cases of mild or moderate injury, this diffuse deafferentation may be followed by adaptive recovery, associated with the sprouting of nearly intact fibers (30); however, in cases (moderate and/or severe), through mechanisms not entirely clear, non-adaptive recovery can ensue (27, 28).

DIFFUSE VASCULAR INJURY

In general, diffuse vascular injury is not a frequent occurrence following traumatic brain injury. It is typically reserved for patients who sustain the most severe forms of traumatic brain injury and who generally die during the first hours post injury. Typically, in these patients, diffuse petechial hemorrhages are found scattered throughout the brain and the brainstem, leading to the suggestion that forces of injury were so severe as to cause widespread, direct mechanical disruption of the microvasculature.

Generalized Changes

NEUROEXCITATION

In addition to these well described, well accepted pathophysiological changes, investigative studies in animals and man over the last decade have also recognized a host of general or widespread responses that occur concomitant with and/or as the result of the above described events. Apparently, the same shear and tensile forces of injury that contribute to axonal damage and other forms of change result in neuronal depolarization with the release of multiple neurotransmitters, resulting in a wave of neuroexcitation (for a review, see Reference 33). Typically, this neurotransmitter storm can participate in multiple abnormal agonist-receptor interactions that result either in neuronal cell dysfunction or death. To date, in acute phases of injury, the glutaminergic systems have received the most attention in both the experimental and clinical settings. In the laboratory and clinical settings, the use of microdialysis probes have provided compelling evidence for the marked elevation of excitatory amino acids immediately following traumatic brain injury (7, 14, 22). In animals, this rise is dramatic yet brief in duration, occurring in minutes/hours of the traumatic episode, depending upon the nature of the injury and the placement of the probe. In man, this acute elevation of excitatory amino acids has not been detected, as patients cannot be monitored in the first minutes of injury. However, experience with microdialysis probes in humans suggests the occurrence of such initial excitatory surge via the routine detection of decreasing glutamate levels in the early posttraumatic period. Additionally, in the same patient population whose posttraumatic course is complicated by contusional expansion and/or a reduction in perfusion pressure to ischemic levels, a secondary rise in excitatory amino acids occurs, and this is believed to participate in additional abnormal agonist-receptor interactions (25, 37). Further evidence of the involvement of excitatory amino acids is also found in various experimental studies, which demonstrate that the use of various receptor antagonists targeting the glutamate NMDA receptor, in particular, translates into anatomic, behavioral, and neurochemical protection (11, 15, 21; for a review, see Reference 20). Although the space constraints of this review preclude a full discussion of the damaging consequences of traumatically induced neuroexcitation, it is important to note that the above described neurotransmitter storm is believed to exert its damaging consequences through receptor-mediated pathology. In the case of the glutamate, its interaction with its various receptor subtypes, including the NMDA, AMPA, and metabotrophic receptors, is believed to contribute to various forms of ionic dysregulation (primarily Na^+ and Ca^{2+}) that can have either lethal or sublethal consequences for the target neurons. In the worst case scenario, the glutamate NMDA and AMPA receptors allow for the influx of sodium and calcium, leading to neuronal swelling and death, a phenomenon not typically seen in vivo. Alternatively, the glutamate NMDA receptor activation may allow for the influx of calcium, which, upon reaching elevated intracellular levels, can elicit the activation or overstimulation of phospholipases, calpains and other proteases, protein kinases, nitric oxide synthases, calcineurin, and endonucleases (for a review, see Reference 34). It is assumed that this excessive stimulation of calcium-dependent processes translates into Ca^{2+}-mediated cell membrane and organelle damage, cytoskeletal disruption, the overproduction of toxic processes, or the activation of genetic signals leading to cell death. These processes may be interrelated and may lead to either a necrotic form of neuronal death and/or the initiation of apoptotic cell death (32). Those intracellular calcium levels, not evoking cell death, may impact upon cell function via secondary pathways including, but not limited to, metabotropic receptor activation leading to the generation of inositol triphosphate, which triggers the release of bound intracellular Ca^{2+}. Typically, in this case, the involvement of the glutamate NMDA and/or the metabotropic receptor alters signal transduction, resulting in impaired electrophysiological responses such as impaired LTP, the synaptic analogue of memory, and altered behavioral and cognitive manifestations (20, 31). In this neuroexcitatory phase, the role of the related nonglutaminergic systems in these pathophysiological changes is unclear. Although it is known that antagonism of the muscarinic receptors does translate into forms of protection, their exact downstream postsynaptic consequences are not fully appreciated. As posited by several investigators, the cholinergic system may interface with the glutaminergic system by evoking depolarization, which removes the magnesium block on the glutamate NMDA receptor complex, allowing for sustained calcium influx, with profound postsynaptic consequences (20, 33). Further evidence for this wave of neuroexcitation is also supported by the finding in animals and humans of a rapid posttraumatic phase of glucose hypermetabolism (1, 2, 12, 13). This hyperglycolysis is assumed to be the result of the brain's attempt to restore the ionic homeostasis disrupted by the neuroexcitatory storm. In traumatically brain-injured patients and animals, this hyperglycolysis is followed over time by a hypoglycolytic phase, which seems to parallel the animals' and patients' clinical course, with the patients'/animals' recovery paralleling the restoration of normal brain glucose utilization.

ROLE OF DAMAGED OXYGEN RADICALS

In addition to the above described pathobiological and physiological responses following traumatically induced agonist-receptor interactions, traumatic brain injury, particularly that of severe intensity, typically involves generalized microvascular change whose pathobiology seems closely linked to the generation of damaging oxygen free radicals. In severely brain-injured humans as well as animals, blood-flow abnormalities have described. Specifically with severe injury, the detection of reduced flow, sometimes reaching ischemic levels, has been reported in a subpopulation of patients (18). In addition to this potential ischemic injury, in the early posttraumatic phase, laboratory and clinical investigations have also reported the finding of other forms of microvascular dysfunction. Typically, traumatically damaged microvessels do not respond to physiological challenges in a normal fashion (6, 36). Arterioles may not respond to changes in blood gas composition as anticipated, and they may not respond to normal endothelia-dependent processes, such as those involving endothelia-dependent relaxation and/or contraction. For example, in experimental animals subjected to severe traumatic brain injury, the normal vasodilatory effect of acetylcholine application is translated into vasoconstriction in the early postinjury phase (5). Similarly, hypocapnic challenges, normally resulting in vasoconstriction, result in vasodilation (36). In the laboratory setting, these and a host of other vascular abnormalities have been directly linked to the production of damaging oxygen free radicals at the time of injury. In the microvascular bed, the source of these damaging radicals can be directly associated with the accelerated metabolism of arachidonic acid via cyclooxygenase and lipoxygenase pathways, whereby oxygen radicals are produced as a byproduct of prostaglandin synthesis (17). The vascular-derived oxygen radicals can also be augmented by those derived from the brain parenchyma, particularly those generated by a glutamate NMDA storm, which evokes calcium dysregulation, and the activation of the same arachidonic acid cascade, which again exerts its damaging consequences via the oxygen free radical-induced lipid and protein oxidation (9). Such radical-mediated lipid peroxidation effects neuronal, glial, and vascular membranes and is further catalyzed by free iron whose release is accelerated by the acidotic conditions commonly seen with traumatic brain injury. Any subsequent lipid peroxidation geometrically progresses in relation to cell membranes, resulting in increased membrane permeability, disruption of ionic homeostasis, and possibly membrane lysis. In the case of traumatic brain injury, many of the abnormal microvascular consequences have been effectively blunted by the use of radical scavengers and/or the antioxidants (9, 17). These agents were assumed to scavenge the superoxide anion in addition to the hydroxyl radical while, in some cases, blocking the downstream oxidation of various lipids and proteins.

IMPLICATIONS

Based upon this new and enhanced appreciation of the pathobiology and pathophysiology of traumatic brain injury, the field has witnessed a burst of Phase III clinical trials targeting many of the above-described mechanisms. Although somewhat contrived, one can categorize the major clinical trials conducted to date around four themes shown in Tables 8.1–8.4, which represent modifications and updating of tables originally prepared by Doppenberg and Bullock (4). As can be seen in *Table 8.1,* one group of clinical trials, which are the least theoretically focused, converges on the concept of cholinergic suppression or the general suppression of brain metabolism. As can be seen in *Table 8.1,* the majority of these trials were well-conducted studies involving double-blind, placebo-controlled randomized trials. As can be seen in *Table 8.2,* another group of clinical trials was clustered around the concept of traumatically induced neuroexcitation, focusing on the excitatory amino acids, with particular emphasis on the glutamate NMDA recep-

TABLE 8.1
Completed "Neuroprotection" Clinical Trials Targeting Brain Metabolism and Cholinergic Suppression in Severe Traumatic Brain Injury January 1998

Investigator/Year	Agent	# Patients/ Country	Outcome/ Comments
Ward et al., 1950	Atropine	20 U.S.	Uncontrolled, "clinical improvement"
Heppner et al., 1958	Biperiden (anticholinergic)	200 Germany	Uncontrolled, shorter hospitalization, reduced duration of coma
Six authors	Corticosteroids	365	Some controlled, no net benefit
Schwartz et al., 1985	Manitol vs. pentobarbital	59 Canada	Randomized crossover permitted, Manitol group had better outcome
Ward et al., 1985	Barbiturates (prophylaxis)	53 U.S.	DBPCRT,[a] no benefit
Eisenberg et al., 1988	Barbiturates (therapeutic)	73 U.S.	DBPCRT, benefit to subset with uncontrolled intracranial pressure
Wolf et al., 1993	THAM (tromethamine buffer)	149 U.S.	DBPCRT, reduced deleterious effects of hyperventilation

[a]IDBPCRT, double-blind, placebo-controlled randomized trial.
Modified from Doppenberg and Bullock. **J Neurotrauma** 14(2): 71–80, 1997.

tor. These trials also involved large patient populations orchestrated into Phase III clinical trials. In *Table 8.3*, one can see the third subset of clinical trials focused primarily upon the direct suppression of radical-mediated damage and/or their sequelae in terms of lipid protein oxidation. Again, these studies involved large numbers of patients in Europe and the U.S. and were performed as well controlled double-blind, placebo-controlled clinical trials. *Table 8.4* illustrates similar well-done clinical trails using calcium channel blockers. Lastly, *Table 8.5* shows those large scale clinical trails still in progress. Regrettably, as is well known to most in the neurosurgical community and discussed in multiple review articles (10), none of these trials has proved successful despite the fact that many of the proposed therapeutic strategies exerted profound neural and vascular protection in traumatically brain-injured animals. Although extensively reviewed in other articles (10) and beyond the scope of this presentation, the failure of these trials does not

TABLE 8.2
Completed "Neuroprotection" Clinical Trials Targeting Traumatically Induced Neuroexcitation In Severe Traumatic Brain Injury
January 1998

Investigator/Year	Agent	# Patients/Country	Outcome/Comments
Bullock et al., 1995	Selfotel (CGS-19755)	266 U.S. and Israel 466 EU and Australia	DBPCRT,[a] both terminated due to excess Mortality in concomitant stroke trials—no benefit (reports awaited)
Bullock et al., 1995	CGS 19755 (NMDA antagonist)	113 U.S. and U.K.	DBPCRT, intracranial pressure lower
Cohadon et al., 1996	Synthelabo Eliprodil (SL 82) Phase II	453 France	DBPCRT, better outcome in "brain swelling" patients ($P < 0.002$)
Gamzu et al., 1997	Cerestat (CNS 1102) non-competitive NMDA antagonist	512 U.S. and EU	DBPCRT, terminated due to excess mortality in concomitant stroke trial—no benefit (reports awaited)
Nichols, 1997	Bradycor (bradykinin receptor antagonist)	133 U.S.	DBPCRT, 10% trend toward better outcome

[a]IDBPCRT, double-blind, placebo-controlled randomized trial.
Modified from Doppenberg and Bullock, **J Neurotrauma** 14(2): 71–80, 1997.

necessarily imply that the underlying therapeutic concepts are fatally flawed. As noted by others, the reasons for failure in clinical trials are many and varied. In some cases, the failure resides in inadequate preclinical studies to assess optimal drug dosage and the therapeutic window of efficacy. Further, in the Phase I and Phase II clinical trials, there has been, in some cases, inadequate attention to the pharmacokinetics of the drug as well as its potential interactions with other agents used in the routine therapeutic management of traumatically brain-injured patients. To further compound the problem, some agents used in clinical trials were not the exact agents used in the laboratory in that some were modified to influence biological impact by increasing their half-life and/or modifying blood-brain barrier permeability. Other potential

TABLE 8.3
Completed "Neuroprotection" Clinical Trials Targeting Oxygen Free Radicals and Lipid and Protein Oxidation in Severe Traumatic Brain Injury January 1998

Investigator/Year	Agent	# Patients/ Country	Outcome/ Comments
Muizelaar et al., 1993	PEG-SOD free radical scavenger (Phase II)	94 U.S.	DBPCRT,[a] ICP lower, outcome better ($P < 0.01$)
Young et al., 1996	PEG-SOD (Phase III) 3 dose levels	463 U.S.	DBPCRT, trend for 8% better outcome ($p < 0.15$)
Alves and Jane, 1995	Tirilizad (aminosteroid antioxidant)	1170 U.S. and Canada	DBPCRT, no benefit (reports awaited)
Marshall, 1995	Tirilizad	1128 EU and Australia	DBPCRT, no benefit (reports awaited)

[a]DBPCRT, double-blind, placebo-controlled randomized trial.
Modified from Doppenberg and Bullock, **J Neurotrauma** 14(2): 71–80, 1997.

TABLE 8.4
Completed "Neuroprotection" Clinical Trials in Severe Traumatic Brain Injury Targeting Calcium Channels January 1998

Investigator/Year	Agent	# Patients/ Country	Outcome/ Comments
Teasdale et al., 1992	Nimodipine (HIT I) L channel CA antagonist	255 U.K. and Finland	DBPCRT,[a] no benefit
Braakman, 1993	Nimodipine (HIT II)	840 EU	DBPCRT, improved outcome in subset of SAH patients
Harders et al., 1996	Nimodipine (Phase II)	123 Germany (only SAH patients selected)	DBPCRT, 55% relative reduction in bad outcome at 6 mo ($P < 0.002$)

[a]DBPCRT, double-blind, placebo-controlled randomized trial.
Modified from Doppenberg and Bullock. **J Neurotrauma** 14(2): 71–80, 1997.

TABLE 8.5
*Ongoing Traumatic Brain Injury Clinical Trials
January 1998*

Company/Organization	Agent Treatment	Phase	# Patients/County	Mechanism/Comments
NIH	Moderate hypothermia (32–33°C,)	III	~500, U.S.	Five supportive pilot studies
Parke-Davis	SNX-111	III	~600, U.S. and EU	N Ca channel blocker
Pfizer	CP-101, 606	II/III	~450, U.S.	NR2B site NMDA antagonist
Sandoz/Novartis	SDZ EAA 494	II/III	~400, EU	NMDA antagonist
Bayer	BAY X 3702	II	~100, EU	5HT1A agonist, ion channel blocker
Pharmos	HU-211 Dexanabinol	I/II	Israel	multifunctional cannabinoid derivative
Janssen	Lubeluzole	II	60–120, EU and U.S.	nitric oxide synthase inhibitor effective in stroke

Modified from Doppenberg and Bullock, **J Neurotrauma** 14(2): 71–80, 1997.

reasons for failure include the fact that the traumatically brain-injured population is relatively heterogeneous, and, unfortunately, most clinical trials have treated this population as a homogeneous group. Lastly, the outcome measures used in clinical trials were extremely labor intensive and involved long-term studies that frequently did not directly target the direct action of the chosen therapeutic agent. Given the fact that these therapeutic studies in traumatic brain injury represent some of the most complex drug studies ever conducted to date in the most complex organ known to man, in retrospect, it seems somewhat puzzling that we did not expect setbacks and/or failures.

FUTURE DIRECTIONS

In view of the above statements, and in view of the fact that many of the remaining ongoing clinical trials (*Table 8.5*) are in the process of being terminated, the question remains where the field should move in terms of new therapeutic opportunities. Although the exact path is unclear, it is important that those involved in the field do not abandon hope and withdraw from the careful preclinical and clinical evaluations of various therapeutic approaches. In fact, shortcomings underlying our past failures should guide us in conduct of future clinical trials. In the general sense, it seems that future clinical trials should move away from attempts to blunt or effectively block the acute immediate consequences of traumatic brain injury, as it is unlikely, because of practical limitations related to patient retrieval and informed consent, that these agents could be given early enough to have profound efficacy. This statement, however, does not mean that many of the previously proposed therapeutic approaches were scientifically or clinically flawed. Rather, now the central issue hinges on whether or not we should consider the downstream/delayed consequences of these traumatically induced factors as targets for therapeutic intervention. Although the use of glutamate antagonists has not proved protective, perhaps targeting their consequences in terms of calcium dysregulation and/or lipase and protease activation may be the more appropriate strategies. For example, preclinical studies using calpain inhibitors have shown significant neuroprotection, suggesting that long-range strategies targeting the sequelae of neuroexcitation should be considered. In terms of these neuroexcitatory-mediated events and general traumatic change, there also should be renewed focus on the somewhat simplistic, yet profound concept of maintaining membrane integrity and the related membrane pumps in concert with the retention of mitochondrial function. These structures are functionally interrelated, in that mitochondrial failure can lead to the lack of energy needed to provide for the maintenance of membrane pumps and cell membrane function. In this context, the continued use of moderate posttraumatic hypothermia seems fully warranted (despite the recent setbacks in the clinical setting), in that recent work from our laboratory has demonstrated that it stabilizes the axolemmal membrane and prevents the progression of those damaging sequelae that result in disconnected and damaged axons (16). Specifically, the use of hypothermia seems to blunt the increase in calpain-mediated spectrin proteolysis and the subsequent in cytoskeletal collapse, suggesting that the hypothermic event is working at the axolemmal and subaxolemmal front. Interestingly, unpublished work from our lab also reveals that such moderate hypothermia results in continuing or prolonged neuroprotection rather than delaying the ultimate pathological demise of these fibers. Equally intriguing are other studies recently generated from our lab which clearly demonstrate that focal preservation of mitochondrial integrity also translates into profound neuroprotection in terms of traumatically induced axonal injury (24). These studies used cyclosporin A to block the mitochondrial permeable transition pore, which is opened in the presence of excessive intracellular calcium. In these studies, we observed that pretreatment with cyclosporin A in traumatically brain-injured rats resulted in local mitochondrial protection, which translated into significantly reduced axonal damage (24). Once again, this protection was directly correlated with a dramatic decrease in calpain-mediated spectrin proteolysis and virtually no loss of any intra-axonal cytoskeletal integrity (23). From our prospective, these studies of cyclosporin A suggest that the maintenance of local mitochondrial integrity is integral to the maintenance of local ATP production, which in turn is integral to the maintenance of the overlying axolemmal membrane. Although studies using cyclosporin A seem somewhat futuristic, we would point out that recent studies using cyclosporin A in stroke have also shown consistent neuroprotection (35).

In sum, new opportunities for therapeutic intervention seem to be on the horizon. New areas for investigation have been identified, and obviously they should be actively pursued. Further, old concepts, particularly those dealing with therapeutic strategies targeting the more delayed sequelae of traumatic brain injury, should be revisited through rigorous preclinical investigations and highly focused and rigorously conducted Phase II clinical trials. In this regard, the use of radical scavengers and antioxidants seems a reasonable approach for continued investigation once issues regarding drug delivery, blood-brain barrier permeability, and overall pharmacokinetics have been addressed. Similarly, the use of calpain antagonists may also constitute another rational course of potential therapeutic intervention.

REFERENCES

1. Andersen BJ, Marmarou A: Post-traumatic selective stimulation of glycolysis. **Brain Res** 585:184–189, 1992.
2. Bergsneider M, Hovda DA, Shalmon E, et al.: Cerebral hyperglycolysis following severe human traumatic brain injury: A positron emission tomography study. **J Neurosurg** 86:241–251, 1997.
3. Buki A, Povlishock JT: Evidence for calpain-mediated spectrin proteolysis in the pathogenesis of traumatically induced axonal injury. **J Neuropathol Exp Neurol** 58:365–375, 1999.
4. Doppenberg EMR, Bullock R: Clinical neuro-protection trials in severe traumatic brain injury: Lessons from previous studies. **J Neurotauma** 14(2):71–80, 1997.
5. Ellison MD, Erb DE, Kontos HA, Povlishock JT: Recovery of impaired endothelium-dependent relaxation after fluid-percussion brain injury in cats. **Stroke** 20:911–917, 1989.
6. Enevoldsen EM, Jense FT: Autoregulation and CO_2 responses of cerebral blood flow in patients with acute severe head injury. **J Neurosurg** 48:689–703, 1978.
7. Faden AI, Demediuk P, Panter SS, Vink R: The role of excitatory amino acids and NMDA receptors in traumatic brain injury. **Science** 244:798–800, 1989.
8. Graham DI: Neuropathology of head injury, in Narayan, RK, Wilberger JE, Povlishock JT (eds): *Neurotrauma*. New York, McGraw-Hill, 1996, pp 43–59.
9. Hall ED: Free radicals and lipid peroxidation, in Narayan RK, Wilberger JE, Povlishock JT (eds): *Neurotrauma*. New York, McGraw-Hill, 1996, pp 1405–1419.

10. Hall ED, Mohberg DN, Poole RM: Development of novel therapies for acute traumatic brain injury: Pharmaceutical industry perspective. **Brain Injury Source** 2(2):19, 20, 40, 1998.
11. Hayes RL, Jenkins LW, Lyeth BG, et al.: Pretreatment with phencyclidine, a N-methyl-D-aspartate antagonist, attenuates long-term behavioral deficits in the rat produced by traumatic brain injury. **J Neurotrauma** 5:259–274, 1988.
12. Hovda DA: Metabolic dysfunction, in Narayan, RK, Wilberger JE, Povlishock JT (eds): *Neurotrauma.* New York, McGraw-Hill, 1996, pp 1459–1478.
13. Hovda DA, Yoshino A, Kawamata T, Katayama Y, Fineman I, Becker DP: The increase in local cerebral glucose utilization following fluid percussion brain injury is prevented with kynurenic acid and is associated with an increase in calcium. **Acta Neurochir Suppl** 52:331–333, 1990.
14. Katayama Y, Becker DP, Tamura T, Hovda DA: Massive increases in extracellular potassium and the indiscriminate release of glutamate following concussive brain injury. **J Neurosurg** 73:889–900, 1990.
15. Kawamata T, Katayama Y, Hovda DA, Yoshino Y, Becker DP: Administration of excitatory amino acid antagonists via microdialysis attenuates the increase in glucose utilization seen following concussive brain injury. **J Cereb Blood Flow Metab** 12:12–24, 1992.
16. Koizumi H, Povlishock JT: Posttraumatic hypothermia in the treatment of axonal damage in an animal model of traumatic axonal injury. **J Neurosurg** 89:303–309, 1998.
17. Kontos HA, Povlishock JT: Oxygen radicals in brain injury. **Cent Nerv Syst Trauma** 3:257–263, 1986.
18. Marion DW, Dabry J, Yonas H: Acute regional/cerebral blood flow changes caused by severe head injuries. **J Neurosurg** 74:407–414, 1991.
19. Maxwell WL, Povlishock JT, Graham DL: A mechanistic analysis of nondisruptive axonal injury: A review. **J Neurotrauma** 14(7):419–440, 1997.
20. McIntosh TK, Juhler M, Wieloch T: Novel pharmacologic strategies in the treatment of experimental traumatic brain injury: 1998. **J Neurotrauma** 1998; 15(10)731–769.
21. McIntosh TK, Vink R, Soares HD, Hayes RL, Simon R: Effect of noncompetitive blockade of N-methyl-D-aspartate receptors on the neurochemical sequelae of experimental brain injury. **J Neurochem** 55:1170–1178, 1990.
22. Nilsson P, Hillered L, Ponten U, Urgerstedt U: Changes in cortical extracellular levels of energy-related metabolites and amino acids following concussive brain injury in rats. **J Cereb Blood Flow Metab** 10:631–637, 1990.
23. Okonkwo DO, Buki A Simon R, Povlishock JT: Cyclosporin A blocks the calpain-mediated spectrin proteolysis and cytoskeletal change associated in traumatic axonal injury. **Neuroreport** 10:353–358, 1999.
24. Okonkwo DO, Povlishock JT: An intrathecal bolus of cyclosporin A before injury preserves mitochondrial integrity and attenuates axonal disruption in traumatic brain injury. **J Cereb Blood Flow Metab** 19:443–451, 1999.
25. Persson L, Valtysson J, Enblad P, et al.: Neurochemical monitoring using intracerebral microdialysis in patients with subarachnoid hemorrhage. **J Neurosurg** 84:606–616, 1996.
26. Pettus EH, Christman C, Giebel ML, Povlishock JT: Traumatically induced altered membrane permeability: Its relationship to traumatically inducted reactive axonal change. **J Neurotrauma** 11(5):507–522, 1994.
27. Phillips LL, Lyeth BG, Hamm RJ, Povlishock JT: Combined fluid percussion brain injury and entorhinal cortical lesion: A model for assessing the interaction between neuroexcitation and deafferentation. **J Neurotrauma** 11:641–656, 1994.

28. Povlishock JT, Christman CW: Diffuse axonal injury, in Waxman SG, Koesis JD, Stys PK (eds): *The Axon*. New York, Oxford University Press, 1995, pp 504–529.
29. Povlishock JT, Jenkins LW: Are the pathobiological changes evoked by traumatic brain injury immediate and irreversible? **Brain Pathol** 5:415–416, 1995.
30. Povlishock JT, Erb DE, Astruc J: Axonal response to traumatic brain injury: Reactive axonal change, deafferentation, and neuroplasticity. **J Neurotrauma** 9:S189–S200, 1992.
31. Reeves TM, Lyeth BG, Povlishock JT: Long-term potentiation deficits and excitability changes following traumatic brain injury. **Exp Brain Res** 106:248–256, 1995.
32. Rink A, Fung KM, Trojanowski JQ, Lee V M, Neugebauer E, McIntosh TK: Evidence of apoptotic cell death after experimental traumatic brain injury in the rat. **Am J Pathol** 147(6):1575–1583, 1995.
33. Smith DH, McIntosh, TK: Traumatic brain injury and excitatory amino acids, in Narayan, RK, Wilberger JE, Povlishock JT (eds): *Neurotrauma*. New York, McGraw-Hill, 1996, pp 1445–1458.
34. Tymianski M, Tator CH: Normal and abnormal calcium homeostasis in neurons: A basis for the pathophysiology of traumatic and ischemic central nervous system injury. **Neurosurgery** 38(6):1176–1195, 1996.
35. Uchino H, Elmer E, Uchino K, Lindvall O, Siesjo BK: Cyclosporin A dramatically ameliorates CA1 hippocampal damage following transient forebrain ischemia in the rat. **Acta Physiol Scand** 155:469–471, 1995.
36. Wei EP, Dietrich WD, Povlishock JT, Kontos HA: Functional, morphologic, metabolic abnormalities of the cerebral microcirculation after concussive brain injury in cats. **Circ Res** 46(1):37–47, 1980.
37. Zauner A, Bullock R: The role of excitatory amino acids in severe brain trauma: Opportunities for therapy—A review. **J Neurotrauma** 12:547–554, 1995.

CHAPTER

9

The Triage and Acute Management of Severe Head Injury

RICHARD J. MEAGHER, M.D., RAJ K. NARAYAN, M.D.

> The mistakes are all there waiting to be made.
> —*Chessmaster Savielly Tartakower, 1887–1956*

Despite substantial reductions in the mortality and morbidity from head injury over the past two decades, neurotrauma remains the most important cause of death and disability in trauma patients. Neurosurgeons are therefore often in the hot seat as trauma systems become increasingly rigorous in their requirements. Such rigor has no doubt contributed significantly to the improvements in outcomes, although this benefit is difficult to document except with historical outcome data. A substantial body of data now suggests that the initial brain injury is but the beginning of a process of cell injury whose evolution can, at least to some degree, be modulated. All secondary insults that are superimposed on the primary injury demonstrably worsen the ultimate outcome. Certainly, the first few minutes and hours after a serious injury are the most critical and offer us the best opportunity for effective and prompt intervention. Conversely, this is the time when much can go wrong, and often does. Several issues relating to the acute management of severe head injury remain controversial, and the published data relating to them are almost entirely Class III (32). Thus, any recommendations relating to these issues are of necessity mostly Options rather than Guidelines or Standards. Nevertheless, we have attempted to briefly review some of the literature pertinent to the triage and acute management of severe head injury to provide the reader with a sense of what is known and to articulate the questions that perhaps deserve further study.

AVAILABILITY OF NEUROSURGEONS

> Eighty percent of success is showing up.
> —*Woody Allen*

Despite that the United States has many more neurosurgeons than virtually any other country in the world, the demands on their time are much greater in a remarkably documentation-driven and litigious society. Furthermore, especially in urban areas there are often many competing hospitals that wish to provide comprehensive services, including neurotrauma. Given the paucity of neurosurgeons relative to other surgical specialties, the availability of neurosurgeons is often cited as a limiting factor in the functioning of trauma systems. In 1992, the Office of the Inspector General of the United States released a report entitled "Specialty Coverage in Hospital Emergency Rooms," in which it was reported that 67% of hospitals surveyed around the country had difficulty in ensuring coverage by at least one specialty in their emergency room (ER) (42). Neurosurgeons were reportedly the most scarce, with 49% of hospitals reporting inadequate neurosurgical coverage. Rural hospitals reported more difficulty than urban facilities. Some of the factors cited by neurosurgeons for this lack of availability included inadequate reimbursement for difficult work, usually inconvenient hours, and the fear of litigation.

In a more recent analysis of the American College of Surgeons Trauma Consultation Program, Mitchell et al. reviewed the reports of consultation visits between 1987 and 1992 for hospitals desirous of being verified as Level I and II Trauma Centers (30). Lack of neurosurgeon availability was the 11th most cited deficiency. In fact, 13 of 52 hospitals (25%) were noted to have a deficiency in neurosurgical coverage. Furthermore, only approximately one-third of hospitals with neurosurgical deficiencies were eventually able to correct this problem and become designated. Commenting on this paper, Blaisdell (30) stated:

> The most common cause of mortality, particularly in those centers that deal with blunt trauma, relates to head injury. A lack of neurosurgical monitoring or immediate availability of neurosurgical decompression has been and remains a major detriment to providing optimal trauma care.
>
> I would suggest that a solution to the problem of neurosurgical availability might well be the training of general surgeons in the simpler neurosurgical procedures which are required for optimal management of head injury. The first of these and the oldest operation that has been documented by man has been cerebral decompression. The second need is cerebral monitoring, which is key to managing the trauma case with head injury in the ICU.

While agreeing with these comments, the authors added:

> Interestingly enough, we found as we survey the country, it varies from community to community. In the past, neurosurgical unavailability was a major problem.... We would agree with your comments and note that there are places in the country where credentials have

been given to general surgeons to practice those techniques that you have described and think this may be something that will have to be considered as a potential solution in the future.

The issue of neurosurgical involvement in the management of head injury has been previously addressed with concern (4). The argument was made that unless neurosurgeons maintained a vigorous presence in neurotrauma care, other specialists would step in to fill any apparent void. Although this would eliminate some of the problems associated with treating trauma patients, it would also entail essentially walking away from a significant population of patients and further shrinking the field of neurosurgery.

The 1993 edition of the Resources for the Optimal Care of the Injured Patient, which serves as the basis for the American College of Surgeons Committee on Trauma reviews, required a "neurosurgeon to be promptly available" (2). This was accepted as meaning that a neurosurgeon should be in the hospital within 30 minutes of the patient's arrival. Furthermore, it required "a reliable on-call schedule with a specific protocol for back-up coverage." The latter requirement met with resistance from the staff of certain smaller trauma centers, who felt that a back-up call schedule was unnecessary and needlessly burdensome.

Lucas et al. recently analyzed the need for back-up neurosurgical coverage (24). They gathered data from 749 patients at 97 trauma centers who required emergency neurosurgical procedures within 24 hours of admission. Based on mathematical modeling, they determined that the probability that a head-injury patient would not be seen promptly because the neurosurgeon was busy with another head-injury patient was 0.23, 0.9, 1.6, and 3.66, respectively in trauma centers that operated on 25, 50, 75, and 100 head-injury patients per year. Thus, not more than one patient per year would have to wait for more than 30 minutes in a trauma center doing 50 trauma neurosurgical procedures per year without a back-up call schedule.

Based on Lucas's study and further discussions, the American College of Surgeons Committee on Trauma revised the requirements in the 1998 edition of the Resources document. The new rule states, "When fewer than 25 emergency neurosurgical procedures, excluding ICP monitor placements, are done per year in any trauma center, a published back-up call list is not necessary. . . . In trauma centers where a neurosurgeon provides simultaneous coverage of two or more hospitals, there must be either an identified back-up neurosurgeon on call or a previously defined, coordinated neurotrauma diversion plan" (3).

In Level III and IV trauma centers, there is often limited or no neurosurgical coverage. Where there is no coverage, the trauma director will determine whether a particular patient will remain at the facility. If so, a quality improvement program must document appropriate care. In Level III or IV trauma centers, a clear transfer agreement must exist with a Level I or a Level II trauma center. The Resource document also states that on rare occasions, burr holes may be undertaken by a nonneurosurgeon after appropriate training by a neurosurgeon (3).

Rinker et al. recently described their success with emergency burr holes in a hospital in Montana (36). These surgeons, who did not have easy access to a neurosurgical team, undertook two 1-day workshops with a neurosurgeon and learned the basic techniques for burr hole decompression of an intracranial mass. They established clear guidelines for patient selection. Among 792 patients admitted to their facility over a 6-year period (1991–97), there were 20 patients with closed head injury and a Glasgow Coma Score (GCS) of 13 or less. All but eight were flown to a Level II trauma center that was a 1-hour flight away. However, burr holes were performed by the general surgeons on eight patients who met the following criteria: subdural or epidural hematoma on computed tomographic (CT) scan, rapid neurological deterioration, nonreactive pupil, GCS of 8 or less, hemiparesis, hypertension, and bradycardia. With the benefit of a phone consultation with the neurosurgeon and with a radiologist in the operating room, the procedures were successful. Good recovery was reported in six patients, moderate disability in one, and death in one patient, who had an admission GCS of 3.

The issue of neurosurgical coverage is a complex one. It seems clear that a single solution is probably not appropriate or feasible for all situations. Neurosurgeons should remain actively involved in the planning and delivery of neurotrauma care. However, when local circumstances make this impossible, they should consider innovative approaches that could save lives and reduce the needless morbidity caused by delayed intervention.

THE INITIAL NEUROLOGICAL EXAMINATION— DEPENDS ON WHOM YOU TALK TO

There are few pieces of information that are as important as the initial neurological examination in planning management, determining prognosis, and assessing the effectiveness of therapeutic interventions. However, the reliability of the data is often questionable, and descriptions of the findings can vary considerably based on the expertise of the examiner, the point at which the examination was conducted, and the confounding effect of various physiological and pharmacological influences.

The initial neurological examination should be conducted soon after the primary survey (i.e., airway, breathing, and circulation). The examination should consist of the elements of the GCS and pupillary reaction to light. Other brainstem reflexes such as corneal responses, oculocephalic or oculovestibular reflex, and cough reflex are generally deferred until later in the resuscitative process. It must be emphasized that the neurological examination can be significantly compromised by hypoxia or hypotension. However, an initial examination can still be valuable. The most reliable examination, however, is the postresuscitation examination, which is obtained after the patient's blood pressure and oxygenation have been normalized.

Marion and Carlier reported a survey of 17 major head-injury centers consisting of a two-page questionnaire with 16 multiple-choice questions (26). They noted that the initial GCS score was most often obtained by the junior neurosurgery resident, the trauma resident, or the ER nurse. Non-neurosurgical personnel were more likely to determine GCS scores at the time of the patient's arrival in the ER, regardless of whether the patient had received sedation or had been adequately resuscitated. Furthermore, 20% of attending neurosurgeons and 24% of non-neurosurgical ER personnel reported using the worst motor response in determining the GCS, although the correct way is to use the best motor response. The residents did better in this regard. Considering how much management and prognosis is based on this initial assessment, it is clear that better education is called for in the assessment of the GCS.

AIRWAY MANAGEMENT—WITHOUT JUMPING THE GUN

In many areas with advanced rescue squads, a patient with an altered sensorium is often intubated in the field and arrives in the hospital already chemically paralyzed. For those patients who arrive breathing spontaneously, the current enthusiasm for intubating and paralyzing them as soon as they enter the ER has added to the difficulty in obtaining an accurate neurological examination, especially if a long-acting paralytic agent is administered. Of course, ensuring adequate oxygenation is a major priority in the management of trauma patients. Hypoxia, defined as apnea or cyanosis in the field, or a PaO_2 of less than 60 mm Hg was noted in 46% of patients in the Traumatic Coma Data Bank and was an independent predictor of increased morbidity and mortality (10).

In addition to their hypoxia, head-injury patients tend to become hypercarbic (46). This respiratory insufficiency may be secondary to depressed consciousness, drug or alcoholic intoxication, airway obstruction, or aspiration. During a two-decade period in the United Kingdom, the proportion of patients who were intubated and mechanically ventilated before being transferred from local hospitals to regional neurosurgical centers increased from 11 to 82% (16). During this period, the incidence of hypoxia decreased from 22 to 8%. The benefits of airway management were also seen in a prospective study of 147 patients with head injury in Germany. The authors showed that 46% of patients who were not initially intubated developed aspiration and that 72% of these patients subsequently developed respiratory insufficiency. In contrast, only 9% of intubated head-injured patients developed aspiration, and 35% of these suffered respiratory insufficiency (41).

The data in support of early intubation are therefore quite convincing. However, when the patient's respiratory function seems adequate, immediate intubation is not always necessary and should be deferred for a few minutes to allow for a reliable neurological examination. The latter should not take more than 3 minutes.

PARALYSIS AND SEDATION—PROS AND CONS

When patients are picked up in the field, chemical paralysis during intubation and transport can help rescue personnel keep patients under control, prevent them from hurting themselves, and reduce the risk of aspiration. Furthermore, agitation and bucking the ventilator may cause surges in intracranial pressure (ICP) at a time when there is no way to monitor this parameter. However, if a long-acting paralytic agent is used, it certainly interferes with the neurological examination. Because an analgesic-sedative should be used along with a paralytic agent, this further complicates the picture. Current Guidelines for the Management of Severe Head Injury state at the level of an Option:

> Sedation and neuromuscular blockade can be useful in optimizing transport of the head injury patient. However, both treatments interfere with the neurological examination. In the absence of outcome-based studies, the choice of sedative is left to the physician. Neuromuscular blockade should be employed when sedation alone proves inadequate, and short-acting agents should be used when possible (17).

A retrospective analysis of 514 patients with severe head injury treated at the centers participating in the Traumatic Coma Data Bank demonstrated that paralysis could have deleterious effects (19). One set of patients had received chemical paralysis (not for ICP control) for at least 12 hours, and another set had not. The group that received paralysis had a significantly higher incidence of pneumonia and showed a trend toward a greater incidence of sepsis. Furthermore, paralyzed patients did not show a better outcome. The authors recommended that neuromuscular blockade be reserved for transport and for the control of ICP rather than used routinely in patients with severe head injury.

Recently, the ultra-short-acting sedative-anesthetic agent propofol has shown promise for the treatment of head-injured patients. Propofol's advantages include its short elimination half-life, its wide dose-response curve, and its neuroprotective effects. This allows the depth of sedation to range from light sedation to burst suppression and permits frequent neurological examinations. The results of a multicenter, double-blinded pilot trial suggested that a propofol-based regimen was a safe and possibly desirable alternative to a morphine-based regimen for sedation and control of ICP (23). Long-term outcome, mean ICP, and mean cerebral perfusion pressure were similar among the two groups despite a significantly higher incidence of poor prognostic indicators in the propofol group. Although there was a trend toward a greater use of vasopressors with propofol, the use of neuromuscular blocking agents, benzodiazepines, and pentobarbital for sedation and ICP control was significantly less frequent in this group. The propofol group also needed significantly less frequent cerebrospinal fluid drainage on therapy Days 2 and 3 (Day 2: 77 ± 74 ml/24 hr versus 191 ± 102 ml/24 hr, $P < 0.002$; Day 3: 75 ± 105 ml/24 hr versus 179 ± 127 ml/24 hr, $P < .05$).

HYPERVENTILATION—TOO MUCH OF A GOOD THING?

Hyperventilation became commonly used in the 1970s when it was noted that it reduced ICP in patients who were undergoing ICP monitoring. Hyperventilation reduces PCO_2 and reduces cerebral blood volume because of vasoconstriction. The reduction in intracranial volume results in a lowering of ICP. This maneuver can be especially useful in patients with a "tight" craniospinal axis, in whom a volume reduction of even a fraction of a milliliter can result in a significant reduction in ICP. However, the cerebral vasoconstriction that forms the basis of its effect on ICP can also reduce cerebral blood flow to ischemic levels. Several studies have shown that during the first day, and especially during the first 6 hours after a severe head injury, cerebral blood flow is less than half of that seen in normal individuals (7, 8, 25). This low cerebral blood flow makes these patients particularly vulnerable to the deleterious effects of hyperventilation. This is also the time during which respiratory parameters are least well regulated and there is often a tendency to "aggressively" hyperventilate a patient. It has been shown by jugular saturation monitoring that patients who have been hyperventilated to PCO_2 levels ≤ 25 mm Hg are at highest risk of oxygen desaturation in the cerebral venous blood.

Levels between 25 and 30 mm Hg are borderline, and levels above this seem relatively safe (40).

Beyond the acute management phase, a prospective randomized clinical trial by Muizelaar et al. showed a deleterious effect of prophylactic hyperventilation (31). Cruz proposed the concept of "optimized hyperventilation" and suggested that for each patient there is a different tolerance to hyperventilation that can be determined by jugular saturation monitoring (12). However, in the acute stages of management, one usually does not have access to either ICP or jugular oxygen saturation data.

At the present time, we do not have enough information to make clear recommendations regarding the use of hyperventilation in the newly injured patient. The data do seem to indicate that hyperventilation to PCO_2 levels of less than or equal to 25 mm Hg can be harmful. However, in a patient with signs of transtentorial herniation, it is well known by anecdotal experience that short periods of hyperventilation can reverse a dilated pupil, presumably by reducing ICP. Therefore, there does seem to be a role for the use of acute hyperventilation in a patient with a herniation syndrome. Based on these limited data, the present recommendation from the Guidelines for the Management of Severe Head Injury at the level of an Option reads as follows:

> The first priority for the head-injured patient is complete and rapid physiologic resuscitation. No specific treatment should be directed at intracranial hypertension in the absence of signs of transtentorial herniation or progressive neurological deterioration not attributable to extracranial explanations.
>
> When either signs of transtentorial herniation or progressive neurological deterioration are present, however, the physician should assume that intracranial hypertension is present and treat it aggressively. Hyperventilation should be rapidly established. The administration of mannitol is desirable, but only under conditions of adequate volume resuscitation (17).

HYPOTENSION—ITS CAUSES AND EFFECTS

Hypotension represents a relatively advanced stage of shock and is an ominous finding in the head-injured patient. It is also fairly prevalent, having occurred in 34.6% of patients in the Traumatic Coma Data Bank (10). Almost never is it caused by an isolated head injury. Rather, the most common culprit is hemorrhage from any of a number of extracranial injuries. In a series of 100 closed-head-injury patients, long bone and pelvic fractures were the most frequently associated extracranial injuries (29). A retroperitoneal hematoma caused by a pelvic fracture can lead to several liters of blood loss. Thoracic and abdominal visceral injuries must also be sought; 4 of the 100 patients had ruptured spleens. Of imminently life-threatening concern are other conditions such as tension pneumothorax and cardiac tamponade. In head-injured patients, it seems that the hypotension caused by many of these conditions, and not the conditions themselves, is the contributing factor to added morbidity and mortality. In fact, when the effects of hypotension are controlled for, the effects of extracranial injuries seem to contribute little to the neurological outcome (10).

Hypotension has devastating effects on head-injured patients, increasing the associated mortality from 27 to 60% (10). In Westmead, Australia, a prospective study of 315 patients with severe head injury found hypotension to be a significant predictor of death in these patients (15). When physiological variables were measured minute by minute in 124 adult head-injured patients in Scotland, the most significant predictor of mortality was the duration of hypotensive episodes (21). In yet another study, 66% of head-injured patients who experienced a hypotensive episode in the ICU setting had poor outcomes based on the GCS compared with 17% who did not (11). When hypotension occurred in the operating room, it increased mortality from 25% seen in normotensive patients to 82% in a series of blunt trauma victims with severe head injury (the GOS in this population inversely correlated with the duration of hypotension) (33). Many other studies have also confirmed the negative effects of hypotension on head injury (18, 20, 27, 28). It is clear that head-injured patients are more vulnerable to the deleterious effects of hypotension than trauma patients without head injuries. It is therefore recommended at the level of a Guideline that hypotension (systolic blood pressure < 90) be "scrupulously avoided, if possible, or corrected immediately" (17).

The harsh consequences of hypotension have implications for the order of treatment of extracranial injuries. For example, Townsend and colleagues found that head-injured patients who underwent early operative fixation of femur fractures were eight times more likely to develop hypotension than patients who had their surgery deferred for 24 hours (43). Among those patients operated on within 2 hours, in whom hypotension caused by intraabdominal or retroperitoneal bleeding could be excluded, 89% experienced hypotension during their procedure, prompting the authors to recommend delayed surgery for long bone fractures.

FLUID RESUSCITATION—HOW MUCH OF WHAT?

Dehydration was commonly used in the past in neurosurgical patients as a strategy to prevent the development of cerebral edema and elevated ICP. In the 1980s and beyond, fluid restriction was largely abandoned because of a perceived risk of hypotension and, perhaps, thrombosis. Current dogma recommends a state of euvolemia.

Advanced Trauma Life Support protocol currently dictates that hypotensive patients initially be resuscitated with a 2-L bolus of lactated Ringer's solution (1). However, isotonic fluids may not necessarily be the fluid of choice in patients with severe head injury. Many animal studies show that volume resuscitation with lactated Ringer's solution may actually increase ICP (37, 39, 51). The optimal fluid for resuscitation is, therefore, still under investigation. Many studies are now beginning to reveal the benefits of hypertonic solutions for this purpose. In patients with head injury, their effects on ICP are of particular interest.

Hypertonic saline solution has been demonstrated to decrease ICP when used for resuscitation in animal studies (5, 13, 14, 34, 35, 37, 39, 47, 51). The mechanism for this effect is not totally clear but seems to be related to its ability to decrease the cortical water content in areas of the brain with an intact blood-brain barrier. It also decreases cerebral vascular resistance by promoting cerebral vascular dilatation. Aside from its ICP reducing effect, it also expands the plasma volume and can be infused in small volumes (13).

Vassar et al. reported a controlled, double-blinded, multicenter trial that compared the efficacy of small volumes of hypertonic saline with lactated Ringer's solution as the initial resuscitation fluid in hypotensive trauma patients (45). Although there was an improvement in survival in the group resuscitated with hypertonic saline versus lactated Ringer's solution, it was not statistically significant. However, in patients with baseline GCS scores of 8 or less, there was a statistically significant improvement in survival to discharge—34% of patients treated with hypertonic saline versus 12% of those treated with lactated Ringer's solution.

Hypertonic solutions show promise for all trauma patients because of their ability to more effectively expand the plasma volume and increase oxygen delivery to peripheral tissues. They may prove to be even more suitable for multiple-trauma patients with head injury because of their cerebrovascular effects and their ability to decrease ICP.

PRIORITIZING—BRAIN VERSUS BODY

The hypotensive multiple-trauma patient with evidence of head injury poses a formidable diagnostic dilemma. Although a significant percentage of these patients will require a general surgical operation, a comparable number of severely head-injured patients will require early neurosurgical intervention. The effects of hypotension on the neurological examination further compound this problem. Neglecting to obtain an early CT scan in this population hinders the identification of those patients requiring placement of ICP monitors or urgent cerebral decompression. In light of the rapidity with which CT scans of the head can be obtained with modern spiral CT scanners, paradigms for the evaluation of hypotensive patients with CT scans must be updated. Although the need for immediate surgery in refractory hypotension is uncontested, less clear is the priority of treatment in patients who show favorable hemodynamic responses to initial resuscitation. One retrospective study of blunt trauma victims with hypotension found that there was no detriment in proceeding to computed tomography before a general surgical operation if the patient responded to fluid resuscitation (49). No patient who responded to initial fluid resuscitation experienced hemodynamic instability in the computed tomography suite, including 15 patients with a positive diagnostic peritoneal lavage (DPL). The rate of craniotomy was 19% for patients with a GCS score of less than 8 and 9% for those with a GCS between 8 and 13. This was comparable to the 19% rate of general surgical procedures. The authors therefore suggested that CT scanning of the head be a high priority in this group.

A DPL has been the usual test of choice in most centers in the evaluation of the multiple-trauma patient with an altered sensorium (6, 9). However, with more rapid CT scanners now available, this may be replaced in some cases with a CT scan of the abdomen performed simultaneously with the head study. Abdominal ultrasound is also used in some centers to rule out abdominal hemorrhage. Thus, all three modalities have their proponents. However, from the neurosurgical perspective, the more difficult question is how to prioritize between an abdominal study and a head CT scan. An algorithm (*Fig. 9.1*) that we had originally suggested has now been adopted by Advanced Trauma Life Support (44).

TIMING OF SURGERY—CAN IT WAIT?

Cerebral decompression for intracranial mass lesions can be life saving. Urgent evacuation has been advocated for acute extra-axial hematomas that are at least 1 cm in thickness. In general, extra-axial hematomas that are at least 5 mm in thickness and associated with 5 mm or more of midline shift should also be quickly removed (22). Although the trauma that produces acute mass lesions may also cause direct, irreversible brain damage, rapid decompression can reduce the likelihood of transtentorial herniation caused by expanding mass lesions and help reduce elevated intracranial pressure. Seelig and col-

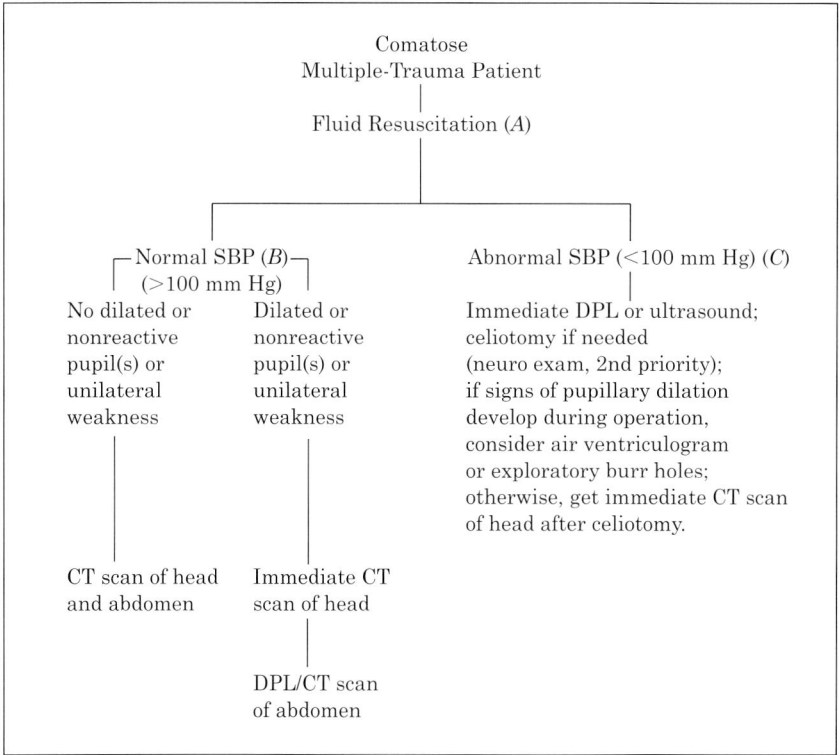

FIG. 9.1 DPL versus ultrasound versus CT scan in head-injured patients. (A) All comatose, head-injured patients will undergo resuscitation (ABCDEs) at the time of arrival in the ER. (B) In borderline cases (i.e., when the SBP can be temporarily corrected but tends to slowly decrease), every effort should be made to get a head CT scan before taking the patient to the operating room for celiotomy. Such cases call for careful clinical judgment and cooperation between the trauma surgeon and the neurosurgeon. As soon as blood pressure is normalized, a minineurological examination is performed (GCS and pupillary reaction). If the blood pressure cannot be normalized, the neurological examination is still performed and the hypotension recorded. (C) If the patient's SBP cannot be brought up to >100 mm Hg despite aggressive fluid resuscitation, the priority is to establish the cause of the hypotension, with the neurosurgical evaluation taking second priority. In such cases, the patient undergoes a DPL or ultrasound in the ER or may need to go directly to the operating room for a celiotomy. CT scan of the head is obtained after the celiotomy. If there is clinical evidence of an intracranial mass, an air ventriculogram, exploratory burr holes, or craniotomy may be undertaken in the operating room while the celiotomy is being performed. If the patient's SBP is >100 mm Hg after resuscitation and the patient has clinical evidence of a possible intracranial mass (unequal pupils, asymmetric motor examination), the first priority is to obtain a CT head scan. A DPL or ultrasound may be performed in the ER, CT area, or operating room, but the patient's neurological evaluation or treatment should not be delayed. Adapted with permission from Reference 44.

leagues performed a review of 82 consecutive comatose patients who underwent craniotomy for evacuation of an acute traumatic subdural hematoma (38). They found that the mortality rate for patients decreased from 90% for those operated on after 4 hours of trauma to approximately 30% for those operated on within 4 hours. Although Wilberger et al. in a subsequent study did not find quite as dramatic an association between early surgical intervention and decreased mortality, a trend toward improvement was nevertheless noted (48). Prompt surgical intervention has intuitive appeal and is recommended for severely head-injured patients who harbor significant traumatic extra-axial hematomas.

CONCLUSIONS

Although much as been learned regarding the pathophysiology of head injury, much remains to be established regarding the acute management of this condition. Much of what we know is based on anecdotal evidence, retrospective data, or expert opinion. Available evidence points to the following broad conclusions:

1. Neurosurgeons should remain actively involved in the planning and delivery of neuotrauma care.
2. In isolated instances, general surgeons may need to perform decompressive surgery. If so, they should become appropriately trained.
3. Every effort should be made to obtain an accurate neurological examination before intubation. The GCS is often inaccurately assessed.
4. Paralysis should be used only when necessary, and short-acting agents should be employed.
5. Hyperventilation should be used only in the face of transtentorial herniation. PCO_2 levels of less than 25 mm Hg should be avoided whenever possible.
6. Hypotension should be detected and corrected very quickly because it is strongly associated with poorer outcomes.
7. Normal saline is the currently recommended resuscitative fluid, although hypertonic saline may have some future role. Hypotonic fluids should be avoided.
8. A CT scan of the head and a CT scan, DPL, or ultrasound of the abdomen should be obtained as quickly as possible after resuscitation of the severe head-injury patient.
9. A significant intracranial mass lesion (typically one causing 5 mm or more of midline shift) should be promptly evacuated.
10. Surgery for long bone fractures should be deferred for at least a few

hours, if not longer, because of a significant risk of intraoperative hypotension and the associated poorer neurological outcomes.

REFERENCES

1. American College of Surgeons Committee on Trauma (ACS COT): Advanced trauma life support—Course for physicians. 1998.
2. American College of Surgeons Committee on Trauma (ASC COT): Resources for optimal care of the injured patient: 1993. Chicago: American College of Surgeons, 1993.
3. American College of Surgeons Committee on trauma (ACS COT): Resources for optimal care of the injured patient: 1998. Chicago: American College of Surgeons, 1998.
4. Andrews BT, Narayan RK: Editorial. **Surg Neurology,** 40:1–2, 1993.
5. Berger S, Schurer L, Hartl R, Messmer K, Baethmann A: Reduction of post-traumatic intracranial hypertension by hyperoncotic/peroncotic saline/dextran and hypertonic mannitol. **Neurosurgery** 37:98–108, 1995.
6. Blow C, Bassam D, Butler K, et al: Speed and efficiency in the resuscitation of blunt trauma patients with multiple injuries: The advantage of diagnostic peritoneal lavage over abdominal computerized tomography. **J Trauma** 44:287–290, 1998.
7. Bouma GJ, Muizelaar JP, Choi SC, et al: Cerebral blood flow and metabolism after severe traumatic brain injury. The elusive role of ischemia. **J Neurosurg** 75:685–693, 1991.
8. Bouma GJ, Muizelaar JP, Stringer WA, et al: Ultra-early evaluation of regional cerebral blood flow in severely head-injured patients using stable xenon-enhanced computed tomography. **J Neurosurg** 77:360–368, 1992.
9. Butterworth JF, IV, Maull KI, Miller JD, et al: Detection of occult abdominal trauma in patients with severe head injuries. **Lancet** 2:759–762, 1980.
10. Chesnut RM, Marshall LF, Klauber MR, et al: The role of secondary brain injury in determining outcome from severe head injury. **J Trauma** 34:216–222, 1993.
11. Chesnut RM, Marshall SB, Piek J, Blunt BA, Klauber MR, Marshall LF: Early and late systemic hypotension as a frequent and fundamental source of cerebral ischemia following severe brain injury in the Traumatic Coma Data Bank. **Acta Neurochir Suppl (Wien)** 59:121–125, 1993.
12. Cruz J: An additional therapeutic effect of adequate hyperventilation in severe acute brain trauma: normalization of cerebral glucose uptake. **J Neurosurg** 82:379–385, 1995.
13. Ducey JP, Mozingo DW, Lamiell JM, Okerburg C, Gueller GE: A comparison of the cerebral and cardiovascular effects of complete resuscitation with isotonic and hypertonic saline, hetastarch, and whole blood following hemorrhage. **J Trauma** 29:1510–1517, 1989.
14. Favre JB, Ravussin P, Chiolero R, Bissonnette B: Hypertonic solutions and intracranial pressure. **Schweiz Med Wochensch** 126:1635–43, 1996.
15. Fearnside MR, Cook RJ, McDougall P, McNeil R: The Westmead Head Injury Project outcome in severe head injury. A comparative analysis of pre-hospital, clinical and CT variables. **B J Neurosurg** 7:267–279, 1993.
16. Gentleman D: Causes and effects of systemic complications among severely head injured patients transferred to a neurosurgical unit. **Int Surg** 77:297–302, 1992.
17. Guidelines for the management of severe head injury. Brain Trauma Foundation,

American Association of Neurological Surgeons, Joint Section on Neurotrauma and Critical Care. **J Neurotrauma** 13:641–734, 1996.
18. Hill DA, Abraham KJ, West RH: Factors affecting outcome in the resuscitation of severely injured patients. **Aust N Z J Surg** 63:604–609, 1993.
19. Hsiang JK, Chesnut RM, Crisp CB, Klauber MR, Blunt BA, Marshall LF: Early, routine paralysis for intracranial pressure control in severe head injury: Is it necessary? **Crit Care Med** 22:1471–1476, 1994.
20. Jeffreys RV, Jones JJ: Avoidable factors contributing to the death of head injury patients in general hospitals in Mersey Region. Lancet 2:459–461, 1981.
21. Jones PA, Andrews JD, Midgley S, et al: Measuring the burden of secondary insults in head-injured patients during intensive care. **J Neurosurg Anesthesiol** 6:4–14, 1994.
22. Kelly DF, Doberstein C, Becker DP: General principles of head injury management, in Narayan RK, Wilberger JE, Povlishock JT (eds): **Neurotrauma.** New York, McGraw-Hill, pp 84–85, 1996.
23. Kelly DF, Goodale DB, Williams J, Herr D, et al: Propofol in the treatment of moderate and severe head injury: A randomized, prospective double blinded pilot trial. **J Neurosurg** 90:1042–1052, 1999.
24. Lucas CE, Dombi GW, Crilly RJ, Ledgerwood AM, Pingyang Y, Vlahos A: Neurosurgical trauma call: Use of a mathematical simulation program to define manpower needs. **J Trauma** 42:818–824, 1997.
25. Marion DW, Bouma GJ: The use of stable xenon-enhanced computed tomography studies of cerebral blood flow to define changes in cerebral carbon dioxide vasoresponsivity caused by severe head injury. **Neurosurgery** 29:869–873, 1991.
26. Marion DW, Carlier PM: Problems with initial Glasgow coma scale assessment caused by prehospital treatment of patients with head injuries: Results of a national survey. **J Trauma** 36:89–95, 1994.
27. Marmarou A, Anderson RL, Ward JD, et al: Impact of ICP instability and hypotension on outcome in patients with severe head trauma. **J Neurosurg** 75:S59–S66, 1991.
28. Miller JD, Becker DP: Secondary insults to the injured brain. **J R Coll Surg Edinb** 27:292–298, 1982.
29. Miller JD, Sweet RC, Narayan RK, Becker DP: Early insults to the injured brain. **JAMA** 240(5):439–442, 1978.
30. Mitchell FL, Thal ER, Wolferth CC: Analysis of American College of Surgeons Trauma Consultation Program. **Arch Surg** 130:578–584, 1995.
31. Muizelaar JP, Marmarou A, Ward JD, et al: Adverse effects of prolonged hyperventilation in patients with severe head injury: A randomized clinical trial. **J Neurosurg** 75:731–739, 1991 (abstr).
32. Narayan RK: Development of guidelines for the management of severe head injury. **J Neurotrauma** 12:907–912, 1995.
33. Pietropaoli JA, Rogers FB, Shackford SR, Wald SL, Schmoker JD, Zhuang J: The deleterious effects of intraoperative hypotension on outcome in patients with severe head injuries. **J Trauma** 33:403–407, 1992.
34. Prough DS, Johnson JC, Poole GV, Stullken EH, Johnston WE, Royster R: Effects on intracranial pressure of resuscitation from hemorrhagic shock with hypertonic saline versus lactacted Ringer's solution. **Crit Care Med** 13:407–411, 1985.
35. Prough DS, Whitley JM, Taylor CL, Deal DD, DeWitt DS: Regional cerebral blood flow following resuscitation from hemorrhagic shock with hypertonic fluid. Anesthesiology 75:319–327, 1991.

36. Rinker CF, McMurry FG, Groeneweg VR, Bahnson FF, Banks K, Gannon DM: Emergency craniotomy in a rural level III trauma center. **J Trauma** 44:984–989, 1998. (Discussion 989–990)
37. Schmoker JD, Zhuang J, Shackford SR: Hypertonic fluid resuscitation improves cerebral oxygen delivery and reduces intracranial pressure after hemorrhagic shock. **J Trauma** 31:1607–1612, 1991.
38. Seelig JM, Becker DP, Miller JD, et al: Traumatic acute subdural hematoma: Major mortality reduction in comatose patients treated within four hours. **N Engl J Med** 304:1511–1518, 1981.
39. Shackford SR, Zhuang J, Schmoker J: Intravenous fluid tonicity: Effect on intracranial pressure, cerebral blood flow, and cerebral oxygen delivery in focal brain injury. **J Neurosurg** 76:91–98, 1992.
40. Sheinberg M, Kanter MJ, Robertson CS, Contant CF, Narayan RK, Grossman RG: Continuous monitoring of jugular venous oxygen saturation in head-injured patients. **J Neurosurg** 76:212–217, 1992.
41. Singbartl G: Eid Bedeutung der praklinischen Notfallversorgung fur die Prognose von Patienten mit schwerem Schadel-Hirn-Trauma. **Anasthiol Intensivmed Notfallmed Schmerzther** 20:251–260, 1985.
42. Specialty coverage in hospital emergency departments. A report by the office of the Inspector General: Washington, DC, Department of Health and Human Services, August 1992.
43. Townsend RN, Lheureau T, Protetch J, Riemer B, Simon D: Timing fracture repair in patients with severe brain injury (Glasgow coma score < 9). **J Trauma** 44:977–983, 1998.
44. Valadka AB, Narayan RK: Emergency room management of the head injured patient, in Narayan RK, Wilberger JE, Povlishock. JT (eds): **Neurotrauma.** New York, McGraw-Hill, 1996, pp 126–127.
45. Vassar MJ, Fischer RP, O'Brien PE, et al: A multicenter trial for resuscitation of injured patients with 7.5% sodium chloride: The effect of added dextram 70. **Arch Surg** 128:1003–1013, 1993.
46. Vicario SJ, Coleman R, Cooper MA, Thomas DM: Ventilatory status after head injury. **Ann Emerg Med** 12:145–148, 1983.
47. Walsh JC, Zhuang J, Shackford SR: A comparison of hypertonic to isotonic fluid in the resuscitation of brain injury and hemorrhagic shock. **J Surg Res** 50:284–292, 1991.
48. Wilberger JE, Harris M, Diamond DL: Acute subdural hematoma: Morbidity and mortality related to timing of operative intervention. **J Trauma** 30:733–736, 1990.
49. Winchell RJ, Hoyt DB, Simons RK: Use of computed tomography of the head in the hypotensive blunt-trauma patient. **Ann Emerg Med** 25:737–742, 1995.
50. Wisner DH, Schuster L, Quinn C: Hypertonic saline resuscitation of head-injury: Effects on cerebral water content. **J Trauma** 30:75–78, 1990.
51. Zornow MH, Scheller MS, Shackford SR: Effect of a hypertonic lactated Ringer's solution on intracranial pressure and cerebral water content in a model of traumatic brain injury. **J Trauma** 29:484–488, 1989.

CHAPTER

10

Contemporary Treatment Paradigms in Head Injury

JACK E. WILBERGER, M.D.

Head injury remains a serious public health problem, occurring at a rate of 150 per 100,000 population per year in the United States. The most current data indicate that head injury accounts for over 20,000 deaths and 50,000 permanent disabilities each year (5, 9). With an understanding of the mechanisms of secondary injury and development of appropriate treatment strategies, there has been a significant decline in head injury mortality over the past two decades (*Fig. 10.1*). Indeed, contemporary multicenter studies are reporting mortality rates as low as 17% (13). In this regard, two important questions remain unanswered: Can such favorable outcomes be achieved outside rigorous scientific studies in routine clinical practice, and can treatment strategies be developed to further improve outcomes?

It is likely that adherence to the management principles enumerated in the *Guidelines for the Management of Severe Head Injury* coupled with the concept of targeted therapy and improved brain monitoring will result in a sustained lowering of mortality after head injury. Such principles and technologies can now be readily applied in most current neurosurgical practice settings. For the future, however, improved outcomes may require refocusing attention on neuroprotective agents and identification of the genetic factors resulting in repair and recovery after head injury.

SECONDARY INJURY

One of the singular advancements in the treatment of head injury has been the understanding of the concept that a large number of patients die not because of the initial injury to the brain but entirely because of additional, secondary insults that occur following injury (4, 11).

The Traumatic Coma Data Bank has clearly shown that hypoxia and hypotension are frequent secondary insults, which, in combination, may more than double mortality. Hypotension (systolic blood pressure

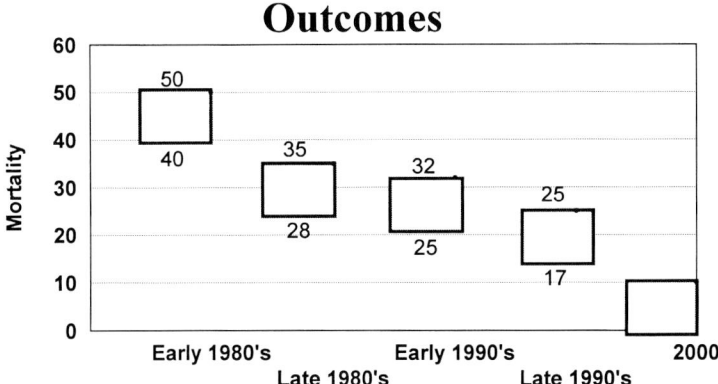

FIG. 10.1 Comparative head injury mortality rates from 1980 to 1998 based on contemporary published studies.

less than 90 mm Hg) occurring one time in the prehospital/emergency room phase will increase mortality by 50%. More recently, it has been shown that hypotension occurring any time during the critical care phase of management of severe head injury will significantly adversely impact outcome (4, 20).

The biochemical substrates of secondary injury have been extensively investigated. A cascade of events is triggered shortly after injury having a variable time course and effect. This cascade is multifactorial, interrelated, and, to some extent, time dependent (1–3, 18).

More recently, investigators have focused on the genetic response to head injury. The research so far has been primarily descriptive in nature; however, a number of genes have been found to be up- or down-regulated after ischemia and trauma (6, 7).

Although the concept of secondary injury is valid and generally applicable in a given head injury patient, it must be borne in mind that head injury is structurally, physiologically, metabolically, and biochemically heterogeneous. Additionally, the factors that may be operative in any one patient may vary from one time period to another. For example, a recent study demonstrated that autoregulation may be present, absent, or altered in the same head-injured patient at various intervals of assessment (12). Such information is vitally important as some forms of current treatment take advantage of the presence (i.e., cerebral perfusion pressure management) or absence (i.e., barbiturates) of autoregulation.

Thus, the heterogeneity of head injury and the patient-dependent features of secondary injury provide a further challenge to develop more sophisticated monitoring systems and to be able to modify treatments based on patient-specific parameters.

TREATMENT STRATEGIES

The treatment principles of the 1980s were based on the concept of preventing/minimizing cerebral edema through fluid restriction, neuroprotection using chronic prophylactic hyperventilation and steroids, and minimizing secondary injury by monitoring and treating elevated intracranial pressure.

A better understanding of the elements of secondary injury have led to a virtually complete revolution in basic treatment tenets. Adequate fluid resuscitation to prevent hypotension, intracranial pressure monitoring as a means of maximizing cerebral perfusion pressure, and avoidance of hyperventilation are now first-line treatment strategies.

A codification of current treatment principles can be found in the *Guidelines for the Management of Severe Head Injury* (10).

GUIDELINES FOR THE MANAGEMENT OF SEVERE HEAD INJURY

The guidelines for the management of severe head injury were developed with an evidence-based approach. All pertinent clinical literature for the past 20 years was assessed, reviewed, and classified on the basis of the following methodology: Class I evidence—prospective, randomized, controlled clinical trials; Class II evidence—clinical studies with prospective data collection, such as case control studies, cohort studies, or retrospective analyses based on reliable data; and Class III evidence—retrospective data collection, such as clinical series, databases, case reviews, and expert opinion.

Each article assessed in this process was then carefully studied with respect to design and methodology to ascertain the reliability of its findings. This evidence was then weighed to determine the level of certainty that could be determined that a particular treatment or intervention in question would positively affect patient outcome. This level of certainty was then expressed as a Standard, Guideline, or Option with respect to patient management strategies: Standard, accepted principles of patient management that reflect a high degree of clinical certainty; Guideline, recommendations that reflect a particular strategy or range of management strategies with a moderate degree of clinical certainty; Option, all remaining strategies for patient management for which there is unclear clinical certainty.

Generally, standards can only be supported by high quality, Class I evidence. The lack of such studies in current neurotrauma literature is reflected in the fact that the guidelines promulgate only three standards in the entire document.

The *Guidelines* have attempted to comprehensively address the clinical management of adult closed head injury from initial resuscitation through the critical care phase of management (*Fig. 10.2*). Fifteen separate sections address individual treatment considerations, and perti-

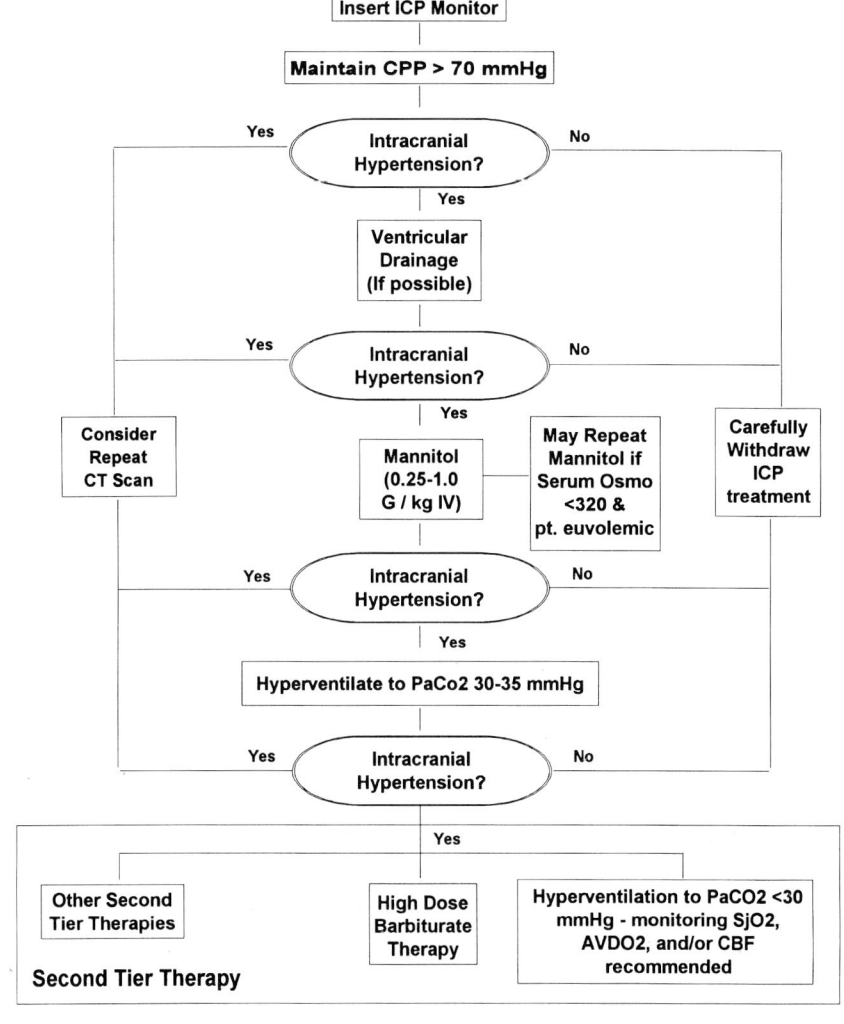

FIG. 10.2 Treatment algorithm for the management of increased intracranial pressure based on the *Guidelines for the Management of Severe Head Injury*.

nent examples are provided for each. Each recommendation is supported by a detailed explanation of the available scientific evidence, evidentiary tables, and recommendations for future research.

The *Guidelines* have recently been revised to reflect new scientific literature that has become available since their publication in 1996. Additional chapters to be added include prognostic indicators and pediatric head injury.

TARGETED THERAPY

A logical extension of the *Guidelines* is the concept of targeted therapy—treating a specific patient's specific pathophysiology. Such an approach requires pertinent and contemporaneous information based on systemic and cerebral monitoring.

An excellent example of this approach is directed management to maintain cerebral perfusion pressure greater than 70 mm Hg (*Fig. 10.3*). Such a goal requires intracranial pressure and systolic blood pressure monitoring. However, once established, a variety of targeted approaches can be brought into play. Preliminary information suggests that this approach improves head injury outcome, and it is one of the most widely used strategies for the treatment of head injury today (22, 23).

Another example of targeted therapy is the avoidance of impaired cerebral oxygenation either due to a decrease in oxygen delivery or an

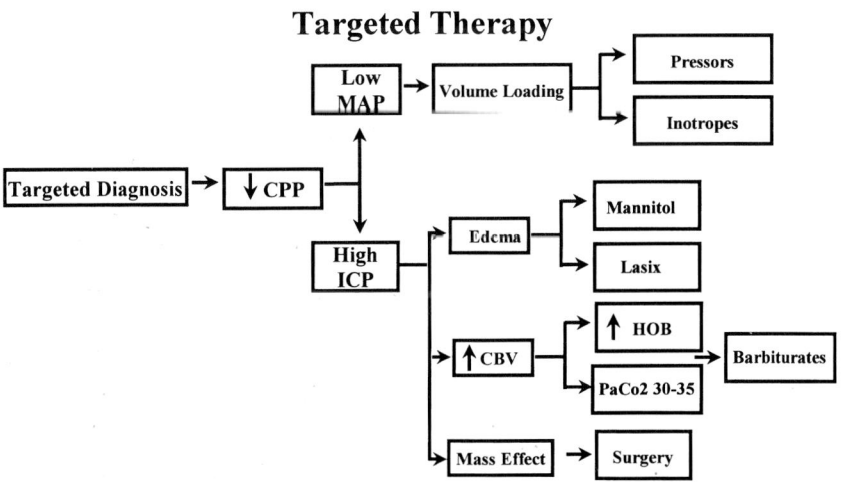

FIG. 10.3 Targeted therapeutic approach to the management of cerebral perfusion pressure.

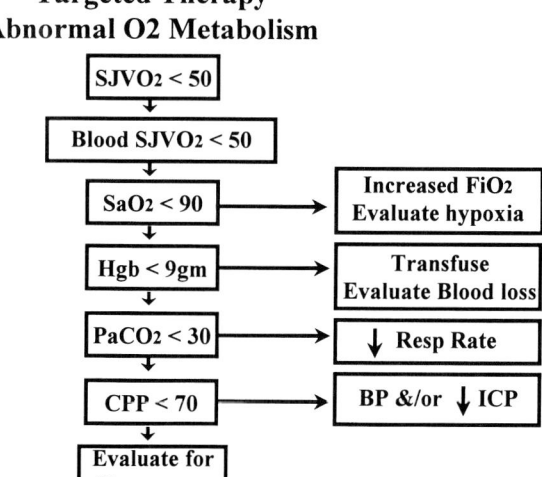

FIG. 10.4 Targeted therapeutic approach for the management of impaired cerebral oxygenation.

increase in oxygen consumption. This approach currently requires monitoring of jugular venous oxygen saturation in addition to a variety of other systemic variables. The identification of oxygen desaturation allows for targeted therapy to correct its source (*Fig. 10.4*). A number of studies have indicated that optimization of blood flow and metabolism through monitoring and normalization of cerebral oxygenation influences outcome (8, 15, 17).

However, it is clear that current clinically available monitoring technology is not sufficiently sensitive to adequately characterize the physiologic, metabolic, and biochemical response to injury in a given patient. New treatment paradigms will require considerably more technological development in this area.

This has led to the concept of multimodality cerebral monitoring. On an experimental and limited clinical basis, it is now possible to measure and monitor brain PO_2 and pH levels, as well as certain biochemical markers using microdialysis (19). Such multimodality monitoring may provide the insight necessary to refine treatment on a patient and time-specific basis. Ultimately, specific neuroprotective strategies may prove more feasible and successful by selectively targeting populations at risk.

NEUROPROTECTION

Considerable effort has been expended in the past decade defining and testing pharmacological agents, which potentially hold great promise in blocking or ameliorating various components of the secondary injury biochemical cascade (14). Despite extremely encouraging experimental animal studies to date, no human trial has proven successful; currently, there is only one ongoing trial in head injury (*Fig. 10.5*). There are a number of speculations as to the reasons for the failure to identify a clinically active compound. The two most pertinent concerns are an inability to appropriately target the population of patients most likely to benefit from such an intervention and the unrealistic pro-

Trial	# pts	Mechanism	Current Status
Triamcinolone	396	Free radical scavenger steroid	Published 1995 Res Exp Med vol 195 (-) overall effect (+) effect contusions
PEG-SOD	463	Free radical scavenger superoxide dismutase	Published 1996 JAMA vol 276 (+) favorable outcome p>0.05
Tirilizad European	1120	Free radical scavenger aminosteroid	Complete, unpublished (-) effect
US	1155		Complete, unpublished (-) effect
Selfotel International	427	NMDA antagonist	Halted 1996 safety concerns efficacy futility
USA	266	NMDA antagonist	Halted 1996
Cerestat	400	NMDA antagonist	Halted 1997 efficacy futility
P-1006	700	N2B NMDA subunit antagonist	ongoing
Hypothermia	800	Multiple	Halted 1997

FIG. 10.5 Current clinical trials in neuroprotection.

jections of the magnitude of benefit that these agents might provide (13, 16, 26).

Nevertheless, if a patient could be identified who clearly had a specific biochemical alteration associated with their head injury pathophysiology (i.e., excess glutamate release in association with a cerebral contusion), s/he could then be targeted for treatment with the appropriate pharmacological agent in the appropriate time frame.

Unless such strategies become practical, it is unlikely that the field of neuroprotection will advance significantly beyond its present state.

GENE THERAPY

The ultimate substrate of CNS response to injury and repair is genetically mediated. Investigators are currently uncovering large amounts of information concerning the central nervous system genetic response to trauma and ischemia (*Fig. 10.6*). Although most studies have been descriptive in nature and their relevance to recovery, if any, unknown, increasing efforts are being expended not only to quantify this response but to manipulate it as well (21, 24, 25).

The ultimate treatment strategy, therefore, would be to down-regulate those genes responsible for the harmful biochemical cascade occurring after injury and to up-regulate those genes responsible for repair and recovery.

Given current research, such seems an attainable goal within the next decade.

Gene	Class	Product Formation	Activation
C-fos / jun	IEG	transcription	neuronal
hsp 70	stress protein	molecular chaperone	neuronal
gfap	intermediate	cytoskeleton	astrocyte
TGF - $B1$	cytokine	neuroprotective	microglia
NGF / FGF	neurotrophins	protection / repair	neurons / glia
B APP	amyloid precursor	membrane stabilization	neurons / glia
Apo E	apolipoprotein	lipid remodeling	glia

FIG. 10.6 Characterization of the genetic response to trauma and ischemia.

STRATEGIES FOR THE MILLENNIUM

Marked improvements have occurred in the recognition and management of severe head injury with concomitant improvements in outcome. The majority of these accomplishments have evolved through greater attention to the details of critical care management of this patient population. More sophisticated monitoring technology has further enhanced the timely identification and reaction to evolving pathophysiology and metabolic derangements. These advancements have been codified in the *Guidelines for the Management of Severe Head Injury*. The concept of targeted therapy is a logical extension of the *Guidelines* to provide for more patient-specific intervention. Ultimately, identification of patient-specific biochemical and genetic responses to injury will allow for a complete understanding of the secondary injury process with the concomitant opportunity to provide the ultimate form of neuroprotection from head injury.

REFERENCES

1. Baker AJ, Moulton RJ, Macmillan VH, et al.: Excitatory amino acids in cerebrospinal fluid following traumatic brain injury in humans. **J Neurosurg** 79: 369–372, 1993.
2. Bullock R, Zauner A, Myseros JS, et al.: Evidence for prolonged release of excitatory amino acids in severe human head trauma: Relationship to clinical events. **Ann NY Acad Sci** 17:290–298, 1995.
3. Bullock R, Zauner A, Woodward JJ: Factors affecting excitatory amino acid release following human head injury. **J Neurosurg** 89:507–518, 1998.
4. Chesnut RM, Marshall LF, Klauber MR, et al.: The role of secondary brain injury in determining outcome from severe head injury. **J Trauma** 34:216–222, 1993.
5. Commission on Professional, and Hospital Activities: The international classification of diseases, ninth revision: Clinical modification (ICD.9.CM). Ann Arbor: Commission on Professional and Hospital Activities, 1986.
6. DeKosky ST, Goss JR, Miller PD, et al.: Up regulation of nerve growth factor following cortical trauma. **Exp Neurol** 130:173–177, 1994.
7. Dutcher SA, Underwood BD, Walker PD, et al.: Patterns of heat shock protein-70 biosynthesis following human traumatic brain injury. **J Neurotrauma** 15:411–419, 1998.
8. Gopinath SP, Robertson CS, Contant CF, et al.: Jugular venous desaturation and outcome after head injury. **J Neurol Neurosurg Psychiatry** 57:717–723, 1994.
9. Graves E: Detailed diagnoses and procedures: National Hospital Discharge Survey, 1990. **Vital Health Stat** 13:113, 1992.
10. Guidelines for the Management of Severe Head Injury. American Association of Neurological Surgeons. Chicago, Illinois, 1996.
11. Jones PA, Andrews PJD, Midgely S, et al.: Measuring the burden of secondary insults in head injured patients during intensive care. **J Neurosurg Anesthesiol** 6:4–14, 1994.
12. Junger EC, Newell DW, Grant GA, et al.: Cerebral autoregulation following minor head injury. **J Neurosurg** 86:425–432, 1997.

13. Marshall LF, Maas AIR, Marshall SB, et al.: A multicenter trial on the efficacy of using tirilazad mesylate in cases of head injury. **J Neurosurg** 89:519–525, 1998.
14. McIntosh TK: Novel pharmacologic therapies in the treatment of experimental traumatic brain injury: A review. **J Neurotrauma** 10:215–222, 1993.
15. Messeter K, Nordstrom CH, Sundbarg G, et al.: Cerebral hemodynamics in patients with acute severe head trauma. **J Neurosurg** 64:231–237, 1986.
16. Murray GD, Teasdale GM, Schmitz H: Nimodopine in traumatic subarachnoid hemorrhage: A reanalysis of the HIT I and HIT II trials. **Acta Neurochir** 138:1163–1167, 1996.
17. Obrist WD, Langfitt T, Jaggi J, Cruz J, Gennarelli TA: Cerebral blood flow and metabolism in comatose patients with acute head injury: Relationship to intracranial hypertension. **J Neurosurg** 61:241–253, 1984.
18. Palmer AM, Marion DW, Botscheller ML, et al.: Increased transmitter amino acid concentration in human ventricular CSF after brain trauma. **NeuroReport** 6:153–156, 1994.
19. Persson L, Hillered L: Chemical monitoring of neurosurgical intensive care patients using intracerebral microdialysis. **J Neurosurg** 76:72–80, 1992.
20. Pietropaoli JA, Rogers FB, Shackford SR, et al.: The deleterious effects of intraoperative hypotension on outcome in patients with severe head injuries. **J Trauma** 33:403–407, 1992.
21. Raghupathi R, Welsh SA, Lowenstein DH, et al.: Regional induction of C-Fos and heat shock protein-72 MRNA following fluid percussion brain injury in the rat. **J Cereb Blood Flow Metab** 15:467–573, 1995.
22. Rosner M: Cerebral perfusion pressure: Link between intracranial pressure and systemic circulation, in Wood JH (ed): *Cerebral Blood Flow.* New York, McGraw Hill, 1987, pp 425–448.
23. Rosner MJ, Coley IB: Cerebral perfusion pressure, intracranial pressure in head elevation. **J Neurosurg** 65:636–641, 1986.
24. Sheng M, Greenberg ME: The regulation and function of C-Fos and other immediate early genes in the nervous system. **Neuron** 4:477–485, 1989.
25. Shohami E, Novikov M, Bass R, et al.: Closed head injury triggers early production of TNFα and IL-6 by brain tissue. **J Cereb Blood Flow Metab** 14:615–619, 1994.
26. Young B, Runge JW, Wilberger JE, et al.: Effect of pegorgotein on neurological outcome of patients with severe head injury: A multicenter randomized controlled trial. **JAMA** 276:538–543, 1996.

CHAPTER

11

Contemporary Treatment Paradigms in Spinal Injury

MICHAEL P. B. KILBURN, M.D., AND MARK N. HADLEY, M.D.

The focus of this article is the neurosurgeon's role in the triage and management of patients who have sustained cranial or spinal trauma, or both. This is an important topic for neurosurgeons. It is especially relevant when we consider the efforts of a variety of other groups in organized medicine, both at local and national levels, to relieve neurosurgeons of these responsibilities, thereby advancing their own agendas and enhancing their own positions as medical providers of trauma care services.

NEUROTRAUMA, INCLUDING BOTH CRANIAL AND SPINAL INJURIES, IS THE NEUROSURGEON'S DOMAIN

No individual group of medical specialists or providers is better trained, experienced, and more able to manage the potential complexities of craniospinal injury. We understand the anatomy and physiology and, because we do the research, the known pathophysiology of these injuries. No one is better equipped to assess and treat brain or spinal cord injury, skull fracture, or vertebral column dislocation than the neurological surgeon. Not only are we uniquely qualified to repair, decompress, realign, and stabilize the myriad of injuries that occur to the skulls and spines, the brains and spinal cords, and the nerves of trauma patients, but we are the only providers who can potentially have a positive impact on neurological outcome following these injuries. Our point here is that *"end-of-workup"* treatment is not all that we should provide. Neurosurgical involvement early in the assessment process, involvement in triage, and the preliminary management of patients with craniospinal injury can facilitate neuroprotective efforts, immobilization, and rapid realignment of the vertebral column. It enables neurosurgeons and can insist on the priority of the central nervous system (CNS) injury in the combined management scheme for an individual patient, often resulting in improved neurological outcome, compared

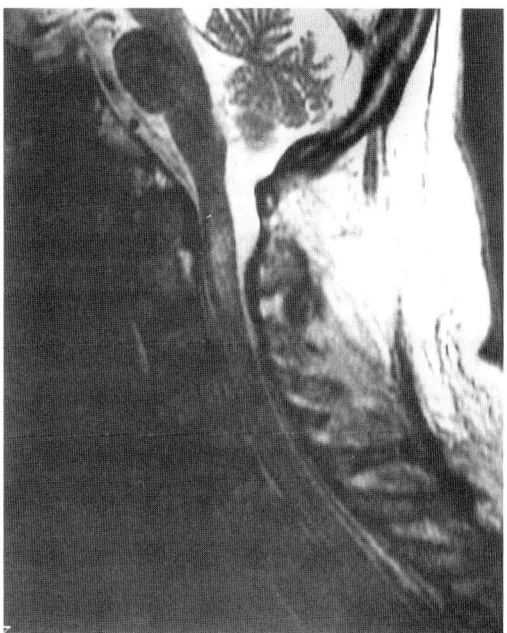

FIG. 11.1 Lateral MR of cervical spine reveals displaced dens fracture and underlying spinal cord injury. The initial lateral cervical spine x-ray revealed normal alignment, but the neurosurgeon in the emergency department was suspicious of a C2 fracture in this before surgery for long bone fractures.

with delayed neurosurgical involvement once the laparotomy is complete or the long bone fractures have been set (*Fig. 11.1*). It is our view that neurological injuries, including skull and spinal trauma, are the responsibility of the neurological surgeon, not the oral-maxillofacial or ear, nose, and throat surgeon, the trauma surgeon, the PM and R physician, the neurologist or the orthopedic surgeon. Our involvement in the management of these patients must be responsible and reliable, comprehensive, and must occur early after injury.

This is bigger than local turf issues, inadequate reimbursement, and demanding call coverage. This is about neurosurgeons stepping up and doing what we must do, not solely for the sake of our profession but also for the sake of our patients.

Neurosurgeons have been at the forefront in the management of spinal injuries since the origin of our profession. We have had a keen interest in spinal cord injury since Hippocrates (14). We developed the means to provide craniospinal traction (halter, Crutchfield, Gardner-

Wells) (5, 18, 60, 61). We performed many of the original operations in an attempt to decompress the spinal cord (7, 37) and reconstruct the human spinal column (4, 27, 44, 49, 59).

Neurosurgeons have been involved in the basic research of spinal cord injury and are presently at work attempting to unlock the complexities of the secondary injury process in the pursuit of effective, timely integrated treatment. A great deal of progress has been made, but we are far from accomplishing our goals. What follows this morning is not so much a "how we do it" approach to the management of patients with spinal and spinal cord injuries but the fundamentals and rationale behind the contemporary management of patients with acute spinal cord injury (SCI). We will not venture into potential therapies or promising research but attempt instead to define the best possible treatment paradigm available to our patients today.

Fractures and Fracture Dislocations

One cannot discuss the management of traumatic spinal cord injury without considering the vertebral column that houses it and, in less severe injury circumstances, protects it. The vertebral column is a mobile, multisegmented skeletal support structure held together by a variety of ligamentous structures, some spanning the length of the spine, others providing local and regional segmental support. Cartilaginous intervertebral discs separate individual bony segment, firmly attached circumferentially by Sharpe's fibers to the body above and the body below. When sufficient traumatic force is applied to the vertebral column, normal range of motion is exceeded, ligamentous structures stretch to failure, intervertebral discs distort and can rupture, and individual bony segments may fracture, collapse, and/or translate one on another. Fractures or fracture-dislocation injuries of the vertebral column cause pain, can result in deformity, and often cause instability, independent of their effect on the spinal cord and nerve roots (*Figs. 11.2 and 11.3*). If the spinal injury has not resulted in a frank cord injury, the potential for the latter is often great, owing to compression of the spinal cord from bone, disc, or hematoma. Spinal instability could also potentially at some later moment result in spinal cord compression (*Fig. 11.4*).

The hallmarks of contemporary spinal column injury management are *rapid detection, immobilization,* and *early reduction of the spinal deformity*. This "contemporary strategy" has not always been so. As recently as 12 years ago, neurosurgeons argued that early reduction, via open or closed means, did not impact outcome (58).

In 1986, Dennis Maiman and Sanford Larson suggested that neurosurgeons reconsider how they manage spine fractures, particularly bi-

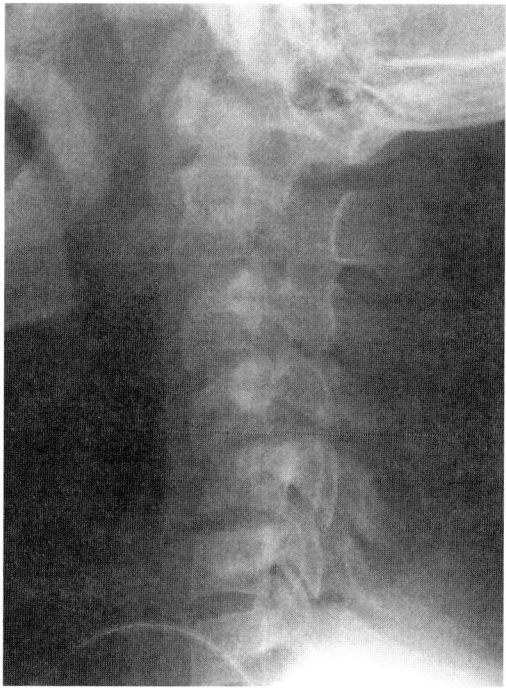

FIG. 11.2 Lateral cervical spine x-ray reveals C4-C5 fracture dislocation in a patient with C5 radiculopathy only.

lateral locked facets. They found that fracture reduction, particularly operative reduction and realignment, may have contributed to important improvement in 6 of 28 patients they managed with bilateral locked facets (43). These results were in contrast with what was "known" about traumatic myelopathy at that time. Most investigators felt that no procedure or maneuver affected the outcome of patients who had sustained a spinal cord injury (21, 36, 65, 69). Ducker et al. reported in 1979 that 6% of patients with complete myelopathy regained useful function at 1-year postinjury, irrespective of the treatment given (22). This dismal outcome furthered the long held opinion that spinal fracture injuries, particularly those with associated spinal cord injuries, were not neurosurgical emergencies. Patients with fracture deformities of the spine were traditionally treated with bed rest, often lengthy periods of craniospinal traction and delayed, elective, spinal reconstructive surgery as indicated. Such was the standard of care, the "contemporary management" of patients with spinal column deformities in the 1970s and 1980s.

In the early 1980s, neurosurgeons and neurosurgical training programs began to emphasize better evaluation and early detection of spinal column injuries, particularly those of the cervical spine (17, 38, 53, 68). In the mid-1980s, the American College of Surgeons developed Advance Trauma Life Support training paradigms, which included the thorough assessment of the cervical spine through the cervicothoracic junction. As radiographic imaging techniques improved and with refinement in computerized tomography (CT), a greater emphasis was placed on the early detection of potential spinal and spinal cord injuries following trauma. As the index of suspicion for spinal injury was raised among emergency medical technicians, emergency department personnel, surgeons, and neurosurgeons nationwide, immobilization of the patient (until a vertebral column injury could be ruled out) became the rule rather than the exception. The halo vest and ring apparatus became recognized as a superb external fixator and immobilization device for a variety of cervical spine fracture injuries. Its use allowed craniospinal traction for potential closed reduction, followed by application of the vest and bar support structures to immobilize and protect, and

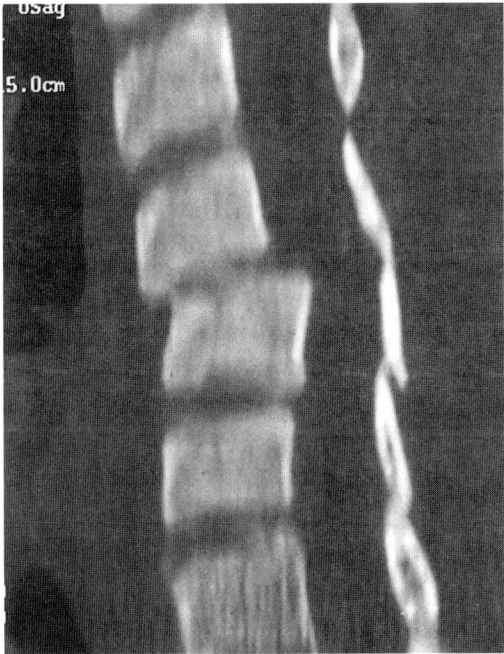

FIG. 11.3 CT reconstruction of injury in Fig. 2 revealing bony compromise of spinal cord.

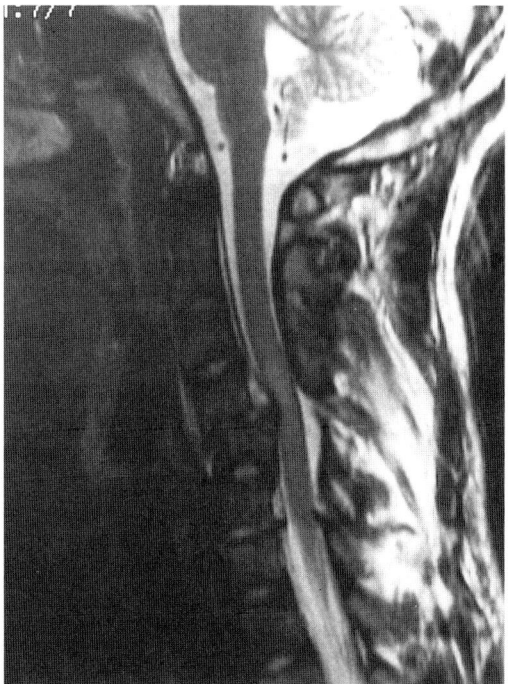

FIG. 11.4 MR of patient in Fig. 2 revealing marked cord compression without overt spinal cord injury.

in many cases, provide bracing for definitive nonoperative treatment. By the mid-1980s and early 1990s, neurosurgeons were increasingly using the halo ring for attempted realignment or closed reduction, rather than Crutchfield or Gardner-Wells tongs, and the halo ring-vest device to provide immobilization and treatment (15, 52, 67).

These three principles (now standard) of the contemporary management of spinal injuries—*detection, immobilization,* and *realignment*—were slow to evolve and have not been verified by randomized, controlled clinical trials. Little of what we in neurosurgery consider to be "standard of care," accepted treatment strategies for patients with spinal disorders has been verified. Despite this, anecdotal data from individual surgeons and evidence from institutional experiences suggest that early detection, protection, immobilization, realignment, and reduction of fracture and fracture-dislocation injuries of the spine, particularly when accomplished by attentive neurosurgeon providers, offer the best possible chance to reduce further injury, protect existing neurological function, and enhance the potential for functional improvement.

The issue of early surgery to decompress the spinal cord, or to realign the dislocated or distorted spinal column, likewise has not been definitively assessed by rigid scientific methods. Neurosurgeons worldwide are interested in this issue, and attempts are ongoing to develop a multicenter study to examine the efficacy of early surgery on spinal and spinal cord injuries. Dozens of neurosurgeons, neurosurgical groups, and non-neurosurgeon spine surgeons have provided retrospective reviews of patients managed with early surgery and describe improved neurological outcomes compared with patients managed by less aggressive, traditional means (6, 20, 23, 29, 32, 47, 50, 71)) (*Table 11.1*). Although we have not proven that early decompression of the spinal cord and realignment of the spinal column preserves function and enhances neurological recovery after fracture and fracture-dislocation injury, the growing body of "soft evidence" suggests that it does (*Fig. 11.5*).

TABLE 11.1
Studies in Support of Surgical Intervention for Traumatic SCI

Year	Investigators	Findings	Type of Study
1978	Rivilin et al. (Toronto)	Early spinal cord decompression is associated with improved neurological outcome.	Experimental animal study
1980	Dolan et al. (Toronto)	Early spinal cord decompression is associated with improved neurological outcome.	Experimental animal study
1987	Benzel et al. (Milwaukee)	Improvement in motor scores following delayed operative decompression.	Retrospective clinical trial
1987	Guha et al. (Toronto)	Significant functional recovery following early decompression.	Experimental animal study
1991	Wolf et al. (Baltimore)	Early operative decompression and stabilization showed improved 1 year postinjury neuro recovery.	Retrospective clinical
1992	Hadley et al. (Phoenix)	Early decompression enhanced neurological recovery in selected patients.	Retrospective clinical
1994	Duh et al. (New Haven)	Surgical decompression does not interfere with pharmacological treatment of SCI. Benefit suggested by early or late decompression.	Retrospective clinical
1996	Schlegel et al. (Salt Lake City)	Early decompression benefited patients with multiple trauma and SCI.	Retrospective clinical

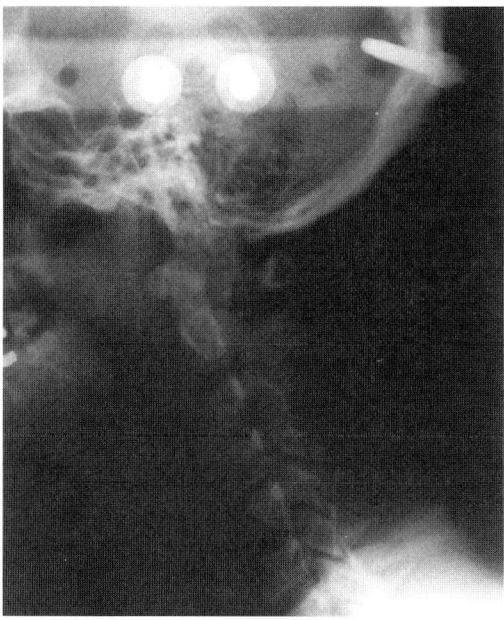

FIG. 11.5 Lateral cervical spine x-ray of patient with C5-C6 fracture-dislocation injury, reduced with 60-pound halo ring craniocervical traction.

Spinal Cord Injury

The spinal cord is a delicate, highly organized portion of the central nervous system. It is made up primarily of axonal pathways with interspersed cell bodies that subserve segmental function. It is housed within the confines of the cervical and thoracic spinal column and receives adequate, although not robust, blood supply from anterior and posterior spinal arteries, which are reinforced by segmental radicular branches. It is protected against modest injury within the central canal of the spine but is vulnerable to crush injury, compression, and/or ischemia if the intensity of the spinal column is distorted or disrupted.

Traumatic injury to the spinal cord results in varying degrees of initial neurological dysfunction, not all of which are permanent or irreversible. Investigators have learned that the primary traumatic injury initiates a complex secondary injury cascade that, if left unchecked, can result in extension of neural damage and lead to worsening neurological injury and permanent complete myelopathy (56).

The cellular and subcellular events that accompany macroscopic injury to the spinal cord have been an area of intense investigation over the last decade (73). Ischemia, membrane destabilization, and deregulation of intracellular calcium homeostasis seem to play major roles in the secondary injury process (24, 62, 63). Researchers have emphasized the maintenance of cellular integrity and function, including intracellular signaling mechanisms, processes that are disrupted after injury (33, 55).

A variety of pharmacological agents have been used in the treatment of human spinal cord injury in an attempt to preserve cellular function after SCI, all of which have shown considerable promise in experimental laboratory animal models (1, 13, 16, 34, 35, 45, 46, 48, 51, 72). Two substances seem to have merit with respect to recovery after acute spinal cord injury: methylprednisolone and the G_{M1} ganglioside known as Sygen (Fidia Pharmaceutical Corporation) (*Table 11.2*). When administered early after acute spinal cord injury, methylprednisolone has been shown to improve neurological outcome compared with placebo in a statistically significant manner. Three subsequent multicenter National Spinal Cord Injury Study trials (NASCIS I, II, and III) (8–12) have confirmed this finding and have defined the timing and amount of loading dose administration and maintenance dose parameters for human patients after acute spinal cord injury. Although the specific mechanisms of action are not completely known, methylprednisolone seems to modulate the secondary injury cascade and improve spinal cord blood flow, maintain membrane integrity, restore electrolyte balance including improving intracellular calcium homeostasis, and inhibit lipid peroxidation. Although not a silver bullet or magical elixir, methylprednisolone has been shown to benefit patients after traumatic SCI.

TABLE 11.2
Mechanisms of Action of Pharmacological Agents of Benefit after Acute SCI

Methylprednisolone
   Augmentation of spinal cord blood flow
   Maintenance of membrane integrity
   Restore electrolyte balance
   Improve intracellular calcium homeostasis
   Inhibition of lipid peroxidation
   Prevention of free radical production
   Attenuation of inflammatory response
GM1 Ganglioside
   Maintenance of membrane and axonal integrity
   Restoration of neuronal function following injury
   Promotion of neurite outgrowth
   Induction of regeneration and sprouting of neurons

G_{M1} ganglioside, a potent nerve growth factor, has been shown to result in improved neurological outcome after spinal cord injury when compared with placebo in both animal studies and initial human trials (28). It remains to be seen if the efficacy of G_{M1} ganglioside will be realized in the larger, recently completed, Phase III Sygen human spinal cord injury trial; these data are not yet ready for release.

Neurosurgeons have led these and other scientific efforts at identifying agents and strategies of benefit to patients after spinal cord injury. As investigation continues into the pathophysiology of SCI, and as we uncover other specific features of the secondary injury process, we will have greater opportunity to modulate and attenuate this destructive injury cascade.

Pharmacological therapy is not the only answer for patients who have sustained spinal cord injury, nor (as we have previously discussed) is surgery (even early surgery), the singular remedy after traumatic spinal cord injury. Although each seems to play a role in selected patients, the primary and secondary injury processes are so variable and so complex that a singular approach, let alone solution to acute spinal cord injury, is inconceivable. Moreover, it is difficult to identify the individual component contribution of a new strategy or pharmacological therapy in the treatment of spinal cord injury because there is no known standardized medical therapy that all investigators follow. Despite the considerable efforts expended in multicenter SCI trials investigating the potential benefits of medication, no study has established or verified a standard best medical therapy for the management of spinal cord injury patients. In each of the above mentioned clinical trials, standard medical therapy varied from one institution to another, depending upon individual surgeon investigator experiences or biases. When one considers this additional confounding detail of spinal cord injury management, it is even more understandable that similar types of injuries can be associated with distinctly disparate neurological outcomes, despite receiving the same drug infusion at the same time interval.

Ischemia remains the final common denominator for a variety of human injury processes, including those that affect the central nervous system. Hypoxia and shock are well established as factors detrimental to the potential recovery from any form of human injury, including SCI. Ischemia is a major component of the secondary injury cascade after SCI. As investigators have learned from the study of cardiac ischemia in the 1980s and cerebral ischemia in the 1980s and 1990s, increased end organ perfusion in the face of ischemia can often eliminate the detrimental effects of hypoperfusion, preserve cellular integrity, and enhance functional recovery and outcome (42). Anthes, Tator, and others have documented sharp reductions in spinal cord blood flow, vasospasm, microvascular sludging, and vascular thrombosis after acute SCI in experimental animal models (2, 3, 26, 39–42, 57, 66) (*Figs. 11.6 and 11.7*). Tator's work depicts the morphological changes in the blood vessels that supply the spinal cord and the time course after injury. It is assumed that similar events occur in humans after spinal trauma. Indeed, the vigorous and immediate resuscitation of patients after acute spinal cord injury has been reported to result in improved and enhanced neurological recovery compared with "traditional methods" of medical management (*Table 11.3*). Our group and others have identified that important relative hypotension exists in patients nearly uniformly after acute SCI, even in those with isolated cord injuries. Although not confirmed by randomized, controlled scientific methodology, restoration of normotensive blood pressure and perfusion with the administration of fluids, colloids, and pressors as necessary can have an important, positive impact on neurological outcome in addition to and/or distinct from any potential benefit provided by surgery or supplemental pharmacological agents (19, 25, 70).

Our perspective of the optimal treatment of patients after acute spinal cord injury is that of comprehensive, multifaceted, simultaneous early attention and treatment, directed by neurological surgeons. We favor a practical management approach that incorporates what we

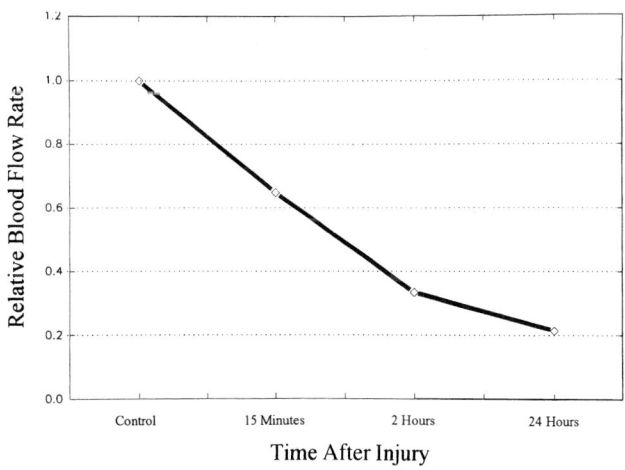

FIG. 11.6 Reduction in spinal cord sulcal anterior blood flow after spinal cord injury in a rat model. Used with permission from Anthes et al. (3).

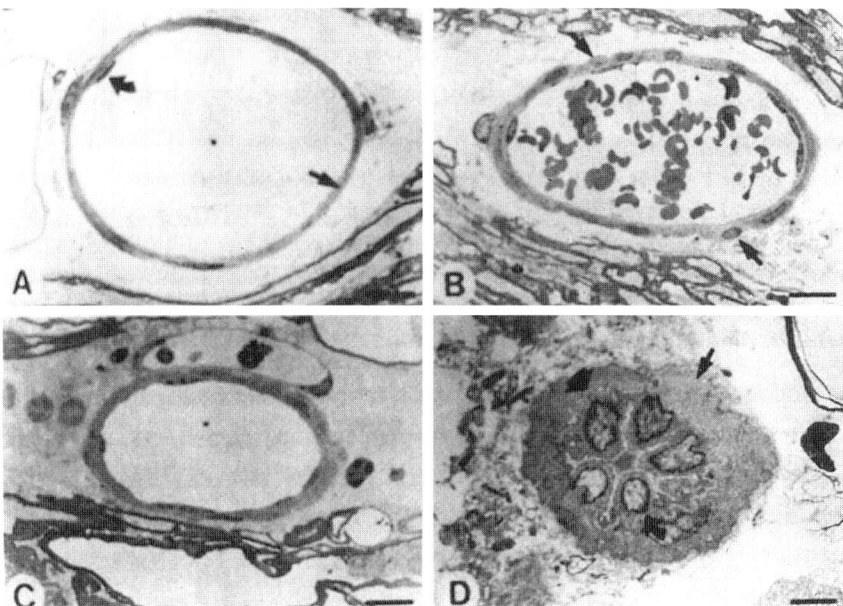

FIG. 11.7 Electron micrographs of spinal cord sulcal arteriotes in rat spinal cord injury model. *A*, control; *B*, 15 minutes after spinal cord injury; *C*, 2 hours after injury; *D*, 24 hours after injury. Note progressive change in smooth muscle morphology, thickened basement membrane due to vasospasm. Used with permission from Anthes et al. (3).

TABLE 11.3
Studies in Support of Aggressive Medical Intervention for Traumatic SCI

Year	Investigators	Findings	Type of Study
1982	Dolan and Tator (Toronto)	Volume resuscitation with blood transfusion improved neurological recovery in acute SCI.	Experimental animal study
1989	Fehlings (Toronto)	Increasing posttraumatic spinal cord blood flow improved function in injured spinal cord axons.	Experimental animal study
1993	Levi et al. (Baltimore)	Improving hemodynamic parameters with fluids, colloids, and vasopressors facilitated neurological recovery in patients with acute SCI.	Prospective clinical
1997	Vale et al. (Birmingham)	Early and aggressive volume resuscitation and blood pressure augmentation contributed independently to 30% ambulation recovery following complete myelopathy at 1 year follow-up.	Prospective clinical

know of the anatomy and physiology of the spinal cord and what we have learned about the pathophysiology of the injury process. We attempt to maximize spinal cord perfusion in the treatment of ischemia early on in the management of these patients, in addition to the administration of pharmacological therapy and the selective use of surgery to decompress the spinal cord (30, 31, 54, 64). Our view is that any contemporary treatment paradigm for SCI must incorporate all known reasonable and beneficial aspects of SCI management in an attempt to provide the patient with the greatest potential for recovery. The combination of *early detection* of spinal cord injury, *immobilization* to prevent further injury, *spinal column realignment/spinal cord decompression* to create the best possible environment for the injured

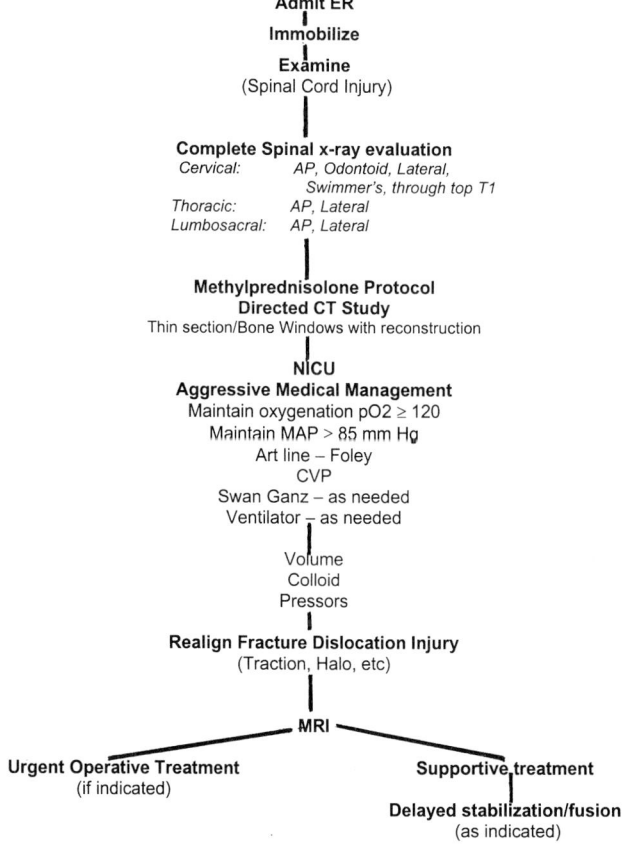

FIG. 11.8 Algorithm for management of patient with spinal column/spinal cord injury.

cord, *pharmacological therapy* to facilitate neuronal protection, and *aggressive medical resuscitation* to reduce spinal cord ischemia offers the best possible strategy for patients who have sustained acute spinal cord injuries (*Fig. 11.8*).

Because most investigators agree that the earlier treatment can be initiated after acute spinal cord injury, the better the opportunity for a good result, it is the neurosurgeon who is most capable to provide this early, comprehensive, contemporary care. We are not just "brain surgeons" or technicians. We are scientists who understand the pathophysiology of neural injury. We are intensivists who can apply the principals of resuscitation and reperfusion. We are orthotists capable of applying halo craniocervical traction and/or immobilization devices. We are craniospinal surgeons well equipped to provide decompression of the spinal cord or spinal column reconstruction as indicated. When we consistently begin to apply this logical and contemporary management paradigm to all patients with acute SCI, we have the potential to dramatically reduce the serious and permanent disabilities associated with these injuries, and we will conclusively and unequivocally secure their management within the domain of the neurosurgeon.

REFERENCES

1. Anderson DK, Hall ED, Braughler JM, McCall JM, and Means ED: Effect of delayed administration of U74006F (Tirilazad Mesylate) on recovery of locomotor function after experimental spinal cord injury. **J Neurotrauma** 8(3):187–192, 1991.
2. Anthes DL, Theriault E, and Tator CH: Characterization of axonal ultrastructural pathology following experimental spinal cord compression injury. **Brain Research** 702:1–16, 1995.
3. Anthes DL, Theriault E, and Tator CH: Ultrastructural evidence for arteriolar vasospasm after spinal cord trauma. **Neurosurgery** 39(4):804–814, 1996.
4. Bailey RW, Badgley CE: Stabilization of the cervical spine by anterior fusion. J **Bone Joint Surg** 422:565, 1960.
5. Baton LG: The reduction of fracture dislocation of the cervical vertebrae by skeletal traction. **Surg Gyn Obs** 67:94, 1938.
6. Benzel EC, and Larson SJ: Functional recovery after decompressive spine operation for cervical spine fractures. **Neurosurg** 20(5):742–746, 1987.
7. Bohlman H: Acute fractures and dislocations of the cervical spine. **J Bone Joint Surg** 61A:1119, 1979.
8. Bracken MB, and Holford TR: Effects of timing of methylprednisolone or naloxone administration on recovery of segmental and long-tract neurological function in NASCIS 2. **J Neurosci** 79:500–507, 1993.
9. Bracken MB, Collins WF, Freeman DF, et al: Efficacy of Methylprednisolone in acute spinal cord injury. **JAMA** 251(1):45–52, 1984.
10. Bracken MB, Shepard MJ, Collins WF, et al: A randomized, controlled trial of methylprednisolone or Naloxone in the treatment of acute spinal cord injury. Results of the second National Acute Spinal Cord Injury Study (NASCIS II). **N Engl J Med** 322(20):1405–1411, 1990.

11. Bracken MB, Shepard MJ, Collins WF, et al: Methylprednisolone or naloxone treatment after acute spinal cord injury: 1-year follow-up data. Results of the second National Acute Spinal Cord Injury Study (NASCIS II). **J Neurosci** 76:23–31, 1992.
12. Bracken MB, Shepard MJ, Holford, TR, et al: Administration of methylprednisolone for 24 or 48 hours or tirilazad mesylate for 48 hours in the treatment of acute spinal cord injury. Results of the third National Acute Spinal Cord Injury randomized controlled trial (NASCIS III). **JAMA** 277(20):1597–1604, 1997.
13. Braughler JM, and Hall ED: Lactate and pyruvate metabolism in injured cat spinal cord before and after a single large intravenous dose of methylprednisolone. **J Neurosci** 59:256–261, 1983.
14. Breasted JH: The Edwin Smith Surgical Papyrus (The University of Chicago Oriental Institute Publications, Vol3). Chicago: University of Chicago Press; 1933.
15. Bucci MN, Dauser RC, Maynard FA, and Hoff JT: Management of post-traumatic cervical spine instability: Operative fusion versus halo vest immobilization. Analysis of 49 cases. **J Trauma** 28(7):1001–1006, 1988.
16. Chen DF, Schneider GE, Martinou J-C, and Tonegawa S: BcI-2 promotes regeneration of severed axons in mammalian CNS. **Nature** 385:434–439, 1997.
17. Cooper PR, and Cohen W: Evaluation of cervical spinal cord injuries with metrazamide myelography-CT scanning. **J Neurosci** 61:281–289, 1984.
18. Crutchfield WG: Skeletal traction for dislocation of the cervical spine. **S Surg J** 2:156, 1933.
19. Dolan EJ, and Tator CH: The effect of blood transfusion, dopamine and gamma-hydroxybutyrate on post traumatic ischemia of the spinal cord. **J Neurosci** 56:350–358, 1982.
20. Dolan EJ, Tator CH, and Endrenyi L: The value of decompression for acute experimental spinal cord compression injury. **J Neurosci** 53:749–755, 1980.
21. Ducker TB, Bellegarrigue R, Salcman M, and Walleck C: Timing of operative care in cervical spinal cord injury. **Spine** 9(5):525–531, 1984.
22. Ducker TB, Russo GL, Bellegarrique R, Lucas JT: Complete sensorimotor paralysis after cord injury: Mortality, recovery, and therapeutic implications. **J Trauma** 19:837–849, 1979.
23. Duh M-S, Shepard MJ, Wilberger JE, and Bracken MB: The effectiveness of surgery on the treatment of acute spinal cord injury and its relation to pharmacological treatment. **Neurosurgery** 35(2):240–249, 1994.
24. Farooque M, Hillered L, Holtz A, and Olsson Y: Changes of extracellular levels of amino acids after graded compression trauma to the spinal cord: An experimental study in the rat using microdialysis. **J Neurotrauma**. 13(9):537–548, 1996.
25. Fehlings MG, Tator CH, and Linden RD: The effect of nimodipine and dextran on axonal function and blood flow following experimental spinal cord injury. **J Neurosci** 71:403–416, 1989.
26. Fried LC, and Goodkin R: Microangiographic observations of the experimentally traumatized spinal cord. **J Neurosci** 35:709–714, 1971.
27. Gallie WE: Fractures and dislocations of the cervical spine. **M J Surg** 486:495, 1939.
28. Geisler FH, Dorsey FC, and Coleman WP: Recovery of motor function after spinal cord injury—A randomized, placebo-controlled trial with GM-1 ganglioside. **N Engl J Med** 324(26):1829–1838, 1991.
29. Guha A, Tator CH, Endrenyi L, and Piper I: Decompression of the spinal cord improves recovery after acute experimental spinal cord compression injury. **Paraplegia** 25:324–339, 1987.
30. Hadley MN, and Argires PJ: The acute/emergent management of vertebral column

fracture/dislocation injuries. Neurological Emergencies The American Association of Neurological Surgeons, Vol II 249–262, 1994.
31. Hadley MN, and Bishop RC: Management of craniocervical junction and upper cervical spine injuries. The Practice of Neurosurgery Williams and Wilkins, Baltimore Volume II, Chapter 111, p1687–1701, 1996.
32. Hadley MN, Fitzpatrick BC, Sonntag VKH, and Browner CM: Facet fracture-dislocation injuries of the cervical spine. **Neurosurgery** 30(5):661–666, 1992.
33. Hall ED, and Wolf DL: A pharmacological analysis of the pathophysiological mechanisms of post-traumatic spinal cord ischemia. **J Neurosci** 64:951–961, 1986.
34. Hall ED, Yonkers PA, Horan KL, and Braughler JM: Correlation between attenuation of posttraumatic spinal cord ischemia and preservation of tissue vitamin E by the 21-aminosteroid U74006F: Evidence for an *in vivo* antioxidant mechanism. **J Neurotrauma** 6(3):169–175, 1989.
35. Hayes KC, Blight AR, Potter PJ, et al: Pre-clinical trial of 4-aminopyridine in patients with chronic spinal cord injury. **Paraplegia** 31:216–224, 1993.
36. Heiden JS, Weiss MH, Rosenberg AW, Apuzzo MLJ, and Kurze T: Management of cervical spinal cord trauma in Southern California. **J Neurosci** 43:732–736, 1975.
37. Howorth B, Petrie G: Injuries to the spine. Baltimore: Williams and Wilkins, 1964.
38. Kalsbeek WD, McLaurin RL, Harris BSH, and Miller JD: The National Head and Spinal Cord Injury Survey: Major findings. **J Neurosci** 53:S19-S31, 1980.
39. Kobrine AI, Doyle TF, and Rizzoli HV: Spinal cord blood flow as affected by changes in systemic arterial blood pressure. **J Neurosci** 44:12–15, 1976.
40. Koyanagi I, Tator CH, and Lea PJ: Three-dimensional analysis of the vascular system in the rat spinal cord with scanning electron microscopy of vascular corrosion casts. Part 1: Normal spinal cord. **Neurosurgery** 33(2):277–284, 1993.
41. Koyanagi I, Tator CH, and Lea PJ: Three-dimensional analysis of the vascular system in the rat spinal cord with scanning electron microscopy of vascular corrosion casts. Part 2: Acute spinal cord injury. **Neurosurgery** 33(2):285–292, 1993.
42. Levy ML, Day JD, Zelman V, and Giannotta SL: Cardiac performance enhancement and hypervolemic therapy. **Neurosurgery Clinics of North America** 5(4):725–739, 1994.
43. Maiman DJ, Barolat G, and Larson SJ: Management of bilateral locked facets of the cervical spine. **Neurosurg** 18(5):542–547, 1986.
44. Mason C, Cozen L, Adelstein L: Surgical correction of flexion deformity of the cervical spine. **Cal Med** 79:244, 1953.
45. McKenzie AL, Hall JJ, Aihara N, Fukuda K, and Noble LJ: Immunolocalization of endothelin in the traumatized spinal cord: Relationship to blood-spinal cord barrier breakdown. **J Neurotrauma** 12(3):257–268, 1995.
46. Qiao J, Hayes KC, Hsieh JTC, Potter PJ, and Delaney GA: Effects of 4-Aminopyridine on motor evoked potentials in patients with spinal cord injury. **J Neurotrauma** 14(3):135–149, 1997.
47. Rivlin AS, and Tator CH: Effect of duration of acute spinal cord compression in a new acute cord injury model in the rat. **Surg Neurol** 10:39–43, 1978.
48. Robertson CS, Foltz R, Grossman RG, and Goodman JC: Protection against experimental ischemic spinal cord injury. **J Neurosci** 64:663–642, 1986.
49. Rogers WA: Treatment of fracture—dislocation of the cervical spine. **J Bone Joint Surg** 24:245, 1942.
50. Schlegel J, Bayley J, Yuan H, and Fredricksen B: Timing of surgical decompression and fixation of acute spinal fractures. **J Orthopaedic Trauma** 10(5):323–330, 1996.
51. Schnell L, Schneider R, Kolbeck R, Barde Y-A, and Schwab ME: Neurorophin-3 enhances sprouting of corticospinal tract during development and after adult spinal cord lesion. **Nature** 367:170–173, 1995.

52. Sears W, and Fazi M: Prediction of stability of cervical spine fracture managed in the halo vest and indications for surgical intervention. **J Neurosci** 72:426–432, 1990.
53. Sonntag VKH: Management of bilateral locked facets of the cervical spine. **Neurosurg** 8(2):150–152, 1981.
54. Sonntag VKH, and Hadley MN: Management of upper cervical spinal instability. In: Wilkins R and Rengachary S (eds) Neurosurgery, Second Edition. McGraw-Hill, 1995.
55. Tator CH: Biology of neurological recovery and functional restoration after spinal cord injury. **Neurosurgery** 42(4):696–708, 1998.
56. Tator CH: Pathophysiology, and Pathology of Spinal Cord Injury. In: Pathophysiology and Pathology of Spinal Cord Injury, Part VIII Cranial and Spinal Trauma. P. 2847–2858:.
57. Tator CH, and Koyanagi I: Vascular mechanisms in the pathophysiology of human spinal cord injury. **J Neurosci** 86:483–492, 1997.
58. Tator CH, Duncan EG, Edmonds VE, Lapczak LI, and Andrews DF: Comparison of surgical and conservative management in 208 patients with acute spinal cord injury. **Can J Neurol Sci** 14:60–69, 1987.
59. Taylor AS: Fracture dislocation of the cervical spine. **Ann Surg** 90:321, 1929.
60. The Halo: A spinal skeletal traction device. **J Bone Joint Surg** 50A:1400, 1968.
61. Treatment of fractures and dislocations of the cervical spine. **Ann Surg** 106:770, 1937.
62. Tymianski M, and Tator CH: Normal and abnormal calcium homeostasis in neurons: A basis for the pathophysiology of traumatic and ischemic central nervous system injury. **Neurosurgery** 38:1176–1195, 1996.
63. Tymianski M, Charlton MP, Carlen PL, and Tator CH: Source specificity of early calcium neurotoxicity in cultured embryonic spinal neurons. **The J Neuroscience** 13(5):2085–2104, 1993.
64. Vale FL, Burns J, Jackson AB, and Hadley MN: Combined medical and surgical treatment after acute spinal cord injury: Results of a prospective pilot study to assess the merits of aggressive medical resuscitation and blood pressure management. **J Neurosci** 87:239–246, 1997.
65. Wagner FC, and Chehrazi B: Surgical results in treatment of cervical spinal cord injury. **Spine** 9(5):523–524, 1984.
66. Wallace MC, Tator CH, and Frazee P: Relationship between posttraumatic ischemia and hemorrhage in the injured rat spinal cord as shown by colloidal carbon angiography. **Neurosurgery** 18(4):433–439, 1986.
67. Walters RL, Adkins RH, Nelson R, and Garland D: Cervical spinal cord trauma: Evaluation and non-operative treatment with halo-vest immobilization. **Contemporary Orthopaedics**. 14(1):35–45, 1987.
68. White AA, and Banjabi MM: The role of stabilization in the treatment of cervical spine injuries. **Spine** 9(5):512–522, 1984.
69. Wilmot CB, and Hall KM: Evaluation of acute surgical intervention in traumatic paraplegia. **Paraplegia** 24:71–76, 1986.
70. Wolf LL, and Belzberg H: Hemodynamic parameters in patients with acute cervical cord trauma: Description, intervention and prediction of outcome. **Neurosurgery** 33(6):1007–1016, 1993.
71. Wolf A, Levi L, Mirvis S, et al: Operative management of bilateral facet dislocation. **J Neurosci** 75:883–890, 1991.
72. Wrathall JR, Teng YD, and Choiniere D: Amelioration of functional deficits from spinal cord trauma with systemically administered NBQX, an antagonist of non-N-methyl-d-asparate receptors. **Experimental Neurology** 137:119–126, 1996.
73. Young W: The post-injury responses in trauma and ischemia: Secondary injury or protective mechanisms? **Central Nervous System Trauma** 4:27–51, 1987.

CHAPTER

12

Neurological Injuries in Infants and Children: An Overview of Current Management Strategies

THOMAS G. LUERSSEN, M.D., F.A.C.S., F.A.A.P.

In the spectrum of all patients suffering neurotrauma, children with serious brain and spinal cord injuries represent a relatively small proportion of the population. However, when one considers this problem only within the pediatric age group, these injuries, especially traumatic brain injury, are now the most common cause of death and disability. For most neurosurgeons, pediatric neurotrauma will represent a relatively small proportion of a practice. Fortunately, most of the general issues related to patient management are not age specific and can be logically applied to any head or spinally injured patient, regardless of the patient's age. However, and as with most of the diseases treated by neurosurgeons, there are specific and important issues that are unique to this patient population. This article will review some of these issues and provide an overview of the management of brain and spinal cord injury in childhood.

BRAIN INJURY

There are many notable differences in the characteristics of traumatic brain injuries between children and adults. Some of these include the expected distribution of injury severities, the occurrence and character of skull fractures, the incidence and type of traumatic mass lesions, the occurrence and characteristics of brain swelling, posttraumatic epilepsy, associated systemic complications, as well as the widely recognized differences in expected outcomes (1, 28). Furthermore, all of these general characteristics of brain injury vary continuously with age, throughout all ages of patients, child or adult. Some, but clearly not all, of these differences may be related simply to the different mechanisms of injury that commonly occur in "children" compared with adults.

On the other hand, there seems to be a small but progressively enlarging literature, both from laboratory experiments and clinical studies, suggesting that some of the injury-related pathophysiological responses of the very immature brain may be different, either in character or in intensity, from those in the more mature brain (2, 4, 16, 47). Investigations such as these are important and are being actively pursued. Ultimately, these research efforts may result in the development of therapies that are unique or specific to certain ages of brain-injured patients. However, at present, the author has concluded that one cannot yet derive from any of the current information a suggestion that the basic management strategies that will be discussed below should be any different for children than for adults.

The advent of large studies of the natural history of traumatic brain injury and the subsequent clinical trials of a variety of therapies, pharmaceutical or otherwise, although yet to result in "new" therapies, have resulted in progressively more rigorous analysis of the applications and efficacy of what might now be called "standard therapies" for traumatic brain injury. Over the years, these sequential studies, commonly performed and analyzed by the same investigators, while not finding efficacy in the treatment being studied, seem to demonstrate a progressive decline in mortality, both in the control groups and in the entire study groups. One reason for this trend may be that the rational and aggressive application of treatments known to be effective, i.e., support of blood pressure and ventilation, control of intracranial pressure, and the prevention of systemic complications, is, in itself, the key to improved outcomes. These standard therapies, along with several other basic issues important to the management of head injury, have recently undergone a fairly extensive and evidence-based review. The resulting document, *Guidelines for the Management of Severe Head Injury* (8), provides a template for the general management of head-injured patients. These guidelines, as the authors point out in the Introduction, are intended for adult patients. Nevertheless, the concepts expressed and the management schemes suggested by these guidelines, using the appropriate adjustments for systemic parameters, weights, fluid volumes, etc., are likely to be as applicable for children as they are for adults.

These issues are being studied, but analyses like this are difficult and time consuming for several reasons. First, the general process of creating satisfactory practice parameters is tedious, involving the review and grading of a large volume of literature. The rules are stringent, and reaching consensus about some issues is difficult (53). Second, there is precious little strong scientific evidence specifically addressing the pediatric patient. Finally, it is difficult to glean from many of the studies cited as applicable to adult patients, the actual ages of the patients involved, and what effect on the outcomes might be due to the ages of patients alone.

A study of the applicability of these particular *Guidelines* to severely head-injured children is being undertaken by organized neurosurgery. Similar projects, aimed at developing guidelines for the evaluation and management of minor head injury and head injury in infants, are in various stages of completion (C Homer and S Schutzman, personal communication). The remainder of this section will be devoted to describing the general conclusions available from these projects.

Severe Head Injury

The *Guidelines* address 14 relevant major topics in neurotrauma management. Within each of the major topics, a variety of subtopics are addressed. Out of all of these, only three "standards," the strongest recommendation based on the strongest scientific evidence, are proposed. These recommendations address the use of prophylactic anticonvulsants, glucocorticoids, and the general application of hyperventilation to head-injured patients. There are 8 "guidelines," which are recommendations that are based on less secure, but still strong scientific evidence, that address issues such as trauma systems, resuscitation, intracranial pressure monitoring, osmotic diuretics, barbiturates, and nutrition. The remaining recommendations are presented as "options," which are based on the least secure scientific evidence, including so-called "expert opinion." Although the analyses of these *Guidelines*—applicability to pediatric patients is still in progress, one general statement about the findings is already clear: The vast majority of the recommendations, as they apply to children, are likely to be downgraded at least one level in degree of certainty. Given that, the review of issues that follows is based on the topics addressed by the *Guidelines*—but do not represent the findings of the review committee nor are they intended to be taken as practice parameters.

RESUSCITATION AND PREHOSPITAL MANAGEMENT

A very limited literature suggests that injured pediatric patients are subject to the same problems in management in the prehospital environment as are traumatized adults. Thus, it seems likely that some type of systematic regionalization of trauma care for children would carry the same benefit as for adults. In a retrospective review of hospital-based pediatric deaths in Australia, it was shown that management errors occur commonly in pediatric patients and that most commonly occurring errors were related to airway management and fluid management, both of which require a certain level of expertise in very young children (52). The available literature seems to suggest that outcomes for injured children are improved if they are treated specifically in a trauma center, especially a pediatric trauma center (19, 21, 22, 31).

There is no basis to suggest that the general principles of support of blood pressure and respiration in the prehospital phase as outlined in the *Guidelines* should be any different for head-injured children. Furthermore, the suggestion that clinical signs consistent with herniation or elevated intracranial pressure should be treated aggressively ought to be true for all ages of patients.

MEASUREMENT AND MANAGEMENT OF INTRACRANIAL PRESSURE

The *Guidelines* recommend the use of intracranial pressure (ICP) monitoring for all severely head-injured patients, except for those patients with a clearly normal computed tomographic (CT) scan (8). In the large volume of literature analyzed to justify this recommendation, it seems that the vast majority of patients who were studied were adults. However, there is no evidence that these findings and conclusions should not apply to children, with the important possible exception of infants who have suffered inflicted brain injuries and show early evidence of widespread infarction on admitting CT scans (14). As with adults, children who present at higher levels of consciousness (i.e., Glasgow Coma Scores of 9 or better) who have evidence of brain swelling, shift, cisternal compression, or traumatic intracerebral hemorrhage are at risk for life-threatening deterioration and are likely to benefit from early monitoring of ICP(27). With the technological advances in ICP monitors, especially the parenchymal pressure transducers, the risk of placement of the monitor is less than the risk of deterioration. Finally, some children with normal admitting CT scans may be considered for ICP monitoring, especially if they exhibit clinical signs indicating severe diffuse brain injury (36) or if it is necessary for them to undergo anesthesia or sedation for prolonged emergency surgical procedures to treat other injuries.

The *Guidelines* recommend that the treatment threshold for ICP is 20 to 25 mm Hg. This recommendation seems to be derived almost completely from studies in adult patients. Normal intracranial pressure in children is lower than in adults and seems to progressively rise throughout childhood to reach normal adult levels (51). Although the limited available literature regarding treatment of elevated ICP and outcome in children supports this threshold recommendation (1, 6, 23, 41), the use of lower values, adjusted for the age of the patient, has not been studied. Considering that the normal ICP in young children is lower than adults, as is the blood pressure, it is possible that a threshold of 20 mm Hg is too high for children. Accordingly, strong consideration should be given to using substantially lower ICP thresholds to begin therapy in young children (13, 25).

BLOOD PRESSURE AND CEREBRAL PERFUSION PRESSURE

In every major study of the effects of systemic blood pressure on the outcome from head injury, the occurrence of even a brief episode of hypotension has had a profoundly negative effect on outcome (9, 29). Some of these studies included children, and there is no indication that pediatric patients react any differently or are in some way protected from this process (38). Despite the large body of evidence, the *Guidelines*' recommendation regarding the prevention of hypotension occurs at a lesser level of certainty, apparently only because a randomized controlled trial has never been undertaken. Although the general concept is completely supportable, the recommendation includes the use of 90 mm Hg for the lowest acceptable systolic blood pressure for head-injured patients. Clearly, this specific portion of the recommendation is not applicable to children. The majority of very young children and a large number of older children have normal systolic blood pressures at or below 90 mm Hg (34). However, one should be able to fully accept this recommendation as a general concept for children, correcting for the absolute definition of hypotension according to the age of the child.

Combining the information from ICP and blood pressure has allowed management strategies to develop that focus on maintaining a certain minimum perfusion state and thereby avoid cerebral ischemia. The most popular recent strategy has been called cerebral perfusion pressure (CPP) therapy (44). Many authorities use the maintenance of CPP as the major focus of therapy, including the early and preferential use of vasopressors to substantially increase systemic blood pressure. Despite this, and for a variety of reasons outlined recently by Chesnut (9, 10), the *Guidelines* only offer this recommendation at the level of an option.

Attention to CPP in children is probably as important as in adults. However, as with ICP, one could surmise that normal CPP should be lower in children by virtue of their lower normal mean arterial pressure and ICP and that this relationship should be age related. Preliminary studies seem to confirm this. A recent report indicates that the critical CPP threshold is indeed lower in children and that the fundamental cerebrovascular physiology may be different between children and adults (32). Considering this, and until more information is available, it is not recommended that "CPP therapy," at least as it is popularly used, be undertaken in children, and under no circumstances should the manipulation of CPP in children be undertaken using the physiologic parameters established for adult patients. Finally, whether one chooses to focus primarily on ICP or CPP to guide therapy, there is overwhelming evidence that any episodes of hypotension, even mild in degree and brief in duration, must be assiduously avoided.

VENTILATION AND HYPERVENTILATION

Early control of the airway and respiration has profoundly beneficial effects for the patient with traumatic brain injury. In the *Guidelines,* the recommendations concerning the importance of maintaining an airway and supporting adequate oxygenation of the injured patient are offered at the level of a "guideline." There is no reason to suggest that pediatric patients should be treated differently in this regard. Mechanical ventilation using adequate sedation and muscular paralysis will allow not only support of normal oxygenation but also control of $PaCO_2$, both of which will prevent fluctuations in cerebral blood volume and provide basic control of ICP.

In contrast, the routine use of hyperventilation as a first line therapy for traumatic brain injury is no longer recommended and may, in fact, be harmful. The *Guidelines* review this issue and describe the studies that led to this conclusion. For pediatric patients, there are some similar studies, notably the recent studies of Skippen et al. and Sharples et al., that completely support this view (46, 48). In all studies, a target $PaCO_2$ of 35 mm Hg has been considered a safe and reasonable physiological parameter for the patient, adult or child, who requires ventilatory support.

Nevertheless, when used in appropriate situations and guided by some sort of physiological monitoring, hyperventilation is a powerful and effective means of reducing elevated ICP while maintaining cerebral perfusion. This therapy is recommended when other standard therapies are not effective. Whenever this therapy is used, it should be for as short a period as necessary, preferably supported by some sort of monitoring that reflects either regional or global cerebral blood flow and oxygen metabolism, and only at an intensity that obtains the desired clinical results.

OSMOTIC THERAPIES, CEREBROSPINAL FLUID DRAINAGE, AND BARBITURATES

Each of these escalated therapies of elevated ICP is discussed in the *Guidelines.* All of these therapies have been shown to be beneficial, especially when used to target a specific pathophysiological response (33). In each case, the available evidence seems to suggest that these therapies are at least equally effective in children, although the literature does not support their use with the same strength as it does in adults. As with all medications, and with escalated therapies in general, the use of these therapies should be based on patient weights and the normally expected physiological parameters according to the age or size of the patient. Escalation of the intensity of physiological monitoring is also recommended.

INTEGRATION AND DESIGN OF THERAPIES

The development of a treatment strategy for a head-injured child should take into account the variety of issues specific to a particular patient and type of injury. In many cases, the appearance of the CT scan will provide some indications of the type of injury and the likelihood of elevated ICP and other complications (30). Continued reassessments of the evolution of the injury and the responses to therapy are used as a guide to the next step or change in management. No one therapy or combination of therapies can be appropriate for all types of injuries, and it is also likely that therapeutic strategies may change during the management of an individual patient.

In view of this, the contemporary management of traumatic brain injury involves an ongoing and fluid analysis of the state of the injured brain to target the available therapies and achieve a specific goal. Escalation of therapy should take place, if possible, before deterioration in status. Accordingly, the author has devised an approach using the so-called standard therapies for the management of traumatically brain-injured patients that focuses on maintaining an acceptable perfusion state while minimizing the associated complications (26). This approach to therapy is offered only as one of a variety of approaches that might be devised or are already in use by others. Many, if not most, of the currently used treatment strategies involve the same concepts outlined in the *Guidelines* and mirror the recommended integration of therapies and the care map provided in that document. This is not surprising, as the concepts of brain injury management derived from the medical literature will be based on well proven and effective therapies that have been used and recommended by experts in head injury management for many years.

As indicated in *Table 12.1,* treatments can occur at three general levels of intensity: basic, escalated, and intensive therapy of refractory ICP. Most severely head-injured children can be effectively treated with basic and escalated therapies. As a general rule, the higher level therapies are added to the existing levels, but this is not required if circumstances dictate. Prior to escalating therapy to any higher level, two

TABLE 12.1
Medical Therapies for Traumatic Brain Injury

Treatments	Monitoring
Basic Level Therapy	
• Elevation of head of bed	• Systemic blood pressure and oxygenation
• Keep head in neutral position	
• Sedation and muscular paralysis	• Intracranial pressure
• Mechanical ventilation to maintain PaCO$_2$ at 35 to 40 mm Hg	• Arterial PO$_2$, PCO$_2$, and pH
	• Weight, urine output, pulse, and pulse pressure
• Maintain normal to slightly increased intravascular volume	
• Normal fluid and electrolyte status (no fluid restriction); avoid anemia, hyperglycemia	• Hemogram, serum electrolytes, glucose, and blood urea nitrogen
	• Monitor and aggressively treat for fever and sepsis
• Body temperature normal to slightly hypothermic	• CT Scan
Escalated Therapy	
• Ventricular CSF drainage	• Ventricular catheter
• Mannitol	• Central venous pressure
• Moderate hyperventilation to maintain PaCO$_2$ at 30 to 35 mm Hg	• Serum osmolality
Intensive Therapy of Refractory ICP	
• High-dose barbiturate therapy	• Continuous EEG, barbiturate levels
• Lumbar CSF drainage if indicated	• Jugular venous oxygen saturation, CBF
• Profound hyperventilation	

things must happen. First, one must confirm that the current therapy is being correctly applied. For instance, it is inappropriate to increase a dose of mannitol or intensify hyperventilation when the external ventricular drainage system is malfunctioning. Whereas this seems obvious, it is easy to see how this can happen if one does not undertake continuous reassessment of the treatments at each level. Accordingly, the use of "PRN" orders for treatment of ICP elevations, is not allowed. This proscription automatically reminds the physician to reassess the current status. Only when it is clear that the current therapy is insufficient despite correct and complete application is additional therapy added. Second, prior to any escalation of therapy, escalation of systemic and neurological monitoring must occur. Each level of therapy is accompanied by an additional array of monitors whose purpose is to guide the therapy at that level and avoid, as much as possible, any complications of the therapies.

Basic level therapy is aimed at maximizing systemic parameters and intracranial dynamics. This includes providing adequate oxygenation and control of respiration and the support of systemic circulation to maintain cerebral perfusion. Temperature control is important to avoid the effects of fever or hyperthermia on ICP. The head of the bed is elevated, and the head is maintained in a neutral position without any restriction or compression of jugular venous flow.

It is essential that the patient's intravascular volume be maintained. Therefore, fluids are administered at rates and concentrations calculated to provide at least normal maintenance requirements. Fluid restriction is never used. Although nutrition is not specifically avoided, care must be taken to avoid hyperglycemia. Finally, the patient is mechanically ventilated using adequate narcotic sedation and muscular paralysis such that the stimulation of intubation, coughing, and straining are avoided.

If basic management is not adequate, second tier therapies are used. If basic management was initially successful, even for several hours, the CT scan should be repeated. If not already in place, ventriculostomy is our first choice for treatment of elevated ICP. In some head-injured children, ventricular access may not be possible, at which point one can increase the hyperventilation or begin osmotherapy. For the latter treatment, intravascular volume must be assiduously maintained, and direct measurement of central venous pressures is usually required. Diuresed volume should be replaced with isotonic fluids or plasma expanders.

A small percentage of patients will require more than the above described "conventional" therapies. The remaining extremely intensive therapies carry considerable risk of complication and should not be undertaken unless absolutely necessary. The selection of a therapy depends upon the treating physicians' understanding of the pathophysiological state of the brain and the attendant general systemic conditions. For any of these very intensive therapies, intensive monitoring is required. Of the three therapies mentioned, the most clearly proven beneficial therapy is the administration of high-dose barbiturates.

One must remember that the cause of elevated ICP may change during the course of therapy. Therefore, hyperventilation may be preferable to osmotherapy at one time, with the reverse being true at another time in the course of treating the same patient. One of the major ongoing problems in ICP management is correctly identifying cause and therapy of elevated ICP at each epoch in the patient's treatment. In the absence of a direct medical therapy for traumatic brain injury, the real time analysis of the pathophysiological state of the injured brain and the selection of a specific treatment to improve that state is the true current frontier of brain injury management for all ages of patients.

Mild or Minor Head Injury

Mild closed head injury is one of the most common reasons for seeking urgent medical attention, representing over 10% of all emergency room visits for pediatric patients (42). Despite the magnitude of this problem, there is, at present, a remarkable lack of consensus about the evaluation and management of these patients. Much of the problem revolves around a lack of uniform definitions of injury severity and a lack of understanding of the prevalence of true brain injury in the population of mildly head-injured children. Therefore, the initial evaluation, the selection of patients for neuroimaging, as well as the type of imaging selected, and the rate of admission to hospital are all highly variable.

Recently, a series of efforts to address this issue has been undertaken. The formation of a multidisciplinary committee spearheaded by the American Academy of Pediatrics and the American Academy of Family Physicians is in the final stages of preparing a practice parameter aimed at children ages 2 through 20 years (C Homer, personal communication). Another group, similarly constituted, is beginning to address the issue in children under the age of 2 years (S Schutzman, personal communication). Pediatric neurosurgeons are intimately involved in both of these efforts.

One of the major goals of evaluating patients with minor head injuries is to reliably detect the subpopulation of these patients that harbor a potentially life-threatening or disabling brain injury. Considering this, it seems likely that an acceptable practice parameter must include the very liberal and early use of CT scanning for mildly head-injured patients. Although a few case series indicate the clinical constellation of the following findings: Glasgow Coma Scale of 15, normal neurological examination, no history of loss of consciousness, no vomiting, no headache, and no subtle changes in mental status, are not associated with abnormal CT findings (12, 18), there are also studies indicating that these clinical indicators may not identify all of the patients at risk (20, 43, 50). These reports should be viewed in light of a larger body of evidence that the finding of a normal CT scan in a mildly head-injured patient is associated with essentially no risk of life-threatening deterioration (11, 49).

SPINAL CORD INJURY

Spinal cord injuries in children are rare. Only about 5% of all spinal cord injuries occur in children (24, 35, 45). Vertebral column injuries that do not cause neurological deficits are much more common. In one large series, only half of the children with vertebral injuries had neurological deficits (17).

The mechanisms and patterns of injury are age related. Approximately one-half of all pediatric spinal injuries occur as the result of motor vehicle accidents. Another one-quarter are related to recreational diving accidents. Clearly, prevention efforts directed at these two mechanisms alone would dramatically reduce the occurrence of spinal cord injury in the pediatric age group. The remaining major mechanisms of injury are falls and sporting events, each of which accounts for about 10% of the reported injuries. Younger children are more likely to be injured in a fall; adolescents are more likely to be injured as the result of a diving mishap or in a sporting event (3, 35).

The pattern of spinal cord injury in children shows a bimodal age distribution. Young children suffer cervical spine injuries almost exclusively, whereas older children suffer injuries in roughly the same distribution as adults. Another way of looking at this is that younger children tend to have extremely rostral spinal cord injuries and that this tendency decreases with increasing age. This phenomenon is independent of the mechanism of injury and is directly attributable to the anatomy of the juvenile spine and the craniocervical disproportion of the young child.

The pediatric spine has several properties that allow significant yet self-reducing displacement of the vertebral elements to a degree that the spinal cord can be completely disrupted. Some of these properties are increased elasticity of the joint capsules and ligaments, shallow and horizontally oriented facet joints, anterior wedging of the vertebral bodies, and poorly developed uncinate processes (5). These properties, coupled with the disproportionate size of the child's head and weak cervical musculature, permit extreme ranges of flexion and extension in young children.

These anatomic properties also predispose the young child to spinal cord injury in the absence of vertebral fracture or dislocation, a syndrome that has been termed SCIWORA (spinal cord injury without radiographic abnormality). Initial reports characterizing this syndrome indicated that SCIWORA represented as much as 67% of the pediatric spinal cord injuries (37). However, a more recent survey of the relevant literature indicates that the incidence may be closer to 35% (39).

The diagnosis of this syndrome is complicated by the frequent occurrence of delayed neurological deficits. Many children with this injury will develop the neurological deficit hours or even days after the traumatic event. However, given the rarity of spinal injury and the attendant difficulty in recognizing or documenting an early transient neurological deficit, it is possible that the delayed presentations that are seen with this syndrome actually represent reinjury and not the first event.

SCIWORA was first described before the widespread availability of spinal magnetic resonance imaging. Therefore, although it is still true that most children with this syndrome show no bony injury on plain spine films and CT scan, most patients will have demonstrable injuries to the spinal cord or the surrounding structures on good quality magnetic resonance imaging studies (15). Therefore, a high index of suspicion is required to make the early diagnosis of this injury. Once the injury is documented or even suspected based on a history, then immobilization of the hypermobile spinal segment effectively prevents the delayed neurological deterioration (40).

The basic approach to the management of a spinally injured child is guided by the same principles as those used to treat spinally injured adults. Thus, aggressive support of systemic perfusion and ventilation is of paramount importance. Because children tend to have more rostral injuries of the cervical spinal cord, impaired respiratory function is likely to be present early after an injury. Furthermore, acute gastric dilatation commonly occurs in injured children, and this reaction can rapidly compromise ventilation. Gastric decompression can improve ventilatory parameters, but early elective intubation should always be considered.

Immobilization of the spine in anatomic alignment will allow healing in over 90% of spinally injured children (35). The halo brace orthoses are available in all sizes and can be successfully used even in very young children. For thoracolumbar injuries, acrylic bracing is usually successful. Instrumentation and segmental spinal fusions are not routinely necessary and should be avoided, if at all possible, to avoid the complications associated with spinal growth. However, some complex injuries will require operative fusion, which should be performed only by surgeons greatly experienced with diseases of the pediatric spine.

It is now recommended that all patients with acute spinal cord injury receive high-dose methylprednisolone for either 24 or 48 hours, depending on the time from injury to medical attention (7). Although all of the randomized trials of the therapy of spinal cord injury have excluded pediatric patients, the author is unaware of any information that suggests that pediatric patients may not benefit at least as much as adults by these therapies, nor of any information that these therapies may, in some way, be uniquely harmful to children. Therefore, all children with a documented or suspected spinal cord injury are administered methylprednisolone using the currently recommended dosing and time parameters.

REFERENCES

1. Alberico AN, Ward, JD, Choi SC, Marmarou A, Young HF: Outcome after severe head injury: Relationship to mass lesions, diffuse injury, and ICP course in pediatric and adult patients. **J Neurosurg** 67:648–656, 1987.
2. Aldrich EF, Eisenberg HM, Saydjari C et al.: Diffuse brain swelling in severely head injured children: A report from the NIH Traumatic Coma Data Bank. **J Neurosurg** 76:450–454, 1992.
3. Anderson JM, Schutt AH: Spinal cord injury in children: A review of 156 cases seen from 1950 through 1978. **Mayo Clin Proc** 55:499–504, 1980.
4. Armstead WM, Kurth CD: Different cerebral hemodynamic responses following fluid percussion brain injury in the newborn and juvenile pig. **J Neurotrauma** 11:487–497, 1994.
5. Bailey DK: The normal cervical spine in infants and children. **Radiology** 59:712–719, 1952.
6. Berger MS, Pitts LH, Lovely M, Edwards MS, Bartkowski HM: Outcome from severe head injury in children and adolescents. **J Neurosurg** 62:194–199, 1985.
7. Bracken MB, Shepard MJ, Holford TR, et al.: Administration of methylprednisolone for 24 or 48 hours or tirilizad mesylate for 48 hours in the treatment of acute spinal cord injury. **JAMA** 277:1597–1604, 1997.
8. Bullock R, Chesnut R, Clifton G, et al.: *Guidelines for the Management of Severe Head Injury*. New York, Brain Trauma Foundation, 1996.
9. Chesnut RM: Avoidance of hypotension: Conditio sine qua non of successful severe head injury management. **J Neurotrauma** 42: S4—S9, 1997.
10. Chesnut RM: Implications of the guidelines for the management of severe head injury for the practicing neurosurgeon. **Surg Neurol** 50:187–193, 1998.
11. Davis RL, Mullen N, Makela M, Taylor JA, Cohen W, Rivara FR: Cranial computed tomography scans in children after minimal head injury with loss of consciousness. **Ann Emerg Med** 24:640–645, 1994.
12. Dietrich AM, Bowman MJ, Ginn-Pease ME, Kusnick E, King DR: Pediatric head injuries: Can clinical factors reliably predict an abnormality on computed tomography? **Ann Intern Med** 22:1535–1540, 1993.
13. Duhaime AC, O'Rourke M: Intensive care management of children with head injuries, in Andrews BT, Hammer GB, (eds): *Pediatric Neurosurgical Intensive Care*. Park Ridge, IL, American Association of Neurological Surgeons, 1997, pp 125–138.
14. Duhaime AC, Christian CW, Rorke LB, Zimmerman RA: Nonaccidental head injury in infants: The "shaken-baby" syndrome. **N Engl J Med** 25:1822–1829, 1998.
15. Grabb PA, Pang D: Magnetic resonance imaging in the evaluation of spinal cord injury without radiographic abnormality in children. **Neurosurgery** 35:406–414, 1994.
16. Grundl PD, Biagas KV, Kochanek PM, Schiding JK, Barmada MA, Nemoto EM: Early cerebrovascular response to head injury in immature and mature rats. **J Neurotrauma** 11:135–148, 1994.
17. Hadley MN, Zabramski JM, Browner CM, Rekate H, Sonntag VK: Pediatric spinal trauma: Review of 122 cases of spinal cord and vertebral column injuries. **J Neurosurg** 68:18–24, 1988.
18. Hennes H, Lee M, Smith D, Sty JR, Losek J: Clinical predictors of severe head trauma in children. **Am J Dis Child** 142:1045–1047, 1988.
19. Hulka F, Mullins RJ, Mann NC, et al.: Influence of a statewide trauma system on pediatric hospitalization and outcome. **J Trauma** 42:514–519, 1997.

20. Jeret JS, Mandell M, Anziska B, et al.: Clinical predictors of abnormality disclosed by computed tomography after mild head trauma. **Neurosurgery** 32:9–16, 1993.
21. Johnson DL, Krishnamurthy S: Send severely head injured children to a pediatric trauma center. **Pediatr Neurosurg** 25:309–314, 1996.
22. Jubelirer RA, Agarwal NN, Beyer FC, et al.: Pediatric trauma triage: Review of 1307 cases. **J Trauma** 30:1544–1547, 1990.
23. Kasoff SS, Lansen TA, Holder D, Filippo JS: Aggressive physiologic monitoring of pediatric head trauma patients with elevated intracranial pressure. **Pediatr Neurosci** 14:241–249, 1988.
24. Kewalramani LS, Kraus JF, Sterling HM: Acute spinal cord lesions in a pediatric population: Epidemiological and clinical features. **Paraplegia** 18:206–219, 1980.
25. Luerssen TG: Intracranial pressure: Current status in monitoring and management. **Sem Pediatr Neurol** 4:146–155, 1997.
26. Luerssen TG, Wolfla CE: Pathophysiology and management of increased intracranial pressure in children, in Andrews BT, Hammer GB (eds): *Pediatric Neurosurgical Intensive Care*. Park Ridge, IL, American Association of Neurological Surgeons, 1997, pp 37–57.
27. Luerssen TG, Hults K, Klauber M, Marshall LF: Improved outcomes as a result of recognition of absent and compressed cisterns on initial CT scans, in Hoff JT, Betz AL (eds): *Intracranial Pressure VII*. Berlin, Springer-Verlag, 1989, pp 598–602.
28. Luerssen TG, Klauber MR, Marshall LF: Outcome from head injury related to patient's age: A longitudinal prospective study of adult and pediatric head injury. **J Neurosurg** 68:409–416, 1988.
29. Marmarou A, Anderson RL, Ward JD, et al.: Impact of ICP instability and hypotension on outcome in patients with severe head trauma. **J Neurosurg** 1991; S59–S66.
30. Marshall LF, Marshall SB, Klauber MR, et al.: A new classification of head injury based on computerized tomography. **J Neurosurg** 75:S14-S20, 1991.
31. McKoy C, Bell MJ: Preventable traumatic deaths in children. **J Ped Surg** 18:505–508, 1983.
32. Mendelow AD, Chambers IR, Kane PJ, et al.: Cerebral perfusion pressure in head injured children, in Nagai H, Kamiya K, Ishii S (eds): *Intracranial Pressure IX*. Tokyo, Springer-Verlag, 1994, pp 450–451.
33. Miller JD, Piper IR, Dearden NM: Management of intracranial hypertension in head injury: Matching treatment with cause. **Acta Neurochirurg** 57(Suppl):152–159, 1993.
34. National Heart Lung, and Blood Institute: Report of the second task force on blood pressure control in children—1987. **Pediatrics** 79:1–25, 1987.
35. Osenbach RK, Menezes AH: Pediatric spinal cord and vertebral column injuries. **Neurosurgery** 30:385–390, 1992.
36. O'Sullivan MG, Statham PF Jones PA, et al.: Role of intracranial pressure monitoring in severely head injured patients without signs of intracranial hypertension on initial computerized tomography. **J Neurosurg** 80:46–50, 1994.
37. Pang D, Wilberger JE: Spinal cord injury without radiographic abnormalities in children. **J Neurosurg** 57:114–129, 1982.
38. Pigula FA, Wald SL, Shackford SR, Vane DW: Effect of hypotension and hypoxia on children with severe head injuries. **J Pediatr Surg** 28:310–316, 1993.
39. Pollack IF, Pang D: Spinal cord injury without radiographic abnormality (SCIWORA), in Pang D (ed): *Disorders of the Pediatric Spine*. New York, Raven Press, 1995, pp 509–516.

40. Pollack IF, Pang D, Sclabassi R: Recurrent spinal cord injury without radiographic abnormalities in children. **J Neurosurg** 69:177–182, 1988.
41. Pople IK, Muhlbauer MS, Sanford RA, Kirk E: Results and complications of intracranial pressure monitoring in 303 children. **Pediatr Neurosurg** 23:64–67, 1995.
42. Rivara FP: Childhood injuries: III. Epidemiology of non-motor vehicle head trauma. **Dev Med Child Neurol** 26:81–87, 1984.
43. Rivara F, Tanaguchi D, Parish RA, Stimac GK, Mueller B: Poor prediction of positive computed tomographic scans by clinical criteria in symptomatic pediatric head trauma. **Pediatrics** 80:579–584, 1987.
44. Rosner MJ, Rosner SD, Johnson AH: Cerebral perfusion pressure: Management protocol and clinical results. **J Neurosurg** 83:949–963, 1995.
45. Ruge JR, Sinson GP, McLone DG, Cerullo LJ: Pediatric spinal injury: The very young. **J Neurosurg** 68:25–30, 1988.
46. Sharples PM, Stuart AG, Matthews DSF, Aynsley-Green A, Eyre JA: Cerebral blood flow and metabolism in children with severe head injury:. Part 1. Relation to age, Glasgow Coma Score, outcome, intracranial pressure, and time after injury. **J Neurol Neurosurg Psychiatr** 58:145–152, 1995.
47. Shaver EG, Duhaime AC, Curtis M, Gennarelli LM, Barrett R: Experimental acute subdural hematoma in infant piglets. **Pediatr Neurosurg** 25:123–129, 1996.
48. Skippen P, Seear M, Poskitt K, et al.: Effect of hyperventilation on regional cerebral blood flow in head-injured children. **Crit Care Med** 25:1402–1409, 1997.
49. Stein SC, Ross SE: The value of computed tomographic scans in patients with low-risk head injuries. **Neurosurgery** 26:638–640, 1990.
50. Stein SC, Spettell C, Young G, Ross SE: Limitations of neurological assessment in mild head injury. **Brain Inj** 7:425–430, 1993.
51. Welch K: The intracranial pressure in infants. **J Neurosurg** 52:693–699, 1980.
52. Wheatley J, Cass D: Pediatric post-injury management: A hospital-based review of deaths. **J Paediatr Child Health** 26:25–30, 1990.
53. Woolf SH: Practice guidelines, a new reality in medicine: II. Methods of developing guidelines. **Arch Intern Med** 152:946–952, 1992.

CHAPTER

13

Evolving Models of Neurotrauma Critical Care: An Analysis and Call to Action

RANDALL M. CHESNUT, M.D., F.A.C.C.M.

THE PERIPATETIC HEAD INJURY

Wide variability in management techniques applied to patients with severe traumatic brain injury (TBI) has been documented. In a 1995 publication, 219 centers that routinely manage severe TBI patients were surveyed as to their routine treatment practices (6). This survey revealed that it would be unlikely that a given TBI patient be managed in a similar fashion at different hospitals (*Table 13.1*). Of the 219 centers, only 50% monitored intracranial pressure (ICP) of patients with Glasgow Coma Scale ≤ 8, only 28% doing so routinely. Despite the irregularity with which ICP was monitored, 83% of the centers routinely administered Mannitol, and 83% of centers routinely hyperventilated. Of these, 29% routinely hyperventilated to a $PaCO_2 < 25$ mm Hg. This latter figure is most distressing in view of the Class I evidence that prophylactic hyperventilation to this extent is strongly associated with worse recovery. Finally, in terms of general approaches to head injury, the practice of fluid restriction is extremely widespread despite a growing body of evidence that hypovolemic hypotension is devastating to the traumatic brain injury patient and that the purported physiological principals underlying the concept of volume restriction in TBI are badly flawed.

Such data would suggest that one would not want to have a severe traumatic brain injury in "Anytown, USA." A review of the literature would suggest, however, that being treated for a brain injury at academic neurotrauma centers would not guarantee less treatment variability. Classic "ICP-based therapy" holds that intracranial hypertension is associated with poor outcome and that maintaining ICP at >20–25 mm Hg improves outcome (2, 9). A TBI patient being treated at a center using this practice philosophy would have the head of the bed elevated to 30 degrees, blood pressure maintained at a normal

TABLE 13.1
Critical Care Management of Severe Traumatic Brain Injury in 219 U.S. Centers that Routinely Manage Such Patients (6)

Management Parameter	% of Centers
Intermittent ICP monitoring	50
Routine ICP monitoring	28
Osmotic diuretics	83
Hyperventilation	83
Severe hyperventilation (25–30 mm Hg (3.3–4.0 kPa))	57
Extreme hyperventilation (25 mm Hg (< 3.3 kPa))	29
Steroids	64
Barbiturates	33

level, be fully fluid resuscitated, intubated, and ventilated, and have a staircase-type of escalating treatment protocol applied to intracranial hypertension. In general, cerebral spinal fluid drainage would be the first step, mannitol administration would be the second step, and hyperventilation would be the third step. Treatment of refractory intracranial hypertension might involve high-dose barbiturate treatment.

The "Cerebral Perfusion Pressure Management School" holds that the critical parameter is cerebral perfusion pressure (CPP), which is defined as [mean arterial pressure] − [intracranial pressure] (10, 11). This treatment philosophy holds that maintaining a CPP of >]70 mm Hg (or higher at some institutions) will prevent intracranial ischemia. Practitioners of CPP-based therapy often hold that CPP is much more important than ICP as a treatment parameter. Being managed at a center following such a philosophy generally involves keeping the head of the bed flat, resuscitating to hypervolemia, endotracheal intubation, and normal ventilation with strict avoidance of hyperventilation, and free use of pressors and inotropes to maintain CPP. Agents such as barbiturates are almost never used despite protracted and refractory elevations of ICP.

The "Optimized Hyperventilation School" holds that a primary cause of intracranial hypertension is increased cerebral blood volume, which results when cerebral blood flow outstrips cerebral metabolic needs (4, 5). This management school hinges upon the drop in cerebral metabolism that commonly follows severe TBI. Optimized hyperventilation management relies on measuring the oxygen saturation in the blood exiting the brain via the jugular vein to reveal the balance between cerebral perfusion and cerebral oxygen metabolism. Management at such a center generally involves elevating the head of the bed to 30 degrees, resuscitation to euvolemia, maintaining the blood pressure at normal levels, and inserting a continuous oxygen saturation monitoring catheter into the jugular vein at the level of the jugular bulb. Control of cerebral blood volume is then accomplished by manipulating cerebrovascular hypocapneic vasoconstriction through the use of hyperventilation targeted at keeping jugular venous oxygen saturation within normal limits.

Finally, a management school commonly known as the "Lund method" believes that a major cause of intracranial hypertension is cerebral vasogenic edema (1, 7). This school holds that the blood-brain barrier becomes leaky after trauma and that the brain becomes swollen as a result of fluid leakage from the vasculature into the brain parenchyma. The Lund method is based on attempting to keep fluid within the cerebral vasculature by lowering the capillary hydrostatic pressure and raising the capillary osmotic pressure. Patients treated according to the Lund method are resuscitated, intubated, and ventilated but not hyperventilated. They are maintained in a state of "negative fluid balance normovolemia," with albumen and plasma comprising a large percentage of administered fluids. Their cerebral perfusion pressure is maintained at 50 mm Hg using a combination of alpha agonists and beta antagonists. They generally receive low-dose steroids. An additional component of therapy may be the administration of dihydroergotamine, a migraine medication that produces vasoconstriction on both the arterial and venous sides.

These four "schools of thought" represent the principal competing philosophies in TBI management. All of them have presented Class III evidence supporting the association between their management strategy and good outcome. Unfortunately, in the absence of comparative studies using internal control groups, it is difficult to understand how such disparate therapies can produce "optimal" results. As demonstrated in *Table 13.2,* however, they do produce impressive variations in individual patient management maneuvers. For instance, the competing manipulations of the head of the bed illustrated when comparing these different schools might be interpreted by the less-informed as suggesting that vestibular stimulation is important in optimizing recovery from TBI.

CRITICAL CARE AS THE *CONDITIO SINE QUA NON* OF SUCCESSFUL TBI MANAGEMENT

Despite such a jarring lack of consensus in treatment, the overall lot of the TBI patient has improved vastly over the last decade. Mortality

TABLE 13.2
Practices Associated with Four Schools of Traumatic Brain Injury Management

Parameter	Management School			
	ICP[a]	CPP	Op Hyp	Lund
Head of bed	↑	↓	↑	↓
Hyperventilation	+	−	+	−
Blood pressure	=	↑	=	↓
Steroid use	±	−	−	+

[a]ICP, management based on intracranial pressure control; CPP, management based on cerebral perfusion pressure control; Op Hyp, management based on optimized hyperventilation using jugular venous saturation monitoring; Lund, management based on minimizing vasogenic edema (Lund Method).

rates reflected in results of multicenter TBI studies from the 1990s range from 18 to 24%, which is significantly better than the 36% mortality documented in the Traumatic Coma Data Bank using data from the 1980s. The issue is, then, how such improvement in outcome has been accomplished in the face of what seems like such clinical discord? A very telling glimpse into what seems to be the answer to this question comes from a quote from an article published in *Neurosurgery* in 1977 by Becker et al., where they stated: "A standardized protocol . . . [with] . . . emphasis on early diagnosis and evacuation of intracranial mass lesions by craniotomy, artificial ventilation, control of increased intracranial pressure, and aggressive medical therapy . . . enables some patients who would have died to make a good recovery" (2). Certainly, the growing rapid availability and experience with computed tomographic scanning of the traumatized brain continues to foster improvements in outcome. This is reflected in their statement, "early diagnosis and rapid evacuation of intracranial mass lesions." In addition, the factor that they quote as "control of increased intracranial pressure" has spurred progress supporting and promulgating ICP monitoring and, indeed, serving as the impetus for the development of the various treatment philosophies that were presented earlier. The two statements reflected as "artificial ventilation" and "aggressive medical treatment," however, may reflect those factors most responsible for the improvement in outcome from TBI. These factors reflect the extraordinary, continuing progress that has been occurring in critical care medicine over the last three decades. This progress is an extremely important but almost universally uncontrolled confounding factor in the vast majority of head injury treatment success reports. Indeed, for instance, it has been argued that the avoidance of in-hospital hypotension alone may account for the majority of improvement in outcome attributed to CPP therapy (3).

Certainly, most of us would readily admit that, in the absence of satisfactory critical care, there is little we could do in a brain-specific fashion to successfully improve recovery from TBI.

The implications of the under-recognized but fundamental role of critical care in improving outcome from TBI are two. First, the essential nature of optimal critical care must be explicitly recognized and formally designed into any system caring for TBI patients. Second, neurosurgery must formally recognize that competency in critical care is a *conditio sine qua non* of managing the TBI patient and that proving this competency will probably soon determine the role of neurosurgery in this field.

Fundamental to all of the treatment protocols outlined previously is aggressive manipulation of the cardiovascular and pulmonary systems in addition to brain therapy. By definition, this requires admission to a competent intensive care unit and familiarity with cardiovascular and pulmonary physiology, including ventilator management. Because of the common association of TBI with extracranial injuries and the often protracted intensive care unit stays, competence in fluid and electrolyte management, infectious disease, nutrition, and other aspects of critical care is also required. As these issues become increasingly complex, the issue of competency and its documentation will continue to grow. In all disciplines outside of neurosurgery, competency in critical care requires some specialized training outside of the normal course of residency and results in specific critical care competency certification. In some hospitals, the ability to be the primary physician in a critical care unit requires certification in critical care and current credentials in advanced cardiac life support management. As the TBI patient cannot be managed outside of an intensive care unit, such issues must be formally recognized by the neurosurgical community. Unfortunately, at present, those interested in special certification in critical care must step outside the discipline of neurosurgery to obtain such recognition.

Models of TBI management range from the neurosurgery service delivering the entire spectrum of care to that of a primary patient management by intensivists with neurosurgical consultation only for insertion of intracranial pressure monitors or removal of surgical mass lesions.

The Neurosurgeon as Team Leader

At the primary end of this spectrum, the neurosurgical service interacts on an equal basis with the trauma service from the admission of the patient. Such a neurosurgery service will assume primary responsibility for critical care TBI patients from the beginning if extracranial injury is minimal or as soon as the other extracranial issues have stabilized. This model requires the neurosurgeon to also function as an intensivist. By definition, a representative of the neurosurgical service with competency in managing critical care issues must be available to intensive care unit patients immediately 24 hours a day, 7 days a week. This is obviously an enormous commitment of both time and critical care specialization for any neurosurgeon and is probably not realistic outside of academic centers, where upper-level residents or fellows can play a significant role in filling these necessities.

The Neurosurgeon as a Team Member

An intermediate TBI practice model would be one in which the neurosurgeon is an active and knowledgeable consultant, primarily determining the therapeutic modalities applied to the injured brain, and interacting with the managing service to accomplish such therapies in consideration of their interactions with extracranial organ systems and multisystem trauma. In such a model, the neurosurgeon may or may not be the primary managing physician, but the treatment will be accomplished by an integrated team that will include someone who serves as the primary intensivist. This person could be part of an independent critical care service or a trauma surgeon with certification in critical care.

Fundamental to such a model is a thorough understanding of and competency in critical care by the neurosurgeon. This is necessary so that the cardiovascular, pulmonary, etc. aspects of TBI management are carefully accomplished and so that they integrate optimally with treatments directed at extracranial organ systems.

This model can vary widely in terms of the neurosurgeon's input. To a great extent, this will depend on the competency and interest of the neurosurgeon in critical care. At the most "neurosurgical" end of the spectrum, the neurosurgeon will manage the majority of critical care issues because most of them will be more or less involved in treating the injured brain. At the least "neurosurgical" end of the spectrum, the majority of interventions will be designed and accomplished by the trauma or intensive medicine service, with the neurosurgeon as a consulting part of the team. If neurosurgery as a discipline wishes to maintain its primacy in managing TBI, it will attempt to maintain a position at the more "neurosurgical" end of the spectrum. If trauma services or intensive medicine services are to become the primary caretakers of TBI patients and managers of brain injury, the less "neurosurgical" end of the spectrum will be satisfactory.

The Neurosurgeon as a Technical Consultant

The most distal end of the spectrum of TBI care will be where the entire continuum of management of these patients is accomplished by an intensivist. Such models already exist in Europe and Latin America and seem to provide exquisite management and excellent outcomes in those specific instances where the intensivists have very strong interests in TBI management. In such models, the neurosurgeon is simply a technical consultant who inserts intracranial pressure monitors or removes intracranial surgical mass lesions (generally as recognized by the intensivist) and has little other input into the care of the patient. Such a model obviously requires little critical care knowledge on the part of the neurosurgeon. This allows neurosurgeons with little interest or sophistication in critical care to fill their minimal role in TBI management. It also allows them to continue their neurosurgical elective practice with minimal disruption by trauma. Finally, it obviates the necessity of formal critical care certification for neurosurgeons.

QUO VADEMUS?

As noted above, critical care is fundamental to the care of TBI patients. It seems, therefore, that the ability to manage the critical care aspects of a patient will increasingly determine the role of the neurosurgeon in TBI management. As previously discussed, models already exist wherein the neurosurgeon is simply a technical consultant and management issues of ICP and cerebral perfusion are entirely accomplished by intensivists. Unpublished prospective data collections on outcomes of TBI patients managed in such systems suggest excellent results. Although these are unusual systems and are directed by intensivists with dominant clinical interests in the area of brain injury, they certainly serve as a harbinger of things to come unless neurosurgery formally addresses the role of the neurosurgeon in TBI management.

Both the American College of Surgeons and the Society of Critical Care Medicine have expressed a powerful and expanding interest in this area. Leaders in both fields have stated that neurosurgeons are underserving the TBI population and that their disciplines (e.g., the American College of Surgeons or the Society of Critical Care Medicine) should be willing to assume more responsibilities for this trauma population. As no intensivists and only rare trauma surgeons in the U.S. are willing to remove intracranial mass lesions, craniotomy will remain in control of neurosurgeons. A growing number of intensivists and trauma surgeons, however, are expressing interest in inserting ICP monitors. In the absence of ready availability of neurosurgeons for such procedures, it may be that ICP monitor insertion will go the way of Swan Ganz catheter insertion and become a procedure that is not limited to the discipline that originated it. At its most extreme, such a course would relegate the neurosurgeon exclusively to a minimal role as a "clotbuster."

Statements and activities coming from surgical and intensive medicine societies in the U.S. and abroad indicate that the gamut has clearly been drawn. The primacy of TBI in determining outcome from trauma and the fundamental role of critical care in managing TBI patients mandates that such questions be explicitly addressed. Approximately three generations ago, neurosurgeons such as Jennett, Jamieson, and Braakman brought the treatment of brain injury into focus. Until recently, the dominance of neurosurgery in TBI management has been unquestionable. Within the last decade, however, the number of publications on the clinical and basic science aspects of TBI management that have appeared in non-neurosurgical journals has grown remarkably. In addition, the appearance of non-neurosurgical "neurointensivists" and of neurocritical care sections within intensive medicine societies has strongly illustrated the increasing focus of non-neurosurgical disciplines upon care for the injured brain. Unfortunately, neurosurgery as a discipline has been distressingly silent during this period.

It would seem that the present is a crucial time for the establishment and maintenance of the proper role of neurosurgery in managing TBI patients. By all indications, if neurosurgery continues as it is going, intensivists will become the primary managers in the future. Preemptive neurosurgical action requires, at the least, a formal analysis of the role of the neurosurgeon in TBI and a policy statement from neurosurgery. If neurosurgery is to maintain its dominant position in this field, neurosurgeons will have to establish and certify their competency in critical care and be available to trauma services and TBI patients as integral members of trauma systems. In addition, situations in which neurosurgical groups charge hospitals exorbitant fees merely to be available cannot be accepted. We need to maintain neurosurgery at the more "neurosurgical" end of the TBI management spectrum.

If this is to be accomplished, neurosurgery must critically evaluate the purported competence in intensive medicine that is claimed by all graduates of neurosurgical residency programs. A neurosurgeon that is truly competent in critical care must be capable of independent management of at least the most fundamental cardiovascular, pulmonary, infectious disease, gastrointestinal, and metabolic issues in the intensive care patient. If we are to claim critical care competency, we must, for instance, be able to prove that we are independently capable of directing proper ventilator management of evolving pathological pulmonary processes.

This may not be possible or desirable for all neurosurgeons. Most neurosurgeons probably do not have the interest or the time to accomplish or maintain competency in critical care. This should be entirely acceptable to the neurosurgical community. For those that are interested in TBI management and do wish to establish competency in intensive medicine, however, the mechanics of accomplishing these ends must be made readily available and recognized. Without such tools, neurosurgeons will be helpless against the rising tide of intensivists, in terms of both professional and clinical-ethical aspects.

The scenario as depicted above suggests that neurosurgery must accommodate the development of a group of neurosurgical neurotraumatologists if neurosurgery is to maintain a predominant role in this area. This will admittedly be a somewhat restricted group as most neurosurgeons did not enter this field to manage brain injury. Because this implies that there will be a limited pool of neurosurgeons willing to serve as "soldiers" in maintaining the role of neurosurgery in TBI management, neurosurgery as a discipline must support them in both training and professional arenas.

TBI management is a highly specialized and somewhat onerous aspect of neurosurgery. In addition, it is the one subspecialty of neurosurgery that cannot exist without significant input from other non-neurosurgical disciplines. Finally, as we have seen above, it is the neurosurgical discipline that is definitely the least "surgical" of all. Because of these constraints, neurotrauma needs to be practiced at specialized centers that possess all of the personnel and physical attributes required by the American College of Surgeons Committee on Trauma for Level I or Level II trauma centers at a minimum. In addition, if selected neurosurgeons are going to be able to focus all or a significant percentage of their practice around neurotrauma management, situations must be developed in which this is possible. Coupled with the high demand of TBI on resource availability, this is a strong mandate for regionalization of TBI care. Trauma systems have been shown to improve the outcome of severe TBI when the trauma system results in the transfer of a patient to a Level I trauma center (8). Clearly, the optimal situation for neurosurgeons would be the development of trauma systems, with a specific focus on neurotrauma, wherein an adequate volume of neurotrauma is seen to support the necessary resource infrastructure, an adequate neurosurgical income stream exists, the hospital's commitment to a neurotrauma service is evident, and neurotrauma research is accomplished. First and foremost should be formal commitment of neurosurgical training programs to support Level I trauma centers in terms of neurotrauma care. The involvement of residents and fellows in neurotrauma benefits the patients, the trauma system, and the training program. Neurosurgery must also support the organiza-

TABLE 13.3
Steps Toward Reinforcing Neurosurgery's Role in Continuing to Lead Traumatic Brain Injury Management

Regionalizing management of severe traumatic brain injury within Level I trauma centers
Optimized resource utilization
Ensures an adequate workload for neurotrauma specialists
Comprehensive training in critical care
Subspecialty certification
Formal actions in support of neurotrauma by organized neurosurgery
Policy statement on the role of neurosurgery in traumatic brain injury
Neurosurgeon as key element
Team leader
Team member
Active recognition of role of other disciplines in team
Statement on fair reasonable financial support for this role
Condemnation of extortion of Level I trauma centers

tion of trauma systems, particularly with respect to the development of neurotrauma specialty centers within the group of Level I centers. In other words, organized neurosurgery must actively recognize the league, supply the players, and support the building of the fields if they are to continue to play ball. An exemplary list of requisite neurosurgical steps to accomplish such ends is presented in *Table 13.3*.

This is an extremely critical time for neurosurgery in TBI management. Most likely, if formal action is not taken soon, neurosurgical predominance in this field will end within a decade. Neurosurgery must recognize that most neurosurgeons do not want to do trauma and should support a system that does not force any neurosurgeon to do so against his wishes. Unless organized neurosurgery is willing to surrender its role in TBI management entirely, however, it must concomitantly optimize practice situations for neurosurgeons who are interested in neurotrauma. Otherwise, it is likely that the role of neurosurgeons in TBI management in the future will be simply that of a technical consultant.

REFERENCES

1. Asgeirsson B, Grande PO, Nordstrom CH: A new therapy of post-trauma brain oedema based on haemodynamic principles for brain volume regulation. **Intensive Care Med** 20:260–267, 1994.
2. Becker DP, Miller JD, Ward JD, Greenberg RP, Young HF, Sakalas R: The outcome from severe head injury with early diagnosis and intensive management. **J Neurosurg** 47:491–502, 1977.

3. Chesnut RM: Avoidance of hypotension: Conditio sine qua non of successful severe head-injury management. **J Trauma** 42:S4—S9, 1997.
4. Cruz J: The first decade of continuous monitoring of jugular bulb oxyhemoglobinsaturation: Management strategies and clinical outcome. **Crit Care Med** 26:344–351, 1998.
5. Cruz J, Raps EC, Hoffstad OJ, Jagg JL, Gennarell TA: Cerebral oxygenation monitoring. **Crit Care Med** 21:1242–1246, 1993.
6. Ghajar J, Hariri RJ, Narayan RK, Iacona LA, Firlik K, Patterson RH: Survey of critical care management of comatose, head-injured patients in the United States. **Crit Care Med** 23:560–567, 1995.
7. Grande PO, Asgeirsson B, Nordstrom C: Aspects on the cerebral perfusion pressure during therapy of a traumatic head injury. **Acta Anaesthesiol Scand Suppl** 110:36–40, 1997.
8. Mullins RJ, Mann NC, Hedges JR, Worral W, Juskovich GJ: Preferential benefit of implementation of a statewide trauma system in one of two adjacent states. **J Trauma** 44:609–616, 1998; discussion, 617.
9. Pacult A, Gudeman SK: Medical management of head injuries, in Becker DP, Gudeman SK (eds): *Textbook of Head Injury*. Philadelphia, WB Saunders, 1989, pp 192–220.
10. Rosner MJ: Pathophysiology and management of increased intracranial pressure, in Andrews BT (ed): *Neurosurgical Intensive Care*. New York, McGraw Hill, 1993, pp 57–112.
11. Rosner MJ, Rosner SD, Johnson AH: Cerebral perfusion pressure: Management protocol and clinical results. **J Neurosurg** 83: 949–962, 1995.

CHAPTER

14

Core Curriculum in Neurosurgical Critical Care

BRIAN T. ANDREWS, M.D., F.A.C.S.

The intensive care unit (ICU) is integral to a neurosurgeon's care of most patients that harbor intracranial disease processes. During the initial period of observation, patients will usually be placed into an intensive care setting to allow for the frequent, detailed neurological observation needed to identify deterioration (8). During the initial medical management of many problems, such as severe head injury (1), acute subarachnoid hemorrhage (5), intracerebral hemorrhage (7), and brain tumors (6), the ICU provides the necessary level of care and ancillary observation needed to apply these therapies safely. Often, initial management requires specialized monitoring, such as for elevated intracranial pressure (ICP), that can only be performed in an ICU setting (1). Following virtually all craniotomies for whatever reason, the ICU has historically been the site of initial postoperative observation and ongoing medical treatment.

Many patients with other problems attended to by neurosurgeons, such as spinal cord injury, also have requirements for care that demand the ICU setting (3). Patients within the pediatric age group also have similar if not more stringent need for specialized pediatric ICU care when facing neurosurgical problems (2).

It is also clear that the quality of neurosurgical management within an ICU can influence patient outcome. As an example, Le Roux et al. (4) showed with Class II evidence that the clinical outcome after rupture of anterior circulation aneurysms improved significantly over the course of a decade (1983–1993). Over this period of time, the surgical management of these patients had not changed, but the incidence of medical complications such as hypoxia, hypotension, and hyperglycemia decreased in a significant way, and vasospasm was treated much more aggressively. Improvements in critical care techniques and in the management of vasospasm seemed to correlate with the improvement seen in clinical outcome. In a similar fashion, improvement in the ICU management of neurogenic hypotension and hypoxia among patients with spinal cord injury in the ICU has been shown to improve outcome (10).

Thus, the great frequency with which neurosurgeons must work within the ICU and the findings that such care when optimized improves patient outcome demand that we be completely facile in the ICU setting. This is not just within the narrow realm of the brain and spinal cord but also as it applies to systemic disease processes.

Over time, and often geographically between different institutions, various models of ICU patient management have evolved. In some hospitals, the patient in the ICU is cared for primarily by the critical care medicine specialist (intensivist), with other specialists acting primarily as consultants. In other settings, particularly trauma centers, trauma surgeons or anesthesiologists are the physicians primarily in charge of the patient. Occasionally, usually in larger academic medical centers, there are specialized neurosurgical ICUs where the neurosurgeon is clearly delineated as the primary physician in charge of the patient, calling in other specialists on an as-needed basis, and managing most problems such as ventilators and cardiovascular management themselves.

THE PROBLEM

The problem facing the neurosurgeon today is that there are numerous competing interests in the care of neurosurgical patients placed into ICUs. Multiple other physician specialists consider such patients within their own realm of specialty, such as the above noted intensivists, trauma surgeons, specialists in pulmonary medicine, anesthesiologists, and, recently, neurologists (9). At times, there are conflicts between these specialists over control of the patient that may hinder the optimal delivery of care and lead to territorial disputes. Indeed, each specialist comes to the bedside with a specific background of training and experience as well as expectations. As one result of the conflicts between specialties, multiple certification examinations and "special qualifications" in critical care from the certifying agencies for anesthesiology, internal medicine, and general surgery have evolved.

From some of these competing interests, there has been voiced skepticism as to the ability of neurosurgeons to handle problems as they arise in the ICU. Indeed, such skepticism may not be unfounded in some cases, where due to a lack of training during residency, or lack of experience following graduation, the neurosurgeon has lost the skills necessary to provide safe management of the patient in the ICU. This may have arisen for no more of a reason than the neurosurgeon having delegated the responsibility of care away to these other physician specialists in their particular practice setting.

Going further, it has become evident that there are some physician specialists who are frankly critical of neurosurgeons remaining responsible for the care of their own patients in the ICU setting (M Rosner, M.D., Ph.D., personal communication). Such specialists feel that it should be the responsibility of their own specialty to administer care, even when the primary problem for which the patient needs the ICU is neurological. In some cases, this has evolved to the point of the intensivists themselves performing neurosurgical procedures, such as the placement of ventriculostomies and other intracranial pressure catheters.

Indeed, it is imperative that neurosurgeons understand that there are many who will gladly fill our role in the ICU if allowed to. This has recently become the focus of attention for some neurologists, who are actively developing a model for the "critical care neurologist" able to manage all aspects of neurological disease in the ICU setting, including the placement of intracranial monitors (9). In the early 1990s, a new section of the American Academy of Neurology began to legitimize these inroads into critical care by collecting consensus guidelines for specific ICU problems, defining the scope of training needed for critical care, and developing academic strength in the area through scientific sessions and practical courses. There is a belief among some neurologists that they are in the best position to direct those units that are occupied by patients with neurological diseases.

This may prove to be an epic step, because until now the neurosurgeon has always had a single, yet insurmountable upper hand over all others interested in our own terrain in the ICU; we have remained the acknowledged expert of intracranial physiology and its assessment. The problems of intracranial pressure elevation, inadequate cerebral perfusion, or oxygen extraction and their treatment have heretofore been ours. This may no longer remain the case unless we take steps to assure that it remains so.

Assuming that the neurosurgeon is adequately trained and prepared for the management of patients in the ICU, there remains the need for adequate documentation of this fact. Some criticism has been lodged against neurosurgeons wishing to remain in charge of their own neurosurgical ICUs for not having specific documentation, or "special qualification" as devised by some other specialties, establishing their intensive care training and credibility. This is particularly true where there are competing interests in the ICU hierarchy.

THE CORE CURRICULUM IN NEUROSURGICAL CRITICAL CARE

As a means to assure the adequacy of training for neurosurgeons in all aspects of patient management in the ICU, an effort has been made by members of the Joint Section on Neurotrauma and Critical Care to establish a Core Curriculum in Neurosurgical Critical Care. This goes well beyond the standard training that most of us received in intracranial physiology, monitoring, and problem solving and includes a broad exposure to the basic principles of intensive care management for each pertinent organ system as well as philosophical issues, such as the withdrawal of care. Such a curriculum is envisioned as one that can be completed during the course of neurosurgical residency or applied or continued during Fellowship. Such a curriculum should also be appropriate and applicable for the practicing neurosurgeon as a component of the "curriculum for life" recently envisioned by the Joint Officers of the AANS/CNS.

Upon completion of the Core Curriculum, the neurosurgeon should be adept at the overall management of patients in the ICU if they so choose to assume such a primary role. It would also establish a baseline of information for co-management, or at a minimum, communicating soundly with other specialists involved in the care of the ICU patient.

THE SYSTEMIC APPROACH

The basic method of the Core Curriculum is a system-by-system approach to the physical diagnosis, pathophysiology, and technical training needed for the care of patients in the ICU. This would include experience in pertinent procedures and techniques. The general systems reviewed include: 1) pulmonary, 2) cardiovascular, 3) neurological, 4) gastrointestinal, 5) genitourinary-renal, 6) hematological, 7) musculoskeletal, and 8) fluids, electrolytes, and acid-base physiology. In addition to these system-by-system reviews, other elements of ICU management will be included, such as 9) infectious disease, 10) pharmacology, 11) psychosocial problems, and 12) ethical and legal issues (e.g., advanced directives, living wills, consent, withdrawal of care).

As an example for the level of detail involved for each system, the core curriculum for the neurological system is described more completely in *Table 14.1*.

To a similar level of detail, the core curriculum will review and include the ICU management of commonly occurring problems such as spinal cord injury, status epilepticus, acute cerebral ischemia and stroke, and hypertensive encephalopathy.

TABLE 14.1
The Neurological System

Cerebral blood flow
  Normal values
  Values for reversible and irreversible ischemia and infarction
  Autoregulation
  Pathological alterations (e.g., vasospasm, head injury, elevations in ICP
  Monitoring techniques (includes methods and analysis of data): xenon-CT, 133-xenon, SPECT, nitrous oxide, transcranial Doppler, thermodiffusion flowmetry; laser-Doppler flowmetry
  Management: volume status, rheology, blood pressure manipulation, pharmacology, neurointerventional, surgical
Cerebral blood volume
  Physiology;
  As a component of increased ICP
  Pathological alterations (e.g., right heart failure)
  Measurement (Yoshino method-rapid sequence contrast CT)
  Management: volume status, cardiopulmonary effects, head of bed elevation
Cerebral oxygen extraction
  Normal physiology and regulation
  Pathological alterations (e.g., ischemia, luxury perfusion)
  Monitoring techniques: arterial-jugular venous oxygen content difference ($AVdO_2$), jugular venous oxygen saturation (SjO_2), cerebral metabolic rate for oxygen ($CMRO_2$), transcutaneous methods; near-infrared spectroscopy
  Pressure management: hypothermia, barbiturate coma
  Management: cardiopulmonary effects, cerebral perfusion
Intracranial pressure
  Normal physiology and regulation
  Pathological alterations (e.g., head injury, brain tumors, hepatic encephalopathy, ischemia)
  Monitoring techniques: ventriculostomy, fiberoptic and strain-gauge techniques, subdural catheters, epidural devices
  Management: cardiopulmonary effects, cerebral perfusion
  Pressure management: hyperventilation, hypothermia, mannitol, corticosteroids, barbiturate coma
Cerebral glucose and energy metabolism
  Normal physiology and regulation
  Pathological alterations (e.g., head injury, ischemia)
  Monitoring techniques: magnetic resonance spectroscopy, cerebral microdialysis (glucose, glycerol, pyruvate, lactate), PET
  Management

CREDENTIALING

Upon completion of the Core Curriculum in Critical Care, it is expected that the neurosurgeon would be equipped, both from a knowledge-base perspective and a technical-skills perspective, to become the primary physician in charge of a patient in the ICU, should they so choose to do so. The documentation of this formalized education may include written and bedside problem solving, documented competence in performing a certain number of technical procedures in the ICU (e.g., endotracheal intubations, jugular-venous catheters, ICP monitors), and completion of a component of the written and oral examinations for the American Board of Neurological Surgeons designed to test such skills.

The provision of a distinct and separate "diploma" or "special certificate" for the completion of this Core Curriculum has already been considered by the American Board of Neurological Surgeons and was rejected on the basis that such a certification might preclude neurosurgeons who don't have such a certificate from caring for patients in the ICU setting. Rather, I suggest that the provision, testing, and completion of such a Core Curriculum within the context of our Residency and Fellowship training programs, and passage of a section of the neurosurgical Boards examination specifically designed to test such skills, can stand on its own as documentation. Thus, the Core Curriculum in Critical Care itself can then be used, for those who might question our abilities in the ICU, to clarify that a high-level standard of education for this purpose has been met.

The members of the Joint Section on Neurotrauma and Critical Care are continuing the development of this Core Curriculum and look forward to its completion within the next year. I call upon all neurosurgeons to embrace this effort.

REFERENCES

1. Andrews BT: The intensive care management of patients with head injury, in Andrews BT (ed): *Neurosurgical Intensive Care.* New York, McGraw-Hill Publishers, 1993, pp 27–242.
2. Andrews BT, Hammer GB (eds): *Pediatric Neurosurgical Intensive Care.* Park Ridge, IL, American Association of Neurological Surgeons Publications, 1997.
3. Dickman CA, Sonntag VKH: The intensive care management of spinal cord injury, in Andrews BT (ed): *Neurosurgical Intensive Care.* New York, McGraw-Hill Publishers, 1993, pp 243–250.
4. Le Roux PD, Elliott JP, Downey L, et al.: Improved outcome after rupture of anterior circulation aneurysms: A retrospective 10-year review of 224 good-grade patients. **J Neurosurg** 83:394–402, 1995.
5. Martin NA, Khanna R, Rodts G: The intensive care management of patients with

subarachnoid hemorrhage. in Andrews BT (ed): *Neurosurgical Intensive Care.* New York, McGraw-Hill Publishers, 1993, pp 291–310.
6. Morita M, Andrews BT, Gutijn PH: The intensive care management of patients with brain tumors. in Andrews BT (ed): *Neurosurgical Intensive Care.* New York, McGraw-Hill Publishers, 1993, pp 372–390.
7. Obana WG, Andrews BT: The intensive care management of nontraumatic intracerebral hemorrhage, in Andrews BT (ed): *Neurosurgical Intensive Care.* New York, McGraw-Hill Publishers, 1993, pp 311–328.
8. Obana WG, Andrews BT: The neurological examination and neurologic monitoring in the intensive care unit, in Andrews BT (ed): *Neurosurgical Intensive Care.* New York, McGraw-Hill Publishers, 1993, pp 31–42.
9. Ropper AH: Neurological intensive care. **Ann Neurol** 32:564–569, 1992.
10. Vale FL, Burns J, Jackson AB, Hadley MN: Combined medical and surgical treatment after acute spinal cord injury: Results of a prospective pilot study to assess the merits of aggressive medical resuscitation and blood pressure management. **J Neurosurg** 87:239–246, 1997.

CHAPTER

15

Outcomes Science and Neurotrauma: A National Database

BEVERLY C. WALTERS, M.D., M.SC., F.R.C.S.C., F.A.C.S.

In recent years, there has been an increased interest in epidemiological, prognostic, diagnostic, and therapeutic research in neurotrauma. As a clinical entity that occupies an inexorable place in neurosurgical practice all over the world, it requires attention that we would sometimes rather spend on other, perhaps more technically challenging clinical areas. However, the population involved—largely men and women at the peak of performance—represents a loss of human potential and resources that is unacceptable in modern society and thus attracts the interest and abilities of some of our finest neurosurgical researchers. To enhance our abilities to effectively manage these patients, evidence-based guidelines were undertaken by the neurosurgical community using a scientific approach (3). This approach requires the evaluation of published literature with respect to its scientific validity according to accepted epidemiological principles (8). In this way, management algorithms can be developed that may increase the precision in our treatment and improve outcome.

In reviewing the literature, it became embarrassingly apparent that there were little data gathered in a truly scientific fashion that could be used to generate practice parameters based upon a high degree of clinical certainty. This would require randomized controlled trials for evaluating therapeutic interventions or large-scale observational studies for determining prognosis. The deterrents to such high quality studies include a lack of appreciation for scientific rigor in human investigation, a lack of energy and time necessary to bring about the successful completion of properly designed studies, and a lack of funding available for such studies. Of these three, the first can be resolved with education and experience, leaving the other two as stumbling blocks to production of good quality evidence from which we might derive strong practice recommendations. Therefore, it might further the cause of clinical research, and thus clinical practice, if there was a way to facilitate implementation of clinical trials and make them less costly to perform.

One possibility might be the creation of a national database on neurotrauma into which randomized trials might be inserted and from which longitudinal studies on outcomes could be derived. In addition, studies on the quality of care could also be carried out using such databases. The purpose of this paper is to discuss concepts of database creation and use and the ways in which databases might further the cause of evidence-based neurotrauma care.

DATABASE CONCEPTS

An understanding of databases in general is a required step in approaching the utilization of databases for neurosurgical research purposes. There are certain aspects of databases that need to be reflected upon before an understanding of databases is possible. These have been best articulated by Pryor and colleagues (7) and can be summarized into the following categories: 1) organization of databases, 2) common characteristics of databases, 3) problems faced by all databases, and 4) characteristics of a successful database. These will be considered in order in the following paragraphs.

ORGANIZATION OF DATABASES

Databases may be organized in various ways, depending upon the focus of the subsequent use of the data, once analyzed. They may be organized by populations or diseases, or specific to particular therapies, devices, or procedures. Therefore, in neurotrauma, they can be developed to examine the process of care or outcomes of the entire population of interest, including all patients admitted to the trauma facility, regardless of age or severity of injury. This would be a *disease-oriented* approach, as it includes all patients with nervous system injury. Patients could be divided into those with brain injury or spinal cord injury, and this would yield two disease-oriented data sets. On the other hand, if an examination were to be undertaken of data pertaining to pediatric or adult patients, this would be *population-oriented* in focus. Examination of data pertaining to patients who had all had early decompressive surgery in spinal cord injury would be an example of *procedure-specific* data. On the other hand, looking at those patients who had been treated with brain tissue pH monitors would provide information that could be considered *device-specific*. If a database was designed to gather information on spinal cord injury or brain injury patients treated with steroids or calcium channel blockers, this would be characterized as *therapy-specific*. If all patients treated for any sort of neurotrauma encountered in clinical practice were included in a national database, divisions of the data could be made in all of the categories listed above, depending upon the focus of the investigation at hand.

COMMON CHARACTERISTICS OF DATABASES

In every database, regardless of organization, all data are collected, entered, stored, retrieved, and analyzed. Data collection and entry should be easy and rapid to accomplish, be exact (precise), contain all relevant variables, be prospectively carried out, and be integrated into clinical practice. This makes a database as usable as possible, and therefore, able to improve the quantity and quality of data collection. Imagine a circumstance in which the information obtained on patients, their clinical condition, the history of their illness, and the process of their treatment was all gathered instantly on a computer keyboard or screen and could be accessed from the moment of input in any form desired. The technology for this is available today and is exemplified in the input of food orders in restaurants—a common occurrence in North America. If this is possible in the food business, surely it is possible in the business of health care. Many clinicians use such databases for clinical practice purposes in the office setting, with the ease of encounter documentation being the primary goal (11). Others use such databases as quality assurance tools feeding back to the practitioner about deficiencies in clinical care (1). It would be a simple process to convert such a database to a research tool (10) or to expand such a database for hospital use on a grander scale. A database was instituted for use in assessing patients in the trauma room in Toronto, including intake sheets that became part of the medical record but that had to be entered separately into a database (*Fig. 15.1*). Institution of these assessment sheets as the record of the patient encounter improved the data collection significantly (12). A newer, "on-line" program is currently being tested as part of a central European neurotrauma effort aimed at gathering data on the process of health care in brain injury following introduction of the severe head injury guidelines. In this demonstration project, data on patients are being sent via the internet to a central data collection center in the United States, including digitized data on imaging studies, principally computerized tomography (*Fig. 15.2*). It is hoped that this program will demonstrate the ease with which data may be collected, entered, stored, retrieved, and analyzed in the busy atmosphere of neurotrauma care.

Also common to all database installation is the difficulty in achieving the appropriate balance between hardware and software requirements. The software needs to be easy to use, with one-touch function wherever possible. It is desirable that the appearance of the computer screen

SUNNYBROOK MEDICAL CENTRE
TRAUMA ASSESSMENT RECORD
NEUROSURGERY

Date: Time:
Age: Male/Female

Incident:

Date: Time:
Place: Referring Hospital:

Trauma History: (circle your choice, comment when necessary)   **COMMENT:**

BLUNT:
AUTO: Driver/Passenger; Front/Rear/Unknown
MOTORCYCLE: Driver/Passenger/Unknown
RECREATIONAL VEHICLE: Driver/Passenger/Unknown;
    Snowmobile/ATV/Pedalbike/Boat/Other
SEAT BELT: Shoulder/Lap/None/Unknown
HELMET: Yes/No/Flew Off
FALL: Recreational/Industrial/Diving/Home/Other
PEDESTRIAN   INDUSTRIAL   ASSAULT

BURN:
Flame
Electrical
Chemical
Explosion

PENETRATING:
Stab/GSW

Alcohol/Drugs: Level: mMol/L   SEIZURE: Yes/No
UNCONSCIOUS: Yes/No; Duration: Since Accid: min;   AMNESIA: Yes/No; Duration: Since Accid: min

Medical History: (circle your choice, comment when necessary)   **COMMENT:**

Alcohol	Auditory disorder	Endocrine (Specify)	Pregnancy	Renal Disease
Anesthetic Problems	Bleeding disorder	Hypertension	Prior Surgery	Seizure Disorder
Angina	Cerebrovascular Disease	Illicit Drugs	Prior Trauma	Visual Disorder
Arthritis	COPD	Malignancy	Prosthesis	NONE
Asthma	Dementia	MI	Psychiatric Hx	UNAVAILABLE

Current Medication: **Allergy:** Environmental / Drug (Specify)

Airway: Adequate (Yes/No) / Nasotracheal tube / Orotracheal tube / Cricothyrotomy / Tracheotomy   SIZE:
    Suspected Hypoxia: Yes/No Duration: min   **Suspected Hypotension:** Yes/No Duration: min

Vital Signs: Heart Rate: Systemic BP: /   Temperature: C (Axillary/Oral/Rectal)
    Respiration Rate: /min   Ventilated: Yes/No

Level of Consciousness: (GCS)

	Incident	Refer Hosp.	SMC Emerg.
Time			
Eyes (4)			
Verbal (5)			
Motor (6)			

Patient: Intubated: Yes/No; Medicated: Yes/No
COMMENT:

Systemic Injury: (circle, comment when necessary)
Face: Indicate on diagram below
Chest: fractured rib(s) flail
    lung contusion
    pneumothorax, hemothorax
    wide mediastinum
Abdomen: minilap: Yes/No Pos/Neg
Pelvis: fracture
Renal: hematuria: Yes/No
    IVP: Pos/Neg
Burns: face/body/extremities
Extremity: fracture, other
Vascular:

Nervous System Examination:
(circle, comment when necessary)

Scalp: Contusion Abrasion Laceration (indicate on diagram)

Skull: Fracture: open/closed/depressed/dura torn
    Basal: Battle's sign/hemotympanum/otorrhagia
    Otorrhea (CSF leak)
    Raccoon eyes, Rhinorrhea (CSF leak)

FIG. 15.1 Both panels depict a type of data collection form for use in the trauma room that may be used to replace the narrative report usually written by the clinician who examines the patient. The data contained in this report can be ultimately stored directly into a database. From Walters and McNeill (Reference 12); used with permission. *(continued)*

SUNNYBROOK MEDICAL CENTRE
TRAUMA ASSESSMENT RECORD
NEUROSURGERY (CONTINUED)

Cranial Nerves: RIGHT   LEFT

Fundi (swollen Closed)
(Normal/Hemorrhage/Papilledema)   C/N/H/P   C/N/H/P
Pupils (swollen Closed)
(Size (mm)/Reaction (+/-))   mm (+ / -)   mm (+ / -)
External Ocular Movements (Comment)
(Voluntary only until C-Spine clear   N/Comment   N/Comment
and tympanic membrane seen)
Corneal Reflex (+/-)   + / -   + / -
Facial Movement
(Normal/Weak/Absent)   N/W/A   N/W/A   COMMENT:
Tympanic Membrane
(Normal/Perforated/Blood/CSF)   N/P/B/C   N/P/B/C

Sensory Examination: (mark on diagrams)   COMMENT:

Normal/Abnormal/Not Done (Paralyzing Agent)

Proprioception: Position Sense Fingers: Yes/No
                Position Sense Toes: Yes/No

Motor System Power: Yes/No
Paralyzing Agent / (R/L) Upper Extremity Fracture / (R/L) Lower Extremity Fracture

(After MRC 0 0/3 overcomes gravity/5 full)   RIGHT   **Limbs:**   LEFT

HAND	TRICEPS	WRIST EXT	BICEPS	DELTOID		DELTOID	BICEPS	WRIST EXT	TRICEPS	HAND
0 1 2 3 4 5	0 1 2 3 4 5	0 1 2 3 4 5	0 1 2 3 4 5	0 1 2 3 4 5		0 1 2 3 4 5	0 1 2 3 4 5	0 1 2 3 4 5	0 1 2 3 4 5	0 1 2 3 4 5

PLANTARFLEX	DORSIFLEX	HAMSTRINGS	QUADRICEPS	ILIOPSOAS		ILIOPSOAS	QUADRICEPS	HAMSTRINGS	DORSIFLEX	PLANTARFLEX
0 1 2 3 4 5	0 1 2 3 4 5	0 1 2 3 4 5	0 1 2 3 4 5	0 1 2 3 4 5		0 1 2 3 4 5	0 1 2 3 4 5	0 1 2 3 4 5	0 1 2 3 4 5	0 1 2 3 4 5

POSTURE LEG EXTENSION/FLEXION | POSTURE ARM EXTENSION/FLEXION | POSTURE ARM EXTENSION/FLEXION | POSTURE LEG EXTENSION/FLEXION

Tendon Reflexes: (2 Normal)   Plantar Response: (Normal/Extensor/Absent)

PLANTAR	ANKLE JERK	KNEE JERK	TRICEPS	BICEPS		BICEPS	TRICEPS	KNEE JERK	ANKLE JERK	PLANTAR
N E A	0 1 2 3 4	0 1 2 3 4	0 1 2 3 4	0 1 2 3 4		0 1 2 3 4	0 1 2 3 4	0 1 2 3 4	0 1 2 3 4	N E A

Rectal Examination: Anal tone: Normal/Reduced/Absent   Bulbocavernosis Reflex: +/-

COMMENT:

Spine:
Cervical: painless/painful, deformity, board, collar   Cleared to T1: yes/no
Thoracic: painless/painful, deformity, board   Cleared to L1: yes/no
Lumbosacral: painless/painful, deformity, board   Cleared: yes/no

Head:
Burr Holes: Yes/No
CT-Head: Yes (Pos/Neg)/No/Pending; Fracture, Space Occupying Lesion, Epidural, Subdural,
Shift, Contusion, Hematoma, Edema, Pneumocephalus, Pneumocranium, Hydrocephalus
Other: List and Describe

Treatment:
Given: Hyperventilation: Yes/No PaCO₂: Other: (Describe)
       Mannitol (20%): Yes/No Volume: cc

Planned: ICP Monitor; Craniotomy for Hematoma; Halo Traction;
Scalp Debridement, suture; Elevate Skull Fracture;   Other: (Describe)

Diagnostic Summary:

Physician Signature: _____ resident for Staff _____

FIG. 15.1 (*Continued*)

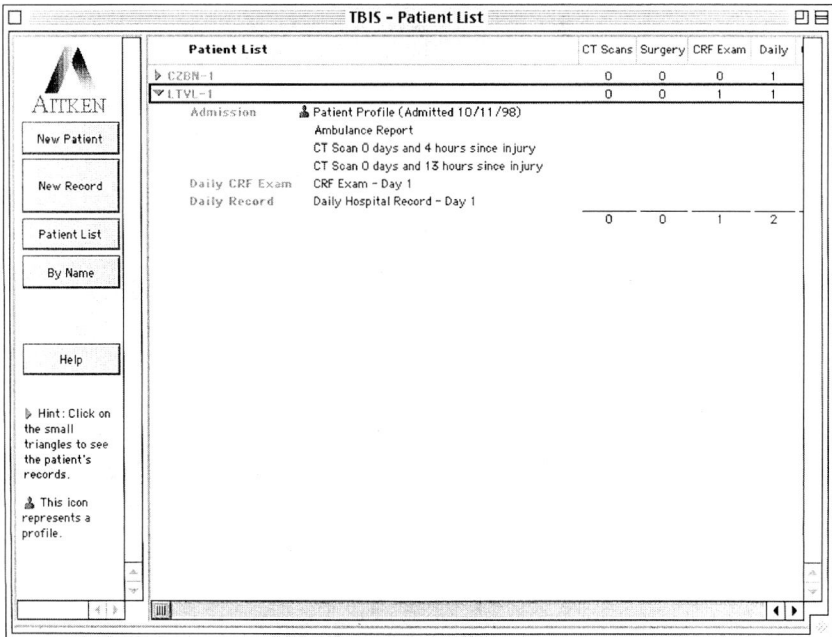

FIG. 15.2 Both panels have been captured from a computer screen and represent the data entry form into which data regarding trauma patients are entered directly, without using a paper representation of the data form. From the Aitken Neuroscience Center, New York, N.Y.; used with permission. (*continued*)

FIG. 15.2 (*Continued*)

mimic, as closely as possible, the intake or output hard copies, if these are separate from the database itself. Ideally, however, the intake document should be the computer screen and not separate from it. The output will almost always be a paper copy of the database in a more standard output form, such as a letter or progress note suitable for placement in the medical record. Hardware needs to reflect the increasing demands of the database, in both quantity and complexity of data. This involves space for the storage of the data and the running of the programs, as well as speed necessary for the quick execution of database searches and the generation of summary statistics. Lastly, the software chosen should facilitate the prospective, "real-time" input of data and be easy for the noncomputer specialist (such as office staff or support personnel in the trauma room, operating suite, or hospital ward) to use.

The storage of information in the database must be easy to use and access, protected from loss, confidential and private, and expandable. The ease of entry and storage of data are closely related, although not necessarily interchangeable. Because of the movement of data in and out of a database, as well as its expansion and modification, a method needs to be built into the database for compacting and reorganizing without losing any important information. This is the purview of the computer scientist, one of the key members of the team needed for database design and support. Likewise, the accessibility of the data must be instantaneous, as soon as its input is complete. This is fairly simple, but does need to be considered ahead of time.

Confidentiality and privacy in the database are essential and ethically challenging (4). There is an inherent conflict between the need for privacy on the part of the patient and the need for information on the part of the health care system. The drive to achieve a high quality of health care will motivate the development of large-scale databases so that quality assurance through outcome measurement can be done. The larger the databases, the more information can be shared, even if the patient wishes for privacy. Although researchers in quality assurance and outcomes are interested primarily in the therapeutic maneuver and its details, there is a great deal of personal information unrelated to the health care issue available within the database. This includes information on demographics, financial details, disabilities, personal and social characteristics, and other private information aside from the strictly medical history and treatment. Computerization in the form of electronic databases can be seen as either a protector or a threat to personal privacy. In the former view, passwords and identifiers, limits to access of certain kinds of data, and various levels of security are all steps taken to preserve confidentiality of the record and the privacy of the patient. In the latter view, however, the electronic record can be available from remote sources via networks and telephone lines so that procurers of database information can be protected from discovery. Because this is possible, the National Research Council has called for the development of "technical and organizational policies, practices, and procedures [such as] authentication of users, access controls, audit trails, disaster recovery, protection of remote access points, and encryption of all patient-identifiable data before transmission on public networks" (4). This sort of policy and technical development will help to protect the patient while enabling the society to benefit from the examination of health care efforts.

COMMON PROBLEMS FACED BY DATABASES

All databases share certain obstructions to adequate design and maintenance. The first, and most important, of these is the requirement for a multidisciplinary team to design and maintain the database. The members of the team include the computer scientist, who can execute the programming necessary to create the database; the statistician, who will ultimately be required to analyze the data in various ways; the clinician, who needs the information; the patients, whose data will make up the database; and ahe link to the scientific community, for dissemination of information derived from the database. Each of these members is key to the success of the database's design, maintenance, and expansion. Finding like-minded individuals with the needed complementary characteristics along with the requisite enthusiasm and experience may not be easy. Occasionally, a clinician may be endowed with abilities in computer science or statistics, but hardly ever with both. In any case, even when these attributes are found in one person, that person is better off in sharing the work with others whose insights into the work may be invaluable.

A second, and often limiting, problem with database design and management is the need for ongoing funding. This funding needs to be available for many functions in the database, including the cost of personnel. Although clinicians will hardly ever expect any payment for time devoted to the database, other personnel, including computer scientists and statisticians, will require the payment for their time, as they are engaged in their primary work activity, unlike the clinician who makes a living doing primarily clinical work. In addition, the database will demand upgrading in software and hardware as time goes on, and this can be quite costly, yet imperative if the database is to be useful over the long term. Unfortunately, the potential sources of funding are few, especially for a large database, such as that which would be required to track patients throughout the entire country. Government funding for such projects does not exist, and the private sector would be interested in such a database only if it helped in the testing of products—devices and drugs. It might be possible to appeal to several companies with the thought that they would all be able to benefit from an ongoing data collection scheme, if they could put their clinical trials more easily into motion as a result of the database's existence.

One of the most difficult problems to overcome is the issue of defining the "value" of the database in light of some achieved goal (or goals). In the general sense that all knowledge is "good," gathering simple epidemiological facts about the trauma population can be useful. For example, if we note that most trauma patients injured in motor vehicle accidents who do poorly were unrestrained, then the enactment of a seatbelt law may be seen to be an approach for preventive strategies. If we then see that the rate of bad outcome decreases after the enactment of such a law, then we are able to evaluate the efficacy of such a change in policy. In addition, any change in treatment strategies for injured patients could be instantly tracked for change in outcome if such a database was in place.

CHARACTERISTICS OF A SUCCESSFUL DATABASE

It should now be clear from the foregoing discussion that the key factors in the achievement of a successful database include a multidisciplinary team and stable funding. In addition, there must be a clear focus in the database of the goals to be achieved, the specific types and scope of the data to be collected, and the overall design of the database. The focus must be, for all three of these areas, on the ultimate use for which the data will be required. This requires the input of all three individuals (or groups) necessary for the design and management of the database: computer scientist, statistician, and end-user or clinician.

No matter how important the above key issues may be, they are not as important as a person or persons to provide leadership for the task. Achieving the commitment and cooperation of many centers, with diverse individuals with substantial expertise in all of the desired areas, is no small assignment. This requires the will, the vision, and the necessary time to seek funding, obtain commitment from other colleagues, and assure momentum for the task. Ideally, this person or group of persons would be from the neurosurgical specialty, as neurosurgeons are uniquely suited to the job.

DATA COLLECTION FOR NEUROTRAUMA

Once the funding is obtained, leadership is in place, and the team is recruited, the database requires careful thought about the variables to be tracked. In general terms, for the neurotrauma population, the variables can be divided into injury, patient, clinical, treatment, and outcome. Injury variables would include type (e.g., head: closed, penetrating; spinal cord: fracture, ligamentous only, missile), mechanism (e.g., industrial, motor vehicle accident, diving), and severity (e.g., Estimated Injury Severity Score, Glasgow Coma Score, complete, incomplete). Patient variables are those pertaining to the patient directly and are unrelated to the injury. These include age, gender, and underlying disease. These are particularly important, as they may be extraneous prognostic variables that must be controlled when calculating risk (or prognosis) (9). Clinical variables refer to assessments of the patient's condition and laboratory or imaging studies that help to determine the scope of the problem. In looking at the patient's clinical condition, it is important to choose examination parameters that are known to be reliable from observer to observer, such as the Glasgow Coma Score. In spinal cord injury, in particular, there need to be two kinds of scales: one for acute and the other for chronic. The acute scale should be quick to execute and should correlate well with a more in-depth scale of final function, thereby being valid as well as reliable. Imaging studies, routinely used to classify injury, include computerized tomography of the brain (traumatic subarachnoid hemorrhage, loss of basal cisterns, midline shift) and many studies of the spine, from plain radiographs to sophisticated three-dimensional studies. All of these require specific detail in data collection.

Treatment variables represent the key aspects of a clinical database. These variables cover everything from stabilization at the scene of the injury, interventions initiated during transport, resuscitation in the trauma room, operative procedures undertaken at any time throughout the hospital stay, and ultimate discharge destination. In this part of the data collection, it would be ideal to insert a treatment protocol, such as a randomized controlled trial, and then evaluate treatment efficacy. It is this aspect of care that prompts us to ask ourselves to what extent we are helping the patients entrusted to our care. This is the essential source of quality of care inquiries, and it must be detailed and exact to be useful.

The last category of information that is essential for a neurotrauma database, and the area in which previous databases have been incomplete, is that pertaining to patient outcome. The outcomes that may be collected can be divided into actuarial, clinical, functional, quality of life, and cost-effectiveness. Actuarial outcomes include those usually tracked by hospitals and insurers and include average length of stay, intensive care utilization, unplanned return to the operating room, and re-admission within 31 days of discharge. They may be indicators of severity of injury or indices of quality of care, but they are rather gross measures at best. However, they are easily accessible from the medical record and are factual in nature, and therefore attractive as first-line measures. Of greater interest to the clinician are the clinical measures, including the physical examination of the patient and imaging studies. Improvement or deterioration in the neurological status of the patient would be exemplary of the first type of measure, and resolution or worsening of abnormalities on imaging studies would be examples of the second. Other outcomes in this group would include mortality and morbidity. However, researchers have begun to realize that these measures alone cannot give a clear idea of patient outcome, certainly not from the patient's perspective. More recently, there has been an interest in measuring treatment success in terms of patient function. The most commonly used measure in neurotrauma is the Glasgow Outcome Scale, which attempts to categorize patient function into large divisions reflecting the scope of outcome in neurotrauma (5). More recently, interest has arisen in more detailed functional measures in neurotrauma, including outcomes in spinal cord injury treatment (2). The next two areas of outcome measures have not yet found their way into the neurotrauma literature, and these include quality of life measures and cost-effectiveness measures. However, these measures will become more important in the future, as money becomes more scarce for health care provision, and those therapies providing the best quality of life for the lowest cost will be the ones reimbursed by payers.

Although we would ideally use a national database as a facilitator for the implementation of randomized controlled trials, we can still obtain extremely usable information from longitudinal studies of patients who present to the trauma room for treatment. Moses has pointed out that databases can be "seriously inaccurate," misleading, and "inscrutable" (6). As long as the ability to adjust for factors that may bias the conclusions reached by database investigation is assured by the database design, the information can be used and understood within its limitations.

By providing the best information about prognosis with treatment in neurotrauma, we will be able to defend our positions regarding treatment maneuvers that the evidence suggests are best for these patients. Unless we can show benefit in terms of relevant and meaningful outcomes beyond survival, there will be doubt about the efficacy and effectiveness of neurotrauma care. A national database would help to provide this information in a short period of time, making both experimental and observational studies feasible and affordable. With the data thus obtained, we could perhaps diminish the drain upon our population, in terms of lost human potential and societal responsibility for long-term care for those disabled by traumatic brain and spinal cord injury.

REFERENCES

1. Barnett GO, Winickoff R, Dorsey JL, Morgan MM, Lurie RS: Quality assurance through automated monitoring and concurrent feedback using a computer-based medical information system. **Med Care** 1978; 16:962–970, 1978.
2. Bracken MB, Shepard MJ, Holford TR, et al.: Administration of methylprednisolone for 24 or 48 hours or tirilazad mesylate for 48 hours in the treatment of acute spinal cord injury: Results of the Third National Acute Spinal Cord Injury Randomized Controlled Trial. **JAMA** 277:1597–1604, 1997.
3. Bullock MR, et al.: Guidelines for the management for severe head injury. **J Neurotrauma** 13:639–734, 1996.
4. Gostin L: Health care information and the protection of personal privacy: Ethical and legal considerations. **Ann Intern Med** 127:683–690, 1997.
5. Jennett B, Bond M: Assessment of outcome after severe brain damage. **Lancet** 1:480–484, 1975.
6. Moses LE: Measuring effects without randomized trials? Options, problems, challenges. **Med Care** 33:AS8—AS14, 1995.
7. Pryor DB, D'Agostino RB, Harell FE Jr, et al.: Clinical data bases: Accomplishments and unrealized potential. **Med Care** 23:623–647, 1985.
8. Rosenberg J, Greenberg MK: Practice parameters: Strategies for survival into the nineties. **Neurology** 42:1110–1115, 1992.
9. Sackett DL, Haynes RB, Tugwell PX: *Clinical Epidemiology: A Basic Science for Clinical Medicine.* Toronto, Little, Brown, 1985.
10. Stillman RM, Mitchell WG, Shaftan GW, Sawyer PN, Kountz SL: The computer as an unbiased medical investigator: Experience on an active surgical service. **Am J Surg** 132:209–213, 1976.
11. Tally PW: The computer workplace, in Bean JR (ed): *Neurosurgery in Transition: The Socioeconomic Transformation of Neurological Surgery.* Baltimore, Williams & Wilkins, 1998, pp 45–60.
12. Walters BC, McNeill I: Improving the record of patient assessment in the trauma room. **J Trauma** 30:398–409, 1990.

CHAPTER

16

Trauma: The Neurosurgeon's Domain

LAWRENCE H. PITTS, M.D., AND MARTIN HOLLAND, M.D.

As we move into the new millennium, neurosurgeons have the opportunity, privilege, and responsibility to define the care of the neurotrauma patient. We have laid an important foundation over the past 30 years on which to build, but clearly there remains much to be done. This chapter will address four areas—prevention, legislation, research, and treatment—in which neurosurgeons have had considerable success, or in which we have had less influence than perhaps we should.

PREVENTION

Effective prevention programs reduce the devastation of traumatic injuries, including neurotrauma, far more than the best possible treatments. Efforts by many people and groups have achieved at least partial success in a number of areas. Unfortunately, prevention programs for traumatic injury do not have as broad-based an appeal or sense of immediacy as other medical problems, such as prevention of childhood diseases or acquired immunodeficiency syndrome, or the complications of hypertension. Trauma causes more years of lost productive life than any other disease; there are over 55,000 head injury deaths per year (6), far fewer than deaths from heart disease, stroke, and cancer, which are generally diseases of older patients. Public health efforts to improve exercise and dietary habits have been better funded and disseminated more widely because of the huge segment of the population at risk. Traumatic injury is unexpected, and people generally feel that it "won't happen to me." Thus, securing substantial and long-range funding for trauma prevention has been difficult and spotty. Some of the more effective programs have come from lay groups, such as Mothers Against Drunk Driving and The American Paralysis Association, where families of trauma patients or the patients themselves have conducted prevention programs that may be having some beneficial effect as noted below.

Numerous reports in the last decade discussed trauma prevention in general and include head injury and spinal cord injury prevention as well. A MEDLINE search (using "prevention" and "trauma" or "head injury" or "spinal cord injury") shows the distribution of prevention articles since 1985 (*Table 16.1*). After spinal cord injury related to aortic or cardiac surgery was eliminated, 163 references remained in 1994 to 1998; 80% of these articles reported prevention of problems after injury and were actually "patient care" rather than "prevention." Partial summaries of the topics appear in *Tables 16.2* and *16.3*. Only 14 references were found that included "prevention, spinal cord injury, and neurosurgery"; about half of these few articles were published by neurosurgeons.

Several trauma organizations currently emphasize trauma prevention. The American College of Surgeons' (ACS) Committee on Trauma

TABLE 16.1
Trauma and Prevention (Number of References)

MEDLINE	1985–1990	1990–1994	1994–1998
Trauma	627	880	1392
Head injury	140	215	352
Spinal cord injury	107	198	245

TABLE 16.2
Head Injury and Prevention

MEDLINE, 1994–1998, 352 References	
Helmet use (bicycle, motorcycle)	87
Pediatric care	79
(helmet use)	(33)
Sports medicine	33
Epidemiology	67
Government, legislative	7
Trauma systems	0

TABLE 16.3
Spinal Cord Injury and Prevention

MEDLINE, 1994–1998, 163 References	%
General patient care	23
Preinjury prevention, epidemiology	18
Experimental treatment	15
Pulmonary emboli, coagulation	10
Surgical treatment	8
Infection and antibiotics	4
Decubiti	4

TABLE 16.4
Trauma and Prevention
American College of Surgeons/Committee on Trauma Prevention Programs

Think First
Safe Kids
Bicycle and motorcycle helmet programs
Handgun violence
Seatbelts and infant car seats—"Buckle Bear"
Teen alcohol, "Teens under Fire"
"Trauma Nurses Talk Tough"
Burn Outreach

(ACSCOT) conducted surveys of the ACSCOT state chairs in 1996 and 1997; 66 regions reported, including military regions and North American regions outside the United States. In 1996, about half had prevention programs, increasing somewhat in 1997. The survey probably is not entirely accurate, but topics that were covered were predictable and interesting (*Table 16.4*). Neurosurgery's Think First program was conducted in a number of states. Another program, Safe Kids, addressed bicycle and motorcycle helmet safety; several other programs were aimed at prevention of handgun violence.

Neurosurgeons should be proud of our involvement in the Think First program. Think First For Teens was started in 1986 and has reached a large number of youngsters across the country. There are more than 200 local programs throughout the United States, Canada, Mexico, and Chile. During the 1996–1997 year, more than 700,000 students were introduced to the Think First program, and almost 6 million people have participated in the Think First program since its inception. Its newest iteration (and now strongly emphasized) is the Think First For Kids curriculum for younger children.

It is difficult to measure the effectiveness of prevention programs, but this is being tried in several areas where Think First For Kids is in place. Two abstracts were presented at the 1998 national Think First meeting. One study in Portland, OR evaluated the program in 55 Grade 1—3 classrooms in seven elementary schools. Pretesting and posttesting showed increased knowledge of injury prevention at all three grade levels, and somewhat greater benefit was measured in lower socioeconomic class students (Green, personal communication). A second study from Southern California evaluated 2,000 Grades 1—3 students and again found significantly improved scores for injury prevention, knowledge, and self-reported behavior (Gresham, personal communication). One other publication evaluated the Think First program in three junior high and three high schools but found no consistent change in knowledge or self-reported behavior; by direct observation, the authors found no rise in seat belt use (15). The program for teenagers may require modification to increase its value; perhaps these programs are more effective when delivered to younger children. It will be extremely important to see if their knowledge will be retained as the students become adults.

LEGISLATION

In the past 15 years, the number of publications describing legislative action regarding trauma has risen modestly (*Table 16.5*). Although neurotrauma benefits from general trauma legislation, CNS trauma itself has commanded too little attention by legislatures. MEDLINE searches may overlook some contributions to a topic, but they indicate that legislative interest in CNS injury is no greater now than a decade ago. *Table 16.6* recounts the most common published trauma issues in

TABLE 16.5
CNS Trauma and Legislation

MEDLINE	1985–1989	1990–1993	1994–1998
Trauma	110	152	172
Brain, head injury, spinal cord injury	13	18	15
Head injury	2	3	2
Spinal cord injury	1	1	2
Pediatrics	3	2	2
Firearms	—	—	2
Brain death, transplantation	1	4	1
Organization of trauma care	2	1	—

TABLE 16.6
Trauma and Legislation

MEDLINE	1994–1998	175 citations
Trauma system organization, EMS, government		23
Sexual assault		12
Pediatrics		11
Malpractice, expert witness		9
Bicycle and motorcycle helmets		8
Alcohol		8
Firearms		7
Psychiatric, memory disturbance		7
Insurance		4
Seatbelts		3

the legislative arena. These have changed in the past decade, with less emphasis on such issues as the need for or effectiveness of seatbelt and helmet laws, and have turned to more global problems such as trauma and EMS legislation, sexual assault, and medical malpractice. Articles related to pediatric trauma legislation are still fairly common; pediatricians and pediatric organizations rather than neurotrauma experts remain the champions in this area.

Neurosurgeons, through the American Association of Neurological Surgeons and Congress of Neurological Surgeons (AANS-CNS) Washington office, have joined with other medical organizations including the American Medical Association, ACS, American College of Emergency Physicians, and American Hospital Association to sponsor and support a number of national legislative efforts. They filed an amicus curiac brief regarding the improper use of federal "antidumping" laws instead of state malpractice laws in instances of inappropriate transfer of some trauma cases from one hospital to another. The AANS and CNS have been partners in the initiative to increase requests for organ donations in appropriate patients near or after death. Neurosurgery has urged that reimbursement for emergency care be reimbursed using a "prudent layperson" judgment instead of more restrictive rules devised by health maintenance organizations (federal bills HR-4250, S-2330). The Health Professions' Education Partnership was passed by the Senate (S-1754) and reauthorizes the Trauma Care System Planning and Development Act of 1992–1995 to facilitate state planning of trauma systems. A Senate bill has been introduced (S-2440) that requests language be included to recognize the importance of trauma and urges the director of the National Institutes of Health to develop a coordinated process for trauma research across the Institutes. Neurosurgery and other medical organizations successfully supported legislation for safer childhood sleepwear.

Funding for trauma research increased in 1998 with the improved economy and budget surplus (*Table 16.7*). The AANS, CNS, and ACS

TABLE 16.7
Trauma Funding Changes Comparing 1997 with 1998

Federal Agency	Proposed House Budget (%)	Proposed Senate Budget (%)
NIH	+9	+15
CDC for Injury Prevention and Control	+29	−2
CDC for Public Health	+4	−19
National Institute for Disability and Rehabilitation	+5	

among others have begun discussions regarding the desirability of an institute specifically for trauma research (National Institute for Trauma). This is a complex issue, and it is unclear whether trauma will receive better funding through current mechanisms or through its own dedicated institute. The latter has the advantage of sharper focus on trauma problems but the disadvantages of the administrative expense of another institute and of probably taking funds from existing institutes. The debate on this issue will continue in the coming years.

Trauma legislation and prevention certainly *can* work. Use of seat belts substantially lowers injuries and costs. In Maryland, seatbelts reduced the total number of injuries by 34%, major injuries by 57%, and minor injuries by 20%. No deaths occurred among the belted group in one study (5). In Colorado, one-half of belted passengers escaped injury, whereas five-sixths of nonbelted passengers were injured. Two-thirds of restrained passengers had no medical costs; only 29% of nonbelted ones had none (8). In Kentucky, more unrestrained drivers were killed or disabled, and the medical care cost was significantly more for unbelted ($18,165) than for belted drivers ($7,634) (4).

Helmet prevention programs and legislation repeatedly have been shown effective in reducing head injury severity, mortality, and cost. In a Canadian study, public education tripled helmet use, particularly in elementary school children (10). In children, use of bicycle helmets reduced the risk of head injury by 63% and coma by 86% (14). In Washington, legislation in 1990 required motorcycle helmet use, and public education at about the same time aimed at increasing bicycle helmet use; helmet use rose from 5% in 1987 to 62% in 1993. Head injuries, severe head injuries, and mortality in both bicyclists and motorcycle riders were significantly reduced during this time, and hospital and ICU stays were shortened for bicyclists (9). After legislation was passed in California, motorcycle helmet use increased from about one-third of injured riders to more than 85%. With more frequent helmet use, head injury rates fell from 38% to 25%. There were fewer skull fractures, cerebral injuries, fewer and shorter periods of coma, and shorter hospital stays (7). Some motorcyclists expressed concern that helmets would increase spinal injuries; head injuries were markedly decreased in one study, whereas spinal injuries were not (11).

RESEARCH

Neurosurgeons have figured much more prominently in neurotrauma research than in preventative or legislative endeavors, with the important exception of the Think First Program. The scope of neurotrauma research is so broad that we cannot cover it all here. Rather, we will describe an example of neurosurgeons' clinical research in neurotrauma that has extended over a number of years and continues still.

Nimodipine was shown to be efficacious in reducing the morbidity of vasospasm after aneurysmal subarachnoid hemorrhage (12), and Bayer Pharmaceuticals initiated trials of nimodipine for patients with severe head injury. A trial in the United Kingdom and Finland with six centers and 350 patients found a slight but not statistically significant difference in outcome comparing nimodipine with placebo administration (13). Because of the slight improvement, a second trial was conducted, again without demonstration of benefit with nimodipine use (1). In examining risk factors for poor outcome, severity of trauma and the presence of traumatic subarachnoid hemorrhage were about equally important as negative predictors of outcome, along with advanced age and the need for surgery. When only patients with traumatic subarachnoid hemorrhage were considered, nimodipine did produce a significant improvement in outcome, and the authors suggested that a clinical trial of nimodipine limited to patients with traumatic subarachnoid hemorrhage was warranted (1). Such a trial has been completed; a West German group has found a significant benefit (3), and another large, international multicenter trial is currently being conducted. Whether it will demonstrate a benefit of nimodipine in traumatic subarachnoid hemorrhage remains to be seen.

Unfortunately, there is a growing list of unsuccessful clinical trials for patients with severe head injury. These expensive ventures have come only after extensive preclinical testing with neuroprotective drugs showed improvement in a number of features of experimental head injuries. These agents affect a wide spectrum of neuropathological processes including inflammatory changes (bradykinin antagonist), free radical damage (tirilazad, superoxide dismutase), presynaptic and postsynaptic calcium channel alterations (CGS-19755, EAA-494, cerestat, lubeluzole SNX-111), and vasospasm (nimodipine) among others. Despite a number of preclinical trials and some limited favorable clinical experience with hypothermia in trauma and ischemia, a recent large multicenter trial of hypothermia for patients with head injury did not show improved outcome. A recent multicenter trial of moderate hypothermia was completed; results will be available shortly (Clifton, personal communication). Because of the importance of finding better treatment for the large number of patients with severe head injury throughout the world, several more agents are being considered or actually being investigated clinically, including the selective NMDA NR2B receptor CP-101, dexanabinol, and a propofol-related anesthetic compound. Despite the frustration of negative trials to date, we must continue to identify and evaluate new agents in preclinical studies and take the most promising of them to clinical trials for eventual widespread use in patients with head injuries.

Because of the public health importance of neurotrauma, and because of their pivotal role in treating patients with nervous system injury, neurosurgeons have continued actively to pursue neurotrauma research. Of the 206 abstracts submitted for presentation at the annual meeting of the Neurotrauma Society meeting in November 1998, neurosurgery departments supported more than half. Of these, over half were submitted by a relatively small number of institutions that are leaders in neurotrauma research, including the University of Pennsylvania, the Medical College of Virginia, the University of Pittsburgh, Baylor University, the University of Texas-Houston, UCLA, and the University of Miami. The range of topics was remarkable, including a number of preclinical neuroprotective agent trials in animals, trying to define the best compounds to take to human trials. Some agents were tested in combination, which is important because occasionally two drugs that appear beneficial when used alone may worsen the outcome when used in combination. If some form of neuroprotective "cocktail" ultimately is required to improve outcome after head injury, careful testing of combined therapies must be done in a preclinical setting before they can safely be tested in humans. Many neuropathological mechanisms were investigated, including the role of inflammation, ionic influences, and changes in blood-brain barrier, blood flow, lactate, and glucose, in some instances using genetically engineered animals or enriched environments. Given the number of both experienced and young well-trained investigators in neurotrauma research, we believe that important and effective advances will be made in treating neurotrauma patients within the next decade.

TREATMENT

Several earlier chapters in this volume discuss current treatment of neurotrauma in considerable detail, and we will not address this further. One additional important topic in the treatment of head-injured patients is the application of treatment protocols and guidelines. The Joint Section on Neurotrauma under the sponsorship of the Brain Trauma Foundation and the auspices of the AANS published *"Guidelines for the Management of Severe Head Injury"* in 1996 (2). These guidelines address a number of vital concerns in treating head-injured patients, including trauma system development, early management, ICP monitoring and treatment, and the use of specific treatments including hyperventilation, mannitol, corticosteroids, barbiturates, anticonvulsants, and nutrition. The guidelines provide specific recommendations for treatment. Some are based on excellent published data ("standards"), others on substantial demonstrated value ("guidelines"), and still others on data insufficient to be of certain efficacy ("options"). Although the options cannot yet be proven to be useful in managing head injury patients, the authors felt that they represent the best treatment and should be used in treating these patients. These guidelines have been adopted as the basis for treating patients in clinical trials conducted by the American Brain Injury Consortium (ABIC); an evaluation of patient management before and after adoption of the guidelines by ABIC is underway. We hope to demonstrate that careful attention to treatment detail as defined in the guidelines will improve outcome after severe head injury.

Despite the major contributions that neurosurgery has made to advances in the treatment of neurotrauma, we still have much work to be done. We hold ourselves as the most prominent contributors to solving neurotrauma problems, but we have to carry our message beyond our neurosurgical colleagues, to other important segments of the trauma care community. Of 62 papers presented during plenary sessions at the 1998 Annual Meeting of the American Association for the Surgery of Trauma (AAST), one of the premier organizations in this country dealing with trauma care, only 4 discussed neurotrauma issues, and only half of those were presented by neurosurgeons. Trauma surgeons and intensivists have begun addressing preclinical and clinical issues in neurotrauma, presumably because they feel that some areas are not being addressed adequately by neurosurgeons or other neurological researchers. We sadly note that only five neurosurgeons have been elected to the AAST in the last decade, and only a dozen in the last 20 years. This is an arena in which neurosurgery could and should exercise an important influence in the way trauma is managed and accentuate the role of the neurosurgeon in the management of neurotrauma.

CONCLUSION

The prevention and treatment of traumatic injuries is a complex issue, requiring knowledge not only of physiology and biochemistry but also of social, political, and financial factors.

Prevention is preferable to treatment, and efforts to maximize this aspect of care should be vigorously pursued. Neurosurgery and trauma outreach programs can and should be coordinated with efforts by lay groups to educate the community at large and focus on "high risk" groups (young men) and activities (handgun use, motorcycle riding, contact sports). Legislative action can enhance prevention programs financially and facilitate the use of mass media (television, radio) for education through public service announcements, for instance. In addition, legislation such as the "seatbelt" and "helmet" laws can be used to curb the incidence of trauma-related injuries.

Unfortunately, trauma cannot be legislated or educated away altogether, highlighting the need for effective treatment programs. As is true of prevention programs, the coordinated efforts of neurosurgery and trauma associations, along with those of city, state, and federal agencies are needed for their optimal development. These should be directed along three avenues: first, through education and information dissemination among health-care professionals; second, through the development of comprehensive city or countywide trauma systems; and third, through intensive neurotrauma research.

Education and information dissemination can take many forms: peer-review publications; presentations at local, regional or national meetings; and development of management guidelines for head and spinal cord injury. By these means, the most up-to-date information regarding treatment options and "standards" can be distributed widely and rapidly to the health care community.

As the treatment of trauma becomes increasingly sophisticated, comprehensive city or countywide trauma systems must develop where resources and expertise can converge to provide the best trauma care possible. Ideally, these systems should include effective Emergency Medical Services, dedicated trauma hospitals, and comprehensive post-hospitalization care facilities (acute rehabilitation hospitals, skilled nursing facilities, and long-term placement centers) so that coordinated treatment protocols can be instituted in the prehospital setting and continued through the acute hospitalization and after discharge.

Over the past fifteen years or so, greater understanding of the pathophysiology of traumatic brain injury has allowed us to change the emphasis of treatment protocols. We have slowly moved away from a primarily mechanical view of trauma to focus more on the biochemical alterations that contribute to cellular injury. This phase shift has come from research, both basic and clinical. Laboratory findings have translated to the clinical situation, and intensive care units have become "clinical laboratories" where physiological parameters are measured and correlated to treatment protocols. Multicenter drug trials and outcome studies addressing not only severe but also moderate and mild traumatic brain injuries have also added to our knowledge, bringing us ever closer to more effective treatments for brain injury.

Unfortunately, the development of prevention and professional education programs, comprehensive trauma systems, and research is expensive, and funding is scarce. Furthermore, the most common sources of funds (governmental agencies, industry and private foundations) have generally been uninterested in trauma. For this to change, we—as neurosurgeons—must establish the need for trauma prevention and treatment programs and emphasize their importance, both to individual patients and to society as a whole.

As we head into the twenty-first century, we must take advantage of our unique position as experts in neurotrauma to educate both the community and government about the physical, emotional, and financial impact of trauma. Without this emphasis, prevention and treatment programs cannot take permanent root and will surely struggle to survive. We have the option to take a back seat to other subspecialties or to take the lead in this worthy crusade.

Acknowledgment

The authors thank Katie Orico in the AANS Washington office, Cindy Brown in the ACS Washington office, Carol Williams in the ACS Chicago office, and Fred Grubbe in the Think First Chicago office for valuable assistance in providing data for this paper.

REFERENCES

1. A multicenter trial of the efficacy of nimodipine on outcome after severe head injury: The European Study Group on Nimodipine in Severe Head Injury. **J Neurosurg** 80:797–804, 1994.
2. Bullock R, Chesnut RM, Clifton G, et al.: Guidelines for the management of severe head injury. **J Neurotrauma** 13:643–734, 1996.
3. Harders A, Kakarieka A, Braakman R: Traumatic subarachnoid hemorrhage and its treatment with nimodipine: German tSAH Study Group (see comments). **J Neurosurg** 85:82–89, 1996.
4. Hooker EA, Danzl DF, Thomas DM, Miller F, Zupances W: Economic impact of motor vehicle restraints in Kentucky: A trauma center's experience. **J Ky Med Assoc** 88:59–61, 1990.
5. Kaplan BH, Cowley RA: Seatbelt effectiveness and cost of noncompliance among drivers admitted to a trauma center. **Am J Emerg Med** 9:4–10, 1991.
6. Kraus JF, McArthur DL: Epidemiologic aspects of brain injury. **Neurol Clin** 14:435–450, 1996.
7. Kraus JF, Peek C: The impact of two related prevention strategies on head injury reduction among nonfatally injured motorcycle riders, California, 1991—1993. **J Neurotrauma** 12:873–881, 1995.
8. Marine WM, Kerwin EM, Moore EE, Lezotte DC, Baron AE, Grosso MA: Mandatory seatbelts: Epidemiologic, financial, and medical rationale from the Colorado matched pairs study. **J Trauma** 36:96–100, 1994.
9. Mock CN, Maier RV, Boyle E, Pilcher S, Rivara FP: Injury prevention strategies to promote helmet use decrease severe head injuries at a level I trauma center. **J Trauma** 39:29–33; discussion 34–25, 1995.

10. Morris BA, Trimble NE, Fendley SJ: Increasing bicycle helmet use in the community: Measuring response to a wide-scale, 2-year effort (see comments). **Can Fam Physician** 40:1126–1131, 1994.
11. Orsay EM, Muelleman RL, Peterson TD, Jurisic DH, Kosasih JB, Levy P: Motorcycle helmets and spinal injuries: Dispelling the myth. **Ann Emerg Med** 23:802–806, 1994.
12. Pickard JD, Murray GD, Illingworth R, et al.: Effect of oral nimodipine on cerebral infarction and outcome after subarachnoid haemorrhage: British aneurysm nimodipine trial. **Br Med J** 298:636–642, 1989.
13. Teasdale G, Bailey I, Bell A, et al.: A randomized trial of nimodipine in severe head injury: HIT I. British/Finnish Co-operative Head Injury Trial Group. **J Neurotrauma** 9[Suppl 2]:S545—S550, 1992.
14. Thomas S, Acton C, Nixon J, Battistutta D, Pitt WR, Clark R: Effectiveness of bicycle helmets in preventing head injury in children: Case-control study (see comments). **Br Med J** 308:173–176, 1994.
15. Wright M, Rivara FP, Ferse D: Evaluation of the Think First head and spinal cord injury prevention program (see comments). **Injury Prev** 1:81–85, 1995.

III

General Scientific Session III

CHAPTER

17

Organizing Cerebrovascular Care Teams

MARC R. MAYBERG, M.D.

Cerebrovascular disease is the third most prevalent cause of death and the leading cause of disability in the United States; there are almost 750,000 cases of stroke in North America annually or approximately 200 cases of cerebrovascular disease per neurosurgeon. Cerebrovascular disease is also a growth industry. Stroke is a disease of the elderly; as the U.S. population ages, the incidence and prevalence of stroke will increase in the future.

For reasons that are not entirely clear, the neurosurgeon's role in the important area of cerebrovascular disease has diminished over the past several years. This is reflected in an analysis that was done as part of the American Association of Neurological Surgeons/Congress of Neurological Surgeons (AANS/CNS) Carotid Endarterectomy Task Force in 1995. The impact of several prospective randomized trials in carotid endarterectomy was immediately felt in the frequency of carotid endarterectomies in the U.S., as reflected in Medicare data. The total number of procedures declined during a period of concern about the operation, then increased sharply when the North American Symptomatic Carotid Endarterectomy Trial (NASCET) (12), Veterans Affairs (9), and Asymptomatic Carotid Atherosclerosis Study (ACAS) (4) trials published (*Fig. 17.1*). However, the neurosurgeon's role in this trend has been relatively minimal. The number of endarterectomies done by neurosurgeons has not changed over this time, whereas the percentage of all endarterectomies has substantially declined (*Fig. 17.1*). In terms of financial impact, this has had a tremendous effect upon reimbursement for neurosurgeons. In 1994, out of nearly 90 million dollars in Medicare reimbursement for this operation, only about 5.5 million dollars went to neurosurgeons. Why is this so? Part of the problem lies in the emphasis in neurosurgical training programs. In a survey by the AANS/CNS Carotid Endarterectomy Task Force, most neurosurgical training programs did less than 25% of carotid endarterectomy procedures within their institution, with a median value of approximately 15 to 20% of cases performed (*Fig. 17.2*). One possible reason for this observation was that neurosurgeons traditionally

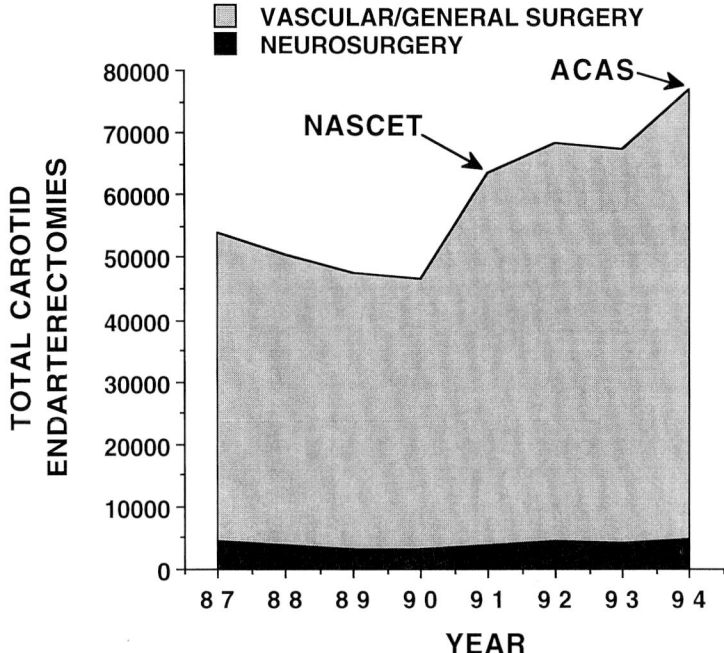

FIG. 17.1 Total Medicare carotid endarterectomies performed in U.S. during 1987–1994.

have not operated on asymptomatic carotid stenosis; in the survey, over half of all neurosurgeons queried responded that they did not operate on patients with asymptomatic stenosis (*Fig. 17.3*).

Neurosurgeons are the ideal practitioners to care for patients with cerebrovascular disease. Neurosurgeons are familiar with the brain and the cerebrovascular circulation, which differentiates us from other specialists involved in treatment of carotid artery disease. We have direct access to the cerebrovascular circulation. In addition, neurosurgeons are microsurgeons and are gaining skills in the field of neuroendovascular surgery, which enables another route of access to the intracranial circulation. Neurosurgeons understand cerebral protection and the concepts of monitoring cerebral function. Finally, neurosurgeons are neurointensivists and often provide medical care for patients with a variety of acute disorders in the intracranial circulation.

Much of the research related to cerebrovascular disease has been done by neurosurgeons. Data from the primate stroke model reported by Jones et al. (6) have become the standard for the understanding of the evolution of stroke in focal ischemia. The concept of ischemic

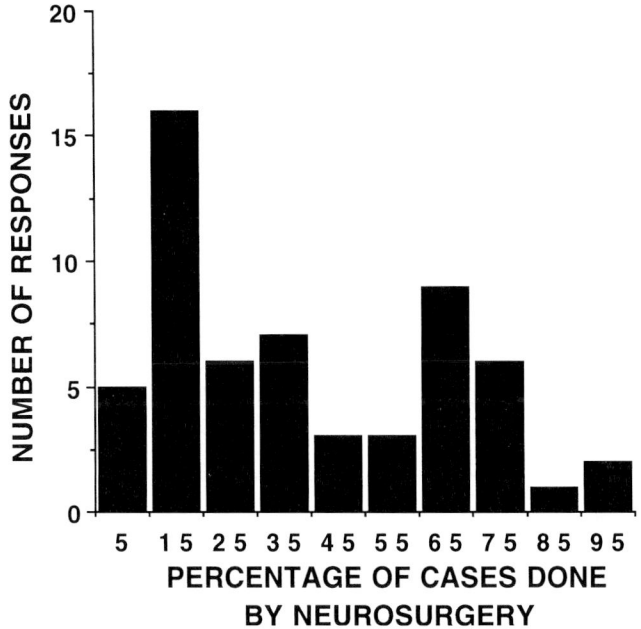

FIG. 17.2 Percentage of carotid endarterectomy cases done by neurosurgeons in academic medical centers. Data derived from survey by Carotid Endarterectomy Task Force.

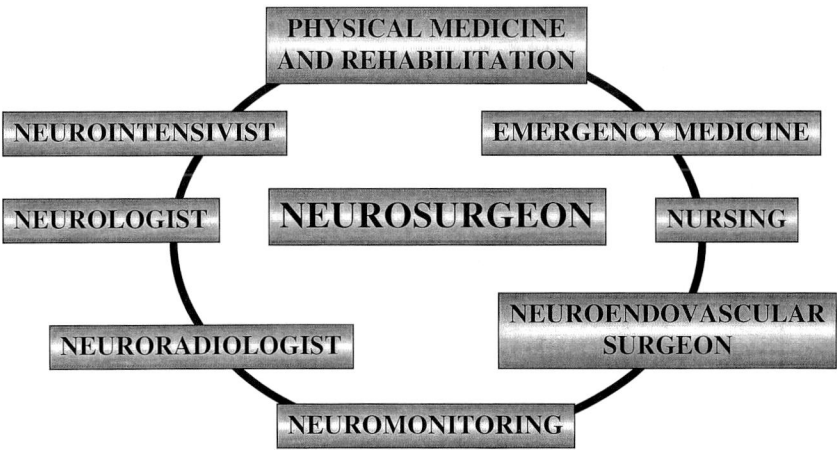

FIG. 17.3 The Stroke Team.

penumbra was derived in part from work from Lindsay Symon's laboratory looking at ischemic thresholds and ionic mechanisms of neuronal death (3). Neurosurgeons have been directly involved in the diagnosis of stroke. For example Newell (11) and Martin (7) have described emboli monitoring and hemodynamic testing to noninvasively determine pathophysiological mechanisms in stroke.

Developing a Stroke Team is an essential first step in providing care for patients with cerebrovascular disease. Neurosurgeons should be at the center of the Stroke Team, which should also involve a neuroendovascular surgeon, a neurologist, a neurointensivist, physical medicine and rehabilitation specialists, and an individual to direct neuromonitoring (*Fig. 17.3*). The Stroke Team, surrounding the neurosurgeon, should be able to care for the entire range of patients with ischemic and hemorrhagic stroke. How does one develop a Stroke Team? The tools are available and readily accessible; it is simply a matter of taking the initiative. At present, there are five direct, practical ways to incorporate existing information into Stroke Team development. These involve the SMART program, involvement in emergency services, the Brain Attack Coalition Tool Box, the Cerebrovascular Section outcomes instruments, and practice guidelines. The Carotid Endarterectomy Task Force developed a brochure that is available to AANS and CNS members. This brochure summarizes data about the carotid endarterectomy trials and introduces the surgeon to the local community as a cerebrovascular expert. The SMART program in cerebrovascular disease has been updated by Warren Selman and Bruce Kaufman and is currently available. The program consists of educational materials for both physicians and patients, a series of brochures, and promotional materials that neurosurgeons can use in their community to promote themselves as cerebrovascular experts. Brain attack is an emergency, and neurosurgeons are well versed in dealing with emergent problems. There have been a variety of solutions to integrating neurosurgeons in the emergency community. For example, Julian Bailes in Orlando recently was named Director of Emergency Services for the surrounding region. He will be at the forefront in organizing the emergency services related to cerebrovascular disease for an entire county. This kind of involvement in stroke programs from the initial evaluation and triage of patients, continuing through diagnosis and therapy, is critical in the development of a Stroke Team. The Brain Attack message was initially promoted by Roberto Heros and ultimately led to formation of the Brain Attack Coalition, a multidisciplinary panel designed to promote the Brain Attack message, coordinate stroke programs, and develop national initiatives. One of these initiatives is the Acute Stroke Toolbox. This is a Web page that includes published guidelines related to stroke, clinical pathways that can be used to design hospital treatment plans, stroke scales that are important in evaluating patients for treatment protocols, and a wide variety of public information materials that the neurosurgeon can use to help promote cerebrovascular disease in the community. These materials are free and immediately available (http://www.stroke-site.org). The AANS and CNS have been extremely active in promoting the Stroke Team concept for neurosurgeons through the Washington Committee. The AANS/CNS joint officers have commissioned two task forces, the Carotid Endarterectomy Task Force and the Neuroendovascular Task Force, both of which are still active. The AANS/CNS Cerebrovascular Section is developing additional educational guidelines and outcomes instruments, which will be useful in the developing stroke teams. Under the direction of Bob Harbaugh, there are currently two outcomes instruments in testing: an aneurysm instrument and a carotid endarterectomy instrument. These outcome data can provide valid information for payers, hospitals, and patients. A variety of guidelines relating to management of cerebrovascular disease are available, including acute stroke (2), transient ischemic attack (5), subarachnoid hemorrhage (8), tissue plasminogen activator therapy for acute stroke (1), and carotid endarterectomy (10). New guidelines relating to management of unruptured aneurysms and arteriovenous malformations are in process.

Neurosurgeons need to look to the future to remain leaders in this field, including awareness of new medical therapies and changing technology, especially in the area of angioplasty and stenting. It is essential that neurosurgeons become involved in clinical trials to demonstrate the safety and effectiveness of new technologies and procedures. In summary, there are a number of imperatives for neurosurgeons to maintain leadership in the role of cerebrovascular disease. Most importantly, each neurosurgeon in his or her own community should reestablish an individual role as the stroke expert in the community. This can be done through the development of Stroke Management Teams using tools that are readily available. All neurosurgeons should be involved and promote basic and clinical research, including participation in ongoing clinical trials. Neurosurgeons need to be able to adapt to the changing environment and incorporate new technologies into the treatment of cerebrovascular disease.

REFERENCES

1. Ad Hoc Committee of the American Heart Association: Guidelines for thrombolytic therapy for acute stroke: A supplement to the guidelines for the management of patients with acute ischemic stroke. **Circulation** 94:1167–1174, 1996.

2. Ad Hoc Committee of the American Heart Association: Management of patients with acute ischemic stroke. **Circulation** 90:1588–1601, 1994.
3. Astrup J, Siesjo BK, Symon L: Thresholds in cerebral ischemia—The ischemic penumbra. **Stroke** 12:6723–6725, 1981.
4. The Asymptomatic Carotid Atherosclerosis Study Group: Endarterectomy for asymptomatic carotid artery stenosis. **JAMA** 273:1421–1428, 1995.
5. Feinberg WM, Albers GW, Barnett HJM, et al.: Guidelines for the management of transient ischemic attacks. **Circulation** 89:2950–2965, 1994.
6. Jones TH, Morawetz RB, Crowell RM, et al.: Thresholds of focal cerebral ischemia in awake monkeys. **J Neurosurg** 54:6773–6782, 1981.
7. Martin NA, Thomas KM, Caron M: Transcranial Doppler: Techniques, application, and instrumentation. **Neurosurgery** 33:4761–4764, 1993.
8. Mayberg MR, Batjer HH, Dacey RG: Guidelines for the management of aneurysmal subarachnoid hemorrhage. **Stroke** 25:2315–2328, 1994.
9. Mayberg MR, Wilson SE, Yatsu F, et al.: Carotid endarterectomy and prevention of cerebral ischemia and symptomatic carotid stenosis. **JAMA** 255:3289–3294, 1991.
10. Moore WS, Barnett HJM, Beebe HG, et al.: Guidelines for carotid endarterectomy. A multidisciplinary statement. **Circulation** 91:566–579, 1995.
11. Newell DW: Transcranial Doppler ultrasonography. **Neurosurg Clin North Am** 5:4619–4631, 1994.
12. North American Symptomatic Carotid Endarterectomy Trial Collaborators: Beneficial effect of carotid endarterectomy in symptomatic patients with high-grade stenosis. **N Engl J Med** 325:445–453, 1991.

CHAPTER

18

Diagnostic Imaging for Stroke

ROBERT H. ROSENWASSER, M.D., F.A.C.S.
ROCCO A. ARMONDA, M.D., M.A.I., M.C., U.S.A.

In recent years, many different approaches to the treatment of acute ischemic stroke have been investigated and undertaken, including recanalization using thrombolytic therapy with associated surgical or endovascular revascularization. In 1995, the recombinant rt-PA stroke study group published their results in the *New England Journal of Medicine,* indicating important positive resultant clinical outcome when this agent was administered within 3 hours of the onset of symptoms in a select group of patients (2, 41). Although the effectiveness of urgent therapy for such patients with profound neurological deficit has not been universally accepted, a new door has been opened through which intervention can perhaps alter the outcome in a disease that, before this, had no therapeutic intervention (11, 19, 20). With the advent of thrombolytics that are administered intraarterially and intravenously, diagnostic imaging for acute ischemic stroke takes on new importance, as misinterpretation of the initial studies can lead to disastrous results with resultant conversion of an ischemic lesion to a lethal hemorrhage event (13). Additionally, assessment of the cerebrovascular reserve is critical for the identification of therapeutic interventions to increase perfusion: induced hypertension, thrombolysis, or reconstructive revascularization process (31, 46, 56). Such evaluations may influence the future success of failure of extracranial/intracranial bypass procedures. This also includes dynamic imaging with a variety of different techniques during balloon test occlusion in an effort to increase the sensitivity of patients who might fail permanent parent vessel sacrifice.

Disclaimer: All views inclosed are the sole opinions of the authors and do not reflect the view of the U.S. Army, Medical Corps, or the Department of Defense.

DIAGNOSTIC STUDIES

Diagnostic studies for cerebrovascular disease include B-mode ultrasound for extracranial carotid circulation and transcranial doppler for the evaluation of the intracranial circulation. These noninvasive studies are often performed on an elective basis and have limited utility in the acute evaluation of a patient who may be a candidate for either intravenous or intraarterial thrombolysis (3, 9, 10, 25, 27, 36–38, 44, 45, 48). More recent innovative forms of noninvasive imaging include regional oxygen saturation monitoring of the brain with near infrared spectroscopy using the INVOS 4100 (Somanectics, Troy MI) (6, 15, 62). Such transcranial imaging allows bedside measurements of regional areas of the anterior circulation of either hemisphere, although it is awaiting full clinical evaluation. Computerized tomographic (CT) scanning and magnetic resonance imaging (MR) form the foundation of diagnostic studies in patients considered for intervention (26, 32). Other modalities, such as positron emission tomography, are extremely valuable in the evaluation of ischemic cerebrovascular disease; however, they are limited by their availability at many institutions (28). Digital subtraction angiography is generally only performed when endovascular intervention is considered for delivery of intraarterial thrombolytics with or without angioplasty and stenting of the affected vessel (53, 56, 57, 61). Digital subtraction angiography may also be valuable in differentiating between vessel occlusion versus preocclusive stenosis with an angiographic string sign (5, 21–24, 60).

Computerized Tomographic Scanning

CT scanning continues to be the mainstay in the acute evaluation of patients suspected of harboring an ischemic vascular lesion (see *Figs. 18.1–18.4*). Extremely important and controversial, however, is the interpretation of such noncontrast scans. vonKummer et al. (54, 55) published the results of early CT findings (within 6 hours) and looked at the sensitivity and prognostic value of early CT scanning in middle cerebral artery (MCA) trunk occlusion. Within 6 hours, there is often loss of definition of the gray/white interface and loss of the insular ribbon, blurring of the lentiform nucleus, and effacement of sulci or slight ventricular compression (50, 51). Also of great utility is the presence of the hyperdense middle cerebral artery (MCA) sign indicating thrombosis in this vessel; combined with clinical correlation, MCA can often be very effective in making a diagnosis and instituting therapy (49).

Based on the European Cooperative Acute Stroke Study, early infarct lesions exemplify the area of irreversible ischemic damage but, more importantly, a hypodensity in more than one-third of the MCA territory is

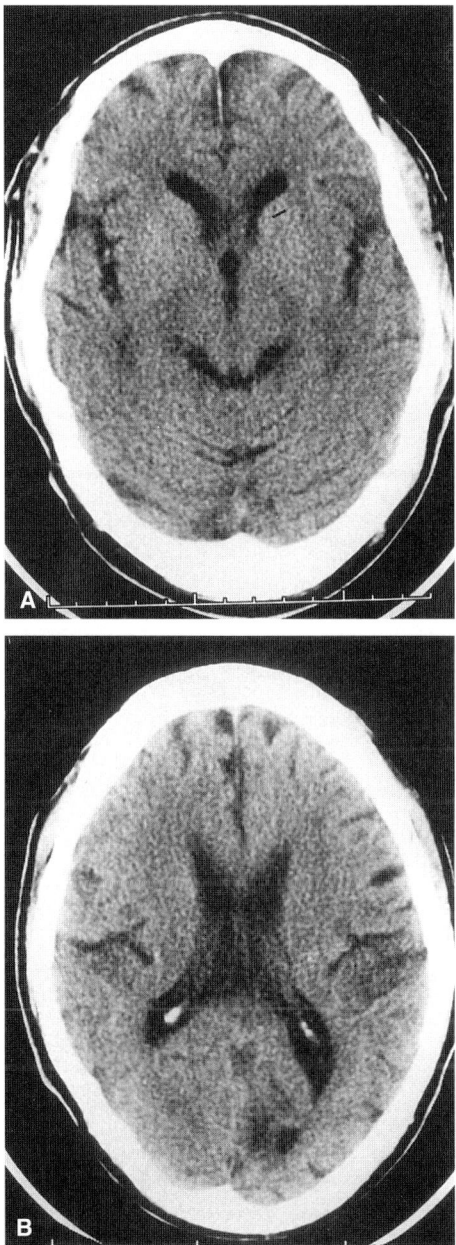

FIG. 18.1 Noncontrast CT scans of a 65-year-old woman with acute right hemiplegia and aphasia between 3 and 6 hours after onset demonstrating evidence of a subtle hypodensity left posterior sylvian superior temporal gyrus with both cortical and subcortical involvement.

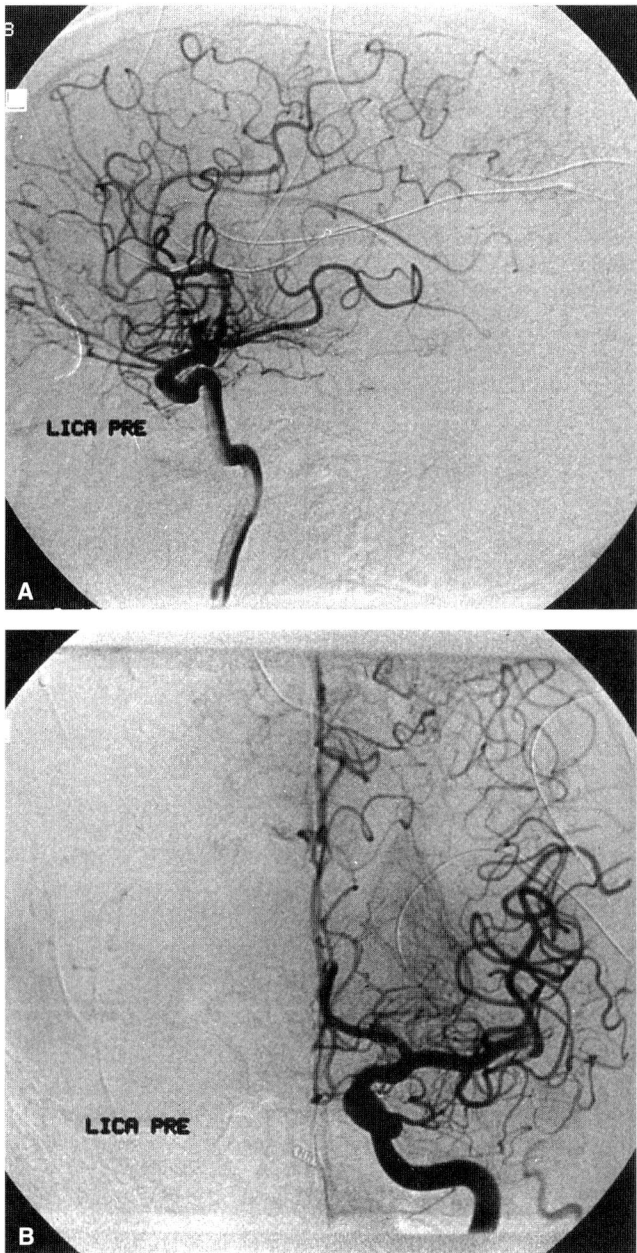

FIG. 18.2 A, Lateral view of an angiogram of the left internal carotid artery with paucity of opercular branches from the superior division of the MCA, absent Rolandic and post-Rolandic branches. B, Anteroposterior view demonstrating nonfilling of the MCA distal to the bifurcation with decreased opercular branches.

a very high predictor of secondary parenchymal hemorrhage and death (19, 20). More recent reports have correlated significantly poorer outcome in patients with more than one-third MCA territory infarcted with a delayed infarction volume of 24 to 33 ml versus more than one-third MCA involvement with infarction volumes of 84.3 to 123.1 ml. Equally important is the interpretation of cranial CT scans in the setting of acute stroke. Schriger et al. (47) reported physician accuracy in determining eligibility for thrombolytic therapy. The objective was to evaluate the physician accuracy, and a pool of 54 CT scans were randomly assigned. There were 38 emergency room physicians, 29 neurologists, and 36 radiologists. Only 67% of emergency room physicians correctly interpreted the studies. Eighty-three percent of neurologists had correct interpretations and 83% of radiologists had correct interpretations; however, the overall average for correct interpretation was only 77%. Obviously, physician education is extremely important, as emergency room physicians are often the initial individuals seeing these patients. Of ever more concern was the detection of hemorrhage; only 17% of emergency room physicians made the correct diagnosis, whereas 40% of the neurologists and 52% of general radiologists correctly interpreted the early acute noncontrast CT scans (47). This obviously has important therapeutic implications in terms of delivery of thrombolytics or commencement of possible intraarterial intervention (see *Figs. 18.1–18.5*).

In summary, CT changes of early acute cerebral ischemia include ill-defined vascular territory hypodensity, subtle mass effect most likely in the insular region, loss of gray/white matter interface or junction, and occasional hyperdense MCA sign.

Magnetic Resonance Imaging

MRI is known to be a much more sensitive indicator of early cerebral ischemia by a ratio of 4.3. MRI findings in early cerebral ischemia include possible loss of vascular flow-related abnormalities or loss of flow void, parenchymal signal changes, and morphological brain swelling. This is best noted on T1 images. Cytotoxic edema occurring in the early stages of cerebral ischemia may not be depicted on early changes in T2-weighted images, which usually occur after 6 to 8 hours of the complete lesion. Also of note is that accumulation of contrast material may occur in the ischemic or infarcted tissue and may be depicted by a strong signal enhancement on T1 images.

MRI PERFUSION TECHNIQUES

In the acute stage of cerebral ischemia, alterations in the vascular flow pattern may be the earliest detectable sign (i.e., the presence or

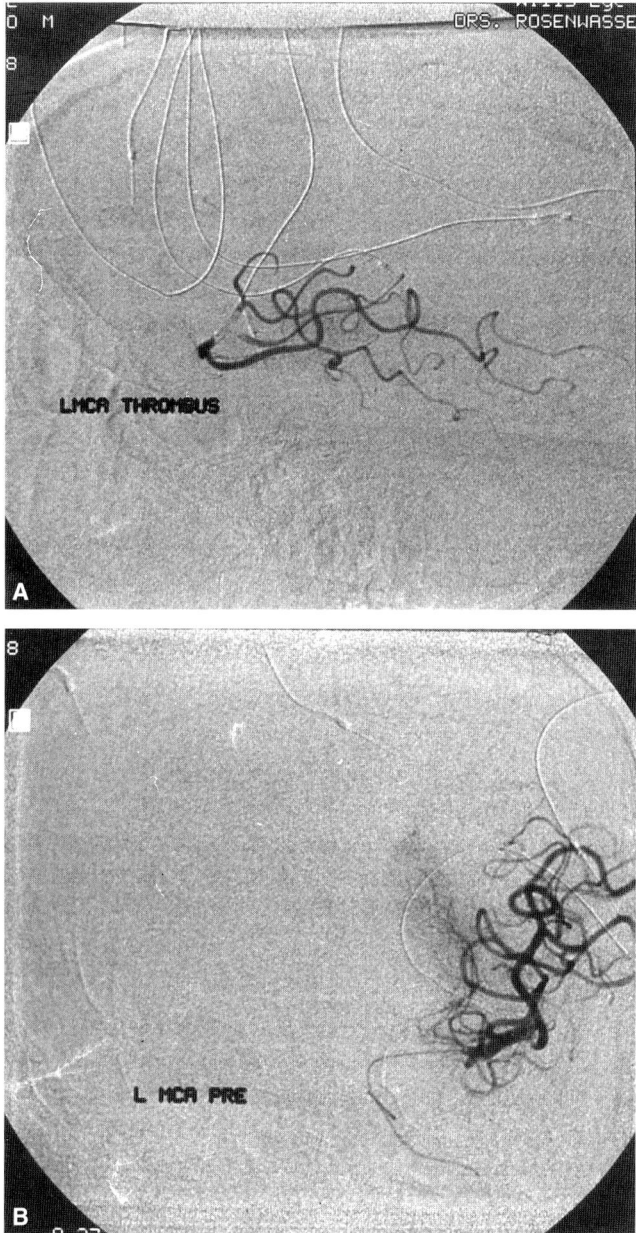

FIG. 18.3 *A*, Anteroposterior and *B*, lateral views of a supraselective injection of the MCA superior division with partial revascularization of the MCA after thrombolysis.

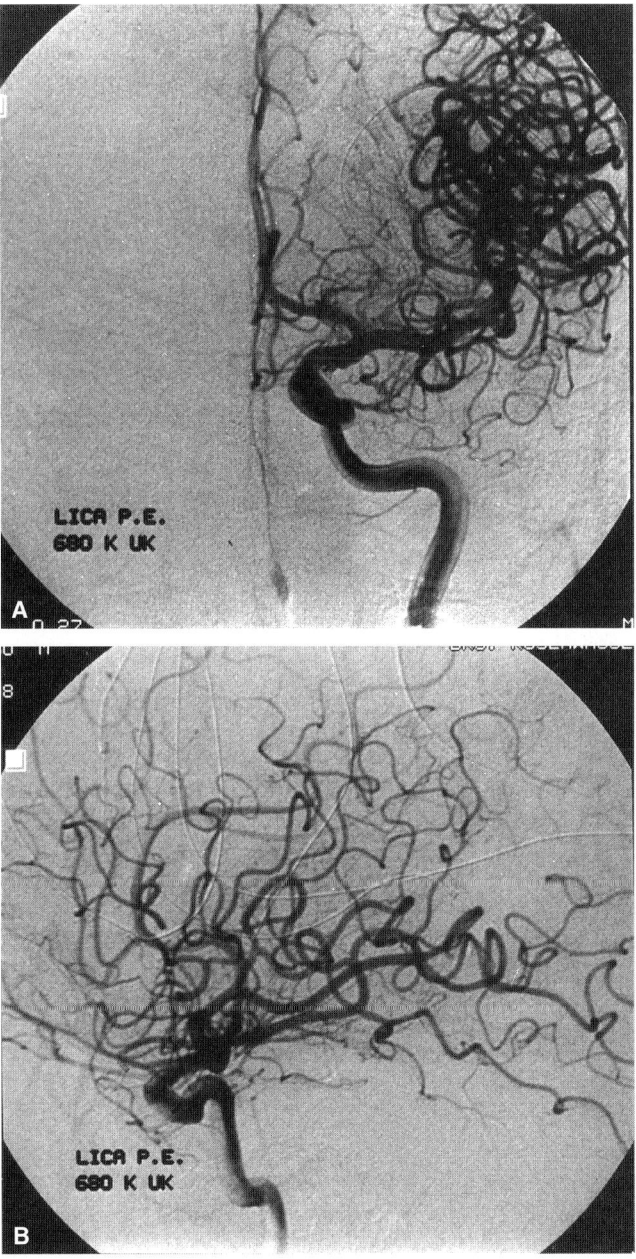

FIG. 18.4 *A*, Anteroposterior and *B*, lateral views of the left internal carotid artery after thrombolysis using 68-kg units of UK. Normal filling of the opercular branches, inferior and superior trunks, luxury perfusion appreciated in the region of the insula.

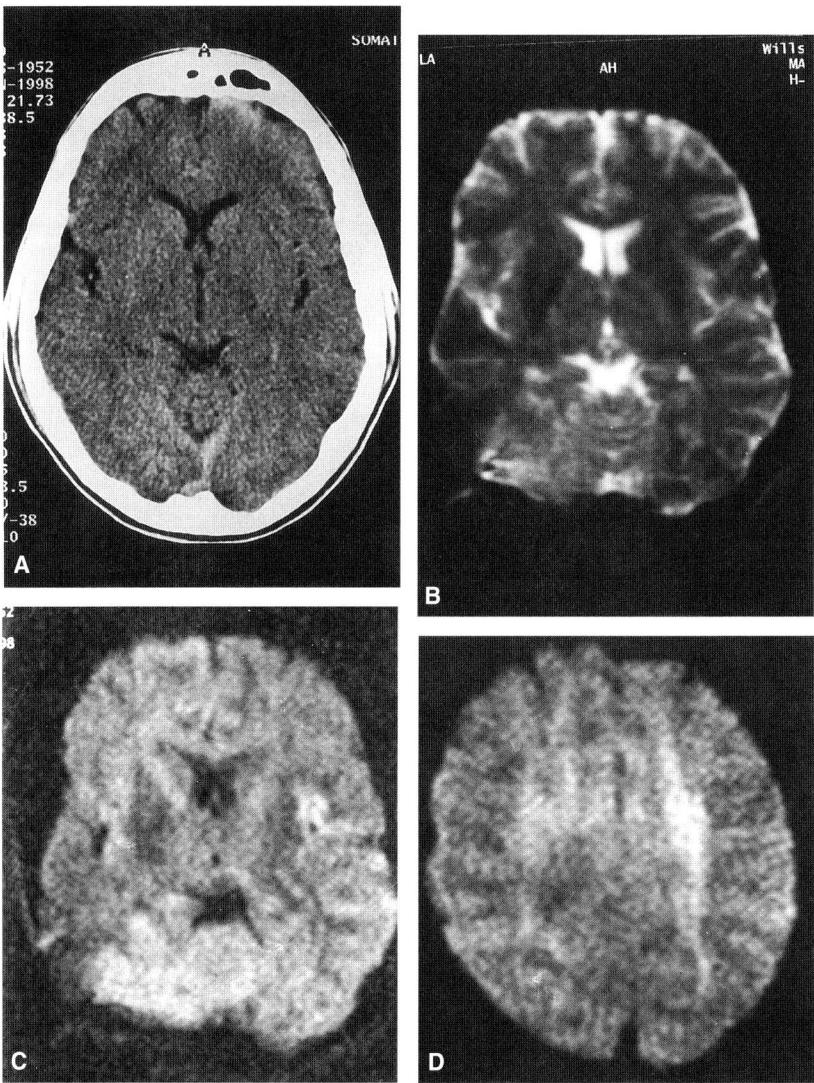

FIG. 18.5 A 47-year-old woman with acute onset hemiplegia and aphasia with *A*, a normal axial CT scan, *B*, normal axial T2-weighted MRI, *C*, abnormal diffusion-weighted MRI with increased signal in the left insular cortex and *D*, increased signal in the centrum semi-ovale.

absence of flow void). Perfusion and diffusion abnormalities, however, may be observed in the first hour after ischemia, and this is currently an optimal study to determine ischemic injury if either intraarterial or intravenous thrombolytic therapy is to be undertaken. The use of perfusion studies combined with diffusion-weighted images described below may also be used to delineate the ischemic penumbra (8, 14). Those regions with a perfusion defect but without a diffusion defect may indicate salvageable ischemic tissue (33). Studies that have combined these two techniques have identified this pattern in up to 61% of patients and 100% of patients presenting acutely less than 3 hours (8). A recent study evaluating the application of perfusion/diffusion imaging evaluated patients treated with t-PA who had this pattern. In this population of patients, the perfusion abnormality reversed after 24 to 36 hours with reversal of clinical deficits and consistent with early reperfusion (35).

MRI DIFFUSION APPLICATIONS

Recently, diffusion imaging of the brain has gained increased attention owing to its usefulness in rapidly detecting acute strokes. Diffusion weighted imaging (DWI) can detect small changes in water diffusion that occur in ischemic brain tissue (36). This works by the identification of random movements of water protons (diffusion), which becomes restricted as cytotoxic edema causes water movement into the cell thereby restricting their movement (intracellular water increasing during the ischemic injury cascade) (1). Current techniques involve the construction of apparent diffusion coefficient (ADC) maps based on a graduated weighting of the diffusion by a b-value. Low b-values indicate no diffusion resulting in bright signal, whereas high b-values indicate high diffusion resulting in dark signal. The differences in the rate of change of signal intensity at different b-values allow calculation of the ADC, which is a quantitative measure of water diffusion. Therefore, high diffusion rates (unrestricted water movement) have a high signal on the ADC map, and low diffusion rates (restricted water movement), as in ischemia, have low ADC values and appear dark on the ADC map (1, 42). On the standard orthogonal-axis diffusion-weighted images, these images appear bright much earlier than T2-weighted changes as early in some cases as 1 to 3 hours, making this tool very applicable to acute stroke intervention (*Figs. 18.5–18.11*). These ischemic volumes closely correlate with the final infarct volume, as seen on the delayed T2-weighted MRIs and tend to be better delineated with sharp margins on diffusion-weighted images. The techniques to obtain the best ADC maps include that of orthogonal-axis diffusion-weighted,

246 CLINICAL NEUROSURGERY

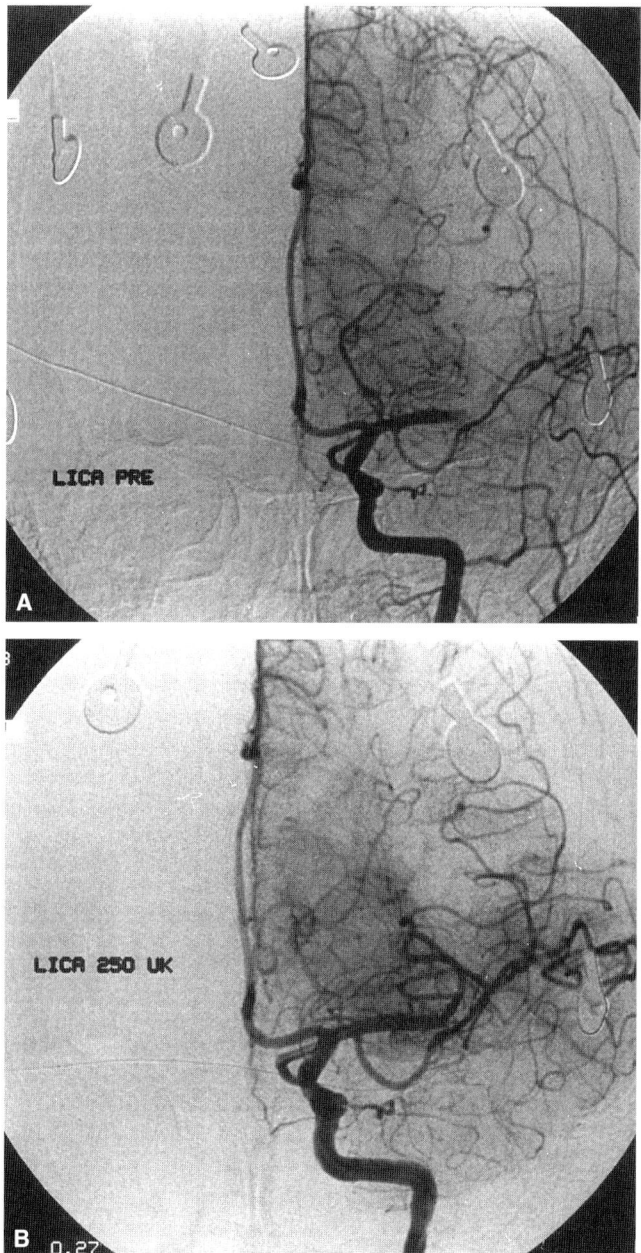

FIG. 18.6 A, Prethrombolysis anteroposterior AP view of the controlled angiogram demonstrating evidence of MCA occlusion proximal to the MCA bifurcation. B, Post-thrombolysis with normal filling of the MCA divisions and the opercular branches.

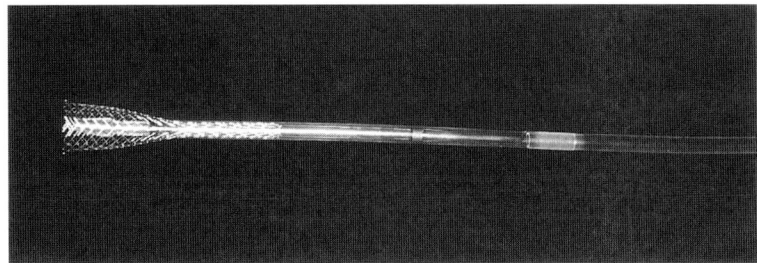

FIG. 18.7 Self-deploying carotid stent (Wal-stent, Schneider) partially deployed, demonstrating stent expansion to present diameter.

isotropic diffusion-weighted, diffusion trace-weighted, and diffusion fusion trace imaging. Results of comparison studies have demonstrated a higher sensitivity, specificity, and accuracy for the simple, orthogonal-axis DWI versus the other three mentioned techniques of postacquisitioned processed images (7). Early detection of irreversible ischemic brain damage is critical in defining strategies that may influence neuronal survival as they relate to intervention, with either intravenous or intraarterial thrombolytic therapy (12, 16, 18, 41). Lutsep et al. (34), in their study of 103 scans obtained a mean of 10.4 days after symptom onset, found that DWI detected six lesions not seen on T2-weighted images and discriminated two new infarcts from old lesions. Their conclusion was that DWI is markedly superior to T2-weighted MRI in detecting acute ischemic events, whereas both techniques assist in determining lesion age. Kidwel et al. (30) reported the results of diffusion-weighted MRI in patients with transient ischemic attacks. They evaluated clinical and MRI data on consecutive patients presenting to their institution over a 6-month period with symptoms of transient ischemic attack (TIA), excluding amaurosis fugax. TIA patient imaging data were compared with a contemporaneous group of 23 patients with completed stroke. Forty-eight percent of the TIA patients demonstrated relevant focal abnormal signals on DWI. Their conclusion was that DWI demonstrates ischemic abnormalities in nearly 50% of clinical TIA patients; in nearly half of these, DWI changes may be fully reversible, whereas in the remainder these findings may herald the development of a parenchymal infarct despite transient clinical symptoms (30). The clinical usefulness of diffusion MRI may also be extended beyond the 3-hour window (4). Albers et al. (1) identified three groups of patients in which diffusion MRI alone identified the following changes that were clinically relevant: 1) the acute symptomatic lesion was confirmed to be in a different vascular territory than had been suspected clinically

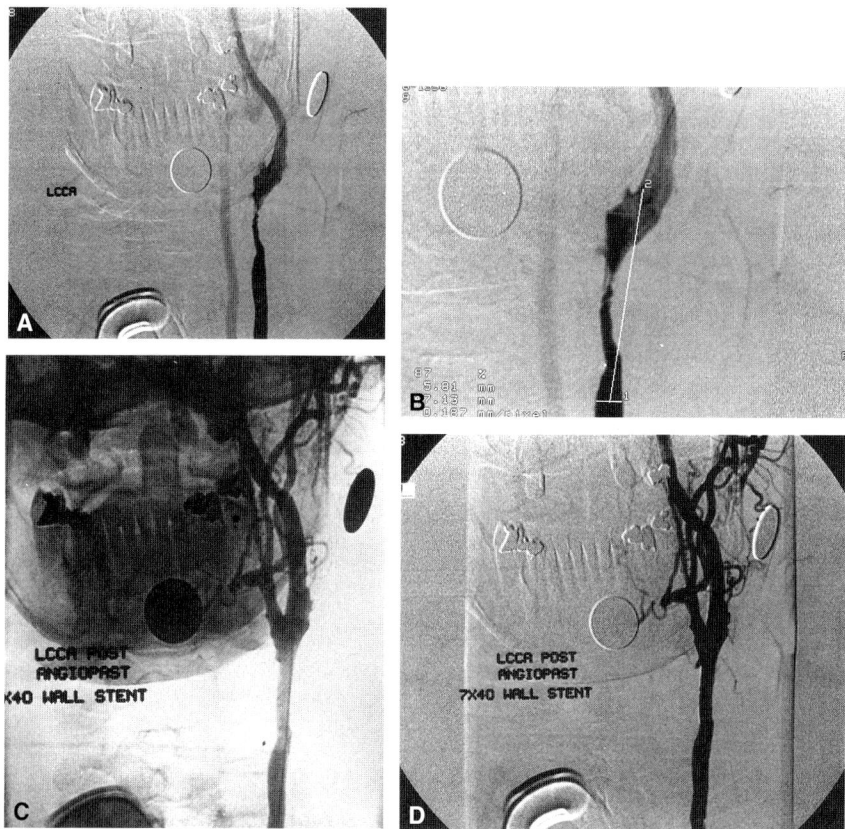

FIG. 18.8 *A*, Anteroposterior common carotid angiogram demonstrating high-grade long segment stenosis of the distal common carotid artery related to postradiation stenosis with nonfilling of the external carotid artery branches. *B*, Axial and longitudinal measurements of the proximal common carotid artery and length of the stenosis taken to select an appropriated stent. *C*, Subtracted angiogram of a postangioplasty and stenting of postradiation stenosis of the common carotid artery. *D*, Nonsubtracted view of the postangioplasty and stent of the same patient demonstrating guidewire across the lesion and the stent extending across the stenosis from the common carotid artery to the internal carotid artery with normal filling of the external carotid artery.

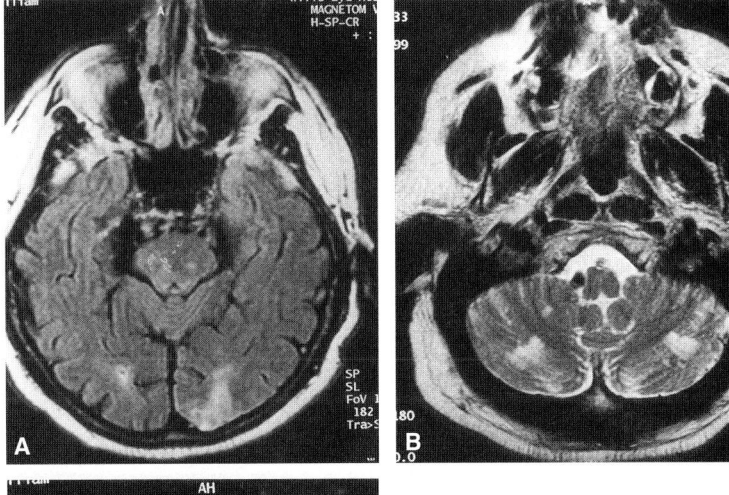

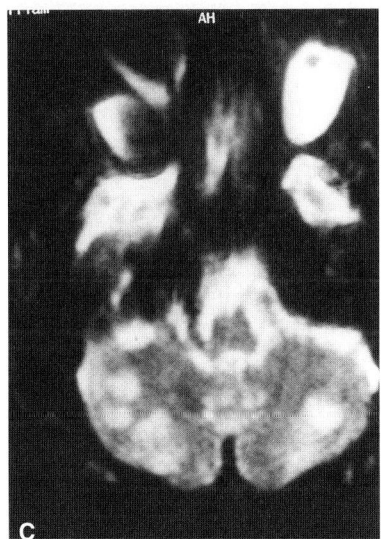

FIG. 18.9 Images from a 64-year-old woman with a history of medically intractable posterior circulation ischemia consisting of loss of coordination, vertigo, dysarthria, and perioral numbness. A, Axial T1-weighted MRI demonstrating evidence of left occipital infarct involving the occipital cortical mantla and subjacent subcortical white matter in a wedge-shaped fashion, representing distal emboli from the vertebral stenosis into the left posterior cerebral artery. B, T2-weighted axial images demonstrating evidence of multiple bilateral cerebellar infarcts and absence of filling of the left vertebral artery with partially thrombosed right vertebral artery. C, Diffusion-weighted MRI with bilateal cerebrellar infarcts seen on the T2-weighted images.

(21%); 2) multiple lesions in different vascular territories suggestive of a proximal source of emboli (8%) were revealed and; 3) it was clarified that a lesion, thought to be acute on conventional imaging, was not acute (29%). This is of particular importance in patients who are about to undergo interventional thrombolytic therapy or require additional studies such as transesophageal echo to identify the source of the proximal emboli (1, 58). Unfortunately, in critically ill patients requiring invasive cardiopulmonary monitoring, MRI is still more cumbersome and

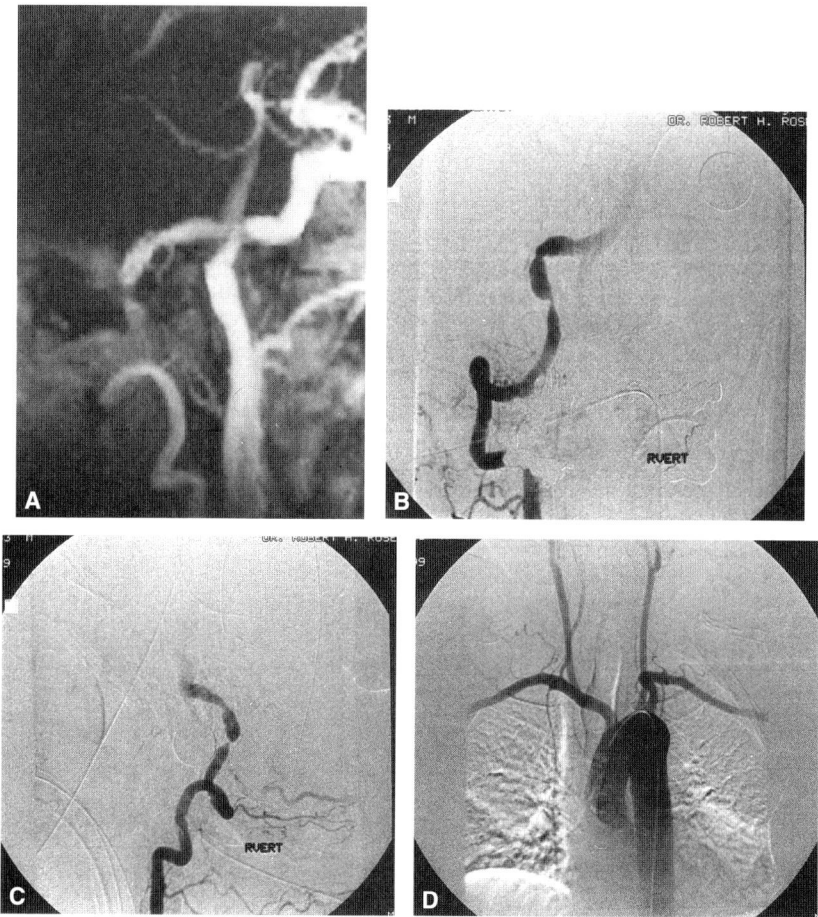

FIG. 18.10 A MRA of patient in *Figure 18.9A, B,* and *C* with evidence of high-grade right intracranial vertebral artery stenosis confirmed on biplane subtraction angiography. *B,* AP and *C,* lateral views, *D,* absence of left vertebral artery from aortic arch injection.

time-consuming than helical-CT augmented with blood flow analysis using Xenon-enhanced computerized tomographic (xe-CT) technology.

Single Photon Emission Computed Tomography

The use of nuclear medicine brain imaging with radiolabeled tracers has allowed the noninvasive measurements of regional cerebral blood flow (CBF), regional oxygen extraction fraction, regional metabolic rate of oxygen, and regional cerebral blood volume and subsequent mapping of regional cerebral perfusion (39, 52).

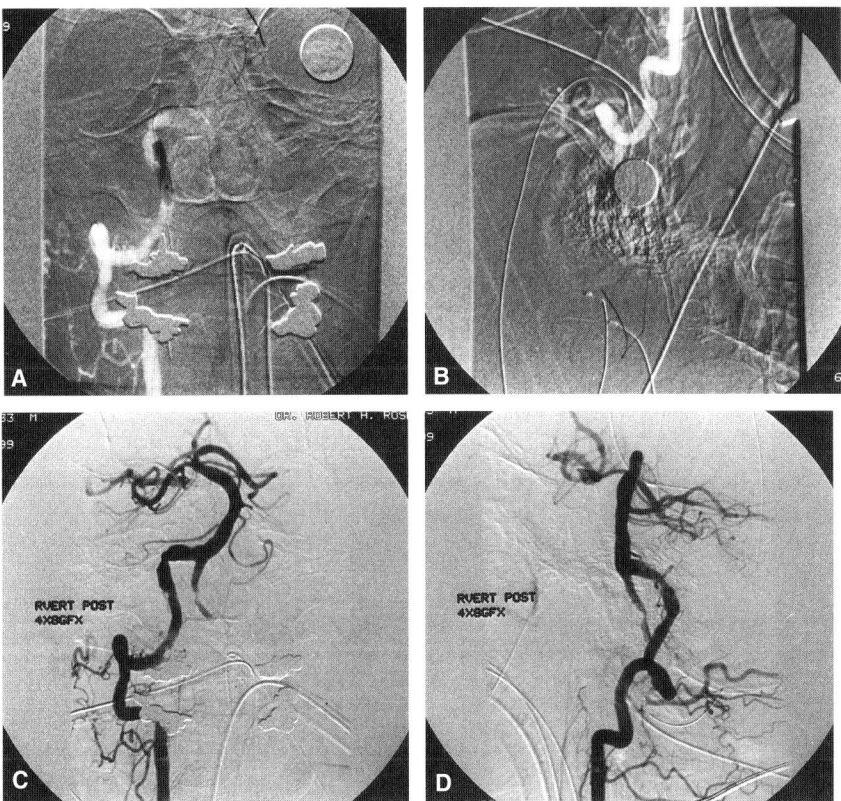

FIG. 18.11 Same patient as in *Figures 18.9* and *18.10* with an over-the-wire balloon mounted coronary stent (GFX stent; AVE, Santa Rosa, CA) being placed into the stenotic intracranial vertebral artery. Note microguidewire anchored into the distal posterior cerebral artery, A, anteroposterior and B, lateral views. Postdilation and angioplasty of the vertebral artery stenosis with marked improvement in the circulation time and filling of the posterior communicating artery and posterior cerebral artery branches. C, anteroposterior and D, lateral views.

The greatest limiting factors remain unchanged: time-consuming, cumbersome, and expensive, as compared with MR spectroscopy (*Fig. 18.12*). One of the most used radiolabeled tracers include Tc-99m HMPAO (hexamethylpropyleneamine oxime). A three-dimensional study is obtained with sagittal, axial, and coronal views. Variable weighting of tracer is obtained by the gamma camera, which can be converted into a 255-value gray-scale map, allowing for a qualitative evaluation of a particular region of interest (*Fig. 18.13*). Regional differences can occur, and variation from one hemisphere to another includes

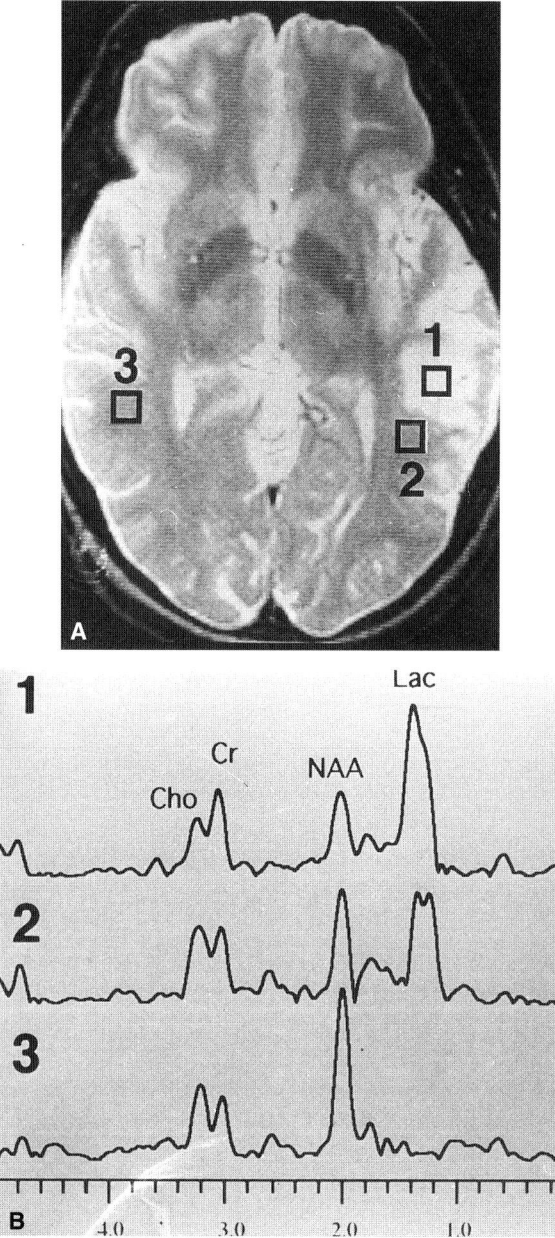

FIG. 18.12 Example of MRI spectroscopy *(A)* and *(B)* of a patient with an infarction of the left temporal lobe. Voxels 1, 2, and 3 demonstrate the three characteristic wave forms associated with the predominant chemical shift in that region: #1 lactate, #2 NAA (neuronal marker on borderzone), and #3 NAA (neuronal marker distal from region of infarction).

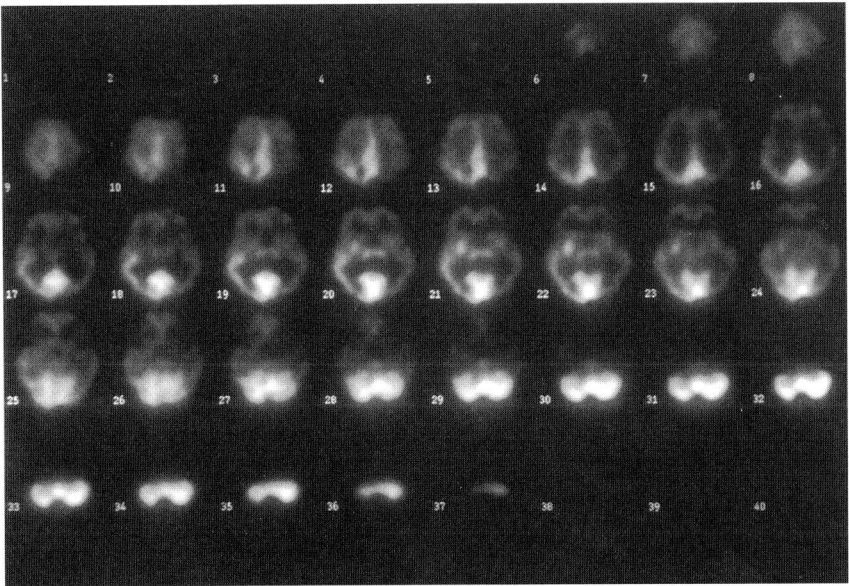

FIG. 18.13 Patient with moyamoya disease demonstrating hypoperfusion of the left cerebral hemisphere by SPECT.

10 to 13% (2). In the evaluation of stroke, single photon emission computed tomographic (SPECT) imaging has been best applied to nonacunar strokes in which the initial anatomic imaging study is negative. One compounding factor is that SPECT imaging cannot discriminate between normal perfusion and luxury perfusion, which may mask an infarct zone (39). Recent applications have included the use of HMPAO SPECT imaging to balloon test occlusion in a series of 16 patients; two patients had deficits after the occlusion without SPECT imaging performed, and five patients had SPECT imaging abnormalities consisting of assymetry of more than 19% without evidence of neurological symptoms during 30 minutes of temporary vessel occlusion. The advantage of the "snap-shot" of the brain perfusion with little redistribution is that it allows evaluation of the regional CBF during balloon inflation, unlike xe-CT, which requires balloon inflation on the CT table and inhalation of the xenon-mixed gas for several minutes, thereby affecting the neurological observations during the balloon test occlusion. Although reports in the literature have included patients in whom the CBF was symmetrical by HMPAO SPECT imaging and who went on to have ischemia, the combined use of regional oxygen saturation of the

brain monitoring has improved the detection of decreased CBF, which also correlated with stump pressures of less than 40 mm Hg (29).

Xenon-Enhanced CT of Cerebral Blood Flow

The use of xe-CT has allowed a quantitative evaluation of CBF previously available only with more cumbersome and expensive positron emission tomography and 133Xe technology. Xenon is lipid soluble and can be injected or inhaled; the absorbed xenon is calculated by measuring the percentage of xenon inhaled versus the amount exhaled. Therefore, the xenon concentration in the brain (measured by CT) and the xenon concentration in the blood (calculated) allow the calculation of the CBF (43, 63). These blood flow calculations are computerized, allowing rapid data generation and the construction of clinically relevant flow maps. The system is designed to err on the high side, so in patients with CBF values less than 5 ml/100 g this is evidence of no flow, at high risk for perfusion hemorrhage (< 10 ml/100 g/min), reversible ischemia 10 to 20 ml/100 g/min, depending on the length of symptoms and absence of hemorrhage. The advantages of xe-Ct is that it serves as a rapid and repeatable procedure taking 5 min preparation time, 6 min of time, 17 min from time of order for review, and 15 to 20 min until time for repeat study. The ability to image xenon on CT, owing to its radiodensity, allows quantitative maps to be constructed for CBF. Xe-CT has evolved with modern CT technology, computerized maps, and lower concentration of xenon associated with fewer side effects, allowing it to be a rapid, less expensive, and more facile tool than the other technologies in the development of quantitative measures of CBF. Applications for its use include the imaging of patients with acute MCA occlusions with identification of the ischemic core and penumbra (30) identifying the likelihood of intraarterial thrombolysis complications (CBF > 10 cc/100 g/min), identifying hypoperfused areas in the chronic phases of a stroke (40), evaluating CBF during balloon test occlusion (59), and accompanying the use of transluminal angioplasty during treatment of symptomatic aneurysmal vasospasm (17, 43).

ENDOVASCULAR THERAPY IN ACUTE STROKE

Nearly 80% of strokes are ischemic in nature, and the vast majority of these lesions result from atherothrombotic or thrombo-embolic occlusion of large vessels supplying cerebral tissue. Most of the emboli responsible for these lesions originate from extracranial carotid circulation or are cardiogenic in origin. If patients are studied angiographically within 6 hours of onset, some studies indicate that an occlusive vascular lesion correlating with the clinical deficit may be found in over

75% of cases. Several studies have looked at the role of intraarterial thrombolysis and angioplasty in the treatment of acute stroke. Urbach et al. (53) reported on a series of 12 patients with combined occlusions of the distal internal carotid artery, anterior cerebral artery, and proximal MCA. The patients were initially evaluated with CT and MR scanning, and the dose of the urokinase administered was limited to 1,000,000 units. They also received a heparin bolus of 50 units per kilogram to achieve a partial thromboplastin time of twice normal. Four of the patients in their study had a good outcome, with a Barthel index greater than 90 at 3 mo, when the treatment was performed at a mean of 121 min after onset of symptoms. Four patients had major deficits with a Barthel index of 40 to 55 when treatment was performed at a mean of 232 min after onset of symptoms. Four patients died with treatment performed at a mean of 203 min to therapy. There was a significant correlation between recanalization and clinical outcome ($P = 0.038$ Kruskal-Wallis test). Multiple regression analysis indicated that there was a significant positive correlation between a short interval to therapy and the presence of leptomeningeal collaterals (53). Endo et al. (16) reported on the results of urgent thrombolysis in patients with major stroke and atherothrombotic occlusion of the cervical internal carotid artery. Their study included 33 patients with NIH Stroke Scale greater than 24 who had a normal CT scan on admission. Angiography with intraarterial or intravenous thrombolytics was performed within a 6-hour window. The results indicated that they were able to achieve recanalization in eight patients; four patients had a good clinical outcome. The two factors that were significant were treatment at less than 3 hours and immediate correction of stenosis after recanalization of the cervical internal carotid system by either percutaneous transluminal angioplasty and stent placement or carotid endarterectomy. This continuing theme of resolution of the embolic event with correction of the offending lesion is extremely important (16).

DelZoppo et al. (12) reported on the PROACT study, a phase-two randomized trial of recombinant pro-urokinase by direct arterial delivery in acute MCA stroke. Inclusion criteria included focal deficit corresponding to MCA territory infarct within a 6-hour window and a minimum NIH Stroke Scale of 4. The age range was 18 to 85 years. Exclusion criteria included presence of blood on initial CT scan, NIH Stroke Scale greater than 30, blood pressure greater than 180/100, or a 6-week history of neurological events, possibility of cardiac source, or coagulopathy. In this group, 180 patients underwent transfemoral cerebral angiography and 49 patients were randomized; 26 patients received recombinant pro-urokinase and 14 patients received placebo. Recanalization with pro-urokinase was significant over placebo; however, hemorrhagic transformation was 15.4% in the pro-urokinase group and 7.1% in the placebo group. Recanalization and hemorrhage complications were influenced by heparin dose, in that patients receiving a large heparin dose of 100 units per kilogram had a higher hemorrhagic transformation rate than those who received lesser doses. The end number of patients randomized was too small to achieve statistical significance; however, there was a 10 to 12% absolute increase in excellent neurological outcome in patients treated with pro-urokinase over placebo at 90 days. The 90-day mortality was 26.9% in the pro-urokinase group and 42.9% in the placebo group, indicating that, in larger groups, this treatment may achieve statistical significance (12). Further studies regarding pro-urokinase are currently under way and are promising.

SUMMARY

With the advent of therapy for acute stroke via in intraarterial or intravenous pathway, early diagnosis with physician education is extremely important. A common theme in all studies is the continued stress on patient and physician education, rapid triage and diagnosis with the use of CT scanning, xenon blood flow or diffusion MRI, cerebral protection, and revascularization with either carotid surgery or percutaneous angioplasty for an offending lesion, if such is identified. Although the current studies are cautiously optimistic, prospective randomized trials are needed for the evaluation of intraarterial thrombolytics as well as percutaneous transluminal angioplasty. It is important that the neurosurgical community be identified as physicians who can diagnose and treat the patient with an acute stroke.

REFERENCES

1. Albers GW, Lansberg MG, Norbash AM, et al.: Yield of diffusion weighted MRI for detection of potentially clinically relevant findings in stroke patients. Presented at the 24th American Heart Association International Conference on Stroke and Cerebral Circulation, Nashville TN, 1999.
2. Alberts MJ: Hyperacute stroke therapy with tissue plasminogen activator. **Am J Cardiol** 80(4C): 29D–34D, 1997.
3. Asalid R, Huber P, Nornes H: Evaluation of cerebrovascular spasm with transcranial Doppler ultrasound. **J Neurosurg** 60:37–41, 1984.
4. Ay H, Buonanno FS, Schaefer PW, et al: Clinical and Diffusion-weighted imaging characteristics of an identifiable subset of TIA patients with acute infarction. Presented at the 24th American Heart Association International Conference on Stroke and Cerebral Circulation. Nashville, TN. 1999.
5. Bluemke DA, Chambers TP: Spiral CT angiography: Alternative to conventional angiography. **Radiology** 197:381–387, 1995.

6. Carlin RE, McGraw DJ, Calimlin JR, Macia MF: The use of near-infrared cerebral oximetry in awake carotid endarterectomy. **J Clin Anaesth** 10:109–113, 1998.
7. Chong J, Lu D, Aragao F, et al.: Diffusion-weighted MR of acute cerebral infarction: Comparison of data processing methods. **Am J Neuroradiol** 19:1733–1739, 1998.
8. Darby DG, Barber PA, Desmond PM, et al.: Patterns and frequency of acute ischemic stroke topography as depicted by combined perfusion- and diffusion-weighted magnetic resonance imaging. Presented at the 24th American Heart Association International Conference on Stroke and Cerebral Circulation. Nashville, TN, 1999.
9. Davies KN, Humphrey PR: Complications of cerebral angiography in patients with symptomatic carotid territory ischaemia screened by carotid ultrasound. **J Neurol Neurosurg Psychiatry** 56:967–972, 1993.
10. Dawson DL, Zierler RE, Strandness DEJ, et al. The role of duplex scanning and arteriography before carotid endarterectomy: A prospective study. **J Vasc Surg** 18:673–680, 1993.
11. DelZoppo GJ, Ferber A, Otis S, et al.: Local intra-arterial fibrinolytic therapy in acute carotid territory stroke: pilot study. **Stroke** 19:307–313, 1988.
12. delZoppo GJ, Higashida RT, Furlan AJ, Pessin MS, Rowley HA, Gent M, et al.: PROACT: A phase II randomized trial of recombinant pro-urokinase by direct arterial delivery in acute middle cerebral artery stroke. **Stroke** 29:4–11, 1998.
13. DelZoppo GJ, Zeumer H, Harker LA: Thrombolytic therapy in stroke: Possibilities and hazards. **Stroke** 17:595–607, 1986.
14. Edelman RR, Siewart B, Darby DG, et al.: Qualitative mapping of cerebral blood flow and functional localization with echo-planar MR imaging and signal targeting with alternating radio frequency. **Radiology** 192:513–520, 1994.
15. Ekelund A, Kongstad P, Saveland H, et al.: Transcranial cerebral oximetry related to transcranial doppler after aneurysmal subarachnoid hemorrhage. **Acta Neurochir (Wien).** 140:1029–1036, 1998.
16. Endo S, Kuwayama N, Hirashima Y, Akai T, Nishijima M, Takaku A: Results or urgent thrombolysis in patients with major stroke and atherothrombotic occlusion of the cervical internal and carotid artery. **Am J Neuroadiol** 19:1169–1175, 1999.
17. Firlik AD, Kaufmann AM, Jungreis CA, Yonas H: Effect of transluminal angioplasty on cerebral blood flow in the management of symptomatic vasospasm following SAH. **J Neurosurg** 86:830–839, 1997.
18. Firlik AD, Yonas H, Kaufmann AM, et al.. Relationship between cerebral blood flow and the development of swelling and life-threatening herniation in acute ischemic stroke. **J Neurosurg** 89(2):243–249, 1998.
19. Hacke W, Kaste M, Fieschi C, et al.: Intraveneous thrombolysis with recombinant tissue plasminogen activator for acute hemispheric stroke. The European Cooperative Acute Stroke Study. **JAMA** 274;1017–1025, 1995.
20. Hacke W, Kaste M, Fieschi C, et al.: Safety and efficacy of intravenous thrombolysis with a recombinant tissue plasminogen activator in the treatment of acute hemispheric stroke. Results of ECASS, the European Cooperative Acute Stroke Study. **JAMA** 274, 1995.
21. Heiserman JE: The role of magnetic resonance angiography in the evaluation of cerebrovascular ischemic disease. **Neuroimaging Clin N Am** 753–767, 1992.
22. Heiserman JE, Dean BL, Hodak JA, et al: Neurologic complications of cerebral angiography. **Am J Neuroradiol** 15:1401–1407, 1994.
23. Heiserman JE, Drayer BP, Fram EK, et al.: Carotid artery stenosis: Clinical efficacy of two-dimensional time-of-flight MR angiography. **Radiology** 182:761–768, 1992.

24. Heiserman JE, Drayer BP, Keller PJ, Fram EK: Intracranial vascular stenosis and occlusion: Evaluation with three-dimensional time-of-flight MR angiography. **Radiology** 185:667–673, 1992.
25. Hennerici M, Mohr JP, Rautenberg W, Steinke W: Ultrasound imaging and Doppler sonography in the diagnosis of cerebrovascular disease, in Barnett HJM, et al.: *Stroke* 241–268, 1992.
26. Hoff DJ, Wallace MC, TerBrugge KG, Gentili F: Rotational angiography assessment of cerebral aneurysms. **Am J Neuroradiol** 15:1945–1948, 1994.
27. Huston J, Lewis BD, Weibers DO, et al.: Carotid artery: Prospective blinded comparison of two-dimensional time-of-flight MR angiography with conventional angiography and duplex US. **Radiology** 186:339–344, 1993.
28. Iwama T, Hashimoto N, Takagi Y, Tsukahara T, Hayashida K: Predictability of extracranial/intracranial bypass function: A retrospective study of patients with occlusive cerebrovascular disease. **Neurosurgery** 40:53–60, 1997.
29. Kaminogo M, Ochi M, Onizuka M, Takahata H, Shibata S: An additional monitoring of regional cerebral oxygen saturation to HMPAO SPECT during BTO. **Stroke** 30:407–113, 1999.
30. Kidwell CS, Alger J, DiSalle F, Starkman S, Villablanca P, Bentson J, Saver JL: Diffusion-weighted magnetic resonance imaging in patients with transient ischemic attacks. Presented at the 24th American Heart Association International Conference on Stroke and Cerebral Circulation. Nashville, TN, 1999.
31. Kleinschmidt A, Steinmetz H, Sitzer M, et al.: Magnetic resonance imaging of regional cerebral blood oxygenation changes under acetazolamide in carotid occlusive disease. **Stroke** 26:106–110, 1995.
32. Knauth von Kummer R, Jansen O, et al.: Potential of CT angiography in acute ischemic stroke. **Am J Neuroradiol** 18:1001–1010, 1997.
33. Lucas TH, Yang SH, Shi J, et al.: Diffusion-weighted and T2-weighted MRI predict ischemic brain injury: Correlation of in vivo cytotoxic and vasogenic edema with histopathology in focal cerebral ischemia-reperfusion injury. Presented at the Joint Meeting of the AANS/CNS Section on Cerebrovascular Surgery and the American Society of Interventional and Therapeutic neuroradiology. Nashville, TN, 1999.
34. Lutsep HL, Albers GW, De Crespigny A, Kamat GN, Marks MP, Moseley ME: Clinical utility of diffusion-weighted magnetic resonance imaging in the assessment of ischemic stroke. **Ann Neurol** 41:574–580, 1997.
35. Marks MP, Tong D, Beaulieu C, Albers G, de Crespigny A, Mosely ME: Effective early reperfusion and intravenous tPA therapy on diffusion and perfusion weighted MRI. Presented at the 24th American Heart Association International Conference on Stroke and Cerebral Circulation. Nashville, TN, 1999.
36. Markus HS, Clifton A, Buckenham T, Brown MM: Carotid angioplasty. Detection of embolic signals during and after the procedure. **Stroke** 25:2403–2406, 1994.
37. Meairs S, Röther J, Neff KW, Hennerici M: New and future development in cerebrosvascular ultrasound MRA and related techniques. **J Clin Ultrasound** 23: 139–149, 1995.
38. Mittl RL, Broderick M, Carpenter JP, et al. Blinded reader comparison of magnetic reasonance angiography and duplex ultrasonography for carotid artery bifurcation stenosis. **Stroke** 25:4–10, 1994.
39. Mullan BP, O'Connor MK, Hung JC: Single photon emission computed tomography brain imaging. **Neurosurg Clin N Am** 7(1);617–651, 1996.
40. Nasel C, Trattnig S, Samec P, Schnaberth G, Schindler E: Stable xenon CT in

patients with chronic cerebrovascular disease. **Neurodiology** 38:S47–S50, 1996.
41. The National Institute of Neurological Disorders and Stroke rt-PA Stroke Study: Tissue plasminogen activator for acute ischemic stroke. **N Eng J Mid** 333:1581–1587, 1995.
42. Oliveria-Filho J, Ay H, Buonanno FS, et al.: Clinical correlates of acute small subcortical or brainstem infarctions detected by diffusion-weighted MRI. Presented at the 24th American Heart Association International Conference on Stroke and Cerebral Circulation. Nashville, TN 1999.
43. Pindzola RR, Yonas H: The xenon-enhanced computed tomography cerebral blood flow method. **Neurosurgery** 43(6):1488–1492, 1998.
44. Ries S, Steinke W, Neff KW, Hennerici M; Echocontrast-enhanced transcranial colorcoded sonography for the diagnosis of transverse sinus venous thrombosis. **Stroke** 28:696–700, 1997.
45. Robinson ML, Sacks D, Perlmutter GS, Marinelli DL: Diagnostic criteria for carotid duplex sonography. **Am J Roentgenol** 151:1045–1949, 198.
46. Schreiber WG, Guckel F, Stritzke P, Schmiedek P, Schwartz A, Brix G: Cerebral blood flow and cerebrovascular reserve capacity: Estimation by dynamic magnetic resonance imaging. **J Cereb Blood Flow Metab** 18:1143–1156, 1998.
47. Schriger DL, Kalafut M, Starkman S, Krueger M, Saver JL: Cranial computed tomography interpretation in acute stroke. **JAMA** 279:1293–1297, 1988.
48. Steinke W, Kloetzsch C, Hennerici M: Carotid artery disease assessed by color Doppler flow imaging: Correlation with standard Doppler sonography and angiography. **Am J Neuroradiol** 11:259–266, 1990.
49. Tomsick T, Brott B, Barsan W, et al.: Thrombus localization with emergency cerebral CT. **Am J Neuroradiol** 12:257–263, 1992.
50. Touho H, Karasawa J, Ohnishi H, et al.: Comparison of dynamic CT and stable Xenon CT in ischemic cerebrovascular disease. **Am J Neuroradiol** 14:655–660, 1993.
51. Ueda T, Hatekeyama T, Kohno K, Kumon K, Sakaki S: Endovascular treatment for acute thrombotic occlusion of the middle cerebral artery: Local intra-arterial thrombolysis combined with percutaneous transluminal angioplasty. **Neuroradiology** 39(2):99–104, 1997.
52. Ueda T, Sakaki S, Kumon Y, Yuh WTC: A role of SPECT in intra-arterial thrombolysis for acute ischemic stroke. Presented at the Joint Meeting of the AANS/CNS Section on Cerebrovascular Surgery and the American Society of Interventional and Therapeutic Neuroradiology Nashville, TN, 1999.
53. Urbach H, Ries F, Ostertun B, Solymosi L: Local intra-arterial fibrinolysis in thromboembolic "T" occlusions of the internal carotid artery. **Neuroradiology** 39: 105–110, 1997.
54. von Kummer R, Meyding-Lamade U, Forsting M, et al.: Sensitivity and prognostic value of early computed tomography in middle cerebral artery trunk occlusion. **Am J Neuroradiol** 15:9–15, 1994.
55. von Kummer R, Weber J: Brain and vascular imaging in acute ischemic stroke: The potential of computed tomography. **Neurology** 49 (Suppl 4):S52–S55, 1997.
56. Warnock NG, Gandhi MR, Bergvall U, Powell T: Complications of intraarterial digital subtraction angiography in patients investigated for cerebral vascular disease. **Br J Radiol** 66:855–858, 1993.
57. Waugh JR, Sacharias N: Arteriographic complications in the DSA era. **Radiology** 182:243–246, 1992.
58. Wijdicks EFM, Nichols DA, Thielen KR, Fulgham JR, Brown RD, Meissner I, Meyer

FB, Piepgras DG: Intra-arterial thrombolysis in acute basilar artery thromboembolism: The initial Mayo Clinic experience. **Mayo Clin Proc** 72:1005–1013, 1997.
59. Witt JP, Yonas H, Jungreis C: Cerebral blood flow response pattern during balloon test occlusion of the internal carotid artery. **Am J Neuroradiol** 15:847–857, 1994.
60. Wolpert SM, Caplan LR: Current role of cerebral angiography in the diagnosis of cerebrovascular diseases. **Am J Radiol** 159:191–197, 1992.
61. Yadav JS, Roubin GS, Iyer S, et al.: Elective stenting of the extracranial carotid arteries. **Circulation** 95:376–381, 1997.
62. Yonas H, Cho H, Nemoto E, Balzer J, Sclabassi RJ: Cerebral oximetry by near-infrared spectroscopy and somatosensory evoked potentials during carotid endarterectomy. **J Neurosurg** 88, 1998.
63. Yonas H, Darby JM, Marks EC, et al.: CBF meaasured by Xe-CT: An approach to analysis and normal values. **Cereb Blood Flow Metab** 11:716–725, 1991.

CHAPTER

19

Contemporary Acute Ischemic Stroke Therapy with Intravenous Recombinant Tissue Plasminogen Activator

JEFFREY I. FRANK, M.D.

Studies clearly demonstrating the feasibility and safety of thrombolytic therapy for acute ischemic stroke served as the foundation for the first clinical trial demonstrating efficacy of intravenous recombinant tissue plasminogen activator (rt-PA) in improving outcome in selected patients with acute ischemic stroke (1, 9, 10). However, the long history of concerns regarding intracerebral hemorrhage as a complication, the poor results of several randomized control trials of intravenous streptokinase (4, 11, 14) and dissapointing results of a European intravenous rt-PA trial (7) have led to the slow entry of intravenous rt-PA into the acute ischemic stroke treatment arena. The European Cooperative Acute Stroke Study (ECASS) (7, 8) and the National Institutes of Neurological Disorders and Stroke (NINDS) rt-Pa trial (15), are the most important contemporary studies on the efficacy of intravenous rt-PA for acute ischemic stroke.

ECASS was a European-based, multicenter, randomized clinical trial that enrolled 620 selected patients and treated them with 1.1 mg/kg of rt-PA within 6 hours of stroke onset (7). The ECASS primary endpoints included 90-day Barthel Index and modified Rankin Scale. The intention to treat analysis showed no benefit with rt-PA in the primary endpoints. However, 109 patients had major protocol violations, and if they were excluded from the analysis there was a statistically significant difference in the 90-day Rankin Scale in favor of rt-PA–treated patients. There was no difference in the 30-day mortality between the treatment groups, but large parenchymal intracerebral hematomas were more common in the rt-PA group.

The NINDS trial had two parts (15). Part 1 ranodmized 291 patients to receive 0.9 mg/kg of rt-PA versus placebo within 3 hours of stroke onset. The inclusion and exclusion criteria were rigorous and maintained (*Table 19.1*). Less than 5% of the screened stroke patients met entry cri-

TABLE 19.1
NINDS Trial Inclusion and Exclusion Criteria

Inclusion criteria
1. Ischemic stroke within 180 min and a clearly defined time of onset
2. A neurological deficit measurable by NIHSS
3. CT scan of the brain showing no intracranial hemorrhage

Exclusion criteria
1. Stroke or serious head trauma within the preceding 3 months
2. Major surgery within 14 days
3. History of intracranial hemorrhage
4. Systolic blood pressure greater than 185 mm Hg or diastolic blood pressure greater than 110 mm Hg
5. Aggressive treatment required to reduce blood pressure to the specified limits
6. Rapidly improving or minor neurological symptoms
7. Symptoms suggestive of subarachnoid hemorrhage
8. Gastrointestinal hemorrhage or urinary tract hemorrhage within the preceding 21 days
9. Arterial puncture at a noncompressible site within the preceding 7 days
10. Seizure at the onset of the stroke
11. Use of oral anticoagulants
12. Prothrombin time greater than 15 seconds
13. Platelet count less than $100,000/mL^3$
14. Heparin within the 48 hours before onset of stroke with elevated partial thromboplastin time
15. Glucose concentration less than 50 mg/dL (2.7 mmol/L) or greater than 400 mg/dL (22.2 mmol/L)

teria. The proposed positive outcome measures were at least a 4-point improvement in the National Institutes of Health Stroke Scale or the resolution of neurological deficit within 24 hours of receiving rt-PA. This predesignated "positive outcome" was not achieved, however, at 3 months after stroke onset, all of the outcome measures were improved more in the rt-PA–treated group relative to placebo.

The NINDS trial Part 2 methodology was the same as for Part 1. The difference was the projected interpretation of positive outcome, focusing on 3-month outcome. Part 2 randomized 333 patients for a total of 624 patients randomized between the two parts. At 3 months, the rt-PA–treated patients were 30% more likely to have minimal or no disability relative to placebo-treated patients, and the odds ratio for favorable outcome was 1.7 (95% CI, 1.2–2.6; $P = 0.008$). The benefit in outcome from rt-PA was observed in all stroke subgroups (stroke mechanisms). The incidence of symptomatic intracerebral hemorrhage within 36 hours of treatment was substantially higher in the rt-

PA–treated patients: 6.4% in the rt-PA group versus 0.4% in the placebo group ($P < 0.001$). However, the overall mortality rate was similar between the two groups: 17% (rt-PA) versus 21% (placebo). In addition, secondary analyses of the NINDS data demonstrated that the rt-PA–treated patients (relative to placebo) had a lower chance of death or severe disability ($P < 0.02$), a shorter acute hospital length of stay, and a greater frequency of patient discharges to home (versus to a rehabilitation setting or nursing home).

The positive results of the well-designed NINDS trial and the ultimate FDA approval of intravenous rt-PA for selected patients with acute ischemic stroke have led to a heightened medical and lay interest in acute stroke treatment. However, the ECASS results have brought about a healthy dose of skepticism and scrutiny (2, 6), ensuring a relatively slow introduction of intravenous rt-PA into the commonly applied stroke treatment armamentarium. In fact, ECASS II was a European translation of the NINDS trial protocol for treatment within 6 hours of stroke onset. These results were just published (11) and again did not demonstrate convincing benefit from intravenous rt-PA for the acute ischemic stroke patients studied. However, the vast majority of patients were treated within the 3- to 6-hour time window in contrast to the < 3-hour treatment window of the NINDS trial.

Perhaps one of the greatest benefits from the positive results of the NINDS trial is the attention brought to the need for an improved system of emergency triage and care for ischemic and hemorrhagic stroke patients. After all, for patients to even potentially benefit from the one approved acute ischemic stroke treatment, intravenous rt-PA, they must clinically present and be treated with a narrow time window at a facility with the infrastructure that can properly determine eligibility and ensure appropriate posttreatment medical care and monitoring. The state of acute stroke care has not yet reached such a level of organization at most centers.

The University of South Alabama Stroke Center reviewed their experience in a system "geared up" for acute stroke management (16). In a 12-month period, they interfaced with 134 ischemic stroke patients brought to attention through a "stroke code" acute intervention system. Forty-eight (36%) presented within 3 hours of stroke onset. Only nine patients (7% of all the ischemic stroke patients) actually received intravenous rt-PA.

A similar experience was described by others at the University of Texas (3). They prospectively monitored the utilization and outcome of consecutive acute ischemic stroke patients during a 1-year period (after the publication of the NINDS trial results) treated at the university hospital and two community hospitals in Houston. They found that only 6% of all patients hospitalized with ischemic stroke received intravenous rt-PA at the university hospital compared with 1.1% at the community hospitals. The safety and efficacy profile was generally in keeping with the NINDS trial results, but only 30 patients were treated with intravenous rt-PA.

Both of these studies defined the limited contemporary utilization of intravenous rt-PA for acute ischemic stroke. Some of this relates to limitations in patient eligibility by exclusions that are independent of time of presentation. However, delays in patient presentation as well as acute stroke evaluation (after hospital arrival) are also important factors that limit patient eligibility for intravenous rt-PA. With respect to acute stroke presentation, one group showed that the time delay for ischemic stroke patient presentation was 0–3 hours in 4%, 4–6 hours in 12%, 7–12 hours in 21%, and greater than 12 hours in 63% (12).

Improving public awareness of the nature of stroke symptoms and responding to the need for emergent evaluation and treatment are essential to globally improving stroke care and investigating more promising therapies. Concurrently, improving stroke emergency triage and management is also critical. Tremendous strides have been made toward these goals with much work still ahead. One of the most important steps was a consensus meeting of 50 organizations in Washington, DC, in December 1996 to establish new standards of care for stroke patients. One of the many accomplishments of this meeting was the development of time goals for stroke treatment (*Table 19.2*) (13). Although some of the details of these guidelines are controversial, they importantly underscore the value of establishing a system of care capable of rapidly evaluating and treating stroke patients.

At the present time, the application of intravenous rt-PA should require

TABLE 19.2
Time Goals for Acute Stroke Treatment

Elapsed time (minutes)	Action
0	Patient arrives at hospital
10	Physician examines patient
15	Neurological consultation made
25	CT scan completed
45	CT scan read
60	rt-PA infusion started
120	Neurosurgeon consulted (phone OK)
180	Patient admitted to monitored bed

strict adherence to the NINDS trial eligibility and treatment protocols. These are delineated in the NINDS publication (15) and other, more recent reviews on the subject (5). The availability of an environment familiar with thrombolytic therapy for close neurological and hemodynamic monitoring of patients is essential. In addition, preparedness for rapid identification and treatment of hemorrhagic complications is critical.

The benefit of intravenous rt-PA for acute ischemic stroke demonstrated by the NINDS trial is very exciting, but it is not for every patient, and the benefit is not so impressive that we should be complacent about the present state of acute stroke management treatment alternatives. We can, however, derive a great deal from the invigorated interest in acute stroke treatment. Improvement in public education and emergency medical and hospital approaches to acute stroke patients will improve care for ischemic and hemorrhagic stroke patients. Defining multidisciplinary stroke teams along the broad definition of ischemic and hemorrhagic stroke will improve care for all stroke patients. In addition, it will promote continuing investigation of other promising stroke treatments on the horizon.

The strengthened partnership between emergency medicine physicians, neurologists, neurosurgeons, neuroradiologists, and neurophysiatrists catalyzed by renewed interest in acute stroke management will undoubtedly lead to important breakthroughs that positively impact on patient outcome. However, only through the valued inclusion (on stroke teams) of nurses, therapists (respiratory, speech, physical, and occupational), social workers, chaplains, bioethicists, and case managers (hospital and insurance) can we truly accomplish the necessary global changes in stroke management that reach into improving and maintaining the quality of survivorship from neurologically disabling stroke. In my opinion, this latter challenge deserves as much attention as acute stroke medical treatment investigations.

REFERENCES

1. Brott TG, Haley EC, Levy DE, et al.: Urgent therapy for stroke: Part 1—Pilot study of tissue plasminogen activator administered within 90 minutes. **Stroke** 23:632–640, 1992.
2. Caplan LR, Mohr JP, Kistler JP, Korschetz W: Thrombolysis: Not a panacea for ischemic stroke. **N Engl J Med** 337:1309–1310, 1997.
3. Chiu D, Krieger D, Villar-Cardova C, Kasner SE, Morgenstern LB, Bratina PL, et al.: Intravenous tissue plasminogen activator for acute ischemic stroke: Feasibility, safety, and efficacy in the first year of clinical practice. **Stroke** 29:18–22, 1998.
4. Donnan GA, Davis SM, Chambers BR, et al.: Trials of streptokinase in severe acute ischemic stroke. **Lancet** 345:578–579, 1995.

5. Furlan AJ: Thrombolysis for acute ischemic stroke: Update on the beginning of a revolution. **Cleve Clin Med** 65:185–190, 1998.
6. Grotta J: t-PA: The best current option for most stroke patients **N Engl J Med** 337:1310–1311, 1997.
7. Hacke W, Kaste M, Fieschi C, et al.: Intravenous thrombolysis with recombinant tissue plasminogen activator for acute hemispheric stroke: The European Cooperative Acute Stroke Study (ECASS). **JAMA** 274:1017–1025, 1995.
8. Hacke W, Kaste M, Fieschi C, von Kummer R, Davalos A, Meier D, Larrue V, et al.: Randomised double-blind placebo-controlled trial of thrombolytic therapy with intravenous alteplase in acute ischaemic stroke (ECASS II). **Lancet** 352:1245–1251, 1998.
9. Haley EC Jr, Brott TG, Sheppard GL, et al.: Pilot randomized trial of tissue plasminogen activator in acute ischemic stroke. The TPA Briding Study Group. **Stroke** 24:1000–1004, 1993.
10. Haley EC, Levy DE, Brott TG, et al.: Urgent therapy for stroke: Part II—Pilot study of tissue plasminogen activator administered 91–180 minutes from onset. **Stroke** 23:641–645, 1992.
11. Hommel M, Boissel JP, Cornu C, et al.: Treatment of trial of streptokinase in severe acute ischemic stroke. **Lancet** 345:57, 1995.
12. International Stroke Trial Collaborative Group: The International Stroke Trial: A randomized trial of aspirin, subcutaneous heparin, both or neither among 19,435 patients with acute ischemic stroke. **Lancet** 349:1569–1581, 1997.
13. Marler JR, Jones PW (eds): Rapid identification and treatment of acute stroke. Proceedings of a national symposium. NIH Publication No. 97-4239, August 1997.
14. Multicentre Acute Stroke Trial-Italy (MAST-I) Group: Randomized controlled trial of streptokinase, aspirin, and combination of both in treatment of acute ischemic stroke. **Lancet** 346:1509–1514, 1995.
15. The National Institute of Neurological Disorders and Stroke rt-PA Stroke Study Group: Tissue plasminogen activator for acute ischemic stroke. **N Engl J Med** 333:1581–1587, 1995.
16. Zweifler RM, Brody ML, Graves GC, Drinkard R, Cunningham S, Rothrock JF: Intravenous t-PA for acute ischemic stroke: Therapeutic yield of a stroke code system. **Neurology** 50:501–503, 1998.

CHAPTER

20

Honored Guest Presentation: Management Strategies for the Treatment of Intracranial Arteriovenous Malformations

JOHN M. TEW, JR., M.D., AND ADAM I. LEWIS, M.D.

Microsurgery is the principal method for the treatment of intracranial arteriovenous malformations (AVMs). Over the past decade, there have been numerous improvements in imaging, endovascular techniques, surgical techniques, and stereotactic radiosurgery. The expanded armamentarium has provided patients with more options and potentially better outcomes. However, these new options have also created controversy as to the best management strategy for many types of AVMs. This controversy has been heightened by retrospective reports lacking randomization, controls, and long-term follow-up. In addition, there has been significant variation in outcome measurements that make direct comparisons difficult. In this chapter, the authors provide a paradigm and a philosophy for the treatment of AVMs that strives to combine all of the treatment options in a complementary fashion, applied by a cooperative team of physicians who complement each other in skill, experience, and perspective.

Eliminating the risk of hemorrhage is the primary goal in AVM decision making. The risk of hemorrhage depends on the angioarchitecture and location of the AVM. In general, small AVMs have higher perfusion pressures and are accompanied with hemorrhage more often than are large AVMs (37). Deep-seated AVMs located in the basal ganglia, thalamus, and posterior fossa usually present with hemorrhage and have a high propensity for repeat hemorrhage (40, 42). Deep venous drainage and a single draining vein are frequently associated with venous hypertension and an increased risk for hemorrhage (22). Associated aneurysms on the feeding arteries (pedicular), in the nidus (intranidal), and on the veins (venous) are frequently the source of hemorrhage (25). It is uncertain whether saccular aneurysms on proximal arteries are flow-related to the AVM.

On the basis of current technology and experience with more than 300 AVMs, the authors have proposed 10 recommendations to eliminate the risk for recurrent hemorrhage and preserve quality of life and functional capacity.

1. The treatment goal is complete angiographic obliteration and preservation of neurological function. Pediatric AVMs may recur despite apparent angiographic cure. The incidence of recurrent AVM despite normal postoperative angiography varies 4 to 9%.
2. Stereotactic radiosurgery and microsurgery are complementary treatment strategies in the treatment of AVMs. Outcome analysis should document effective treatment and cost comparison.
3. AVMs with a Spetzler-Martin grade 1 to 3 convexity are best treated with microsurgery (12, 38). Large, complex AVMs frequently require a combination of embolization and microsurgery.
4. Embolization of AVMs eliminates associated aneurysms, reduces operative blood loss, reduces operative time, and serves as a road map to the AVM to avoid injury to normal arteries of passage.
5. Arterial aneurysms associated with AVMs are frequently the source of hemorrhage and should be obliterated before stereotactic radiosurgery or delayed microsurgery.
6. The presence of a single draining vein, a venous aneurysm, or venous restrictive disease are important risk factors for hemorrhage and a relative contraindication for stereotactic radiosurgery.
7. Stereotactic radiosurgery is best suited for small, unruptured AVMs in eloquent brain tissue such as the basal ganglia, thalamus, and brainstem. Radiosurgery may be used to treat small residual AVMs after microsurgery.
8. Fractionated radiotherapy is an attractive treatment option for large (>3 cm), deep-seated unruptured AVMs.
9. Surgery is the only proven treatment for cavernous malformations. Stereotactic radiosurgery is associated with a high rate of radionecrosis for cavernous malformations in the brainstem.
10. Venous malformations have a benign natural history. Surgical removal may cause a venous infarction, and stereotactic radiosurgery is associated with a high rate of radiation injury.

Proper patient selection is the key to successful treatment outcomes. In this chapter, we describe a management strategy that emphasizes a multidisciplinary team approach, complementary treatment options, measuring outcomes in terms of quality and cost, and achieving patient satisfaction.

OBSERVATION

The current options for the treatment of AVMs include continued observation, embolization, stereotactic radiosurgery, and microsurgery. The safety and efficacy of any management strategy is measured against the natural history of the disease. One of the best reports on the natural history of AVMs is a 24-year prospective study by Ondra et al. (24). In that report, the annual risk of bleeding for symptomatic AVMs was 4%, the combined rate of major morbidity and mortality was 2.7% per year, and the annual mortality rate was 1%.

When there is an associated arterial aneurysm, a recent study shows that the risk of bleeding is increased to 10% per year (35). The Cooperative Study on AVMs documented a 20% risk of major stroke and 10% risk of death after each bleeding episode (26). These figures are conservative estimates for morbidity and mortality. A recent report by the University of Toronto Cerebrovascular Group indicates that the rates of major morbidity and mortality from AVM bleeding may be markedly higher (34).

For some AVMs, observation is the preferred treatment. We advocate observation for thalamic and basal ganglia AVMs that are larger than 6 cm (Spetzler-Martin grade 5) and intrinsic brainstem AVMs that are more than 2.5 cm in diameter. Observation is also recommended for elderly patients with AVMs that are Spetzler-Martin grade 4 and 5 convexity. All venous malformations and asymptomatic brainstem cavernous malformations should be observed. Outcome analysis should be employed to document that observation is the preferred treatment option.

EMBOLIZATION

Embolization is rarely curative and remains predominantly an adjunct to microsurgery and stereotactic radiosurgery. Embolization achieves its greatest utility in large AVMs (Spetzler-Martin grade 4–6). When the flow and nidus size are reduced by more than 50%, there is a significant reduction in operative blood loss and operative time (*Fig. 20.1*). Embolization is not performed on most small-to-medium convexity AVMs (Spetzler-Martin grades 1–3), because they can be removed surgically with minimal blood loss and low morbidity. For AVMs in critical brain regions, embolization creates an intraoperative road map for the surgeon to distinguish vessels of passage from feeding arteries. The best embolization strategy is to obliterate the deep arterial supply from the lenticulostriate and thalamoperforate arteries. These penetrating arteries have little smooth muscle within the wall and are difficult to eliminate with bipolar electrocautery (13). However, the deep arterial supply is also the most difficult to catheterize because the arteries are extremely small and branch off the parent artery at acute angles (*Fig. 20.2*). Embolizing these penetrating arteries also poses a high risk for cerebral infarction. Intranidal embolization can be performed, but oc-

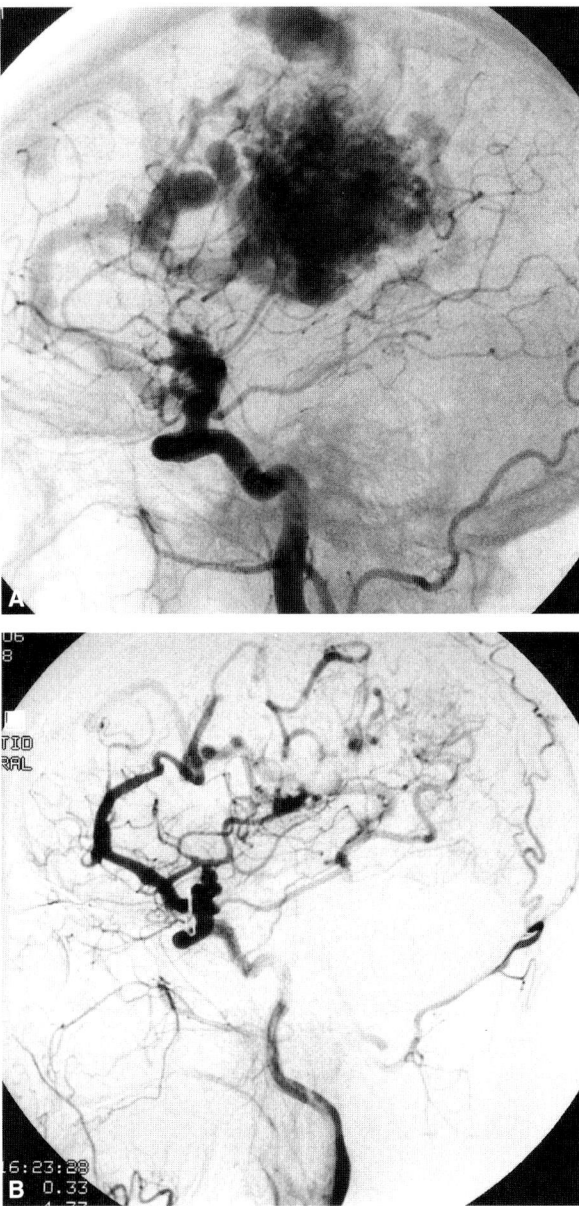

FIG. 20.1 Embolization is used to reduce the flow to large, high-flow AVMs before surgery. (A) The preoperative angiogram shows a large, posterior temporal AVM. (B) After embolization, over 90% of the AVM has been obliterated.

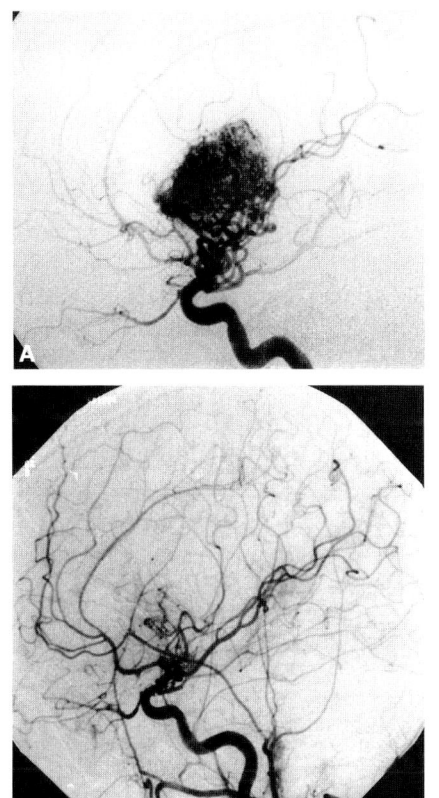
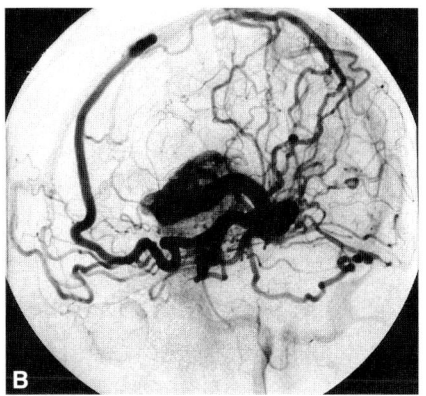

FIG. 20.2 Deep-seated AVMs usually have arterial supply that is too small to embolize, and venous hypertension is often present. (A) The angiogram shows a large left basal ganglia-thalamic AVM with a myriad of small feeding arteries and occlusion of the straight sinus. (B) Occlusion of the straight sinus leads to dilated, tortuous veins that cause obstructive hydrocephalus at the foramen of Monro. (C) The postoperative angiogram shows complete removal of the AVM.

cluding the draining veins before the arterial supply is eliminated increases the risk of AVM rupture significantly. Similarly, embolization of small AVMs with a single draining vein can lead to a high risk if the vein is occluded too early. Long-term cure with embolization is unlikely because delayed recanalization of the AVM can occur even with acrylic glue.

Embolization is effective for obliterating pedicular aneurysms that are located on proximal arteries or in the nidus of the malformation. Hemorrhage associated with AVMs is frequently due to a ruptured arterial aneurysm on a proximal feeding artery to the AVM. Occluding the feeding artery to the AVM leads to elimination of the flow-related aneurysm. More rarely, intranidal aneurysms within an arteriovenous fistula can be embolized selectively. Saccular aneurysms of the circle of Willis are treated with Guglielmi detachable coils or are clipped surgi-

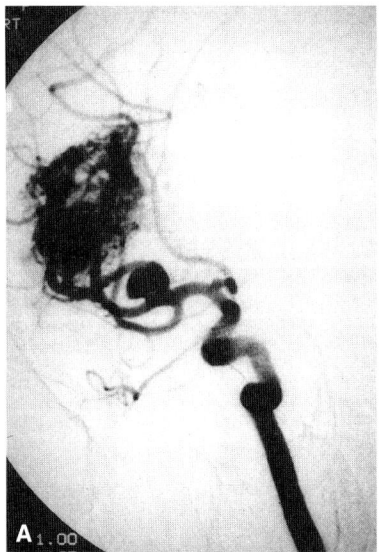
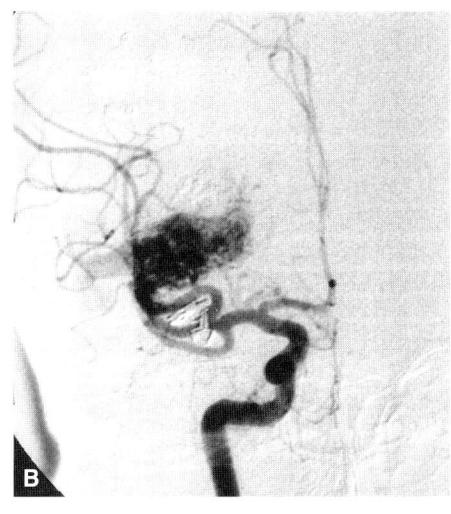
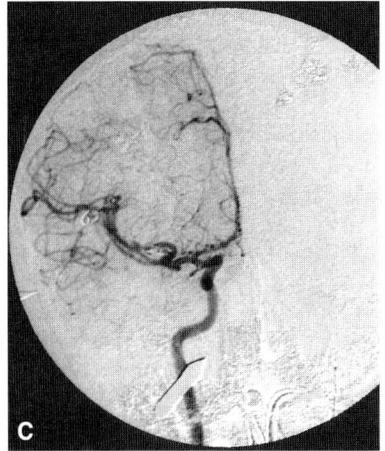

FIG. 20.3 Associated aneurysms are frequently the source of hemorrhage and must be treated acutely to avoid rebleeding. They are best treated by preoperative embolization. (A) The preoperative angiogram shows a ruptured middle cerebral artery aneurysm and a large sylvian AVM. (B) The middle cerebral artery aneurysm has been clipped and the AVM embolized partially. (C) The postoperative angiogram shows clipping of the aneurysm and removal of the sylvian AVM.

cally (*Fig. 20.3*). Proximal and pedicular aneurysms should be eliminated before treatment of the AVM with microsurgery or stereotactic radiosurgery (41). However, some of the lesions may regress after the high-flow AVMs have been eliminated.

The role of embolization before stereotactic radiosurgery is controversial. Because the AVM may recanalize after embolization, the radiation collimator must cover the entire nidus. Stereotactic radiosurgery may fail to obliterate the nidus in patients who undergo embolization and receive radiosurgery to the remaining portion of the nidus (5, 30).

Therefore, embolization may add unnecessary risk before stereotactic radiosurgery. The section on stereotactic radiosurgery (later in this chapter) discusses this controversy.

Hemispheric AVMs frequently cause seizures because of vascular steal or venous hypertension. Pedicular, intranidal, or venous aneurysms may rupture, resulting in intraparenchymal hemorrhage or, rarely, subarachnoid hemorrhage. Global hemispheric AVMs are inoperable; however, embolization can palliate the symptoms and reduce the risk for hemorrhage. Patients may live for many years with a good quality of life. Reducing flow to the nidus can eliminate headaches, seizures, and reverse neurological deficits. Liquid adhesives are more permanent than particles and are preferred for palliative treatment.

Embolization has many benefits and can have a major impact on the treatment of AVMs. However, there are no randomized trials or prospective studies that document the efficacy of embolization. It is difficult to quantify the added benefit of embolization because of the variance that exists in embolic agents, catheters, and operator experience. In a meta-analysis of 1246 patients in 32 series, the risk of minor complications associated with embolization was approximately 15%, major complications 5%, and mortality 2% (11). The added risk of cerebral infarction, hemorrhage, cost, and discomfort must be factored into the treatment plan. It is likely that the rate of embolic complications is lower for Spetzler-Martin grade 1 to 3 AVMs than grade 4 to 6 AVMs. Nevertheless, embolization should not be performed simply because a feeding artery is accessible to a microcatheter. Embolization should be used only to significantly improve the success of microsurgery or stereotactic radiosurgery.

MICROSURGERY

Microsurgery remains the mainstay for treatment of most convexity AVMs. Over the past decade, the technologies with the greatest impact have been magnetic resonance imaging for treatment planning, self-retaining micro-retractors to dissect the AVM, use of induced hypotension during removal of the AVM and postoperatively to reduce hemorrhage and perfusion breakthrough, and intraoperative angiography to document complete removal. Our management of intracranial AVMs is considerably more aggressive than it was 10 years ago. In the past, we would not have operated on Spetzler-Martin grade 3 AVMs unless they had ruptured. Today, improved operator skill, improvements in technology, and a better understanding of the pathophysiology have led us to operate on more complex AVMs with results that compare favorably with the natural history. We recommend surgery when there is a major hemorrhage, progressive neurological deficit, inadequately controlled seizure disorder, medically intractable headaches, or venous restrictive disease. Asymptomatic AVMs may be removed if any substantive risk factors are discovered, or to meet the patient's wishes.

Clinical series show that microsurgery is the best option for unruptured convexity AVMs that are smaller than 3 cm and have superficial venous drainage (12, 36, 38). As shown by mathematical models, surgical removal of convexity AVMs provides longer life expectancy and a better quality of life than would occur with the natural history (2, 7). Microsurgery is superior to stereotactic radiosurgery in the treatment of small convexity AVMs because the angiographic obliteration rate is 100% and there are significantly fewer postoperative hemorrhages ($P = 0.001$), neurological deficits ($P = 0.013$), and deaths ($P = 0.019$) (27). Microsurgery is also more cost effective than stereotactic radiosurgery (23, 33) for convexity AVMs because surgery protects against hemorrhage earlier and with greater success. Cerebellar and pial brainstem AVMs should also be removed because the majority (90%) occur with hemorrhage and there is a high risk of repeat hemorrhage. Ruptured thalamic and basal ganglia AVMs have a high risk of recurrent hemorrhage and should be removed surgically (17, 40). Intrinsic brainstem AVMs are supplied by perforators from the basilar artery and cannot be removed surgically. These lesions should be treated with stereotactic radiosurgery. Stereotactic radiosurgery is performed in patients with operable AVMs who have major medical problems, patients who refuse surgery, and in patients with occipital AVMs (32). In a series of 37 patients with postgeniculate pathway AVMs, only 6% develop visual loss after stereotactic radiosurgery compared with more than 50% in most published surgical series (*Fig. 20.4*) (31).

Most patients with ruptured AVMs undergo surgery in the subacute period to recover from the ictus, reduce brain swelling, consolidate the hematoma, and permit time for embolization of the AVM. Early surgery is indicated when the hematoma causes significant mass effect, the hematoma is located in the posterior fossa, or there is a ruptured aneurysm and subarachnoid hemorrhage. Ruptured aneurysms associated with an AVM should be treated like ruptured intracranial aneurysms because of the high risk of rebleeding. In addition, the subarachnoid hemorrhage may cause severe cerebral vasospasm and delayed ischemic deficits. Hypertensive, hypervolemic, and hemodilutional therapy are generally contraindicated because of the risk of postoperative hemorrhage and swelling in the surrounding brain. Instead, percutaneous transluminal angioplasty and intraarterial papaverine are used to dilate the spastic arteries (*Fig. 20.5*).

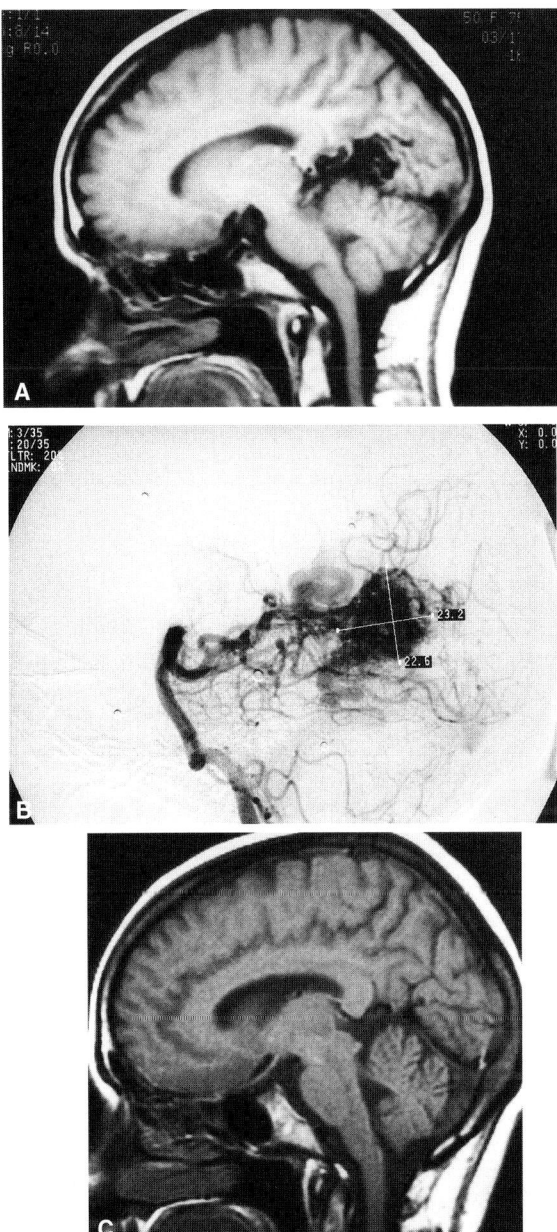

FIG. 20.4 Stereotactic radiation is an excellent option for postgeniculate pathway AVMs, because the risk of vision loss is low compared with microsurgery. (A) The sagittal T1-weighted magnetic resonance image shows an unruptured AVM of the occipital lobe. (B) The angiogram shows the AVM nidus measures 23 × 22 mm. (C) Postradiation elimination of the AVM.

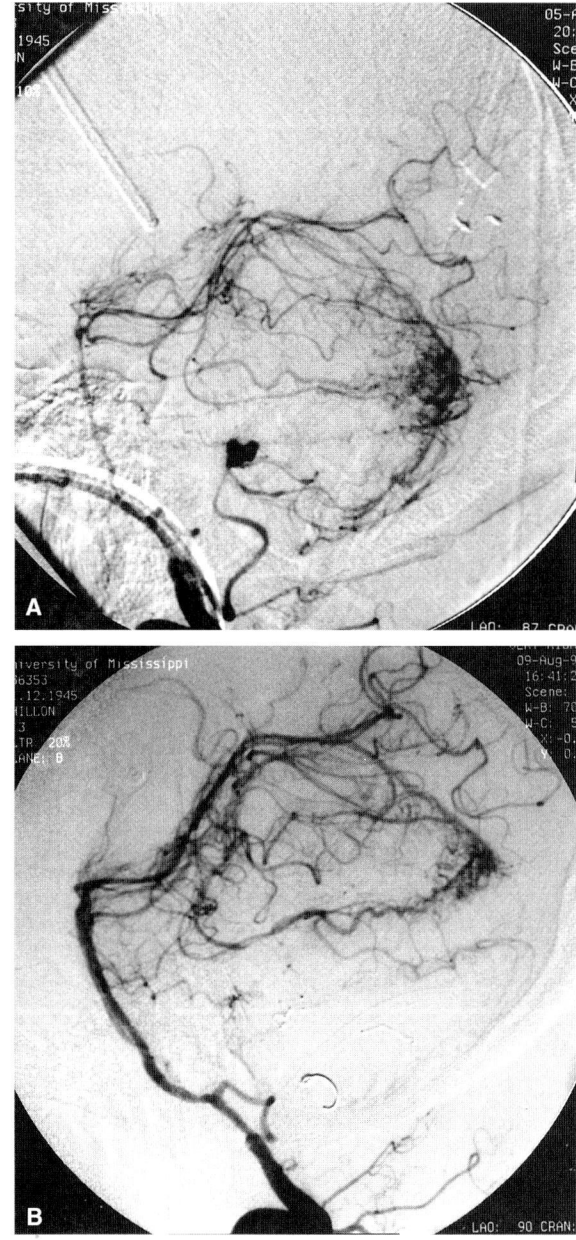

FIG. 20.5 Cerebral vasospasm may occur after an associated aneurysm has ruptured. (A) The preoperative angiogram shows a ruptured distal posterior inferior cerebellar artery aneurysm with vasospasm of the basilar artery. (B) Postoperative angiogram shows obliteration of the aneurysm after coiling and increased caliber of the basilar artery after transluminal angioplasty and intraarterial papaverine.

When there is intraventricular hemorrhage, the AVM is removed acutely, the associated aneurysm is clipped, and a ventricular catheter is placed. Urokinase 10,000 units b.i.d. is injected into the ventricles for 3 days to lyse the subarachnoid and intraventricular clot. Lysis of the intraventricular clot relieves obstructive hydrocephalus, reduces the risk of cerebral vasospasm, and may prevent communicating hydrocephalus.

Microsurgery remains the standard of care for intracranial cavernous malformations (*Figs. 20.6–20.8*). Stereotactic radiosurgery of brainstem cavernous malformations is associated with a high rate of radiation injury, and there are no imaging studies that effectively document obliteration (1). Among 22 patients with cavernous malformations treated with radiosurgery, Karlsson et al. (14) documented 9 (41%) who experienced a hemorrhage and 6 (27%) who developed radiation complications. The annual rate of hemorrhage after radiosurgery was 8%. Dumas et al. (4) reported a 27% incidence of transient complications and 18% permanent complications after stereotactic radiosurgery for brainstem cavernous angiomas. Chang et al. (3) showed that the rebleed rate remains high (9.4% per year) for 3 years after radiosurgery but decreases to 1.6% per year thereafter. Kondziolka et al. (16) also showed an annual decreasing hemorrhage rate from 8.8% during the first 2 years after radiosurgery to 1.1% per year thereafter. Whether there is a protective effect after stereotactic radiosurgery or a delayed reflection of the natural history of cavernous malformations after rupture is unknown.

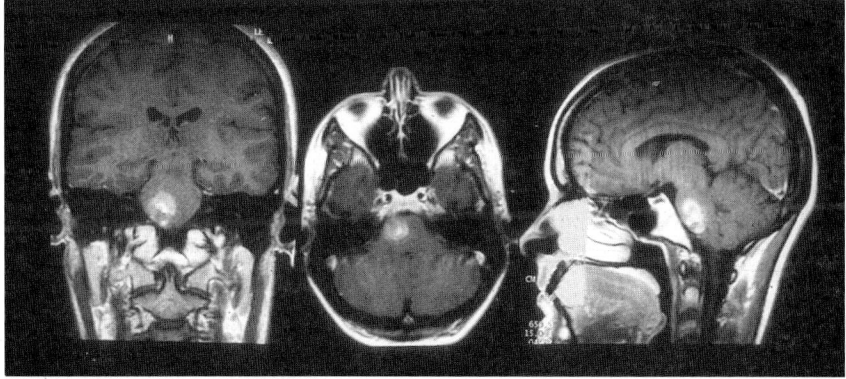

FIG. 20.6 Coronal, axial, and sagittal T1-weighted magnetic resonance images show a large cavernous malformation in the right ventral pons. The patient presented with progressive left hemiparesis and sixth nerve palsy.

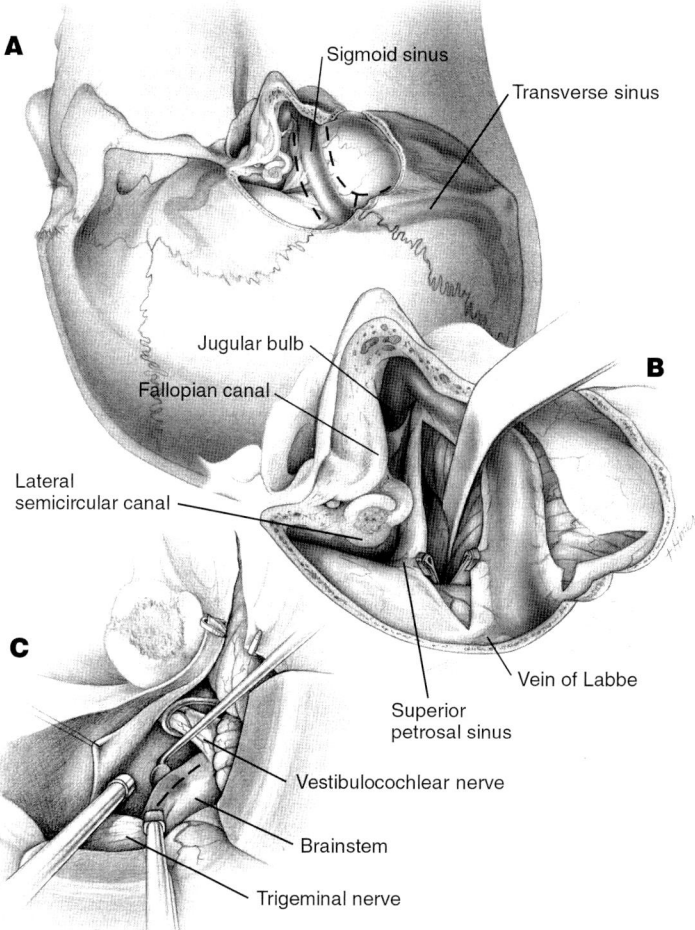

FIG. 20.7 (*A*) Posterior petrosectomy with preservation of the labyrinth and skeletonization of fallopian canal. The mastoidectomy is expanded to expose the temporal lobe to facilitate sacrifice of the superior petrosal sinus, section of the tentorium cerebelli, and placement of relaxing incision above the transverse sinus, along with a small suboccipital (retrosigmoid) craniotomy. Dashed lines represent dural incisions. (*B*) The superior petrosal sinus is sacrificed between two titanium clips. Also shown is a possible opening of the retrosigmoid dura for possible exploration from a conventional suboccipital approach. (From Tew JM Jr, van Loveren HR, Keller JT: *Atlas of Operative Microneurosurgery,* Vol. 2. Philadelphia, Saunders, in press.) (*C*) The surgeon gently applies 10-mm self-retaining retractors to the posterior temporal lobe and lateral cerebellar hemisphere to expose the lateral pons, basilar artery, and cranial nerves V through VIII. A longitudinal incision is made in the brainstem between the V and VIII nerve root entry zones to expose the malformation. (Modified from Tew JM Jr, van Loveren HR, Keller JT: *Atlas of Operative Microneurosurgery,* Vol. 2. Philadelphia, Saunders, in press.)

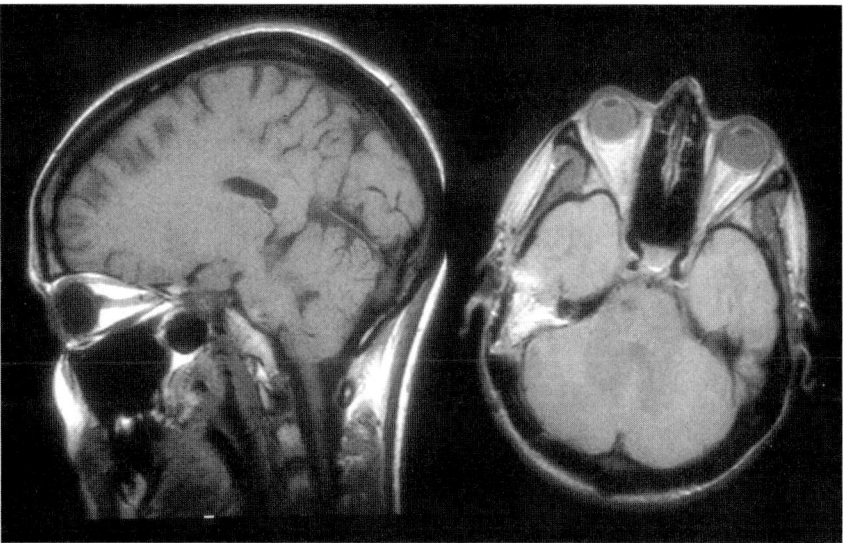

FIG. 20.8 Postoperative sagittal and axial T1-weighted magnetic resonance images show complete resection of the pontine cavernous malformation. The fat placed in the right mastoidectomy defect creates a high signal on the axial view.

Venous malformations are an abnormal collection of veins that drain normal brain tissue. When computed tomography was used for diagnosis, venous malformations were frequently identified as a cause of intracranial hemorrhage (20). With the development of magnetic resonance imaging, the source of hemorrhage can usually be identified as an associated cavernous malformation. Because venous malformations do not have an arterialized shunt, they rarely cause hemorrhage and they have a benign natural history (21). Surgical removal of a venous malformation may cause venous infarction of the surrounding brain. Venous malformations have a high rate of radiation injury after stereotactic radiosurgery (18), perhaps in excess of that associated with radiosurgery of cavernous venous malformations. Mixed malformations, i.e., venous and cavernous, occur in more than 30% of patients.

STEREOTACTIC RADIOSURGERY

Stereotactic radiosurgery is reserved for patients with small, unruptured AVMs in deep and functional locations. These include AVMs of the basal ganglia, thalamus, tectum and intrinsic brainstem. The obliteration rate ranges from 65 to 85% after 2 years for AVMs smaller than 3 cm in diameter and less than 10 cm^3 in volume (19, 39). With increasing size, there is a decrease in the obliteration rate (8). Arteriovenous malformations in or adjacent to functional brain tissue have a higher risk of radiation injury (10). Presumably, the tiny perforating arteries that supply the surrounding brain are more susceptible to the effects of radiation (40). After stereotactic radiosurgery and until the AVM is obliterated, the risk of hemorrhage remains the same as the natural history. There is a 6 to 8% rate of rebleeding during the 2-year latency interval. An increased risk of bleeding occurs when there is an associated intracranial aneurysm (9, 28). The risk of radiation injury ranges from 3 to 10%, depending on the location of the AVM (19, 39). Stereotactic radiosurgery can be repeated after 2 years if the AVM has not thrombosed completely. However, the overall complication rate increases from 3 to 14% for repeat stereotactic radiosurgery (15).

Stereotactic radiosurgery can be used to obliterate residual small AVMs after microsurgery (17). With the use of intraoperative angiography, however, the incidence of postoperative residual AVMs is uncommon. Stereotactic radiosurgery is a good option for elderly patients with Spetzler-Martin grade 3 AVMs. This, too, is an uncommon situation, because most patients with AVMs are young and have few medical problems. Stereotactic radiation is a relative contraindication for AVMs with venous restrictive disease or perinidal aneurysms, because there is a high rate of hemorrhage during the latency interval.

Controversy exists regarding the use of embolization as an adjunct to stereotactic radiosurgery. As the size of the AVM increases, the rate of obliteration with stereotactic radiosurgery decreases and the risk of radiation injury to the surrounding brain increases. To increase the obliteration rate and avoid the risk of radiation injury, embolization is performed to reduce the size of a large AVM so that stereotactic radiosurgery can be performed on a smaller nidus. However, follow-up imaging studies show recanalization of the AVM in the areas that were embolized and not covered by the radiosurgery collimator (30). In addition, previous embolization was shown to be a negative predictor of successful AVM radiosurgery ($P = 0.02$) after radiosurgery (29). These observations have led some investigators to conclude that embolization is contraindicated before stereotactic radiation unless for palliation of symptoms such as medically intractable headaches and seizures. Furthermore, the radiosurgery collimator must cover the entire nidus. Fractionation of radiosurgery is being evaluated as an alternative therapy for AVMs judged too large for single fractionation. Other causes of incomplete obliteration after stereotactic radiosurgery include errors in

AVM targeting, low radiation dosage, reopening of arteries compressed by hematoma, and resistance of blood vessels to the effects of radiation. The strategy of embolizing a portion of the nidus and radiating the remaining portion may no longer be valid. There is still a role for embolization of associated aneurysms in patients who undergo radiosurgery for AVMs to reduce the higher rate of hemorrhage during the latency interval to obliteration.

There is no perfect treatment strategy for large and giant, unruptured deep-seated AVMs (grades 4 and 5). Surgery is associated with transient neurological deficits in nearly 100% and permanent neurological deficits range from 16 to 27% after surgery (38). In the future, large AVMs may be treated with staged stereotactic radiosurgery in which segments of the nidus are obliterated. A recent report by Firlik et al. (6) showed that a combination of staged stereotactic radiosurgery and surgery was effective in obliterating a giant AVM. Alternatively, fractionated radiosurgery may be applied to the entire nidus; however, the safety and efficacy have not been established. We are observing increasing evidence that multimodal therapy is effective in obliterating longer and previously untreatable malformations.

OUTCOME ANALYSIS

Decision making in AVM surgery requires continual refinement, innovation, and evaluation of outcomes. We have developed an AVM outcome scale that measures four independent but related factors. These include physical assessment, functional assessment, angiographic obliteration, and a comparison of pre- and postoperative symptoms. In addition, all patients undergo postoperative neuropsychological testing. The patients with unruptured AVMs undergo preoperative neuropsychological testing, including measures of general intelligence, verbal fluency, naming ability, memory processing, attention tasks, abstract thinking, manual motor skills, and psychosocial status. It is important to monitor outcomes carefully and prospectively to ensure that treatment decisions are correct and remain current with new advances in the field of neurosurgery.

CONCLUSIONS

A decade of improvements in imaging studies, endovascular techniques, surgical techniques, and stereotactic radiosurgery planning has led to more options and better outcomes for patients. Although the additional treatment options have created controversy as to the best management strategy, consensus is beginning to develop. Our approach has been to combine these treatment modalities in a complementary fashion to achieve the best possible outcome for the individual patient. Multimodal therapy should improve outcome and be cost effective. In our experience, microsurgery remains the mainstay for treatment of most convexity AVMs. Embolization is an important adjunct for microsurgery, especially in the treatment of large and complex AVMs. Radiosurgery is reserved for the small, unruptured AVMs in functional locations. The pattern of venous drainage with venous restrictive disease must be considered a primary factor in the treatment planning. Associated aneurysms are frequently the source of hemorrhage and should be obliterated before treatment of the AVM. Management strategies for removal of AVMs have changed over the past decade. With continued improvements and refinements in imaging, radiosurgery planning, endovascular techniques, and microsurgery, management strategies will undoubtedly continue to evolve along with improved outcome expectations.

References

1. Amin-Hanjani S, Ogilvy CS, Candia GJ, Lyons S, Chapman PH: Stereotactic radiosurgery for cavernous malformations: Kjellberg's experience with proton beam therapy in 98 cases at the Harvard cyclotron. **Neurosurgery** 42:1229–1238, 1998.
2. Auger RG, Wiebers DO: Management of unruptured intracranial arteriovenous malformations: A decision analysis. **Neurosurgery** 30:561–569, 1992.
3. Chang SD, Levy RP, Adler JR, Martin DP, Krakovitz PR, Steinberg GK: Stereotactic radiosurgery of angiographically occult vascular malformations: 14-year experience. **Neurosurgery** 43:213–221, 1998.
4. Dumas CM, Lunsford LD, Kondziolka D, Bissonette DJ, Somaza S, Flickinger JC: Radiosurgery for vascular malformations of the brain stem. **Acta Neurochir Suppl (Wien)** 58:92–97, 1993.
5. Ellis TL, Friedman WA, Bova FJ, Kubilis PS, Buatti JM: Analysis of treatment failure after radiosurgery for arteriovenous malformations. **J Neurosurg** 89:104–110, 1998.
6. Firlik AD, Levy EI, Kondziolka D, Yonas H: Staged volume radiosurgery followed by microsurgical resection: A novel treatment for giant cerebral arteriovenous malformations: Technical case report. **Neurosurgery** 43:1223–1228, 1998.
7. Fisher WS III: Therapy of AVMs: A decision analysis. **Clin Neurosurg** 42:294–312, 1995.
8. Friedman WA, Bova FJ: Linear accelerator radiosurgery for arteriovenous malformations. **J Neurosurg** 77:832–841, 1992.
9. Friedman WA, Blatt DL, Bova FJ, Buatti JM, Mendenhall WM, Kubilis PS: The risk of hemorrhage after radiosurgery for arteriovenous malformations. **J Neurosurg** 42:912–919, 1996.
10. Friedman WA, Bova FJ, Mendenhall WM: Linear accelerator radiosurgery for arteriovenous malformations: The relationship of size to outcome. **J Neurosurg** 82:180–189, 1995.

11. Frizzel RT, Fisher WS: Cure, morbidity, and mortality associated with embolization of brain arteriovenous malformations: A review of 1246 patients in 32 series over a 35-year period. **Neurosurgery** 37:1031–1040, 1995.
12. Hamilton MG, Spetzler RF: The prospective application of a grading system for arteriovenous malformations. **Neurosurgery** 34:2–7, 1994.
13. Hurst RW, Berenstein A, Kupersmith MJ, Madrid M, Flamm ES: Deep central arteriovenous malformations of the brain: The role of endovascular treatment. **J Neurosurg** 82:190–195, 1995.
14. Karlsson B, Kihlstrom L, Lindquist C, Ericson K, Steiner L: Radiosurgery for cavernous malformations. **J Neurosurg** 88:293–297, 1998.
15. Karlsson B, Kijlstrom L, Lindquist C, Steiner L: Gamma knife for previously irradiated arteriovenous malformations. **Neurosurgery** 41:1–6, 1998.
16. Kondziolka D, Lunsford LD, Flickinger JC, Kestle JRW: Reduction of hemorrhage risk after stereotactic radiosurgery for cavernous malformations. **Neurosurgery** 83:825–831, 1995.
17. Lawton MT, Hamilton MG, Spetzler RF: Multimodality treatment of deep arteriovenous malformations: Thalamus, basal ganglia, and brain stem. **Neurosurgery** 37:29–36, 1995.
18. Lindquist C, Guo WY, Karlsson B, Steiner L: Radiosurgery for venous angiomas. **J Neurosurg** 78:531–536, 1993.
19. Lunsford LD, Kondziolka D, Flickinger JC, et al: Stereotactic radiosurgery for arteriovenous malformations of the brain. **J Neurosurg** 75:512–524, 1991.
20. Malik GM, Morgan JK, Boulos RS, Ausman JI: Venous angiomas: An underestimated cause of intracranial hemorrhage. **Surg Neurol** 30:350–358, 1988.
21. McLaughlin MR, Kondziolka D, Flickinger JC, Lunsford S, Lunsford LD: The prospective natural history of cerebral venous malformations. **Neurosurgery** 43:195–201, 1998.
22. Miyasaka Y, Yada K, Ohwada T, Kitahara T, Kurata A, Irikura K: An analysis of the venous drainage system as a factor in hemorrhage from arteriovenous malformations. **J Neurosurg** 76:239–243, 1992.
23. Nussbaum ES, Heros RC, Camarata PJ: Surgical treatment of intracranial arteriovenous malformations with an analysis of cost-effectiveness. **Clin Neurosurg** 42:348–369, 1995.
24. Ondra SL, Troupp H, George ED, Schwab K: The natural history of symptomatic arteriovenous malformations of the brain: A 24-year follow-up assessment. **J Neurosurg** 73:387–391, 1990.
25. Perata HJ, Tomsick TA, Tew JM: Feeding artery pedicle aneurysms: Association with parenchymal hemorrhage and arteriovenous malformations in the brain. **J Neurosurg** 80:631–634, 1997.
26. Perret G, Nishioka H: Arteriovenous malformations. An analysis of 545 cases of cranio-cerebral arteriovenous malformations and fistulae reported in the Cooperative Study. Report of the Cooperative Study of Intracranial Aneurysms and Subarachnoid Hemorrhage. Section VI, in **J Neurosurg** 25:467–490, 1966.
27. Pikus HJ, Beach ML, Harbaugh RE: Microsurgical treatment of arteriovenous malformations: Analysis and comparison with stereotactic radiosurgery. **J Neurosurg** 88:641–646, 1998.
28. Pollock BE, Flickinger JC, Lunsford LD, Bissonette D, Kondziolka D: Hemorrhage risk after stereotactic radiosurgery of cerebral arteriovenous malformations. **Neurosurgery** 38:652–661, 1996.
29. Pollock BE, Flickinger JC, Lunsford LD, Maitz A, Kondziolka D: Factors associated

with successful arteriovenous malformation radiosurgery. **Neurosurgery** 42: 1239–1247, 1998.
30. Pollock BE, Kondziolka D, Lunsford LD, Bissonette D, Flickinger JC: Repeat stereotactic radiosurgery of arteriovenous malformations: Factors associated with incomplete obliteration. **Neurosurgery** 38:318–324, 1996.
31. Pollock BE, Lunsford LD, Kondziolka D, Bissonette DJ, Flickinger JC: Stereotactic radiosurgery for postgeniculate visual pathway arteriovenous malformations. **J Neurosurg** 84:437–441, 1996.
32. Pollock BE, Lunsford LD, Kondziolka D, Maitz A, Flickinger JC: Patient outcomes after stereotactic radiosurgery for "operable" arteriovenous malformations. **Neurosurgery** 35:1–8, 1994.
33. Porter PJ, Shin AY, Detsky AS, Lefaive L, Wallace MC: Surgery versus stereotactic radiosurgery for small, operable arteriovenous malformations: A clinical and cost comparison. **Neurosurgery** 41:757–766, 1997.
34. Porter PJ, terBrugge KG, Montanera W, et al: Outcome following hemorrhage from brain arteriovenous malformations at presentation and during follow up: Is it worse than we think? Proceedings of the First Joint Meeting of the ASITN and AANS/CNS Cerebrovascular Section, February 1–4, 1998, p. 36 (abstr).
35. Redekop G, terBrugge K, Montanera W, Willinski R: Arterial aneurysms associated with arteriovenous malformations: Classification, incidence, and risk of hemorrhage. **J Neurosurg** 89:539–546, 1998.
36. Sisti MB, Kader A, Stein BM: Microsurgery for 67 intracranial arteriovenous malformations less than 3 cm in diameter. **J Neurosurg** 79:653–660, 1993.
37. Spetzler RF, Hargraves RW, McCormick PW, Zabramski JM, Flom RA, Zimmerman RS: Relationship of perfusion pressure and size to risk of hemorrhage from arteriovenous malformations. **J Neurosurg** 76:918–923, 1992.
38. Spetzler RF, Martin NA: A proposed grading system for arteriovenous malformations. **J Neurosurg** 65:476–483, 1986.
39. Steiner L, Lindquist C, Adler JR, Torner JC, Alves W, Steiner M: Clinical outcome of radiosurgery for cerebral arteriovenous malformations. **J Neurosurg** 77:1–8, 1992.
40. Tew JM Jr, Lewis AI, Reichert KW: Management strategies and surgical techniques for deep-seated supratentorial arteriovenous malformations. **Neurosurgery** 36: 1065–1072, 1995.
41. Thompson RC, Steinberg GK, Levy RP, Marks MP: The management of patients with arteriovenous malformations and associated intracranial aneurysms. **Neurosurgery** 43:202–212, 1998.
42. Turjman F, Massoud TF, Vinuela F, Sayre JW, Guglielmi G, Duckwiler G: Correlation of the angioarchitectural features of cerebral arteriovenous malformations with clinical presentation. **Neurosurgery** 37:856–862, 1995.

CHAPTER

21

Controversies in Neurosurgery: Microsurgery versus Radiosurgery for Arteriovenous Malformations— The Case for Microsurgery

DANIEL L. BARROW, M.D.

Microsurgical resection and radiosurgical obliteration are now recognized as time-honored methods for managing selected arteriovenous malformations (AVMs) of the brain. Initially reserved for "inoperable AVMs, the indications have been liberalized in many centers and radiosurgery is now considered by some proponents as an appropriate therapeutic option for "resectable" AVMs. Each of these treatment modalities is associated with risks, and each has distinct advantages and disadvantages. The primary advantages of microsurgical resection are the high cure rate and the immediate elimination of the risk of hemorrhage. The primary detractor is that it is an invasive treatment, associated with the general risks of a craniotomy and specific risks related to the particular AVM. These risks vary from lesion to lesion and range from nearly no risk to an unacceptably high risk (inoperable).

The primary attraction of radiosurgery is its noninvasive appeal. The primary and most significant disadvantage is the long interval from treatment to therapeutic effectiveness (1–3 yr), during which time the patient is not protected from hemorrhage. Other liabilities include lack of therapeutic effectiveness for all lesions, the risk of radiation injury, and the need for long-term follow-up, including repeat angiography.

Although zealots remain in both the microsurgical and radiosurgical camps, I believe most experienced neurovascular teams are in agreement on many issues including the following: 1) surgery results in higher cure rates than radiosurgery; 2) surgery is associated with fewer posttreatment hemorrhages than radiosurgery; 3) some AVMs are unable to be surgically resected without an unacceptable risk; 4) smaller AVMs (≤3 cm) respond better than larger ones to radiosurgery, both in terms of lesion obliteration and radiation complications; 5) AVM obliteration is not a certain consequence of radiosurgery; 6) the interval between radiosurgery and AVM obliteration is a concern; 7) hemorrhage during the latent period is not a benign event; 8) for most small AVMs, both radiosurgery and microsurgery have high rates of success. However, some unresolved areas of controversy remain, including comparative morbidity and mortality of these two treatment options, cost effectiveness of treatment, patient preference, and determination of "inoperability."

In the absence of a true randomized clinical trial comparing the results of microsurgical resection with radiosurgery, it is difficult to compare the efficacy of these two treatment modalities for similar cases. A number of factors contribute to these difficulties, including selection biases for both treatment options, a tendency to minimize transient postoperative complications (urinary tract infections, pneumonia, pulmonary emboli, infections), and the increasing number of radiosurgery centers that are relying on magnetic resonance imaging as a replacement for angiography to determine the obliteration rates for AVMs. Furthermore, a review of the existing literature may be misleading, because neither microsurgery nor radiosurgery has reached the limits of their potential.

Several series (1, 2, 3, 6, 9, 14) documented that smaller AVMs respond better to radiosurgery than larger ones, both in terms of success and risk of treatment. Likewise, microsurgical series demonstrated superior results for smaller AVMs. Hamilton and Spetzler (4) prospectively used the Spetzler-Martin grading system to predict morbidity in 120 consecutive patients with AVM. This simple system grades AVMs on the basis of size, the pattern of venous drainage, and the functional importance of adjacent brain tissue (13). They found that the grading system correlates well with transient and permanent postoperative neurological deficits (4, 13). Heros et al. (5) reviewed 153 patients undergoing surgery for AVM of all grades and also found a correlation between outcome and Spetzler-Martin grade. They also found at follow-up that early morbidity resolved significantly. A regression analysis demonstrates that age, lesion size, and preoperative neurological status were predictive of outcome in a series of 72 consecutive microsurgically treated AVMs (8). Spetzler-

Martin grade and the patient's age predicted adverse outcome. Each component of the Spetzler-Martin grading system (size, location, and presence of deep venous drainage) was a predictor of new postoperative neurological deficits.

Comparisons of microsurgery with radiosurgery in the treatment of small AVMs should optimize the outcome statistics for both populations. Sisti et al. (12) reported the results of microsurgical treatment of 67 AVMs that were smaller than 3 cm in diameter, 45% of them being deep-seated in fundamentally important areas. All but one patient underwent control angiography, and 94% of all AVMs were totally removed. Only one patient (1.5%) developed a permanent, significant neurological deficit postoperatively. There were no postoperative hemorrhages and no deaths in this series. Sisti et al. (12) compared their results with several radiosurgical series, concluded that microsurgery was advantageous over radiosurgery with regard to safety and efficacy, and recommended radiosurgery be reserved for lesions that are determined to be "surgically inaccessible, as judged by neurosurgeons experienced in the surgery of AVMs.

Schaller and Schramm (11) analyzed a consecutive series of 62 patients treated by microsurgery for AVMs up to 3 cm in diameter. Thirty-three (53%) AVMs were located in functionally important regions, and all patients underwent control angiography. These authors achieved a 98.4% rate of total excision. Seventeen (27.4%) of the group developed early, new, significant postoperative neurological deficits, with only 3.2% being permanent. Management mortality was 0%, and surgical morbidity (non-neurological) was 9.7%. These authors reviewed the literature for results of radiosurgery and embolization and concluded that microsurgery is superior.

Comparisons of three radiosurgical series with microsurgical series demonstrated that microsurgical resection was statistically significantly more likely to provide definite or probable AVM obliteration (8). Furthermore, microsurgically treated patients were significantly less likely to die, to develop new posttreatment neurological deficits, or to hemorrhage post-treatment. Product-limit estimates of hemorrhage-free survival statistically favor microsurgery over radiosurgery. The results of microsurgical treatment of small AVMs from several centers are outlined in *Table 21.1*.

One of the perceived benefits of radiosurgery over microsurgery is reduced cost because of shorter hospitalization and the minimal invasiveness of this procedure. Cost analysis comparisons of radio-

TABLE 21.1
Microsurgical Treatment of Small AVMs (< 3cm)

Series	Number	Definite Obliteration	Probable Obliteration	Postoperative Hemorrhage	Death	New Permanent Neurlogical Deficit (%)
Hamilton and Spetzler (4)	71	71 (100%)	71 (100%)	0	0	0
Heros et al. (5)	91	79 (87%)	91 (100%)	0	0	nr
Sisti et al. (12)	67	63 (94%)	63 (94%)	0	0	1.5%
Pikus et al. (8)	54	54 (100%)	54 (100%)	0	0	1.9%
Schaller and Schramm (11)	62	61 (98.4%)	61 (98.4%)	0	0	3.2%
Sundt et al. (15)	84	84 (100%)	84 (100%)	0	0	2.2%

nr=not reported

surgery with microsurgery for small AVMs performed, however, by Nussbaum et al. (7) and Porter et al. (10) demonstrated that microsurgery confers a large benefit over radiosurgery. This is because surgery protects the patient from hemorrhage earlier and with greater success than radiosurgery. Nussbaum et al. used a Markov decision analysis model to examine the cost-effectiveness of treating cohorts of 100 patients with small AVMs with observation, surgical resection, or radiosurgery. For surgical resection, the lifetime treatment cost was $25,495.41 per patient, which yields cost savings to society of $7,642.23 and extends quality-adjusted life expectancy by 15 years. Although microsurgery was more expensive than radiosurgery by $6,834.59, quality-adjusted life expectancy was extended by 6 ears. Therefore, the cost-effectiveness of surgical excision compared with radiosurgery is $1,139.09 per quality-adjusted life year gained. The cost and life expectancy for each treatment paradigm is outlined in *Table 21.2*.

In the Canadian study by Porter et al. (10), surgery conferred a 0.98 quality-adjusted life year advantage over radiosurgery at an additional cost of $6,937 per patient. The gain of 0.98 quality-adjusted life years for an additional cost of $6,937 is highly economically attractive and

TABLE 21.2
*Treatment of AVMs: Cost-effectivesness
Comparison of Treatment Modalities for Small AVMs**

Treatment	Cost	Life-Expectancy (years)
Observation	$33,137.64	29
Radiosurgery	$18,660.82	38
Microsurgery	$25,495.41	44

*Data from Nussbaum et al (7).

equates to an incremental cost-effectiveness ratio of $7,100 per quality-adjusted life years for a patient treated surgically. The preferred treatment strategy changes to favor radiosurgery only when surgical morbidity exceeds 12% or mortality 4% (*Table 21.3*).

Patient preference is often cited as an indication for selecting radiosurgery over microsurgery for an AVM that may be safely removed surgically. Although the minimal invasiveness of radiosurgery is very appealing to patients, I have found that the *overwhelming* majority of patients with AVMs follows the advice of their neurosurgeons. In my experience with the management of more than 300 AVMs, I have had only two patients refuse surgery after it was recommended as the optimal treatment option. I have had only one patient refuse radiosurgery when it was recommended. If the advocate of radiosurgery emphasizes the need for general anesthesia, haircut, scalp incision, a hole in the skull, and hours of brain surgery, even the ideal candidate for surgery can be convinced to accept a treatment that is painless, leaves no scar, and can be performed on an outpatient basis. Conversely, the surgical zealot is able to influence patients to accept his or her prejudices by emphasizing the long delay to therapeutic success, the risk of hemorrhage after treatment, and the dangers of radiation associated with radiosurgery. The physician, in most cases, guides patient preference, and it is the obligation of the treating physician to make an appropriate and responsible recommendation for treatment.

Perhaps the most common indication for radiosurgery in the AVM population is the inoperable AVM, which also represents one of the most controversial issues in this debate. The determination of the risk

TABLE 21.3
Treatment of AVMs: Cost-Effectivesness
Baseline Cost-Effectiveness Analysis*

Treatment	Cost	QALYs	Incremental C/E Ratio ($/QALY)
Microsurgery	$33,022.46	22.06	$7,100.65
Radiosurgery	$26,085.12	21.08	
Difference	$6,937.34	0.98	

*Data from Porter et al. (10).

of surgical resection of an AVM depends on a careful analysis of many factors related to the individual patient, the individual AVM, and the individual surgeon. Characteristics of the patient that are important in analysis include age and health, mode of presentation, preexisting neurological deficits, occupation, and psychological reaction to the knowledge that they harbor a lesion that presents a risk to their health and life. The important characteristics of the AVM include size, location, vascular supply, compactness of the AVM, and anatomy of the venous drainage which may influence the risk of hemorrhage. Paramount is the individual surgeon's *personal* experience with similar AVMs.

Appropriate analysis of these multiple factors requires considerable experience. Given the benefits of surgical resection of AVMs, I believe that the determination of operative risk of a particular AVM should be made by a neurosurgeon with experience and interest in the management of these complex lesions. My personal impression is that some AVMs have been labeled inoperable by physicians with limited experience, who find it easier to declare the AVM unfit for surgery and recommend alternative treatments rather than obtaining an opinion from an experienced surgeon. Despite the demonstrated advantages of microsurgical extirpation of AVMs, several areas of controversy persist.

What is the Definition of Inoperable?

Virtually all AVMs can be surgically removed. The issue is whether a particular AVM can be removed surgically with an acceptable risk.

"Acceptable" risk is a risk that is less than the risk of the natural history and a risk that is less than that associated with alternative treatment options. In my opinion, this critical decision requires experience if it is to be accurate. Much of the literature comparing microsurgical with radiosurgical treatment of AVMs has focused on small AVMs because this optimizes the outcome for both treatments. All experienced vascular neurosurgeons and radiosurgeons recognize that there are "good" small AVMs and "bad" small AVMs. An experienced team is usually able to make this distinction before the initiation of treatment. Based on current data, it is appropriate to resect "good" small AVMs microsurgically and use radiosurgery for "bad" small AVMs.

What is the Cost of Minor Unreported Complications of Surgery?

Some of the surgical series advocating the benefits of microsurgical resection of AVMs have failed to address the minor misadventures of surgery, including urinary tract infections, pneumonia, pulmonary emboli, and unrecognized neurological sequelae. This may be a valid criticism of the surgical literature because many surgical series are retrospective and this information may not have been recorded. It is certainly incumbent on all physicians to report accurately and honestly on the outcome of treatment, including major or transient complications, durability of treatment, and long-term complications. Most patients undergoing treatment for AVMs are young and healthy, with long life expectancies, and the primary goal of therapy is to eliminate the risk of future hemorrhage. Minor transient sequelae may well be an acceptable price to pay for immediate and permanent elimination of the future risks of hemorrhage. Those risks, however, must be known and borne in mind.

Can the Neurosurgeon Who Operates on an Occasional AVM Achieve Acceptable Results?

One of the criticisms of the literature that supports the clinical and economic advantages of microsurgical treatment of AVMs over radiosurgical treatment is that these reports are based on the surgical experience of a few outstanding and experienced neurosurgeons. This also may be a valid criticism. Resection of an AVM, however, is rarely an emergency. Even if the patient requires urgent evacuation of an intracranial hemorrhage, this can usually be accomplished without removal of the AVM. It is often best to delay microsurgical resection of the AVM to a later time when the patient has recovered from the acute effects of the hemorrhage rather than attempting to perform a complex microsurgical procedure as an emergency under less than optimal conditions. Therefore, most patients have the opportunity to be transferred to one of a variety of centers in which an experienced neurosurgeon can provide a surgical opinion and surgical treatment comparable with that reported in the literature.

Can the Neurosurgeon Who Treats an Occasional AVM with Radiosurgery Achieve Acceptable Results?

I would submit that experience is equally important in the radiosurgical treatment of AVMs. Those centers with a team of experienced individuals specializing in microsurgical, endovascular, and radiosurgical treatment are most capable of providing optimal decision making and therapy.

Is It Ethical to Offer Radiosurgery as a Treatment Option to a Patient with a Small AVM that has Been Determined to be "Operable" by an Experienced Surgeon?

Despite my surgical bias, I do not view microsurgery and radiosurgery as competitive treatment options for AVMs but rather as complimentary alternatives that can be provided by an experienced team. I believe it is important for the neurosurgeon to present all treatment options to the AVM patient, including no treatment, microsurgical resection, endovascular therapy, radiosurgery, and combinations of these options. Anything less than a full and honest discussion of the risks and benefits is inappropriate. In my opinion, the majority of small AVMs can be removed surgically with a risk that is less than the risks of the natural history of the lesion and the risks of radiosurgery when one considers the delay to therapeutic effect and risk of hemorrhage, lack of therapeutic effectiveness in 10 to 15% of even small AVMs, and the low risk of radiation injury. There are, however, a number of AVMs for which I believe that either microsurgery or radiosurgery is a reasonable option. In this select group, I believe the decision for optimal treatment is made after a careful and honest presentation of the facts and consideration of the patient's preference.

The management of intracranial AVMs presents some of the most complex challenges in clinical decision making. The treating neurosurgeon must have a clear understanding of the natural history of the disorder and the factors that influence that natural history. Furthermore, the surgeon must understand the risks and benefits of all therapeutic options to determine whether to treat a particular AVM and which therapeutic strategy is best for an individual patient. In my opinion, these decisions are best made and therapeutic plans best implemented by an experienced team of physicians with expertise in endovascular therapy, radiosurgery, and the microsurgical resections of AVMs.

REFERENCES

1. Betti OO, Munari C, Rosler R: Stereotactic radiosurgery with the linear accelerator: Treatment of arteriovenous malformations. **Neurosurgery** 24:311–321, 1989.
2. Colombo F, Pozza F, Chierego G, Casentini L, De Luca G, Francescon P: Linear accelerator radiosurgery of cerebral arteriovenous malformations: An update. **Neurosurgery** 34:14–21, 1994.
3. Friedman WA, Bova FJ, Mendenhall WM: Linear accelerator radiosurgery for arteriovenous malformations: The relationship of size to outcome. **J Neurosurg** 82:180–189, 1995.
4. Hamilton MG, Spetzler RF: The prospective application of a grading system for arteriovenous malformations. **Neurosurgery** 34:2–7, 1994.
5. Heros RC, Korosue K, Diebold PM: Surgical excision of cerebral arteriovenous malformations: Late results. **Neurosurgery** 26:570–578, 1990.
6. Lunsford LD, Kondziolka D, Flickinger JC, Bissonette DJ, Jungreis CA, Maitz AH, Horton JA, Coffey RJ: Stereotactic radiosurgery for arteriovenous malformations of the brain. **J. Neurosurg** 75:512–524, 1991.
7. Nussbaum ES, Heros RC, Camarata PJ: Surgical treatment of intracranial arteriovenous malformations with an analysis of cost-effectiveness. Proceedings of the Congress of Neurological Surgeons, 94, in **Clin Neurosurg** 42:348–369, 1995.
8. Pickus HJ, Beach ML, Harbaugh RE: Microsurgical treatment of arteriovenous malformations: Analysis and comparison with stereotactic radiation. **J Neurosurg** 88:641–646, 1998.
9. Pollock BE, Lunsford DL, Kondziolka D, Maitz A, Flickinger JC: Patient outcomes after stereotactic radiosurgery for "operable" arteriovenous malformations. **J Neurosurgery** 35:1–8, 1994.
10. Porter PJ, Shin AY Detsky AS, LaFaive L, Wallace MC: Surgery versus stereotactic radiosurgery for small, operable cerebral arteriovenous malformations: A clinical and cost comparison. **Neurosurgery** 41:757–764, 1997.
11. Schaller C, Schramm J: Microsurgical results for small arteriovenous malformations accessible for radiosurgical or embolization treatment. **Neurosurgery** 40:664–675, 1997.
12. Sisti MB, Kader A, Stein BM: Microsurgery for 67 intracranial arteriovenous malformations less than 3 cm in diameter. **J Neurosurg** 79:653–660, 1993.
13. Spetzler RF, Martin NA: A proposed grading system of arteriovenous malformations. **J Neurosurg** 65:476–483, 1985.

14. Steinberg GK, Farbrikant JI, Marks MP, Levy RP, Frankel KA, Phillips MH, Shuer LM, Silverberg GD: Stereotactic heavy-charged-particle bragg-peak radiation for intracranial arteriovenous malformations. **N Engl J Med** 323:96–101, 1990.
15. Sundt TM Jr, Piepgras DG, Stevens LN: Surgery for supratentorial arteriovenous malformations. Proceedings of the Congress of Neurological Surgeons 1989, **Clin Neurosurg** 37:49–115, 1991.

CHAPTER

22

Therapeutic Embolization of Arteriovenous Malformations: The Case For and Against

NEIL A. MARTIN, M.D., ROHIT KHANNA, M.D.,
CURT DOBERSTEIN, M.D., AND JOHN BENTSON, M.D.

HISTORICAL PERSPECTIVE

In 1960, Alfred Leussenhop, a neurosurgeon, first reported in the *Journal of the American Medical Association* the therapeutic use of embolization for the treatment of a brain arteriovenous malformation (AVM) (20). Since that time, remarkable technological advances have occurred in the field of endovascular therapy. The embolization techniques for cerebral arteriovenous malformations have evolved; from flow-directed silastic beads injected into the cervical carotid artery, to catheter-introduced detachable balloons for AVM feeder occlusion, to microcatheterization of intracranial arteries for embolization using microparticles or rapidly polymerizing acrylics (1, 3, 15, 16, 28, 31 to 33, 36, 39, 40, 43). With these technical advances, endovascular embolization has become widely employed as a standard technique for the management of cerebral arteriovenous malformations over the past 10 years. Embolization joins microsurgical excision and stereotactic radiosurgery as the principal strategies for the management of AVMs. Embolization is now employed for sole treatment of small AVMs, as palliative treatment for symptomatic AVMs, and as a preprocedural adjunct before surgical excision or stereotactic radiosurgery. The dramatic increase in the use of embolization in the treatment of AVMs, however, poses the risk of indiscriminate and excessive use. The fact that this is a "minimally invasive" technique for AVM treatment makes it a seductive choice for both patients and physicians. When choosing embolization as a component of the management strategy for an individual AVM, it is important to understand current technological capabilities, to appreciate the anatomic and physiological effects of embolization, and to keep in mind the potential for complications. Most importantly, despite the astounding technical virtuosity of many contemporary endovascular therapists, it is important to realize that not all arteriovenous malformations can, or should be, embolized. This chapter is intended to review briefly the current technical state of the art, to review the applications for endovascular therapy in the comprehensive treatment of cerebral arteriovenous malformations, and to review the assets and liabilities of this technique.

AVM EMBOLIZATION: WHAT IS POSSIBLE NOW?

Over the past 15 years, there have been dramatic improvements in neuro-angiographic imaging capability, in microcatheter technology, and in embolic materials. Digital angiographic equipment permits rapid, high resolution, real-time subtraction and vascular "road mapping," which have facilitated and made safer the full range of intracranial endovascular techniques (10, 31). Superselective catheterization of relatively small intracranial AVM feeding arteries can be achieved with over-the-wire or flow-guided microcatheters. The flow-guided microcatheters have become small and supple enough to reach distal cortical and deep perforating cerebral arteries with minimal risk of vessel injury (*Fig. 22.1*) (18, 40). Arteries as small as the lenticulostriate, thalamoperforating, and anterior choroidal arteries can be entered in some cases. Once the microcatheter is positioned in the feeding artery, close to the nidus, the specific component of the AVM supplied by that vessel can be defined precisely by superselective contrast injection (*Fig. 22.1*). The safety of embolic occlusion of the individual vessel can be determined by amytal testing (31). Rapidly polymerizing liquid embolic agents can be injected through the microcatheter, with polymerization custom-timed to allow solidification within the AVM nidus. Larger, high-flow fistulas can be occluded with detachable coils. Arterial aneurysms, located remotely on the circle of Willis or close to the AVM on feeding arteries, can also be occluded with the Guglielmi detachable coil system (11–13). Intranidal aneurysms, which may be a source of recurrent hemorrhage, can be defined clearly by superselective angiography and targeted for superselective embolic occlusion (21, 22). Relatively simple AVMs, generally those with one or two feeding arteries, may be cured by complete and permanent embolic occlusion (10, 40). Substantial nidus occlusion by multifeeder selective embolization can greatly facilitate subsequent microsurgical excision or stereotactic radiosurgery.

AVM Embolization: What Are the Remaining Problems?

There are two key problems that currently limit the use of embolization for the management of AVMs. First, embolization is not truly noninvasive, innocuous, or risk-free (24). The procedure is often long and uncomfortable (even painful) and, in many cases, requires general anesthesia to facilitate optimum technique. Although the possibility

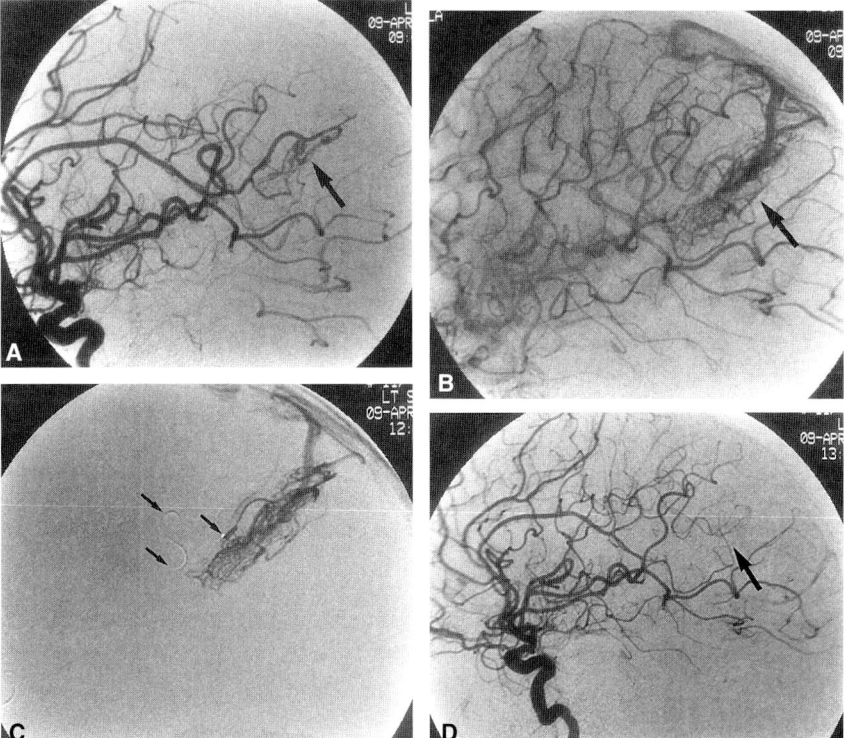

FIG. 22.1 Complete AVM occlusion by embolization alone. *A* and *B*, the pretreatment lateral carotid angiogram demonstrates a small arteriovenous malformation fed by a distal branch of the pericallosal artery. *C*, the superselective, distal catheterization of the feeding artery is demonstrated on this superselective contrast injection. *D*, the postembolization angiogram demonstrates apparently complete occlusion of the arteriovenous malformation following AVM embolization with a new rapidly polymerizing embolic agent. (However, a small fraction of the AVM nidus was seen on the 3-month follow-up angiography to have recanalized).

has been minimized by modern supple microcatheters, feeding artery perforation remains a risk, especially when guidewires are employed in small, fragile arteries (14, 29, 40). Inadvertent deposition of embolic material into feeding arteries "en passage," which supply normal brain in addition to the AVM, may cause ischemic cerebral injury and permanent neurological deficit (2, 18, 40). Ischemic injury can also occur due to reflux of embolic material proximally into normal vessels originating from the feeding artery or as a result of delayed retrograde thrombosis in the feeding artery proximal to the site of embolic occlusion. Control of the site of polymerization of the embolic agent remains imperfect. When the embolic material travels through the AVM nidus and polymerizes in the draining veins, the resulting outflow obstruction may result in a dramatic increase in pressure within the nidus and disastrous rupture (*Fig. 22.2*) (6, 14).

Various quantitative complication rates have been reported for endovascular embolization; a reasonable estimate is that complications occur in 5 to 10% of cases (18). Viñuela and associates, in describing the clinical outcome in 465 patients, reported an incidence of procedure-related ischemic complications of 2.7% and hemorrhagic complications in 4.3% of patients (40). The overall mortality rate in this series, which includes many patients treated years ago with now-outdated technology, was 3.8%. Gobin and associates reported on the complication rate in the course of embolization of 125 patients with AVMs; 5.6% of the patients had "mild" complications, 7.2% of the patients had "moderate or severe" complications, and the mortality rate was 1.6% (10).

The second major problem associated with AVM embolization, is that nidus occlusion is in most cases, to a greater or lesser degree, incomplete (6, 40). Because of the difficulties in timing the polymerization of liquid embolic agents and the critical need to avoid late polymerization in the draining veins, embolic occlusion often occurs primarily within the feeding arteries rather than deep within the nidus. This is also due to the complex nature of the arterial supply to most AVMs. In addition to the large, superficial feeding arteries, which are relatively easy to enter and embolize, the majority of complex AVMs (those in which embolization is most needed to facilitate treatment) have additional sources of arterial supply that are not amenable to embolization. These include small branches of perforating arteries such as the lenticulostriate and anterior choroidal arteries; small leptomeningeal collateral vessels, which travel over eloquent cortical areas before they enter the AVM; and the tiny deep transmedullary arteries that typically supply a large AVM nidus. The small size of such feeding arteries may prevent catheterization and advancement of the microcatheter to the margin of the nidus. The tiny transmedullary arteries are generally so small that they are virtually invisible on angiography.

Viñuela and associates were able to achieve complete AVM occlusion by embolization alone in 9.7% of cases, and Gobin and associates completely occluded 11.2% of their cases (10, 40). Most of these cases were quite small. When we reviewed a series of 18 large AVMs (>6 cm in largest diameter) treated at UCLA, less than one-third of the nidus was occluded in 7 cases, between one-third and two-thirds of the nidus was occluded in 8 cases, and more than two-thirds of the nidus was occluded

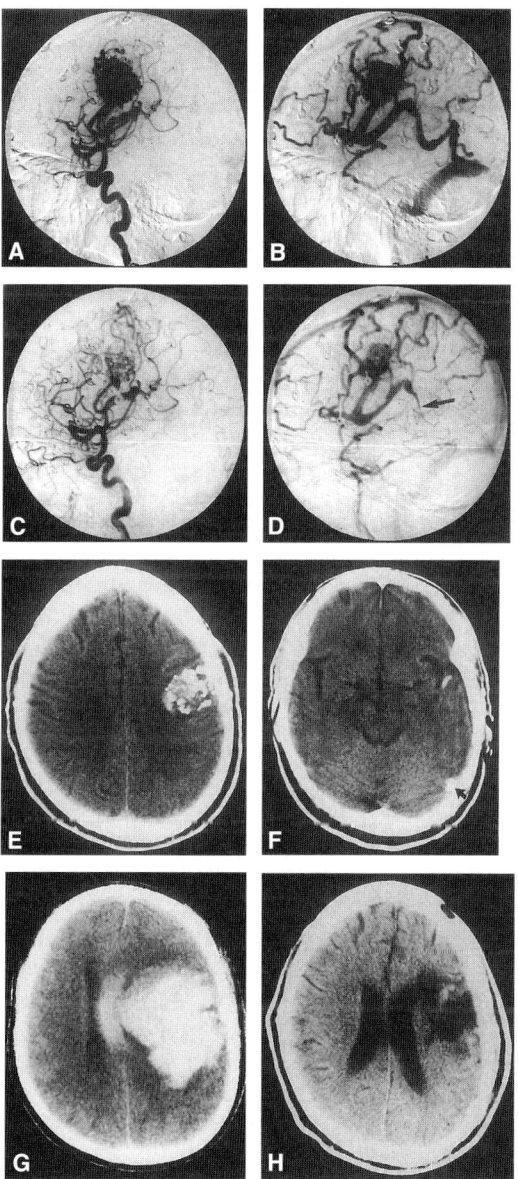

FIG. 22.2 Embolization complicated by inadvertent draining vein occlusion and subsequent AVM rupture: A, the preembolization lateral carotid angiogram demonstrates a posterior frontal arteriovenous malformation supplied by middle cerebral artery branches. B, the venous phase of the carotid angiogram demonstrates a complex venous drainage pattern, with primary drainage through an enlarged vein of Labbé. C, the postembolization arterial phase demonstrates extensive nidus occlusion. D, the postembolization venous phase, however, demonstrates unintended occlusion of the vein of Labbé (*arrow*). E, the postembolization computed tomographic (CT) scan demonstrates extensive embolization within the AVM nidus. F, the postembolization CT scan demonstrates the reason for draining vein occlusion; liquid embolic material has passed through the AVM nidus to polymerize in the vein of Labbé (*black arrow*). G, a cranial CT scan done 3 days later after acute severe neurological deterioration demonstrates postembolization AVM rupture. H, a CT scan done after surgical evacuation of the hematoma and resection of the AVM demonstrates the residual parenchymal damage related to the hemorrhage. This patient was left with a permanent hemiparesis.

in only 3 cases. Incomplete nidus occlusion is a disadvantage, not only because a portion of the AVM remains patent, but also because partially embolized AVMs rapidly and aggressively recruit new sources of arterial supply. All too often, the embolization results in occlusion of the large cortical vessels, which can be easily controlled surgically, only to have this supply replaced by collateral flow from many tiny subcortical arteries, which are thin-walled, fragile, and distended. As any surgeon with extensive AVM experience knows only too well, the particular challenges of removing large AVMs come not from the need to occlude even very large superficial feeding arteries but rather from the frustration of trying to control bleeding from these tiny, dilated subcortical feeding vessels, which requires careful, delicate bipolaring and rebipolaring.

A further disadvantage of AVM embolization is that delayed refilling or recanalization occurs in a certain number of cases (7, 10, 30, 41). This is in part due to the fact that even almost completely embolized AVMs rapidly recruit collateral supply. Viñuela and associates observed that this was particularly true for collaterals arising from posterior cerebral, choroidal, and lenticulostriate arteries (41). Furthermore, pathological studies done on resected AVMs have demonstrated evidence of recanalization of embolized vessels (38). Viñuela et al. demonstrated recanalization in 33% of AVMs in which 50 to 99% nidus occlusion had been achieved by embolization with isobutyl-2-cyanoacrylate (41). Gobin and associates demonstrated an 11.8% revascularization rate, evident by 1 year after embolization in AVMs partially embolized with n-butyl-cyanoacrylate (10).

AVM Embolization: Overview of Indications

Endovascular embolization of AVMs has been advocated for several specific, clinical indications (*Table 22.1*). 1) Embolization may be attempted in small, relatively simple AVMs as primary treatment in an attempt to achieve a permanent cure (this requires total angiographic obliteration). 2) Embolization may be used as an adjunctive, preparatory therapy before definitive microsurgical excision or stereotactic surgery. 3) In large, complex AVMs, for which definitive excision or radiosurgical treatment would be associated with excessive risk, a pallia-

TABLE 22.1
Applications for AVM Embolization

Complete AVM occlusion (cure)
Preparation for surgical excision
Reduce size before radiosurgery
Palliative flow reduction

tive partial embolization may be indicated. The following sections consider the positive and negative aspects of AVM embolization for each of these indications.

AVM Embolization: As Cure

In large clinical series, approximately 10% of AVMs have been obliterated completely by embolization. Viñuela et al. at UCLA reported that long term, complete AVM occlusion was achieved in 9.7% of 465 patients (40). Gobin and associates reported that complete occlusion was accomplished in one-third of small AVMs with a single feeding vessel, one-quarter with two feeding arteries, and 10% of AVMs with three feeding arteries (10). Only 2 of 66 patients with more than three feeding arteries had complete obliteration by embolization alone. None of the patients in the series of Gobin et al., who demonstrated complete occlusion, demonstrated recanalization on follow-up angiography (10). However, at UCLA, we have seen three patients with initial apparent complete embolic occlusion who demonstrated recanalization on followup. One of these patients presented several weeks after apparently complete embolization with recurrent hemorrhage, and angiography demonstrated refilling of approximately 15% of the AVM (*Fig. 22.3*).

When considering embolization for small, simple AVMs with a single feeding artery, one must keep in mind that only a minority are successfully completely occluded and presumably cured. In comparison, microsurgical excision has virtually a 100% success rate for complete occlusion and a very low complication rate in the case of small superficial AVMs. Stereotactic radiosurgery, an alternative to embolization for small deep AVMs, has a cure rate in excess of 80% (9). Given the fact that even embolization of a small, simple, single feeding artery AVM is associated with modest risk as a result of periprocedural ischemia and hemorrhage, an attempt at embolization as definitive treatment of an AVM probably should be recommended only for patients with the most favorably configured small AVMs or for those for whom there is some contraindication to microsurgical excision or stereotactic radiosurgery.

Preoperative AVM Embolization

Preoperative embolization can be a remarkably useful preparatory step in advance of microsurgical excision, particularly when there is an associated aneurysm, a deep surgically inaccessible feeding artery, or a large, multifeeder AVM (15, 23, 39).

Feeding Artery Aneurysm Embolization

Aneurysms arising from AVM feeding arteries, particularly when they arise some distance from the AVM nidus, can be difficult or im-

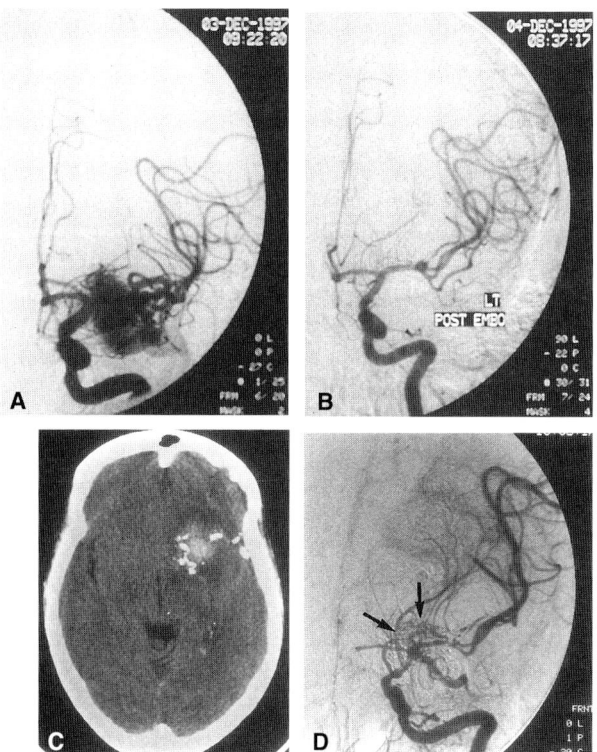

FIG. 22.3 Recanalization after "complete" AVM embolization, with delayed AVM rupture. A, The pre-embolization A-P carotid angiogram demonstrates this deep dominant hemisphere arteriovenous malformation supplied by perforating branches of the internal carotid and middle cerebral arteries. B, the A-P carotid angiogram after embolization with n-butyl-cyanoacrylate demonstrates apparently complete AVM occlusion. C, 2 weeks later, after the patient developed severe headache and aphasia, a cranial CT scan demonstrates evidence of hemorrhage at the site of the embolized AVM. D, a follow-up A-P carotid angiogram performed after the patient presented with delayed hemorrhage demonstrates evidence of recanalization of a portion of the AVM (arrows). Surgical resection of the residual AVM was required (in addition to evacuation of the intracerebral hemorrhage).

possible to access through the craniotomy employed for AVM excision. Such aneurysms are placed at risk of rupture following AVM excision because of the sudden increase in cerebral arterial pressure that accompanies elimination of the AVM shunt flow (25). To eliminate the risk of rupture, aneurysms on the circle of Willis or on feeding arteries should be secured prior to occlusion of the AVM. Whereas a separate surgical approach for clipping of the aneurysm is possible, endovascular occlusion of favorably configured (i.e., narrow neck) proximal aneurysms using the Guglielmi detachable coil system allows the patient to avoid the need for two craniotomies (11–13).

Occlusion of Deep or Inaccessible Feeding Arteries

It is common in large AVMs that, in addition to supply from superficial feeding arteries, there is also supply from deep subcortical perforating arteries (such as the anterior choroidal or lenticulostriate arteries) or from centrally originating feeding arteries (such as those branching from the posterior cerebral artery). Such deep or relatively inaccessible feeding arteries cannot be controlled during the initial phase of dissection of the AVM, and are exposed only when the subcortical apex or the deep medial aspect of the malformation is exposed. These feeding arteries, therefore, provide substantial flow to the malformation and drive intraoperative bleeding right up to the last moments of the resection. Preoperative embolization, specifically targeted at deep or relatively inaccessible feeding arteries, therefore preemptively removes these vessels as a source of troublesome bleeding during the late stages of removal of the AVM nidus, and shifts the bulk of the arterial supply to more superficial and easily controlled feeding arteries (*Fig. 22.4*) (39). This is clearly one of the most valuable applications for AVM embolization.

Stepwise Preoperative Flow Reduction to Prevent Perfusion Pressure Breakthrough and Perioperative Hemodynamic Complications

As initially measured by Nornes, and later confirmed by Spetzler and Duckwiler and their associates, the high arterial flow rates associated with arteriovenous shunting through a large AVM results in abnormally low pressure within the feeding arteries (5, 25, 35, 36). Because the AVM feeding arteries are derived from the normal cerebral circulation, the low pressures in AVM feeders are transmitted to vessels in adjacent normal brain regions. The resulting decrease in local cerebral perfusion pressure is further exacerbated by the relatively high, shunt-induced venous pressures. Local compromise in perfusion pressure results in a compromise in regional blood flow to intact tissue, and the chronicity of the disturbance may result in impairment in local cerebral vascular reactivity. This impairment in normal tissue perfusion surrounding a large AVM can be seen as poor filling of normal cortical arteries adjacent to high-flow lesions, and has been confirmed by cerebral blood flow studies of patients with large AVMs (36). The sudden shutdown of high-flow arteriovenous shunting that occurs with feeding artery occlusion causes a dramatic, immediate rise in pressure in the

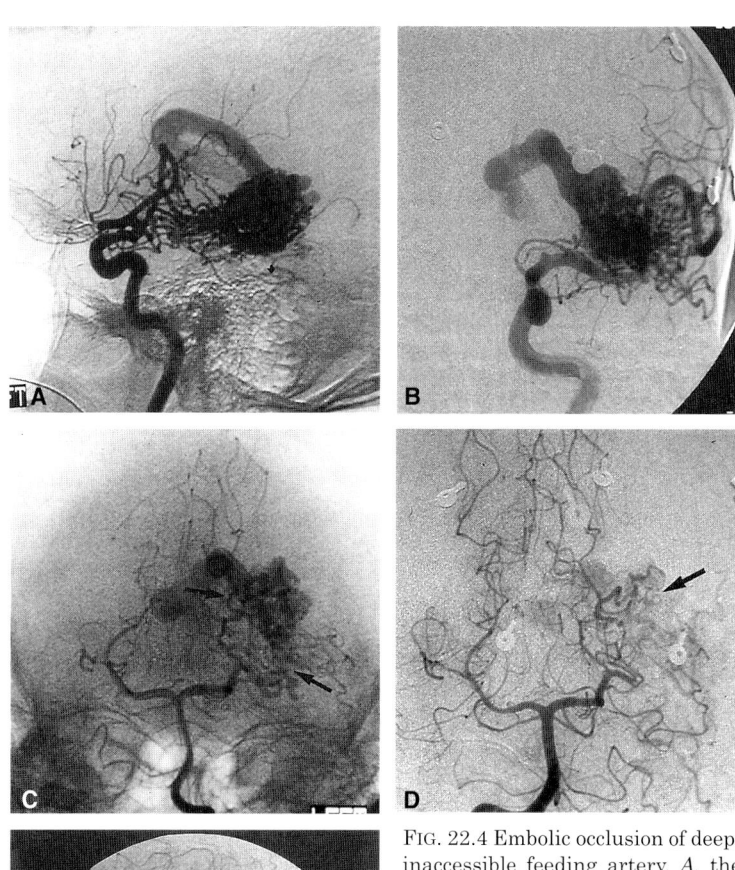
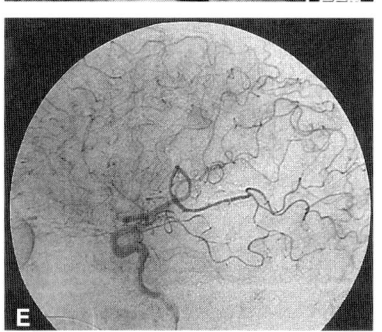

FIG. 22.4 Embolic occlusion of deep, inaccessible feeding artery. *A,* the lateral carotid angiogram demonstrates a large arteriovenous malformation supplied by middle cerebral artery branches. *B,* the A-P carotid angiogram demonstrates the location of this medial temporal lobe arteriovenous malformation and the deep venous drainage. *C,* the Towne's vertebral artery injection demonstrates substantial supply to the medial aspect of the AVM via temporal branches of the left posterior cerebral artery (*arrows*). These deep feeding arteries would be surgically accessible only during the final stage of resection of this AVM. *D,* postembolization vertebral angiogram demonstrates near-complete occlusion of the AVM feeding branches arising from the posterior cerebral artery (*arrow*). *E,* postsurgical angiogram demonstrates complete resection of the arteriovenous malformation, with preservation of normal dominant temporal lobe middle cerebral artery branches. Surgical resection of the arteriovenous malformation, which was approached through the inferior aspect of the temporal lobe, was greatly facilitated by preoperative embolization of the deep feeding arteries.

proximal feeding artery and in the arteries supplying normal brain tissue. Decreased AVM flow also results in a drop in cerebral venous pressure. The combined effect abruptly exposes the brain to a much higher cerebral perfusion pressure, which may be poorly compensated for because of chronic impairment of local vascular reactivity. In a number of cases reported in the literature, it seems that the abrupt hemodynamic alterations precipitated by the sudden arrest of shunt flow has resulted in cerebral edema or frank hemorrhage into surrounding normal brain areas. Overall, this complication is relatively rare: it occurred in 2 of 166 cases reported by Drake, in 2 of 65 cases described by Wilson et al., and 3 of 90 cases reported by Leussenhop and Rosa (4, 19, 42). In a seminal article published in 1978 in *Clinical Neurosurgery,* Spetzler et al. described this phenomenon and termed it "normal perfusion pressure breakthrough" (37). It has been proposed that certain AVM characteristics are associated with risk for this complication. These include: 1) large nidus size with high shunt flow, 2) paucity of filling of normal brain arteries, 3) extensive collateral flow (steal) from vertebrobasilar or contralateral carotid circulation, 4) collateral contribution from the external carotid artery, and 5) clinical symptoms of progressive or fluctuating, nonepileptic neurological deficit (36, 37).

Although the details of the pathophysiology in such cases remains controversial, it is clear that "hemodynamic complications" (edema and hemorrhage) are more commonly seen in the patients with large, high-flow AVMs. A number of clinical groups have recognized that large, high-flow AVMs present unique challenges for treatment and have employed various strategies for staged, stepwise flow reduction before complete AVM resection is attempted. In 1987, Spetzler and associates described the results of surgical management of 20 large AVMs by staged preoperative and intraoperative embolization, followed by operative excision (36). In this report, measurements of intraoperative feeding artery pressures, and preoperative and intraoperative cerebral blood flow measurements provided support for the assumptions underlying the normal perfusion pressure breakthrough theory. Eighteen of the 20 patients in this series ultimately underwent complete AVM excision following multistaged embolization. There were no deaths in this series, and only 3 patients sustained significant postoperative neurological deficits. This work set the standard for current practice and articulated the principles upon which contemporary treatment of large, high-flow AVMs are based.

Using pre-embolization and postembolization measurements of cerebral blood flow and cerebral autoregulation, our group has confirmed that large AVMs induce an impairment in cerebral vascular reactivity in normal surrounding brain regions and that AVM shunt-flow reduction through endovascular embolization has the potential to improve autoregulatory function (*Fig. 22.5*). The improvement in normal brain perfusion has also been graphically illustrated by the demonstration of progressive improvement in angiographic opacification of normal brain arteries in a stepwise fashion following sequential endovascular embolization (*Fig. 22.6*). It seems that progressive, staged reduction in arteriovenous shunting results in gradual restoration of normal cerebral

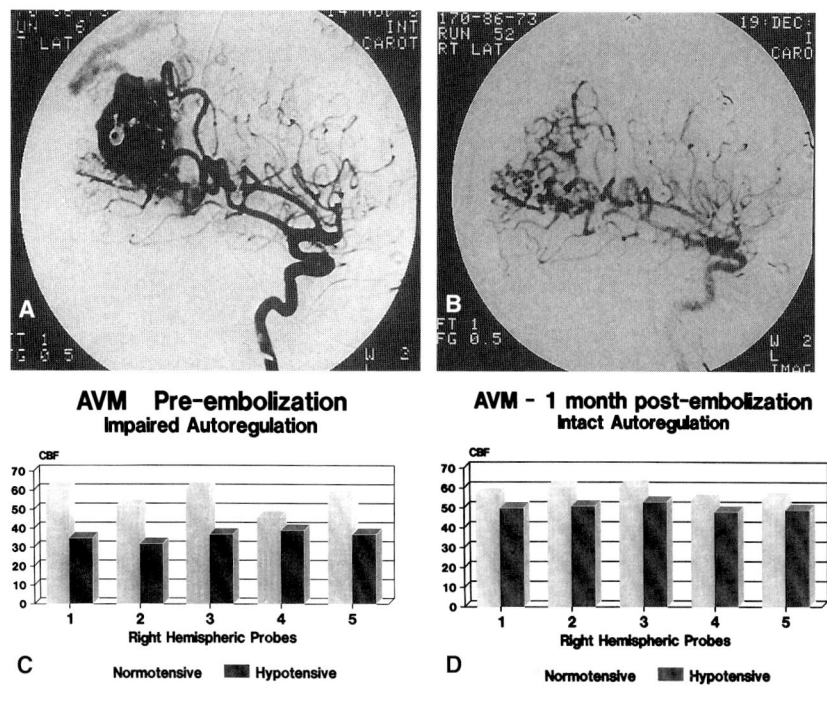

FIG. 22.5 Restoration of normal cerebral autoregulation following embolization. *A*, the lateral carotid angiogram demonstrates a large, high-flow parietal arteriovenous malformation. Note the somewhat poor filling of the frontal middle cerebral artery branches. *B*, the lateral carotid angiogram following the embolization demonstrates substantial AVM occlusion (a portion of the nidus filled during a later angiographic phase) and improved perfusion in the normal right middle cerebral artery branches. *C*, graphic demonstration of the cerebral blood flow (measured by xenon-[133] clearance technique) at five different sites over the right cerebral hemisphere adjacent to (probes 1–3) and remote from (probes 4 and 5) the AVM. The unusually large decrease in cerebral blood flow following induction of arterial hypertension is abnormal and demonstrates impaired autoregulation. *D*, repeat cerebral blood flow evaluation performed 1 month after embolization demonstrates restoration of near-normal autoregulation, with minimal decrease in cerebral blood flow during induced arterial hypertension.

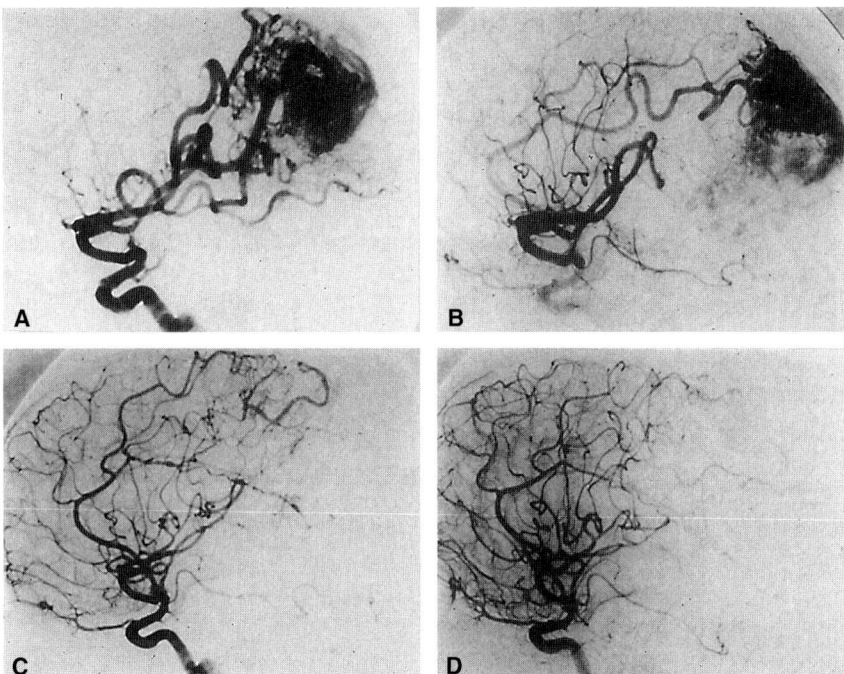

FIG. 22.6 Stepwise AVM flow reduction by staged preoperative embolization. *A*, the preoperative lateral carotid angiogram demonstrates a large, high-flow parietal arteriovenous malformation. Note the poor filling of normal, frontal middle cerebral artery branches. *B*, the lateral carotid angiogram after embolization of the middle cerebral artery branches demonstrates new visualization of the anterior cerebral artery feeding branches (which previously had filled from the contralateral carotid) and much improved visualization of the normal frontal middle cerebral artery branches. *C*, lateral carotid angiogram after the final stage of embolization of the anterior cerebral artery feeding branches demonstrates restoration of near-normal middle and anterior cerebral artery territory filling. *D*, postresection angiogram demonstrates complete AVM obliteration (this was an intraoperative embolization with particles). Courtesy of Robert Spetzler, M.D.; reproduced with permission).

perfusion and vascular reactivity and that this strategy reduces the potential for the perioperative complications of brain swelling and hemorrhage (36, 39, 40). This may be one of the most compelling indications for endovascular embolization of brain AVMs.

Embolization to Decrease AVM Flow, Reduce Nidus Pressure, and Decrease Intraoperative Hemorrhage

Separate from the issue of "normal perfusion pressure breakthrough," embolization has also been advocated as a means of facilitating hemostasis and nidus dissection during AVM resection (18). Although this is the most commonly considered indication for preoperative AVM embolization, it is, in my view, the most often inappropriately applied indication. Based on a personal observation of the referral patterns of AVM patients for endovascular embolization, it seems that preoperative embolization has become virtually a community standard in the protocol for managing virtually all AVMs that are considered for surgery. However, some surgeons with a large experience in managing AVMs have expressed reservations regarding the efficacy of embolization for facilitating AVM excision. For instance, in 1982, Peerless wrote "even major obliteration of the malformation with bucrylate does not, to the surgeon's eye, significantly reduce the technical difficulty of sealing the small [AVM] vessels, nor does it reduce the risk of troublesome intra-operative and postoperative bleeding" (27). My personal observations, now with a series of more than 100 embolized AVMs brought to surgery, are in some cases consistent with that of Peerless. Although preoperative AVM embolization is possible in the vast majority of cases, my sense is that in many cases embolization does not substantially facilitate surgical removal of the lesion. This impression is in large part highly subjective, but it is also based on a very careful review of the results of preoperative embolization in a series of patients with large AVMs treated at UCLA (*Tables 22.2 and 22.3*).

Preoperative embolization designed to reduce intraoperative bleeding and facilitate surgical excision might be expected to be related to the degree of both nidus occlusion and shunt flow reduction. Experience has demonstrated that near-complete nidus occlusion greatly assists in the resection of an AVM; this degree of thorough embolization changes a pulsating, hemorrhagic, vascular mass into something akin to a solid, benign tumor (*Fig. 22.7*). Excision of a near-completely thrombosed AVM is quite straightforward and is a gratifying experience for the surgeon. Unfortunately, this degree of comprehensive embolic occlusion is often not achieved with current techniques for a variety of reasons: 1) it is difficult to penetrate and fill the AVM nidus with rapidly polymerizing acrylic without risking inadvertent and potentially dangerous occlusion of the venous drainage; 2) leptomeningeal collateral supply to the AVM from adjacent cortical vessels is difficult to embolize without risking the occlusion of arteries overlying and supplying normal brain; 3) feeding arteries "en passage," which travel beyond the AVM to supply normal brain tissue, are difficult to embolize safely; 4) branches from perforating arteries may be too small to catheterize selectively for embolization; and 5) large AVMs are supplied subcortically by numerous, tiny transmedullary arteries that are angiographically invisible (yet all too apparent during surgery) and therefore inaccessible to em-

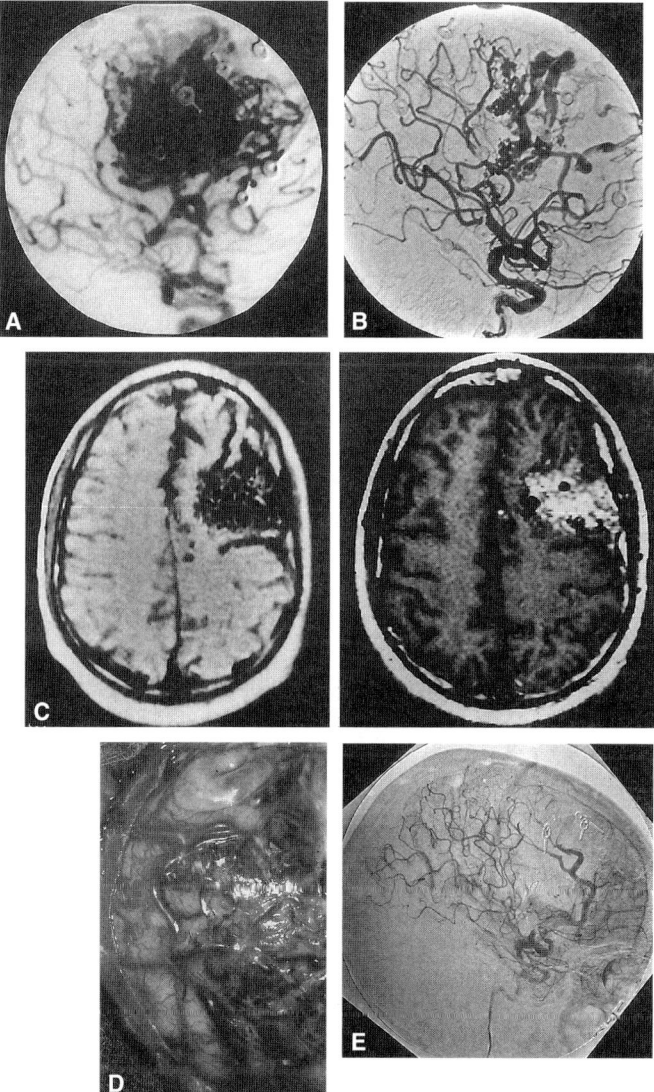

FIG. 22.7 Near-complete AVM nidus occlusion during preoperative embolization. *A,* the lateral carotid angiogram demonstrates a very large frontal arteriovenous malformation. *B,* after two stages of preoperative embolization employing isobutyl cyanoacrylate, more than 85% of the nidus has been occluded. *C,* pre-embolization (*left*), and postembolization (*right*) MRI scans demonstrate the great degree of AVM nidus embolization and thrombosis. *D,* intraoperative view of the large cortical AVM demonstrates near-complete AVM thrombosis. *E,* postoperative lateral carotid angiogram demonstrates complete AVM excision. Surgical removal of this very large AVM was accomplished with minimal blood loss in a 6 to 7-hour operation. The patient, who initially had a moderate hemiparesis following surgery, had recovered normal function by 6 weeks after the procedure.

TABLE 22.2
*Effect of Nidus Size Reduction of Large AVMs (>6 cm)
by Preoperative Embolization on the Ease of Surgical Reduction*

Factors	Nidus Size Reduction			Significance Level (P)
	<34%	34–66%	>66%	
Intraoperative EBL (ml)	1686 ± 663	1094 ± 1267	400 ± 180	<0.05
Intraoperative PRBCs transfused (units)	3.6 ± 2.4	1.5 ± 1.8	0.3 ± 0.6	<0.05
Surgery time (hours)	16.4 ± 3.3	12.8 ± 3	9.6 ± 1.5	<0.05
Degree of surgical difficulty	3.9 ± 0.9	3.0 ± 0.7	1.7 ± 0.6	<0.05
Intraoperative hemorrhage (no. pts.)	2/7 (28.5%)	1/8 (12.5%)	0/3 (0%)	NS
Postoperative hemorrhage (no. pts.)	3/7 (42.9%)	0/8 (0%)	0/3 (0%)	<0.05
Postoperative morbidity (no. pts.)				
Minor	2 (28.6%)	3 (37.5%)	0 (0%)	NS
Major	2 (28.6%)	0 (0%)	0 (0%)	<0.05
Total patients	7	8	3	

bolization. When these conditions prevent a near-complete occlusion of the nidus, embolization only of the larger, catheterizable feeding arteries results in an appreciable slowing of flow into and through the AVM nidus. The delay in nidus opacification, and the presumed decrease in flow rate, is in many cases quite impressive, with the nidus only filling during the early or mid-venous phase (*Fig. 22.8*).

It has been suggested that this angiographically apparent postembolization decrease in flow rate might reduce vascular pressure and distention within the nidus and consequently decrease intraoperative difficulties with dissection and hemostasis (18). To test the presumption that a reduction in flow rate (with delayed nidus filling) facilitates surgical excision of AVMs, we conducted a retrospective review of 18 patients with preoperative embolization of large AVMs (>6 cm in maximum diameter), treated at UCLA between 1986 and 1992. All of these AVMs were Spetzler-Martin Grade IV or V (34). Transfemoral embolization, using isobutyl-cyanoacrylate or *n*-butyl-cyanoacrylate, was carried out in each case over multiple stages. The pre- and postembolization angiograms were reviewed retrospectively and graded for the degree of nidus occlusion (<34%, 34 to 66%, >66%) and for the degree of flow reduction (50 to 66%, >66%). The degree of nidus occlusion and flow reduction were then compared with a number of parameters

TABLE 22.3
*Effect of Flow Reduction in Large AVMs (>6 cm)
by Preoperative Embolization on the Ease of Surgical Resection*

Factors	Flow Reduction 50–66%	>66%	Significance Level (P)
Intraoperative EML (ml)	1658 ± 819	892 ± 1076	NS
Intraoperative PRBCs transfused (units)	3.5 ± 2.4	1.4 ± 1.9	<0.05
Surgery time (hours)	14.8 ± 2.8	13.0 ± 4.3	NS
Degree of surgical difficulty	3.8 ± 1.0	2.8 ± 1.0	NS
Intraoperative hemorrhage (no. pts.)	2/12 (16.7%)	1.6 (12.5%)	NS
Postoperative hemorrhage (no. pts.)	3/12 (25%)	0.6 (0%)	NS
Postoperative morbidity (no. pts.)			
Minor	1/12 (8.3%)	4/6 (66.7%)	<0.05
Major	2/12 (16.7%)	0.6 (0%)	NS
Total patients	12	6	

designed to assess ease of surgical resection, including 1) intraoperative estimated blood loss, 2) amount of intraoperative transfusion, 3) surgical time, and 4) subjective degree of surgical difficulty judged by the operating surgeon. The incidence of intraoperative poorly controlled hemorrhage, postoperative hemorrhage, and postoperative morbidity were also correlated to the results of embolization (see *Tables 22.2 and 22.3*). As seen in *Table 22.2*, in 7 of the cases, less than one-third of the nidus was occluded, and in only 3 of the 18 cases was more than two-thirds of the nidus occluded. In contrast, when flow reduction was used as the criterion for grading the efficacy of the embolization, all of the patients were judged to have at least 50% flow reduction, and 6 of the 18 patients had flow reduction in excess of two-thirds (*Table 22.3*). As can be seen from the Tables, the only specific postembolization result that strongly and significantly predicted easier, safer, and a quicker AVM resection was nidus size reduction in excess of 66%. The patients judged to have a moderate but appreciable degree of flow reduction (flow reduction of 50 to 66%) had the same high degree of difficulty and prolonged surgical time as did the subgroup with minimal (<33%) nidus occlusion. It has been my subjective impression, supported by this case review, that even a substantial degree of flow reduction, in the absence of occlusion of the majority of the nidus, does not significantly facilitate surgical excision of the lesion. In fact, as indicated above, flow reduction alone (which implies occlusion primarily of the lesion on the feeding artery side) may actually make resection of

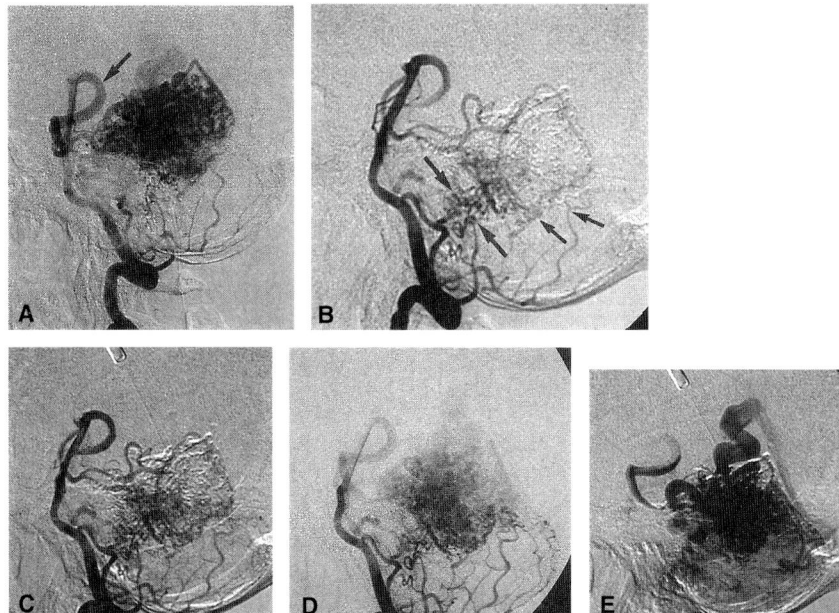

FIG. 22.8 Collateral refilling of a large AVM following extensive embolization of the primary feeding artery. *A,* the pre-embolization lateral vertebral angiogram demonstrates a very large cerebellar arteriovenous malformation supplied primarily by markedly dilated superior cerebellar artery (*arrow*). *B,* following extensive embolization through the superior cerebellar artery, there is markedly retarded filling of the AVM nidus on the early arterial phase. *C,* The mid-arterial phase shows additional filling of the AVM nidus through collateral vessels. *D,* the late arterial phase shows extensive AVM nidus supply through multiple dilated collateral branches arising from the anterior inferior cerebellar artery and the posterior inferior cerebellar artery. Note that all of these vessels have enlarged markedly when compared with the pre-embolization angiogram (see *A*). *E,* the venous phase of the postembolization angiogram demonstrates stasis within the embolized superior cerebellar artery feeder but delayed filling of the majority of the AVM nidus. Note: embolization of the largest feeding artery in this case resulted in dramatic delay in the filling of the AVM nidus, and the early and mid-arterial phases (see *B* and *C*) suggest that much of the AVM nidus has been obliterated. However, the late arterial and venous phases demonstrate that there has only been retardation in the nidus opacification without extensive total nidus occlusion. Surgery in this case was very difficult, and control of bleeding from the multiple small, dilated collateral vessels required many hours of tedious repetitive high magnification bipolaring. Complete surgical resection of the AVM in this case required an operation of almost 20 hours in duration. The patient was left with disabling brainstem and cerebellar deficit.

the lesion more difficult by promoting the recruitment of tiny, difficult-to-control transmedullary or perforating feeding arteries (*Fig. 22.8*).

Should preoperative embolization be recommended for small and medium-sized AVMs? It is the author's personal impression that small and medium-sized AVMs, especially those that are cortically based and that do not have deep or inaccessible feeding arteries, are not made much easier for surgical resection by preoperative embolization. In fact, as noted above, partial embolization of the easily accessible cortical feeding arteries results in the recruitment of collateralization through the more difficult-to-control transmedullary feeders. Some of the easiest AVM resections that I have carried out involved superficial medium-sized, nonembolized lesions (*Fig. 22.9*). In summary, it seems that AVM embolization is strongly indicated to control deep or relatively inaccessible feeding arteries and to attempt maximal staged preoperative occlusion of large, high-flow AVMs to reduce the potential for hemodynamic complications. To facilitate hemostasis and resection of the AVM nidus, the appropriate goal of presurgical embolization is maximal nidus occlusion rather than flow reduction alone.

EMBOLIZATION AS AN ADJUNCT TO RADIOSURGERY

Stereotactic radiosurgery is a viable option for AVMs that are not suitable for microsurgical excision. However, for medium-sized and large AVMs (>3 cm maximal diameter or >10 cubic cm volume), the efficacy and safety of this form of treatment is somewhat diminished (9). Gobin and associates cited three potential advantages of embolizing a large AVM before treating with radiosurgery: 1) embolization can reduce residual nidus size and, therefore, the radiosurgical target volume; 2) embolic occlusion of associated arterial or intranidal aneurysms might reduce the risk of hemorrhage while awaiting delayed, radiosurgically induced AVM obliteration; and 3) embolization enables the occlusion of large fistulous components of AVMs that might be refractory to the action of radiosurgery (10). In their 1996 report, they described the results of treatment in 125 patients with brain AVMs. Most of these were Spetzler-Martin Grade 3 or greater, and approximately half of these lesions had a diameter of greater than 4 cm. In this group, 11% of the patients were cured by embolization alone, and 77% of the patients were deemed suitable for radiosurgery following embolization. More than 10% of the patients with AVMs with diameters 4 to 6 cm, and more than 50% of the AVMs with diameters greater than 6 cm, did not have sufficient nidus size reduction to make radiosurgery suitable. In the patients with AVMs less than 4 cm in diameter, the overall cure rate (by embolization alone or embolization followed by radiosurgery) was 76 to 78%. The cure rate for the smallest

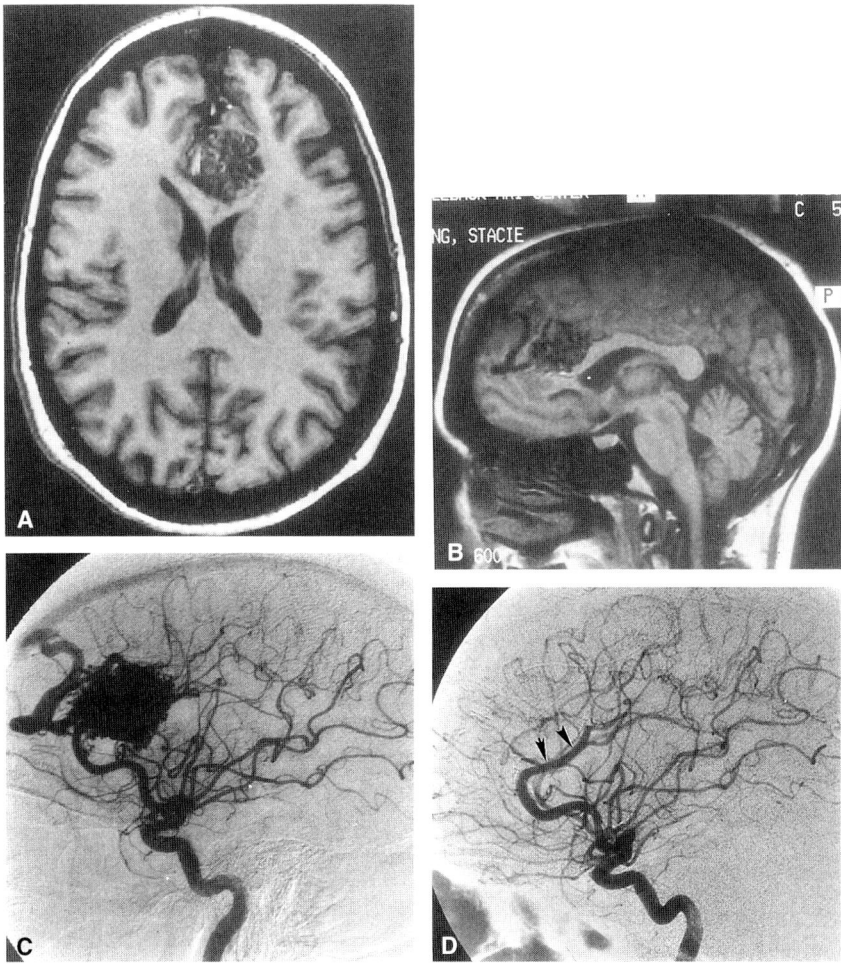

FIG. 22.9 AVM resection without embolization. *A*, the axial MRI scan demonstrates a medium-sized arteriovenous malformation involving the medial aspect of the dominant frontal lobe and the corpus callosum. *B*, the sagittal MRI scan demonstrates the relationship of the AVM nidus to the corpus callosum. *C*, the later arterial phase of the carotid angiogram demonstrates the entire AVM nidus and the draining vein. *D*, the postsurgical carotid angiogram demonstrates complete resection of the AVM, with preservation of the pericallosal artery (*arrows*).

group of embolized AVMs (<3 cm) was 78%, and it is not clear whether embolization improved the results of treatment in this group. This cure rate is virtually the same as that reported for radiosurgery alone (without embolization) for small AVMs (9). The cure rate for embolization and radiosurgery in patients with AVMs between 4 and 6 cm in diameter was

59%, and this probably represents an improvement in the rate of complete occlusion over that achievable by radiosurgery alone. The combination of embolization plus radiosurgery resulted in the cure of only 1 of 15 patients with AVMs larger than 6 cm in diameter.

Gobin points out the fact that "permanent" embolic material should be employed in these cases because the radiosurgical target volume generally excludes the embolized, angiographically occluded portion of the AVM nidus (9). This nonradiated, embolized portion of the AVM remains liable to recanalization, particularly if nonpermanent embolic material (such as polyvinyl alcohol particles) is used. However, even in those patients embolized with cyanoacrylate (a presumably permanent agent), revascularization of occluded portions of the nidus has been observed (7, 10, 30, 38).

Does partial embolization reduce the risk of hemorrhage during that 1 to 3-year latent period between the administration of radiosurgical treatment and ultimate AVM obliteration? In the patients with partially embolized AVMs, Gobin and associates observed a bleeding rate of approximately 3% per year—not significantly different from that for untreated AVMs (10, 26). This was somewhat disappointing, because the embolizations in this series focused on the occlusion of putatively high-risk, angio-architectural features such as associated aneurysms. Furthermore, no data were presented in this paper that suggested that embolic occlusion of a large arteriovenous fistula within an AVM nidus improved the results of radiosurgical treatment.

In summary, adjunctive embolization seems to improve the efficacy of radiosurgical treatment for lesions of approximately 3 to 6 cm in diameter. When embolization was performed in lesions smaller than this, there was no convincing advantage over radiosurgery alone. Embolization of lesions larger than 6 cm did not reduce the residual nidus and radiosurgical target volume sufficiently to result in a significant cure rate. Preradiosurgical embolization did not seem to convey a substantial, significant, protective effect for interval hemorrhage during the latent period while awaiting ultimate postradiosurgical occlusion. Furthermore, late follow-up angiography is required to be certain that delayed recanalization does not occur in embolization-occluded portions of the nidus.

PALLIATIVE PARTIAL EMBOLIZATION

Incomplete endovascular embolization, with the goal of AVM flow reduction, has been proposed as a palliative treatment for presumptively flow-related symptoms such as intractable headache or intermittent or progressive nonhemorrhagic neurological deficit (8, 17, 18, 44). Embolization, particularly of posterior cerebral artery feeding vessels or of external carotid artery feeding vessels, seems to have a beneficial effect in a significant proportion of patients with intractable headache. There have been reports of reversal of neurological deficits, presumably due to arterial "steal" or venous hypertension, by embolization (17). However, the benefit may only be temporary until new collateral circulation is recruited by the AVM. Given the promising nature of some reports regarding palliative embolization to control flow-related symptoms, this strategy seems to be reasonable in patients with progressive or refractory symptoms, in whom a more definitive treatment is judged impractical or unsafe.

Does Partial Embolization Reduce the Risk of Future Hemorrhage?

Certain angiographic features of AVMs, such as the presence of intranidal aneurysms or stenosis of draining veins, have been associated with the occurrence of AVM hemorrhage (10, 18, 21, 22). This has led to the suggestion that partial embolic occlusion specifically targeting, for instance, an intranidal aneurysm might reduce the risk of future hemorrhage. In cases in which repetitive focal hemorrhage seems to have been associated with an intranidal aneurysm, it is reasonable to consider such directed, partial embolization (22). However, the efficacy of this strategy (or of any type of incomplete embolization) for reducing the risk of future rupture remains to be demonstrated. In fact, data such as that presented by Gobin and associates (described above) suggest that incomplete AVM obliteration is not successful in reducing the risk of bleeding (10).

SUMMARY

The field of endovascular therapy has demonstrated stunning technical achievements in AVM embolization. Embolization has the potential to enhance the safety and efficacy of AVM treatment when applied in carefully considered cases. The utility of embolization, at the present time, is limited by the fact that the procedure may be associated with disabling or fatal complications, and because complete or near-complete AVM nidus occlusion can be achieved only in a minority of cases. Because of these factors, embolization should not be considered a "standard-of-care" for the management of all cerebral AVMs, and careful case selection for embolization, with well-defined treatment goals in mind, is essential. Finally, not all AVMs that can be embolized should be embolized.

REFERENCES

1. Bank WO, Kerber CW, Cromwell LD: Treatment of intracerebral arteriovenous malformations with isobutyl 2-cyanoacrylate: initial clinical experience. **Radiology** 139:609–616, 1981.
2. Berenstein A, Choi JS, Kupersmith M, et al.: Complications of endovascular embolization in 182 patients with cerebral AVMs. **Am J Neuroradiol** 10:876, 1989.

3. Debrun G, Viñuela F, Fox A, et al.: Embolization of cerebral arteriovenous malformations with bucrylate: Experience in 46 cases. **J Neurosurg** 56:615–627, 1982.
4. Drake CG: Cerebral arteriovenous malformations: Considerations for and experience with surgical treatment in 166 cases. **Clin Neurosurg** 26:145–208, 1979.
5. Duckwiler G, Dion J, Viñuela F, et al.: Intravascular microcatheter pressure monitoring: Experimental results and early clinical evaluation. **Am J Neuroradiol** 11:169–175, 1990.
6. Duckwiler GR, Dion JE, Viñuela F, et al.: Delayed venous occlusion following embolotherapy of vascular malformations in the brain. **Am J Neuroradiol** 13:1571–1579, 1992.
7. Fournier D, Terbrugge K, Rodesch G, et al.: Revascularization of brain arteriovenous malformations after embolization with bucrylate. **Neuroradiology** 21:497–501, 1990.
8. Fox AJ, Girvin JP, Viñuela F, et al.: Rolandic arteriovenous malformations: Improvements in limb function by IBC embolization. **Am J Neuroradiol** 6:575–582, 1985.
9. Friedman WA, Bova FJ, Mendenhall WM: Linear accelerator radiosurgery for arteriovenous malformations: The relationship of size to outcome. **J Neurosurg** 82:180–189, 1995.
10. Gobin YP, Laurent A, Schlienger M, et al.: Treatment of brain arteriovenous malformations by embolization and radiosurgery. **J Neurosurg** 85:19–28, 1996.
11. Guglielmi G: Endovascular treatment of aneurysms: History, development, and application of current techniques. **J Stroke Cerebrovasc Dis** 6:246–248, 1997.
12. Guglielmi G, Viñuela F, Dion J, et al.: Electrothrombosis of saccular aneurysms via endovascular approach: Part 2. Preliminary clinical experience. **J Neurosurg** 75:8–14, 1997.
13. Guglielmi G, Viñuela F, Sepetka I, et al.: Electrothrombosis of saccular aneurysms via endovascular approach: Part I. Electrochemical basis, technique and experimental results. **J Neurosurg** 75:1–7, 1997.
14. Jafar JJ, Rezai AR: Acute surgical management of intracranial arteriovenous malformations. **Neurosurgery** 34:8–12, 1994.
15. Jafar JJ, Davis AJ, Berenstein A, et al.: The effect of embolization with N-butyl cyanoacrylate prior to surgical resection of cerebral arteriovenous malformations. **J Neurosurg** 78:60–69, 1993.
16. Kerber C: Balloon catheter with a calibrated leak: A new system for superselective angiography and occlusive catheter therapy. **Radiology** 120:547–550, 1976.
17. Kusske JA, Kelly WA: Embolization and reduction of the "steal" syndrome in cerebral arteriovenous malformations. **J Neurosurg** 40:313–321, 1974.
18. Latchaw RE, Madison MT, Larsen DW, et al.: Intracranial arteriovenous malformations: Endovascular strategies and methods, in HH Batjor HH (ed): *Cerebrovascular Disease*. New York, Lippincott-Raven, 1997, pp 707–725.
19. Leussenhop AJ, Rosa L: Cerebral arteriovenous malformations: Indications for and results of surgery, and the role of intravascular techniques. **J Neurosurg** 60:14–22, 1984.
20. Leussenhop AJ, Spence WT: Artificial embolization of cerebral arteries: Report of use in a case of arteriovenous malformation. **JAMA** 172:1153–1155, 1960.
21. Marks MP, Lane B, Steinberg GK, et al.: Hemorrhage in intracerebral arteriovenous malformations: Angiographic determinants. **Radiology** 176:807–813, 1990.
22. Marks MP, Lane B, Steinberg GK, et al.: Intranidal aneurysms in cerebral arteriovenous malformations: Evaluation and endovascular treatment. **Radiology** 183:355–360, 1992.
23. Martin NA: Treatment of arteriovenous malformations: Indications, grading, and techniques. **J Stroke Cerebrovasc Dis** 6:272–276, 1997.

24. Martin NA, Duckwiler GR: Complications of interventional neuroradiology: Neurosurgical management, in Wilkins RH and Rengachary SS (eds): *Neurosurgery*. New York, McGraw-Hill, 1996, vol 1, pp 645–652.
25. Nornes H, Grip A: Hemodynamic aspects of cerebral arteriovenous malformations. **J Neurosurg** 53:456–464, 1980.
26. Ondra SL, Troupp H, George ED, et al.: The natural history of symptomatic arteriovenous malformations of the brain: A 24-year follow-up assessment. **J Neurosurg** 73:387–391, 1990.
27. Peerless SJ: Successful treatment of the normal perfusion pressure breakthrough syndrome (comment). **Neurosurgery** 11:629–630, 1982.
28. Pelz DM, Fox AJ, Viñuela F, et al.: Preoperative embolization of brain AVMs with isobutyl-2-cyanoacrylate. **Am J Neuroradiol** 9:757–765, 1988.
29. Purdy PD, Batjer HH, Samson D: Management of hemorrhagic complications from preoperative embolization of arteriovenous malformations. **J Neurosurg** 74:205–211, 1991.
30. Rao VRK, Mandalam KR, Gupta AK, et al.: Dissolution of isobutyl 2-cyanoacrylate on long-term follow-up. **Am J Neuroradiol** 10:135–141, 1989.
31. Rauch RA, Viñuela F, Dion J, et al.: Preembolization functional evaluation in brain arteriovenous malformations: The superselective Amytal test. **Am J Neuroradiol** 12:303–308, 1992.
32. Samson D, Ditmore QM, Beyer CW Jr: Intravascular use of isobutyl 2-cyanoacrylate: Part 1. Treatment of intracranial arteriovenous malformations. **Neurosurgery** 8:43–51, 1981.
33. Serbinenko FA: Balloon catheterization and occlusion of major cerebral vessels. **J Neurosurg** 41:125–145, 1974.
34. Spetzler RF, Martin NA: A proposed grading system for arteriovenous malformations. **J Neurosurg** 65:476–483, 1986.
35. Spetzler RF, Hargraves RW, McCormick PW, et al.: Relationship of perfusion pressure and size to risk of hemorrhage from arteriovenous malformation. **J Neurosurg** 76:918–923, 1992.
36. Spetzler RF, Martin NA, Carter LP, et al.: Surgical management of large AVMs by staged embolization and operative excision. **J Neurosurg** 67:17–28, 1987.
37. Spetzler RF, Wilson CB, Weinstein P, et al.: Normal perfusion pressure breakthrough theory. **Clin Neurosurg** 25:651–672, 1978.
38. Vinters HV, Lundie MJ, Kaufmann JC: Long-term pathological follow-up of cerebral arteriovenous malformations treated by embolization with bucrylate. **N Engl J Med** 314:477–483, 1986.
39. Viñuela F, Dion JE, Duckwiler G, et al.: Combined endovascular embolization and surgery in the management of cerebral arteriovenous malformation: Experience in 101 cases. **J Neurosurg** 75:856–864, 1991.
40. Viñuela F, Duckwiler G, Guglielmi G: Contribution of interventional neuroradiology in the therapeutic management of brain arteriovenous malformations. **J Stroke Cerebrovasc Dis** 6:268–271, 1997.
41. Viñuela F, Fox AJ, Pelz D, et al.: Angiographic follow-up of large cerebral AVMs incompletely embolized with isobutyl-2-cyanoacrylate. **Am J Neuroradiol** 7:919–925, 1986.
42. Wilson CB, Domingue J: Microsurgical treatment of intracranial vascular malformations. **J Neurosurg** 51:446–454, 1979.
43. Wolpert SM, Stein BM: Catheter embolization of intracranial arteriovenous malformations as an aid to surgical excision. **Neuroradiology** 10:73–85, 1975.
44. Wolpert SM, Barnett FJ, Prager RJ: Benefits of embolization without surgery for cerebral arteriovenous malformations. **Am J Roentgenol** 138:99–102, 1982.

CHAPTER

23

Treatment Decisions in Brain AVMs: The Case For and Against Surgery

H. HUNT BATJER, M.D.

Arteriovenous malformations (AVMs) of the brain remain a group of fascinating congenital malformations capable of producing disability or death to afflicted individuals in the prime of life. At this juncture, there is clearly good news and bad news for victims of this disease. The good news is that major developments in microsurgery, endovascular techniques, and radiosurgery over the past decade have dramatically expanded the percentage of patients who can be cured of their malformation and have decreased the risk of treatment. The bad news is that as our menu of potential treatment alternatives expands, the decision-making process becomes much more difficult for the treatment team. This chapter will attempt to summarize a single neurosurgeon's thoughts, prejudices, and preferred therapeutic strategies in articulating the case for and against microsurgical treatment of AVMs.

NATURAL HISTORY

In absence of a life-threatening intracranial hematoma, treatment strategies directed at the cure of an AVM are essentially prophylactic in nature and are directed at reducing the risk of future complications. Only in rare circumstances of massive arterial-to-venous shunting and resulting brain ischemia could the surgeon hope to actually *improve* the neurological condition of a patient with this condition. Because treatment of an AVM has little hope of making the patient better, and certainly carries the potential of making the patient worse, a thorough understanding of the natural history of this disease process is absolutely essential to render appropriate advice and counseling to patients and their families. Perhaps the most important information available comes from the report by Ondra et al., in which the experience of Professor Troupp in Finland was carefully studied (3). 160 patients who presented with symptomatic AVMs were followed for a mean follow-up of 24.7 years. The average age of this population was 33 years. The authors found that without treatment, the patients were subject to a 4% yearly risk of bleeding regardless of the type of presentation. The interval between presentation and subsequent hemorrhage was 7.7 years on average. Thus, a composite yearly morbidity of 1.7% and yearly mortality of 1.0% was defined.

This is an extraordinarily important study, as we will never again have the opportunity to survey a large group of untreated patients. The finding that the future of the patient was identical regardless of the mode of presentation is counterintuitive, and I find myself continuing to recommend much more aggressive treatment strategies to patients who have presented with hemorrhage. I suspect that most cerebrovascular surgeons share this approach, but it is critical that patients be informed that we have very little to go on in this regard.

Unfortunately, the Troupp data were acquired during an era where subgroup analysis of potentially important variables was not possible. For instance, what is the significance of intranidal aneurysms? Do patients with AVM drainage with obvious stenotic lesions have a higher risk of initial or recurrent bleeding? These and many other questions remain unanswered, and therefore critical data for individual treatment planning are not available. Nevertheless, it is crystal clear that the risk of recurrent hemorrhage from even a ruptured AVM is lower than the risk of rebleeding from a ruptured aneurysm by an order of magnitude. Thus, a very different philosophical approach is appropriate.

PRINCIPLES

To make judgments and recommendations that are tailored to the individual patient and circumstance, a number of basic concepts should be understood. Brain AVMs are in fact a multidisciplinary disease. Partners in the team that must be intimately involved in the evaluation, strategic planning, and implementation of a plan include, but are not limited to, the following members: one or more neurosurgeons, diagnostic and interventional neuroradiologists, a radiosurgeon, a neuro-anesthesiologist, and a critical care specialist. Individual circumstances such as pre-existing heart disease, pulmonary disease, etc. may expand this team membership substantially. It is my firm opinion that although the initial analysis of a case should be performed in a multidisciplinary gathering, final decision making is not a committee exercise. The microsurgical neurosurgeon is in fact the "captain of the ship." Advice and recommendations are solicited from all team partners, but ultimately the final decision is not a vote. Once a strategic plan is developed that may include all or only a portion of the evaluation team, it is critical that effective communication and dialogue be maintained among all treating physicians as the plan becomes implemented. Each member of the treatment team carries responsibility to the patient and maintains a supporting relationship with the primary neurosurgeon (1, 4).

TREATMENT STRATEGIES

As mentioned above, the menu of treatment options has fairly dramatically expanded during the past several years. I would list the following as potential options, and this list could arguably be expanded: 1) no therapy, 2) primary embolization for cure, 3) palliative embolization, 4) radiosurgery, 5) staged radiosurgery (overlapping fields), 6) embolization followed by radiosurgery, 7) embolization followed by microsurgery, 8) microsurgery alone, 9) microsurgery plus radiosurgery for residual, and 10) embolization plus microsurgery followed by radiosurgery.

In light of the natural history data quoted above, it is critical to keep in mind that *no therapy* is a very rational and reasonable approach in some patients. Primary embolization for cure remains a controversial topic. In my 17 years of cerebrovascular surgical practice, I am aware of two patients who have potentially been cured by embolization alone. The relatively unique single pedicle malformations may be candidates. The long-term rate of recanalization in these "cures" remains unknown. I am aware of two cases within the past few months in which cure was attempted, only to be followed by immediate hemorrhage despite what appeared to be an obliterated malformation angiographically.

Embolization can be used palliatively in a number of circumstances. Patients with severe headaches and malformations that have external carotid-derived feeding can often benefit by embolizing the external carotid branches. This certainly does not cure the malformation, but it should not destabilize the hemodynamics and often eliminates their headaches. This is especially helpful in the elderly.

Certain high-flow malformations that are diagnosed with progressive ischemic symptoms in elderly patients may also be candidates for sequential embolization without plans for resection. Staged radiosurgery is being actively investigated and may offer the potential to treat some deep malformations that are larger than the traditional size acceptability for primary radiosurgery. A highly controversial area concerns the use of radiosurgery for residual malformation following surgical resection. In almost all circumstances, immediate reoperation is indicated, as the hemodynamics have been disturbed, and often venous drainage has been sacrificed. Nevertheless, there are certain cases with preserved venous outflow in which the residual is located in eloquent brain tissue. We have treated rare patients with residual in the thalamus with subsequent radiosurgery rather than reoperation.

Regardless of the strategy selected, successful patient management in my opinion is predicated on the following items, listed in order of importance: 1) case selection, 2) case selection, 3) case selection, 4) strategic planning, 5) technical proficiency, 6) critical care, and 7) patient expectations.

The issue of case selection will be discussed below. Patient expectations must be considered in great detail. Patients who are essentially neurologically intact have no basis for truly understanding a neurological deficit unless they have had a deficit in the past. This is important for the counseling physician to remember. What may appear to the surgeon to be an outstanding result with only minor cortical hand dysfunction may be a result that requires months of physical therapy and time to achieve. If the patient happened to be a practicing surgeon or involved in any other occupation requiring a very high level of dexterity, the surgeon may have failed to provide a cure at an acceptable expense for that individual.

CASE SELECTION

Perhaps the most widely used AVM grading scale employed by neurosurgeons worldwide is the one proposed by Drs. Spetzler and Martin (5). This grading scale considers three key variables and assigns a point scale for each parameter. The three variables felt to have the most predictive significance are size, eloquence, and pattern of venous drainage. Although no one could dispute the negative prognostic significance of increasing size, one might question issues of eloquence and the pattern of venous drainage. The issue of eloquence is now being redefined by physiologic neuroimaging. Functional magnetic resonance imaging studies can now detect evidence of displacement of key brain functions, as one might expect from a congenital malformation. Thus, traditional anatomic landmarks may be imprecise in defining whether a malformation is eloquent or not. Confirmation of these early observations might well redefine the concepts of suitability for treatment. Analysis of my own operative experience has not suggested evidence of increasing risk of surgery with deep venous drainage. In fact, I actually prefer that drainage is deep as it does not encumber the early phases of dissection and is not in the way during the deep periventricular dissection.

Rather than a point system or a formalized grading scale, I favor a more descriptive method of case selection. The issues that I think should definitely be included are the following: 1) size, 2) presentation (?) (Troupp data), 3) hemorrhage with intranidal aneurysm (?), 4) eloquence (?) (anatomic versus physiologic), 5) embryonal nidus (compact), 6) angiomatous change, 7) irrigation by numerous perforators, 8) presence of intranidal aneurysms, 9) venous stenosis, and 10) patient and family.

With regard to the final consideration, patient and family, it is my sincere belief that this might well be the most important element to consider. Embarking upon a highly complex treatment strategy dedicated solely to the prophylaxis against potential future adverse events requires detailed understandings between the patient, physician, and the patient's family. Included in this dynamic is the patient's sense of his or her own disease, a detailed education about known natural history data, detailed information about the surgeon's own results (not published data), and their ability to carry on with their life and occupation if some neurological disability results. Failure to achieve detailed understandings in each of these areas can set the stage for serious unhappiness on the part of all parties. It is also appropriate to ensure that the patients realize that if a neurological deficit results, the chances for improvement over time are very high (2).

THE CASE FOR MICROSURGERY

In my opinion, the case for surgery can be argued as follows:

1. Protection from future hemorrhage is immediate.
2. Symptomatic recurrence of a surgically obliterated (angiographically proven) malformation is exquisitely rare. I am aware of one such case in a pediatric patient in my own experience of approximately 725 operative AVM cases. Any subsequent retreatment expense for residual AVM must be added to the primary modality.
3. The definition of eloquent cortex is changing. Functional magnetic resonance imaging and intraoperative mapping techniques offer the potential to expand surgical therapy to subgroups of patients previously denied such possibilities.
4. Strategic embolization can substantially lessen morbidity. It is essential that this modality be deployed in a very strategic fashion. In certain large high-flow lesions, progressive throttling of inflow can prevent life-threatening hemodynamic disturbances postoperatively. In some patients, embolization of deep-feeding pedicles, particularly the posterior cerebral artery or perforating distributions, can clearly be of great benefit to the surgeon. In patients suffering significant intracranial hemorrhage, the early embolization of intranidal aneurysms might well diminish the risk of early rebleeding. Finally, in certain circumstances, the endovascular devascularization of an eloquent plane might be of substantial benefit.

5. Microsurgical resection of arteriovenous malformations has become much safer in the last few years.
6. Embolization is rarely curative (two cases over a 17-year practice experience).
7. Radiosurgery, when performed with appropriate case selection, can achieve a high rate of cure (approximately 90%), but this cure rate is possible only in small lesions that would be cured in approximately 100% of surgical cases.
8. Postoperative deficits, if present, tend to improve over time.
9. Subgroups may have a worse natural history than reported in the Troupp series (intranidal aneurysm, venous stenosis).

THE CASE AGAINST MICROSURGICAL TREATMENT

There are many circumstances in which surgery is clearly contraindicated. In the following summary, I will attempt to provide a balancing argument against surgical therapy in general.

1. Surgical therapy is "invasive."
2. Surgical therapy is "expensive." It is also clear that primary embolization requires repetitive follow-up angiography, as does radiosurgery, thus significantly adding to the expense of the primary therapy. Any subsequent retreatment expense for residual AVM must be added to the primary modality.
3. There is always a risk of perioperative hemorrhage as a result of residual AVM, venous infarction, or hyperemia.
4. "Minor" deficits may be disastrous for certain patients.
5. High-level experience and skill are required to achieve good outcome (surgeon-specific).
6. Each component of therapy has risk. Embolization carries a 5 to 10% risk of ischemic or hemorrhagic complication.
7. Poor case selection is disastrous.
8. Intact patients tolerate postoperative deficits and extended rehabilitation very poorly.
9. Surgery probably carries a higher risk of producing some deficit than other treatment modalities.
10. The natural history of many patients is benign.

SUMMARY

Thus, it is clear that intracranial AVMs are a complex and heterogeneous condition, as are the patients they afflict. There is no true single strategy that is successful in even a majority of patients. The process of evaluation and management of AVM patients is a very strong argument for the creation of a "stroke center" in which a multidisciplinary team of cerebrovascular practitioners interacts collegially and effectively on a day-to-day basis for the management of the gamut of ischemic and hemorrhagic stroke problems.

REFERENCES

1. Batjer HH, Samson DS: Surgery of arteriovenous malformations, in Dudley H, Carter DC, Russell RGC (eds): *Operative Surgery*. London, Butterworth, 1989, ed 4, pp 219–230.
2. Heros RC, Korosue K, Diebold PM: Surgical excision of cerebral arteriovenous malformations: Late results. **Neurosurgery** 26:570–578, 1990.
3. Ondra SL, Troupp H, George ED, Schwab K: The natural history of symptomatic arteriovenous malformations of the brain: 24 year follow-up assessment. **J Neurosurg** 65:387–391, 1990.
4. Samson DS, Batjer HH: Preoperative evaluation of the risk/benefit ratio for arteriovenous malformations of the brain. In Williams RH, Rengachary SS (eds): *Neurosurgery Update II: Vascular, Spinal, Pediatric and Functional Neurosurgery*. New York, McGraw-Hill, 1991, pp 129–133.
5. Spetzler RF, Martin NA: A proposed grading system for arteriovenous malformations. **J Neurosurg** 65:476–483, 1986.

CHAPTER

24

Honored Guest Presentation: Therapeutic Carotid Occlusion

MICHAEL J. LINK, M.D., THOMAS A. TOMSICK, M.D., AND JOHN M. TEW, JR., M.D.

Therapeutic carotid occlusion has a long history in the treatment of unclippable cerebral artery aneurysms. The indications and techniques for performing this procedure have evolved significantly during the past 30 years. Advances in microsurgical techniques for direct repair or to perform trapping and bypass procedures have greatly expanded the available treatment options for many previously inoperable aneurysms. Improvements in endovascular techniques to occlude the parent vessel temporarily or permanently, as well as clinical and quantitative measures to assess collateral cerebral blood flow, have likewise helped develop safer treatment strategies for these difficult lesions. Significant controversy continues to exist regarding the use of universal versus selective revascularization. At the University of Cincinnati, temporary balloon occlusion (TBO) testing is performed when therapeutic carotid occlusion is considered. Bypass, usually a saphenous vein from the external carotid to middle cerebral artery, is reserved for patients who are unable to tolerate parent vessel occlusion. We have found this protocol to be very safe and the most cost-effective approach.

HISTORY

Proximal or Hunterian ligation for treatment of cerebral aneurysms was reported more than 100 years ago. In 1907, Beadles reported that Horsley discovered a right internal carotid artery (ICA) aneurysm during an intracranial exploration that he subsequently treated by ligating the common carotid artery (5). Five years after the operation, the patient was "in extremely good health" (5). Nattrass, in 1928, presumed an aneurysm in the cavernous sinus was causing cranial nerve palsies and performed ICA ligation with improvement in the patient's clinical symptoms (42). Matas, in 1911, probably deserves credit for the first trial occlusion of the carotid artery to test collateral circulation using an aluminum metal band (34). The concept of staged or slow occlusion of the carotid artery to allow development of collateral circulation prompted Dandy in 1942 to recommend ligation of the ICA in two separate stages, 1 week apart (11). This also heralded the development of the adjustable clamp by Selverstone and White (56) and Crutchfield (10) in the 1950s. Most patients treated during this time did not undergo a trial occlusion, and many were treated following subarachnoid hemorrhage (SAH). Not surprisingly, the ischemic complication rate was substantial. The cooperative study reported a 41% complication rate with ICA ligation and a 24% complication rate with common carotid artery ligation (44). Although carotid occlusion did provide some protection against further SAH, as evidenced by the 8% incidence of recurrent SAH among 567 patients treated in the cooperative study (44), clearly further advances in treatment options and patient selection were required. The adoption of the operating microscope and development of microsurgical techniques have made nearly all intracranial aneurysms amenable to direct repair. Currently, the principal controversy surrounding treatment of unclippable intracranial aneurysms involves the necessity of revascularization following parent vessel sacrifice.

The indications for therapeutic carotid occlusion have likewise expanded in recent decades. Initially, this treatment was reserved for unclippable aneurysms of the anterior circulation. Currently, most unclippable carotid aneurysms are located partially or entirely within the cavernous sinus. Most intracavernous carotid aneurysms are asymptomatic and require no surgical treatment unless there is substantive subarachnoid extension of the dome of the aneurysm. Symptomatic intracavernous aneurysms usually present with signs of cranial neuropathy as a result of partial thrombosis or enlargement of the aneurysm. Treatment is then recommended.

Tumors may invade the cavernous sinus, and meningiomas are the most common type. The carotid artery may be encircled or constricted by the invasive process. Surgical attempts to achieve a total removal of these tumors are seldom associated with cure and result in high morbidity, largely as a result of cranial nerve palsies and other neurologic complications. For these reasons, we believe that carotid sacrifice and bypass grafting is not indicated for the treatment of these lesions. Radical resection followed by postoperative radiation is the treatment of choice (46).

In the treatment of carotid-cavernous (C-C) fistulas, preservation of ICA flow is the goal in every procedure. However, patency is maintained in only 70 to 85% of cases of direct C-C fistulas in major series (4, 6, 7, 9, 12, 24, 28, 29, 31, 38, 43, 47, 54, 55). Neurologic complications, largely related to age, are seldom the result of ischemic complications associated with carotid occlusion. In our series, purposeful occlusion of the carotid artery was associated with no incidence of cerebral ischemia (62). It is important to note that occlusion of the ostia of the fistula must accompany proximal carotid occlusion to avoid steal or shunting of blood from the hemisphere (62).

QUESTIONS

There are many concerns regarding selective revascularization when therapeutic carotid occlusion is being considered. These include:

- Is TBO safe? That is, does the information provided by the test outweigh its risk?
- Can TBO accurately predict which patients are at risk for ischemic complications from permanent balloon occlusion (PBO)?
- When compared with universal revascularization without preoperative TBO, does selective revascularization carry less morbidity and mortality?
- Is selective revascularization cost-effective?

UNIVERSITY OF CINCINNATI PROCEDURE AND RESULTS

One of the principal concerns regarding selective revascularization is the ability to predict which patients will tolerate therapeutic carotid occlusion without immediate or delayed ischemia. At the University of Cincinnati, patients undergo a TBO test using a nondetachable silicone balloon catheter (NDSB) (*Fig. 24.1*) (63). The balloon is inflated to occlude the ICA following heparin anticoagulation. Collateral blood flow is evaluated by selective angiography, and the mean arterial pressure is reduced 25 to 30%. During the time the artery is occluded, the patient undergoes continuous clinical neurologic testing of motor, sensory, cognitive, and visual function. Previously, technetium hexylmethyl-propylene amineoxine (TcHMPAO) single photon emission computed tomography (SPECT) imaging was performed to assess qualitative asymmetries in cerebral blood flow (CBF) during carotid occlusion. More recently, xenon-enhanced CT, which allows for a quantitative measure of CBF, has been used. This is likely a better predictor of hypoperfusion and risk of stroke with sacrifice of a carotid artery (32, 68).

This diagnostic and treatment paradigm has proven to be very safe when a nondetachable silicone balloon is used. Between 1993 and 1998, 103 TBOs of the ICA were performed (37). No ICA dissections or permanent ischemia due to the balloon were encountered. One patient (0.97%) developed confusion, agitation, and left hemiparesis 36 hours after TBO testing of the left ICA for a giant aneurysm. Repeat arteri-

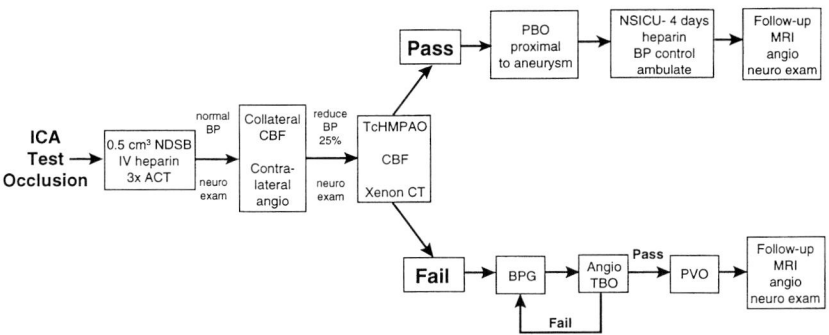

FIG. 24.1. Temporary balloon occlusion test protocol used at the Departments of Neurosurgery and Neuroradiology, University of Cincinnati Medical Center.

ography showed long-segment intimal dissection of the right carotid artery with near occlusion of the vessel lumen, presumably secondary to intimal injury during the diagnostic right common carotid artery injection, which had been performed at the time of the left TBO. The patient underwent an urgent right superficial temporal to middle cerebral artery bypass graft with some resolution of deficits over 2 months. Another patient experienced transient confusion and agitation 20 to 30 minutes following deflation of the balloon and before SPECT scanning could be performed. Neurological examination was nonfocal. The patient regained normal mental status within several hours with supportive care only.

Combining clinical neurologic examination with qualitative cerebral perfusion evaluation via TcHMPAO SPECT during TBO has also proven very reliable in predicting which patients will tolerate permanent ICA occlusion. No acute or delayed ischemia has occurred in the past 6 years in 19 (of 29) patients evaluated with symmetric perfusion on SPECT during TBO testing who then went on to have PBO of the ICA. Of 10 patients with asymmetric perfusion, bypass grafts were performed prior to PBO in 5 patients. Five patients underwent occlusion despite asymmetric perfusion, having passed 30 minutes of TBO, including hypotensive challenge. Infarcts developed in 2 patients because of hypoperfusion. Both were maintained after vessel occlusion with systolic blood pressure greater than 180 mm Hg and full anticoagulation (3× accelerated clotting time) for 48 hours after the procedure. One became ischemic at 12 hours, and the other became ischemic at 60 hours. Both received emergency bypass grafts. One other patient with minimal asymmetry on SPECT and no neurologic deficits during trial occlusion developed a likely thromboembolic stroke at 52 hours (63). Thus, PBO can be safely performed after TBO without clinical deterioration and symmetrical SPECT scan or xenon-enhanced CT CBF greater than 30 cm^3/100 g/min. For patients with asymmetric SPECT studies or CBF less than 30 cm^3/100 g/min, the risk of ischemic complications is increased, and careful individual patient selection is required.

Long-term sequela of permanent vessel occlusion without revascularization is also a concern. Most notably, the risk of delayed stroke and SAH as a result of de novo aneurysm formation has been examined. Seventy-six patients were treated at the University of Cincinnati with PBO of the ICA for unclippable aneurysms between 1978 and 1997. Sixty patients surviving at least 6 months have been followed-up (mean 94 months, median 112 months). Total follow-up for the 60 patients is 468 patient-years. Four delayed infarcts occurred (0.8/100 patient-years follow-up) at 6, 24, 30, and 60 months after treatment. Three of the four infarcts occurred in patients treated for clinoidal or ophthalmic segment ICA aneurysms, wherein the aneurysm neck was not trapped. The incidence of stroke for extradural ICA aneurysms was 0.3 per 100 patient-years follow-up. SAH, as a result of new anterior communicating artery aneurysms, have occurred in two patients (0.4/100 patient-years follow-up). An additional asymptomatic, unruptured posterior communicating artery aneurysm has been discovered and treated. Therefore, delayed stroke and de novo aneurysm formation are rare and not prohibitive when PBO of the ICA is considered for unclippable aneurysms (64).

Finally, in the current medicoeconomic environment, the issue of cost-effectiveness deserves consideration. Acute treatment cost analysis, derived from a population of eight patients treated with PBO and four patients treated with saphenous vein bypass graft and parent vessel occlusion (BPG-PVO) for symptomatic extradural ICA aneurysms between March 1995 and July 1996 at the University of Cincinnati, was performed. Actual acute treatment hospital costs, theoretical costs of complications, quality of life changes, and follow-up costs were considered. For PBO with symmetric SPECT perfusion scan, expected treatment costs are $30,723. For the BPG-PVO paradigm without any surgical complications, treatment costs are $36,438. When quality-adjusted life years (QALYs) are calculated, the expected treatment charges for PBO are $2,226 per QALY. For BPG-PVO, the treatment charges are $2,791 per QALY. In this subgroup of patients with symptomatic extradural ICA aneurysms, the most economical and effective treatment is PBO of the ICA if the following conditions are met: (1) no neurological deficit is elicited during TBO testing, (2) symmetric blood flow to both hemispheres is seen during TcHMPAO SPECT, or (3) CBF is greater than 30 cm³/100 g/min as documented with xenon-enhanced CT (63).

DISCUSSION

TBO with clinical testing and qualitative or quantitative assessment of CBF, followed by PBO in appropriately selected patients, is a safe, reliable, effective, and cost-effective treatment paradigm when therapeutic carotid occlusion is considered for a wide range of pathologies. The greatest experience to date is in treating unclippable aneurysms of the anterior circulation. However, the same principles apply in considering treatment for other vascular or neoplastic lesions.

Mathis et al. reported their experience with 500 TBO tests using a variety of balloon catheters (36). Clinical examination during a 15-minute TBO was combined, when possible, with xenon-enhanced CT CBF analysis. A total of 16 (3.2%) complications occurred. Eight patients (1.6%) remained asymptomatic from six dissections, one middle cerebral artery embolus, and one pseudoaneurysm. These complications were discovered on follow-up angiography or at the time of surgery. In the symptomatic group (n = 8), six (1.2%) neurologic deficits were transient and two (0.4%) were permanent. There were no deaths in this series (36). Several other much smaller series also reported low complication rates from TBO testing of 0 to 8.3%, with an average of 2.2% neurologic complications for 181 procedures performed (2, 17, 20, 40, 41, 48, 57). Horowitz et al. recently reported their experience with 88 TBOs over a 4-year period, noting a 4.5% incidence of carotid dissections with 1.1% permanent neurological deficits and a 1.1% mortality (25).

A recent review of 103 patients who underwent TBO testing at the University of Cincinnati using an NDSB catheter revealed no carotid artery injury or complication, including cerebral infarction related to the TBO itself (37). Thus, TBO testing seems safe and carries a risk comparable with that of conventional angiography (13, 16). Further experience with the NDSB will likely reduce reported complication results even further, as this catheter system is the most compliant and generates minimal pressure on the vessel wall when inflated beyond the volume needed to occlude the vessel (35).

Long-term complications are likewise rare when considering permanent carotid occlusion. Rates for delayed infarct after ICA or common carotid artery occlusion to treat unclippable aneurysms ranged from 0.1 to 1.9 infarcts per 100 years follow-up in various series reported over the last 33 years (19, 27, 33, 45, 50, 52, 64) (*Table 24.1*). SAH as a result of de novo aneurysm formation is also uncommon, occurring at a rate of 0.4 per 100 years follow-up in 510 patients reported in 11 publi-

TABLE 24.1
Delayed Infarct after PVO

Reference	Aneurysms Treated (n)	Infarcts	Mean Follow-up (years)	Infarcts/100 years Follow-up
German and Black (19)	14 ICA	1	10.8	0.1
Kak et al. (27)	89 ICA, CCA[a]	1	6.7	0.6
Love and Dart (33)	22 ICA	2	13.0	0.7
Oldershaw and Voris (45)	21 ICA	2	5.2	1.9
Polin et al. (50)[b]	34 ICA	1	2.7	1.1
Roski et al (52)	18 ICA	2	12.5	1.1
Tomsick et al. (64)[c]	60 ICA	4	7.3	0.8
TOTAL	258	13	8.3	0.9

[a]CCA, common carotid artery.
[b]Two instances of delayed blindness were not included.
[c]Technetium hexylmethylpropylene amineoxine single photon emission computed tomography cerebral blood flow testing was performed in 24 of these cases.

cations. SAH occurred an average of 9.6 years after treatment (64) (*Table 24.2*). These low cumulative incidences are insufficient to support the recommendation of universal revascularization. Also note that extracranial-intracranial (EC-IC) bypass is not a guarantee against significant hemodynamic changes occurring in the cerebral circulation following carotid sacrifice. There is at least one report of a contralateral giant cavernous ICA aneurysm enlarging after a partial ligation of the ICA combined with an EC-IC bypass on the other side (18).

In addition to being safe, TBO is also reliable in predicting which patients will be best served by revascularization and which will tolerate permanent vessel occlusion. ICA sacrifice without TBO testing carries a high rate of morbidity. Linskey et al. found a cumulative stroke rate of 26% and mortality of 12% in their literature review (32). A literature review of ICA sacrifice after clinical passage of a TBO test revealed a 4.7% stroke rate and no mortality in 192 patients (1, 2, 17, 23, 65). Whether adding qualitative or quantitative assessment of CBF during the test adds to its predictability has not been proved, but CBF assessment carries little to no risk, depending on the test used (SPECT versus xenon-enhanced CT) and may detect patients who will tolerate acute carotid occlusion but still be at slightly higher risk of ischemic complications.

Lawton et al. promote universal revascularization for patients with complex aneurysms treated by PVO (30). In their series of 61 patients treated over 9 years with a variety of revascularization techniques, 93% experienced good outcomes and 2% died. Specifically, 1 patient experi-

TABLE 24.2
New Aneurysm Development after PVO

Reference	Aneurysms Treated (n)	New Aneurysms (n)	SAH Occurrence (years after PVO)	Incidental Aneurysms (years after PVO)	SAH Occurrence/ 100 years Follow-up
Clark and Ray (8)	NA	3	3 (14, 16, 18)	0	NA
Fujiwara et al. (18)	27 ICA	2	2 (8,9)	0	0.7
German and Black (19)	14 ICA	2	1 (15.5)	1 (20)	0.5
Kak et al. (27)	25 ICA	0	0	0	0
Miller et al. (39)	72 ICA	2	2	0	NA
Oldershaw and Voris (45)	21 ICA	0	0	0	0
Roski et al. (52)	18 ICA	1	1 (3)	0	0.4
Salar and Mingrino (53)	126[a]	2	2 (9, 15)	0	NA
Somach and Shenkin (58)	6 ICA	2	1 (7)	1 (8)	NA
Wright and Sweet (66)	144[a]	2	2 (6, 9)	0	NA
Tomsick et al. (64)	59 ICA	3	2 (2,3)	1 (6)	0.4
TOTAL	509	19	16	3	0.4

[a]ICA and common carotid artery were not distinguished.

enced early graft occlusion with hemiparesis and stroke, and 3 patients had strokes of presumed thromboembolic etiology in the perioperative period, 2 of whom died within 2 months of the operation. Epidural hematoma was the most common surgical complication (n = 5) (30). Overall, these are outstanding results in an extremely challenging patient population. However, there is some concern that these results would be difficult to duplicate at many neurosurgical centers (21, 49). In fact, by their own literature review, in the past, cervical carotid artery ligation and EC-IC bypass resulted in excellent or good outcome in 77% of patients (range 40–89%), fair or poor outcome in 14% (range 0–50%), and mortality averaged 9% (range 0–20%) (14, 22, 26, 59, 60, 67). They believe the results are better and more comparable with their own in more recent series (3, 15). However, it must also be considered that bypass is performed infrequently as the results of the EC-IC bypass study failed to show a benefit for ischemic stroke (61) and the widespread technical experience may not be available to maintain low morbidity and mortality for this challenging procedure. The only long-term analysis of bypass graft durability revealed a 1.7% per year rate of delayed occlusion, with 20% of these producing symptoms owing to the occlusion (51). This result certainly must be included when the efficacy of a universal revascularization paradigm is considered.

Most notably, the series of Lawton et al. demonstrates that the majority of ischemic complications (75% in their series) (30) following PVO likely result from embolic events rather than poor perfusion. Bypass has never been shown to reduce the risk of embolic complications following proximal vessel occlusion, probably explaining why no benefit could be demonstrated for the population studied in the EC-IC bypass trial (61). Instead, more careful consideration of where the vessel is occluded in relation to collateral circulation, as well as the judicious use of anticoagulation therapy after occlusion, cannot be overemphasized. Anticoagulation therapy must be limited around the time of craniotomy, and careful planning is necessary when considering the timing of PVO following bypass.

CONCLUSION

We favor TBO testing followed by therapeutic carotid occlusion if the patient has no clinical changes during 30 minutes of test occlusion. We have used TcHMPAO SPECT with a hypotensive challenge in the past and, more recently, xenon-enhanced CT to assist in assessing patients who might be at slightly increased risk of future ischemia. We reserve revascularization in cases of therapeutic carotid occlusion for the following clinical situations: 1) patients who clinically fail their TBO testing or have CBF less than 30 cm^3/100 g/min based on xenon-enhanced CT (we consider revascularization in patients who clinically pass their TBO but have asymmetry on SPECT scanning if xenon-enhanced CT has not been performed); 2) patients following SAH because of the increased risk of aggravating vasospasm with PVO alone; 3) patients who have contralateral carotid aneurysms that would be subject to increased hemodynamic stress potentially with contralateral carotid occlusion; 4) patients with isolated middle cerebral artery circulation on their initial diagnostic angiogram in our experience rarely tolerate trial occlusion and are best served by proceeding with EC-IC bypass. Typically, for all of these scenarios, we prefer the high-flow saphenous vein bypass from the external carotid artery to an M2 branch of the middle carotid artery. In our experience, TBO testing followed by selective revascularization is safe, reliable, and cost-effective.

REFERENCES

1. Andrews JC, Valvanis A, Fisch U: Management of the internal carotid artery in surgery of the skull base. **Laryngoscope** 99:1224–1229, 1989.

2. Anon VV, Aymard A, Gobin YP, et al.: Balloon occlusion of the internal carotid artery in 40 cases of giant intracavernous aneurysm: Technical aspects, cerebral monitoring and results. **Neuroradiology** 34:245–251, 1992.
3. Ausman JI, Diaz FG, Sadasivan B, Gonzeles-Portillo M Jr, Malik GM, Deopujari CE: Giant intracranial aneurysm surgery: The role of microvascular reconstruction. **Surg Neurol** 34:8–15, 1990.
4. Barrow D, Fleischer AS, Hoffman JC: Complications of detachable balloon catheter technique in the treatment of traumatic intracranial arteriovenous fistulas. **J Neurosurg** 56:3967–4003, 1982.
5. Beadles CF: Aneurysms of the larger cerebral arteries. **Brain** 30:285–386, 1907.
6. Benati A, Maschio A, Penni S, Beltramello A: Treatment of post-traumatic carotid-cavernous fistula using a detachable balloon catheter. **J Neurosurg** 53:784–786, 1980.
7. Berthelsen B, Svendsen P: Treatment of direct carotid-cavernous fistulas with detachable balloons. **Acta Radiol** 28:683–691, 1987.
8. Clark WC, Ray MW: Contralateral intracranial aneurysm formation as a late complication of carotid ligation. **Surg Neurol** 18:458–462, 1982.
9. Corradino G, Gellad FE, Salcman M: Traumatic carotid-cavernous fistula. **South Med J** 81:660–663, 1988.
10. Crutchfield WG: Instruments for use in the treatment of certain intracranial vascular lesions. **J Neurosurg** 16:471–474, 1959.
11. Dandy WE: Results following ligation of the internal carotid artery. **Arch Surg** 45:521–533, 1942.
12. Debrun G, Lacour P, Vinuela F, et al.: Treatment of 54 traumatic carotid-cavernous fistulas. **J Neurosurg** 55:678–692, 1981.
13. Dion JE, Gates PC, Fox AJ, Barnett HJM, Blom RJ: Clinical events following neuroangiography: A prospective study. **Stroke** 18:997–1004, 1987.
14. Drake CG: Giant intracranial aneurysms: Experience with surgical treatment in 174 patients. **Clin Neurosurg** 26:12–95, 1979.
15. Drake CG, Peerless SJ, Ferguson GG: Hunterian proximal arterial occlusion for giant aneurysms of the carotid circulation. **J Neurosurg** 81:656–665, 1994.
16. Ernest F, Forbes G, Sandok BA, et al.: Complications of cerebral angiography: Prospective assessment of risk. **Am J Roentgenol** 142:247–253, 1984.
17. Fox AJ, Vinuela F, Pelz DM, et al.: Use of detachable balloons for proximal artery occlusion in the treatment of unclippable cerebral aneurysms. **J Neurosurg** 66:40–46, 1987.
18. Fujiwara S, Fujii K, Fukui M: De novo aneurysm formation and aneurysm growth following therapeutic carotid occlusion for intracranial internal carotid artery (ICA) aneurysms. **Acta Neurochir** 120:20–25, 1993.
19. German WJ, Black SPW: Cervical ligation for internal carotid aneurysm: An extended follow-up. **J Neurosurg** 23:572–577, 1965.
20. Gonzalez CF, Moret J: Balloon occlusion of the carotid artery prior to surgery for neck tumors. **Am J Neuroradiol** 11:649–652, 1990.
21. Heros RC: Revascularization and aneurysm surgery (comment). **Neurosurgery** 38:93–94, 1996.
22. Heros RC: Management of giant paraclinoid aneurysms, in Kikuchi H, Fukushima T, Watanabe K (eds): *Intracranial Aneurysms*. Niigata, Nishimura Co., 1986, pp 273–282.
23. Higashida RT, Halback VV, Dowd C, et al.: Endovascular detachable balloon embolization therapy of cavernous carotid artery aneurysm: Results in 87 cases. **J Neurosurg** 72:857–863, 1990.

24. Higashida R, Halbach V, Tsai FY, et al.: Interventional neurovascular treatment of traumatic carotid and vertebral artery lesions. **Am J Roentgenol** 153:577–582, 1989.
25. Horowitz MB, Dutton K, Purdy PD: Assessment of complication types and rates related to diagnostic angiography and interventional neuroradiologic procedures: A four year review (1993–1996). **Int Neuroradiol** 4:27–37, 1998.
26. Hosobuchi Y: Giant intracranial aneurysms, in Wilkings RH, Rengachary SS (eds): *Neurosurgery*. New York, McGraw-Hill, 1985, pp 1404–1414.
27. Kak VK, Taylor AR, Gordon DS: Proximal carotid ligation for internal carotid aneurysms. **J Neurosurg** 39:503–512, 1973.
28. Kendall B: Results of treatment of AVF with the Debrun technique. **Am J Neuroradiol** 4:405–409, 1983.
29. Kupersmith MJ, Berenstein A, Flamm E, Ransohoff J: Neuroophthalmologic abnormalities and intravascular therapy of traumatic carotid cavernous fistulas. **Ophthalmology** 93:906–912, 1986.
30. Lawton MT, Hamilton MG, Morcos JJ, Spetzler RF: Revascularization and aneurysm surgery: Current techniques, indications and outcome. **Neurosurgery** 38:83–94, 1996.
31. Lewis AI, Tomsick TA, Tew JM: Management of 100 direct carotid-cavernous fistulas: Results of treatment with detachable balloons. **Neurosurgery** 36:239–245, 1995.
32. Linskey ME, Jungreis CA, Yonas H, Hirsch WL, Sekhar LN, Horton JA: Stroke risk after abrupt internal carotid artery sacrifice: Accuracy of preoperative assessment with balloon test occlusion and stable xenon-enhanced CT. **Am J Neuroradiol** 15:829–843, 1994.
33. Love DG, Dart LH: Results of carotid ligation with particular reference to intracranial aneurysms. **J Neurosurg** 27:89–93, 1967.
34. Matas R: Testing, the efficiency of the collateral circulation as a preliminary to the occlusion of the great surgical arteries. **Ann Surg** 53:1–43, 1911.
35. Mathis JM, Barr JD, Horton JA: Physical characteristics of balloon catheter systems used in temporary cerebral artery occlusion. **Am J Neuroradiol** 15:1831–1836, 1994.
36. Mathis JM, Barr JD, Jungreis CA, Yonas H, et al.: Temporary balloon test occlusion of the internal carotid artery: Experience in 500 cases. **Am J Neuroradiol** 16:749–754, 1995.
37. Meyer PM, Thakur GA, Tomsick TA: Temporary endovascular balloon occlusion of the internal carotid artery with a non-detachable silicone balloon catheter: Analysis of technique and cost. *Am J Neuroradiol* 20:559–564, 1999.
38. Mickle JP, Quisling RG: Balloon embolization of highflow traumatic arteriovenous fistulae to the brain. **J Fla Med Assoc** 69:767–774, 1982.
39. Miller JD, Jawad K, Jennett B: Safety of carotid occlusion and its role in the management of intracranial aneurysms. **J Neurol Neurosurg Psychiatry** 40:64–72, 1977.
40. Monsein LH, Jeffery PJ, VanHeerden BB, et al.: Assessing adequacy of collateral circulation during balloon test occlusion of the internal carotid artery with 99MTc-HMPAO SPECT. **Am J Neuroradiol** 12:1045–1051, 1991.
41. Moody EB, Dawson RC, Sandler MD: 99MTc-HMPAO SPECT imaging in interventional neuroradiology: Validation of balloon test occlusion. **Am J Neuroradiol** 9:533–538, 1988.
42. Nattrass FJ: Aneurysm of carotid artery in cavernous sinus: Ligature of internal carotid artery; recovery. **Edinb Med J** 35:30–32, 1928.

43. Negoro M, Kageyama N, Isiguchi T: Cerebrovascular occlusion by catheterization and embolization. **Am J Neuroradiol** 4:362–365, 1983.
44. Nishioka H: Report on the cooperative study of intracranial aneurysms and subarachnoid hemorrhage. Section VIII, Part 1: Results of the treatment of intracranial aneurysms by occlusion of the carotid artery in the neck. **J Neurosurg** 25:660–682, 1966.
45. Oldershaw JB, Voris HC: Internal carotid ligation: A follow-up study. **Neurology** 16:351–363, 1966.
46. O'Sullivan MG, van Loveren HR, Tew JM Jr: Surgical resectability of meningiomas of the cavernous sinus. **Neurosurgery** 40:238–247, 1997.
47. Peeters FLM: Treatment of 20 direct carotid cavernous fistula. **Diagn Imaging** 52:137–140, 1983.
48. Peterman SB, Taylor A, Hoffman JC: Improved detection of cerebral hypoperfusion with internal carotid balloon test occlusion and 99MTc-HMPAO cerebral perfusion SPECT imaging. **Am J Neuroradiol** 12:1035–1041, 1991.
49. Piepgras DG: Revascularization and aneurysm surgery (comment). **Neurosurgery** 38:92, 1996.
50. Polin RS, Shaffrey ME, Jensen ME, et al.: Medical management in the endovascular treatment of carotid-cavernous aneurysms. **J Neurosurg** 84:755–761, 1996.
51. Regli L, Piepgras DG, Hansen KK: Late patency of long saphenous vein bypass grafts to the anterior and posterior cerebral circulation. **J Neurosurg** 83:806–811, 1995.
52. Roski RA, Spetzler RF, Nulsen FE: Late complications of carotid ligation in the treatment of intracranial aneurysm. **J Neurosurg** 54:583–587, 1981.
53. Salar G, Mingrino S: Development of intracranial saccular aneurysm: Report of two cases. **Neurosurgery** 8:462–465, 1981.
54. Santhosh J, Rao VRK, Ravimandalam K, Gupta AK, Madhavan Unni N, Srinvasa Rao A: Endovascular management of carotid cavernous fistula: Observation on angiographic and clinical result. **Acta Neurol Scand** 88:320–326, 1993.
55. Scialfa G, Valsecchi F, Scotti G: Treatment of vascular lesions with balloon catheters. **Am J Neuroradiol** 4:395–398, 1983.
56. Selverstone B, White JC: A method for gradual occlusion of the internal carotid artery in the treatment of aneurysm. **Proc N Engl Cardiovasc Soc** 9:24, 1952.
57. Simonson TM, Ryals TJ, Yuh WTC, Farrar GP, Rezai K, Hoffman HT: MR imaging and HMPAO scintigraphy in conjunction with balloon test occlusion: Value in predicting sequelae after permanent carotid occlusion. **Am J Roentgenol** 159:1063–1068, 1992.
58. Somach FM, Shenkin AH: Angiographic end-results of carotid ligation in the treatment of carotid aneurysm. **J Neurosurg** 24:966–974, 1966.
59. Spetzler RF, Carter LP: Revascularization and aneurysm surgery: Current status. **Neurosurgery** 16:111–116, 1985.
60. Sundt TM Jr, Piepgras DG, Marsh WR, Fode NC: Saphenous vein bypass grafts for giant aneurysms and intracranial occlusive disease. **J Neurosurg** 65:439–450, 1986.
61. The EC/IC Bypass Study Group: Failure of extracranial-intracranial arterial bypass to reduce the risk of ischemic stroke. **N Engl J Med** 313:1191–1200, 1985.
62. Tomsick TA: Type A direct CCF: Transarterial balloon occlusion, in Tomsick TA (ed): *Carotid Cavernous Fistula*. Cincinnati, Digital Educational Publishing, Inc., 1997, pp 115–144.
63. Tomsick TA, Auffrey C, van Loveren H, Tew JM Jr: Cost-effectiveness of treatment of unclippable extradural internal carotid artery aneurysm. **J Neurovasc Dis** 2:149–162, 1997.
64. Tomsick TA, van Loveren H, Tew JM Jr, Larson J: Delayed complications of balloon

occlusion of the internal carotid artery for unclippable aneurysm. **J Neurovasc Dis** 2:64–67, 1997.
65. Weil SM, van Loveren HR, Tomsick TA, Quallen BL, Tew JM: Management of inoperable cerebral aneurysms by the navigational balloon techniques. **Neurosurgery** 21:296–301, 1987.
66. Wright RL, Sweet WH: Carotid or vertebral occlusion in the treatment of intracranial aneurysms. **Clin Neurosurg** 9:163–192, 1961.
67. Yasargil MG: Giant intracranial aneurysms, in Yasargil MG (ed): *Microneurosurgery,* Stuttgart, George Thieme, 1984, vol 2, p 304.
68. Yonas H, Linskey ME, Johnson DW, et al.: Internal carotid balloon test occlusion does require quantitative CBF. **Am J Neuroradiol** 13:1147–1148, 1992.

CHAPTER

25

Therapeutic Carotid Occlusion: The Case for Prophylactic Bypass

A. GIANCARLO VISHTEH, M.D., CARGILL H. ALLEYNE, JR., M.D., AND ROBERT F. SPETZLER, M.D.

> A carotid is a terrible thing to waste. . . .
> —O. Al-Mefty

Management of the internal carotid artery (ICA) in the setting of involvement by complex pathologies (aneurysm, tumors, dissection) remains controversial. Historically, Hunterian ligation of the common carotid artery (CCA) and the cervical ICA was used to treat aneurysms and carotid-cavernous fistulas of the ICA. The literature is replete with reports of successful ICA ligation in such settings. Contemporary experience, however, suggests that *acute* ligation of the ICA is associated with a relatively high rate of stroke. In the Aneurysm Cooperative Study, this rate was 30 to 37% (15).

With the awareness that acute carotid ligation is not as benign as once thought, it became imperative to determine which patients could potentially tolerate occlusion of the ICA before its actual sacrifice. With the explosion of technology in the fields of neuroimaging, neurophysiological monitoring, and neuroendovascular therapy, a number of tests (e.g., balloon occlusion test [BOT]) were designed. Advances in the fields of microsurgery and revascularization, which paralleled those in the fields of neuroimaging and endovascular therapy, also provided neurovascular surgeons with the added option of bypassing a diseased ICA segment if primary surgical management was deemed impossible.

With the development of these sophisticated testing and revascularization techniques, two schools of thought have evolved regarding the sacrifice of the ICA. One recommends *selective* revascularization based on results of BOT. The other favors *universal* (prophylactic) bypass for all who are to undergo ICA sacrifice. Controversies revolve around how sensitive ICA occlusion tests are in predicting who can tolerate ICA sacrifice and the feasibility of prophylactic bypass for all who are to undergo elective ICA sacrifice. This article reviews the issues surrounding each management scheme.

PATHOLOGIES THAT MAY REQUIRE ICA SACRIFICE

Disease processes can arise from the ICA or involve it indirectly. "Inoperable" aneurysms have been the major primary pathology for which ICA sacrifice has been recommended. Today, however, it is important that an experienced neurovascular surgeon or neuroendovascular specialist determine whether a lesion is inoperable, because advances and expertise in both fields may render direct surgical or endovascular intervention feasible. Furthermore, although some purely cavernous segment ICA aneurysms may be labeled as inoperable, no intervention may be required unless the patient is symptomatic (e.g., has worsening cranial nerve deficits). The term "inoperable" in such cases, therefore, is moot. Other than aneurysms, primary pathologies of the ICA that may require its sacrifice include symptomatic medically refractory dissections as well as carotid cavernous fistulas that are unamenable to direct surgical or endovascular therapies.

Frequently, head, neck, and cranial-base tumors can encroach on or encase the ICA or CCA. In the case of benign cranial-base tumors (meningiomas), it has long been our philosophy to attempt to preserve the ICA or any other major parent vessel involved with the tumor. If an arachnoidal dissection plane is discernible between the tumor and the artery, preservation of the vessel may be feasible with microsurgical techniques. This strategy, however, can be very dangerous, especially in perforator-rich segments of intracranial arteries. Because meningiomas cannot truly be cured, we favor leaving small amounts of tumor on a vessel if it cannot be easily dissected off the vessel and avoid revascularization for these benign tumors. The single exception to this rule, however, would be a meningioma that completely encases and occludes the ICA in a patient with ischemic symptoms. In such cases, a distal revascularization procedure is performed after documentation of compromised blood flow on a testing modality (e.g., xenon computed tomography cerebral flow ([Xe CT CBF], single photon emission computed tomography [SPECT], or positron emission tomography) followed by tumor resection.

When the ICA is involved with a malignant tumor, the strategy of ICA preservation during aggressive tumor resection is virtually impossible and frankly dangerous (1, 5). With no true arachnoidal plane between malignant tumors and arteries, aggressive resection of such tumors off the ICA vessel wall can potentially lead to disastrous complications (e.g., pseudoaneurysms or blowouts). If, however, radical resection of the tumor and involved vessel segment can prolong a patient's meaningful life expectancy, ICA sacrifice with *en bloc* resection of the tumor is recommended.

ICA SACRIFICE: MANAGEMENT PARADIGMS

"Selective Revascularization": Balloon Occlusion Test

Inoperable aneurysms as well as cranial-base, head, and neck tumors that involve the carotid artery represent the major diseases that can necessitate sacrifice of the parent vessel. Contemporary ICA management revolves around the effective identification of patients who can tolerate sacrifice of their ICA. Matas (11) formulated one of the earliest tests that attempted to identify this subset. During the Matas test, patients would undergo percutaneous compression or surgical occlusion (temporary) of the ipsilateral carotid artery. Based on the absence or presence of neurological symptoms, they would be considered for permanent ICA sacrifice or ICA preservation, respectively. The question remained, however, as to whether those who did not develop symptoms during the Matas test would consistently tolerate parent vessel sacrifice. In fact, the Matas test proved unreliable.

Neurovascular surgeons also devised techniques to determine who could tolerate ICA sacrifice. One such technique was the gradual occlusion of the ICA using a clamp (Selverstone, Crutchfield, Poppen). Theoretically, gradual occlusion would diminish the risk of stroke associated with acute carotid occlusion. Furthermore, collaterals would be able to match cerebral demands more gradually. Once again, however, consistent predictability was lacking. Landolt and Millikan (6) reported ischemic complications with this technique at 38%.

To increase the sensitivity of the noninvasive carotid compression tests, Miller et al. (14) added electroencephalography and CBF tests to this modality. Shortly thereafter, based on the pioneering work of Serbineko (23), endovascular balloons were introduced. They provided a more effective way to occlude the ICA during test parameters and could also be used for permanent occlusion. With the advent of formal BOTs and the availability of CBF tests [e.g., Xe CT-CBF, SPECT, positron emission tomography], more sophisticated management schemes could be applied in the hope of increasing the sensitivity of test.

A management algorithm was developed based on the individual outcomes of ICA BOT, and Xe CT-CBF tests (26,27). Patients undergoing this protocol were divided into three groups. Group III patients "failed" the test by developing symptoms immediately (within a 15-min clinical test period) after inflation of the ICA balloon. Group II patients were asymptomatic during vessel occlusion but showed evidence of compromised blood flow on their Xe CT-CBF study (less than 30 to 35 ml/100 gm/min). Therefore, group II patients were considered at moderate risk for ischemic complications if the ICA was sacrificed. These patients also "failed" the BOT. Group I patients "passed" the clinical test and the Xe CT-CBF portion of the BOT and were thought to be at low risk for developing ischemic complications.

To estimate the overall feasibility of this test, several factors must be considered: the risks inherent to the procedure itself (e.g., endovascular complications), the short-term risks of stroke in patients with false-negative BOTs who undergo permanent balloon occlusion (PBO), and the long-term risks of ischemia and de novo aneurysm formation in the same group after PBO.

Early experience from the Pittsburgh group revealed a BOT procedure-related neurological complication rate of 3.7%, 0.7% of which were permanent (12,27). A later editorial by the same group alerted neurosurgeons to this test's potential lack of predictability (i.e., false-negatives) (21). Of patients who had undergone BOTs and Xe CT-CBF studies for cranial-base tumor resection, four of nine patients (44%) who had "passed" the BOT and had undergone PBO followed by tumor resection developed major strokes. The incidence of stroke (minor and major) for patients who had undergone surgical sacrifice or PBO of the ICA after "passing" the BOT was 13.3% (4 of 30). The overall risk for all patients "passing" the BOT and undergoing ICA occlusion was 20.5% (8 of 39). In a similar follow-up study of Origitano et al. (18), the risk for ischemic complications after passing a BOT (supplemented with a SPECT and Doppler blood flow studies) and undergoing a PBO followed by cranial-base tumor resection was 22%.

In a study by Larsen et al. (7) of strictly "inoperable" ICA aneurysms, the short-term risks of BOT included transient ischemic attacks in 6 of 55 patients (10%). The morbidity associated with false-negative BOTs were one death (1.8%) and two early strokes (3.6%). The overall morbidity and mortality rate as the result of false-negative BOT tests, therefore, was 5.4%. In studying the long-term risks of permanent balloon ICA occlusion in these patients, the same authors (8) reported 66 patients who tolerated the BOT and then underwent PBO. Two of 66 patients died early on and follow-up was unavailable on another four. Long-term follow-up was available in 60 of these 66 patients. Two of 60 patients had delayed strokes and another two had subarachnoid hemorrhage from de novo aneurysms. Overall long-term risks, therefore, were 6.7% (0.8%/year) for cerebrovascular accidents and 3.3% (0.4%/year) for subarachnoid hemorrhage from de novo aneurysms.

In addition to the risks associated with BOT and PBO, a number of contraindications must be considered before opting for ICA sacrifice, including the presence of a contralateral ICA or anterior communicating artery aneurysm. Furthermore, sacrifice of the ICA is not recommended in the setting of aneurysmal subarachnoid hemorrhage with coexistent vasospasm.

Universal Revascularization

When irrigation of the ICA territory is planned in conjunction with elective ICA sacrifice, we have favored high-flow (vein) bypasses. Other high-flow conduits (radial artery) are also available. Although we do not routinely recommend low-flow (superficial temporal artery pedicle) bypasses, necessity sometimes dictates its use. In such cases, we have performed a "double-barrel" superficial temporal artery-to-middle cerebral artery bypass where possible. In the rare case of a meningioma encasing the ICA leading to the gradual occlusion of the vessel and resultant ischemia, we recommend a blood flow study (Xe CT-CBF or SPECT) to distinguish between the need for a high- or low-flow bypass. Because of the chronicity of parent-vessel occlusion, collateral vessels may develop, obviating the need for a higher flow bypass. When de novo ICA sacrifice is planned, however, these additional collaterals are not yet present.

Bypass pedicles available for revascularization of the intracranial ICA territory include the cervical and petrous (*Fig. 25.1*) portions of the ICA, the external carotid artery (ECA), the CCA, and the subclavian artery. In patients with head and neck cancers, scarring from radiation, and/or tumor involvement of the ipsilateral extracranial carotid circulation, the contralateral ECA or branches can be used (so-called "bonnet bypass"; *Fig. 25.2*) (25). Although some surgeons routinely use the ECA to revascularize the ipsilateral ICA territory (while keeping the ICA patent), we prefer to use the ICA pedicle unless an extenuating circumstance exists. Using the ECA as the bypass pedicle permits delayed endovascular occlusion of the ICA and theoretically avoids the risks of stroke associated with early postoperative graft occlusion. Maintaining blood flow through the ICA, however, diminishes the impetus for blood to flow preferentially through the bypass and may actually increase the risk of graft thrombosis. Artificially created partial ICA occlusion may therefore be needed to shunt the blood preferentially to the brain via with the ECA pedicle bypass. This artificial stenosis itself can lead to complications (e.g., dissection). Furthermore, if the ECA is used as the "donor" bypass pedicle and the ICA is occluded, an ECA collateral to the brain would no longer be available in the future should the bypass pedicle thrombose. We therefore continue to prefer the ICA pedicle for our

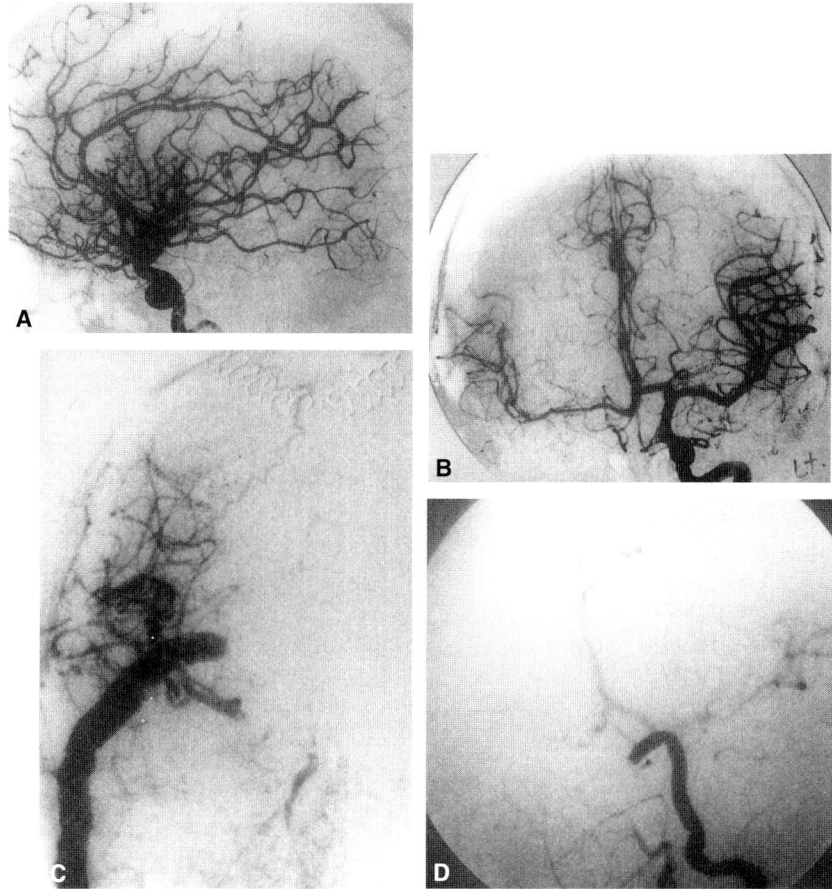

FIG. 25.1. De novo aneurysm formation after carotid artery occlusion. A 12-year old girl involved in a motor vehicle accident 2 years earlier had suffered a depressed cranial fracture, which was elevated, and a right ICA dissection that progressed to complete occlusion. No abnormalities were found in the left ICA. She presented to our institution 2 years later with progressive left retro-orbital pain and diplopia. Left lateral (A) and anteroposterior (B) CCA angiograms show a new left cavernous ICA aneurysm and cross-filling of the right anterior circulation via the anterior communicating artery. A left petrous-to-supraclinoid ICA bypass with aneurysm trapping was planned, but first a right ICA-to-middle cerebral artery (MCA) saphenous vein bypass was performed to enable temporary occlusion of the left carotid artery during that anastomosis. (C) Right ICA-to-MCA bypass is shown on a right anteroposterior CCA angiogram. (D) Left C3-to-C5 bypass is shown on a left anterior oblique CCA angiogram. The patient had an excellent outcome. *Reprinted with permission from Lippincott Williams & Wilkins.*

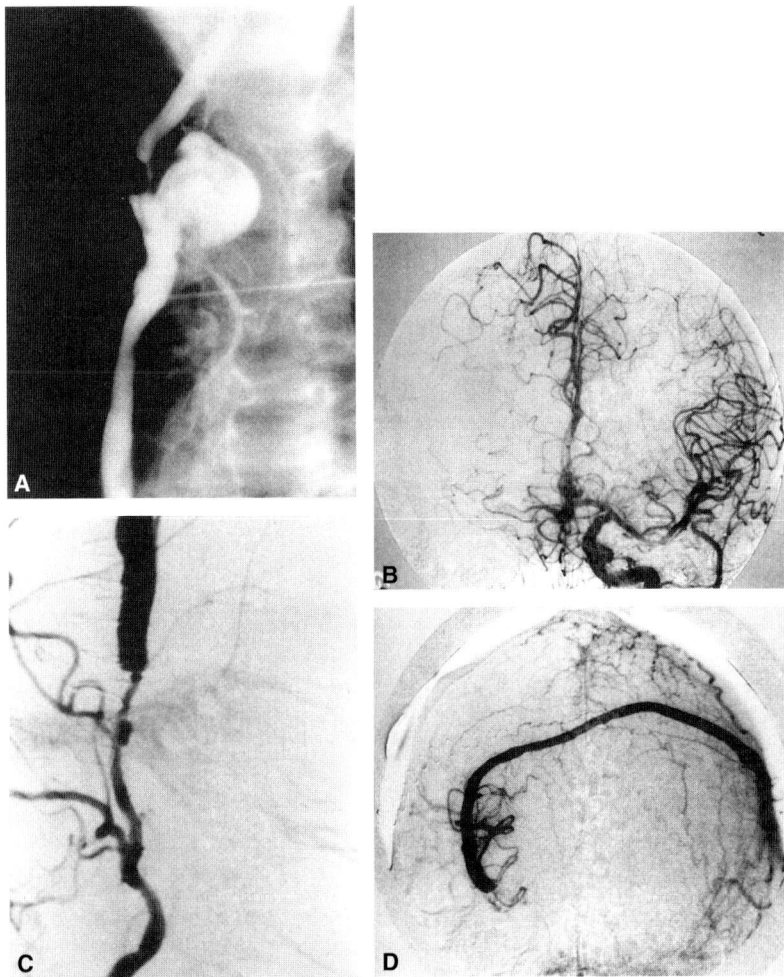

FIG. 25.2. Skull base tumor with carotid encasement and pseudoaneurysm. A 55-year-old man with a history of head and neck (squamous cell) carcinoma underwent resection of the tumor with postoperative irradiation of the neck as well as intraarterial methotrexate chemotherapy. He presented later with a hemorrhagic neck fistula. Angiography (right CCA) revealed an internal carotid artery pseudoaneurysm (A), given the residual disease in the neck as well as poor cross flow (left internal carotid artery digital subtraction angiogram). (B) The patient underwent a "bonnet bypass" from the superficial temporal artery bifurcation to the contralateral M_2 segment of the MCA. Postoperative left external carotid artery injection (C) shows the proximal anastomsis site and (D) the distal anastomosis site, with good filling of MCA proximally and distally. (From Spetzler RF, Koos WT (eds) (with contributions from Richling B): *Color Atlas Microneurosurgery,* 2nd Ed. Vol. II: *Intracranial Neurovascular Lesions,* 1997. Reprinted with permission from Georg Thieme Verlag, Stuttgart.

high-flow vein bypass. Recipient intracranial vessels for irrigation of the ICA territory include the supraclinoid segment of the ICA and the M_2 segment of the middle cerebral artery. Bypass to the M_2 segment tends to be least tedious.

Intraoperative adjuncts that we routinely use during bypass and temporary clipping include barbiturate (electroencephalographic) burst suppression and monitoring of somatosensory evoked potentials. Pharmacologically, we elevate the patient's blood pressure and administer a bolus of heparin just before revascularization (9, 10, 20, 25, 28). Some have argued that tolerance of longer temporary clipping in such cases signifies that the patient would have tolerated ICA occlusion or potentially a lower flow bypass pedicle. This reasoning, however, is moot. As noted, these patients are under a general anesthetic, supplemented with barbiturate (burst) suppression, with pharmacological elevation of their blood pressure and they are also mildly hypothermic. Therefore, tolerance of temporary clipping in such a setting in no way predicts tolerance of ICA sacrifice or hemispheric flow needs in a normal setting.

An objective comparison of the selective ICA sacrifice paradigm with universal revascularization must also include an analysis of the risks of revascularization, including both short-term and the potential long-term risks of symptomatic graft occlusion. Based on previous studies, approximately 10 to 15% of patients who undergo the BOT "fail" the clinical portion of the test. Approximately another 10% do not meet CBF criteria for ICA sacrifice (12). These patients (20–25%) will ultimately require a bypass. This subset of patients therefore incurs not only the procedural risks of BOT but also those of surgery.

At the Barrow Neurological Institute, the rate of neurological complications as related to surgical bypass has been approximately 6.8%, whereas the bypass-unrelated surgical complication rate has been approximately 3.4% (*Table 25.1*) for the treatment of aneurysms (9), cranial-base tumors (10), and refractory traumatic ICA dissections (28). If early successful graft salvage procedures are considered (e.g., surgical thrombectomy or endovascular thrombolysis), the early graft-related complication rate of 6.8% would be even lower. Other surgical experiences (morbidity and mortality rates) have been similar to ours (21, 22).

In the Mayo Clinic series of more than 200 vein grafts followed for a mean of 6.5 years, the *long-term* graft occlusion rate was 1 to 1.5% per year with a 20% morbidity rate associated with each event (19). Therefore, the overall annual morbidity rate after a long vein bypass was calculated at 0.2 to 0.3% per year.

TABLE 25.1
Published Barrow Neurological Institute Experience with 87 Bypasses for Aneurysms (9), Skull Base Tumors, (10) and ICA Dissections (28)

Surgical Risks	No. %
Bypass-related neurological morbidity	5 (5.7)
Bypass-unrelated neurological morbidity	3 (3.4)
Bypass-related mortality	1 (1.1)
Overall morbidity and mortality rate	9 (10.2)

Selective Versus Universal Revascularization

When comparing selective versus universal bypass, both short-term and long-term risks must be evaluated for both modalities (*Table 25.2.*). For BOT, the short-term risks include the risks associated with the BOT as well as the rate of false-negatives. Long-term risks include ischemia, de novo aneurysm formation, and hypertension. For universal revascularization, these risks include both the short- and long-term complications related to bypass surgery. The procedural risks for BOTs range between 0 and 10% (2, 7–9). The BOT false-negative rate, however, varies greatly between patients who undergo PBO for inoperable aneurysms (no subsequent surgery) and those who undergo surgical resection of a cranium-base tumor after PBO. The false-negative rate for inoperable aneurysms ranges between 2 and 14% (2, 7–9, 21) and between 22 and 44% for cranial-base tumors (18, 21). The long-term incidence of ischemia and embolism is 0.8 to 1.9% per year (6, 8, 9, 16, 17, 20, 29), and the per year risk of de novo aneurysm formation is 0 to 2.5% (3, 4, 7,–9, 13, 16, 17, 24) for both subsets of patients who "pass" the BOT (*Table 25.2*). Unknown is the incidence of iatrogenic hypertension after sacrifice of the ICA without bypass (29). As noted, patients who do not "pass" the BOT (groups II and III) incur both the BOT procedural risks and the risks associated with bypass.

The overall neurological morbidity rates associated with short-term surgical bypass range between 10 and 15%. Long-term risks include a 1 to 1.5% risk of graft occlusion per year with a 20% morbidity rate with each event. The annual risk of morbidity (ischemia) as the result of graft occlusion is therefore 0.2 to 0.3% (*Table 25.2*).

RECOMMENDATIONS

Based on the expertise of the individual neurosurgical center and the medical condition of the patient, either approach can be considered. BOT followed by endovascular PBO is attractive in this era of mini-

TABLE 25.2
Relative Risks of Selective and Universal Revascularization[a]

Approach and ICA Pathology	Treatment	BOT: Procedural Neurological Morbidity Rate[b]		Acute Complications		Delayed Complications	
		Permanent (%) (7,8,18,27)	Transient (%) (7,8,18,27)	BOT False Negatives[c] (%) (2,7,8,18,21)	Surgical Morbidity Rate[d] (%) (9,10,28)	Ischemia/ Embolism (%/yr) (6,8,9,16,17,20,29)	Aneurysm[e] (%/yr) (3,4,7-9,16,17,24)
Selective							
Group I ("Pass BOT")							
Aneurysms	PBO of ICA	0 to 0.7	1 to 10	2 to 14	0	0.8 to 1.9	0 to 2.5
SB tumors	PBO of ICA	0 to 0.7	1 to 10	22 to 44	0	0.8 to 1.9	0 to 2.5
Groups II and III ("Fail BOT")							
Aneurysms	Bypass	0 to 0.7	1 to 7	0	10.2[f]	0.2 to 0.3	0
CB tumors[g]							
Universal							
Aneurysms	Bypass	0	0	0	10.2[f]	0.2 to 0.3	0
CB tumors[g]							
Dissections							

[a] Adapted from Lawton MT et al. (9). Reprinted with permission from Lippincott Williams & Wilkins.
[b] Does not include risks of catheter angiography per se.
[c] Stroke after ICA Occlusion.
[d] BNI Experience.
[e] De novo aneurysm formation or enlargement of existing aneurysms.
[f] Includes both bypass-related (6.8%) and unrelated (3.4%) neurological complications.
[g] CB, cranial base

mally invasive therapies to spare the patient major surgery. Both short- and long-term risks, however, remain. Although patients undergoing revascularization incur the majority of short-term risks at surgery, long-term risks are minimized. For inoperable ICA aneurysms, for example, BOT followed by PBO (in a patient who passed the BOT) is a reasonable approach. In experienced hands, however, revascularization may prove less risky when the short- and long-term morbidity and mortality rates of both BOT and PBO are considered, especially in younger patients. When a patient requires surgical resection of a cranial-base tumor, we favor elective revascularization and do not recommend the BOT. In this specific subset of patients, the BOT is least predictive, and patients are left with a high risk of developing a stroke after tumor resection.

REFERENCES

1. Brennan JA, Jafek BW: Elective carotid artery resection for advanced squamous cell carcinoma of the neck. **Laryngoscope** 104:259–263, 1994.
2. Drake CG, Peerless SJ, Ferguson GG: Hunterian proximal arterial occlusion for giant aneurysms of the carotid circulation. **J Neurosurg** 81:656–665, 1994.
3. Dyste GN, Beck DW: De novo aneurysm formation following carotid ligation: Case report and review of the literature. **Neurosurgery** 24:88–92, 1989.
4. Forster DMC, Steiner L, Hakanson S, et al: The value of repeat pan-angiography in cases of unexplained subarachnoid hemorrhage. **J Neurosurg** 48:712–716, 1978.
5. Kennedy JT, Krause CJ, Loevy S: The importance of tumor attachment to the carotid artery. **Arch Otolaryngol** 103:70–73, 1977.
6. Landolt AM, Millikan CH: Pathogenesis of cerebral infarction secondary to mechanical carotid artery occlusion. **Stroke** 1:52–62, 1970.
7. Larson JJ, Tew JM Jr, Tomsick TA, et al: Treatment of aneurysms of the internal carotid artery by intravascular balloon occlusion: Long-term follow-up of 58 patients. **Neurosurgery** 36:23–30, 1995.
8. Larson JJ, Tew JM Jr, van Loveren HR, et al: Delayed complications after permanent balloon occlusion of the internal carotid artery (ICA) for treatment of aneurysms of the ICA. Presented at the 65th Annual Meeting of the American Association of Neurological Surgeons, Denver, CO, April 12–17 paper #747:228, 1997 (abstr).
9. Lawton MT, Hamilton MG, Morcos JJ, et al: Revascularization and aneurysm surgery: Current techniques, indications, and outcome. **Neurosurgery** 38:83–94, 1996.
10. Lawton MT, Spetzler RF: Internal carotid artery sacrifice for radical resection of skull base tumors. **Skull Base Surg** 6:119–123, 1996.
11. Matas R: Testing the efficiency of the collateral circulation as a preliminary to the occlusion of the great surgical arteries. **Ann Surg** 43:1–43, 1911.
12. Mathis JM, Barr JD, Horton JA: Temporary and permanent occlusion of major cerebral vessels: Indications and techniques, in Maciunas RJ (ed): *Endovascular Neurological Intervention*. Park Ridge, IL, American Association of Neurological Surgeons, 1995, p 59–73.
13. McKissock W, Richardson A, Walsh L, et al: Multiple intracranial aneurysms. **Lancet** 1:623–626, 1964.

14. Miller JD, Jawad K, Jennett B: Safety of carotid ligation and its role in the management of intracranial aneurysms. **J Neurol Neurosurg Psychiatry** 40:64–72, 1977.
15. Nishioka H: Results of the treatment of intracranial aneurysms by occlusion of the carotid artery in the neck. **J Neurosurg** 25:660–704, 1966.
16. Odom GL, Tindall GT: Carotid ligation in the treatment of certain intracranial aneurysms. **Clin Neurosurg** 15:101–116, 1967.
17. Oldershaw JB, Voris HC: Internal carotid artery ligation: A follow-up study. **Neurology** 16:937–938, 1966.
18. Origitano TC, Al-Mefty O, Leonetti JP, et al: Vascular considerations and complications in cranial base surgery. **Neurosurgery** 35:351–363, 1994.
19. Regli L, Piepgras DG, Hansen KK: Late patency of long saphenous vein bypass grafts to the anterior and posterior cerebral circulation. **J Neurosurg** 83:806–811. 1995.
20. Roski RA, Spetzler RF, Nulsen FE: Late complications of carotid ligation in the treatment of intracranial aneurysms. **J Neurosurg** 54:583–587, 1981.
21. Sekhar LN, Patel SJ: Permanent occlusion of the internal carotid artery during skull-base and vascular surgery: Is it really safe? **Am J Otol** 14:421–422, 1993.
22. Sen C, Sekhar LN: Direct vein graft reconstruction of the cavernous, petrous, and upper cervical internal carotid artery: Lessons learned from 30 cases. **Neurosurgery** 30:732–743, 1992.
23. Serbinenko FA: Balloon catheterization and occlusion of major cerebral vessels. **J Neurosurg** 41:125–145, 1974.
24. Somach FM, Shenkin HA: Angiographic end-results of carotid ligation in the treatment of carotid aneurysm. **J Neurosurg** 24:966–974, 1966.
25. Spetzler RF, Roski RA, Rhodes RS, et al: The "bonnet bypass": Case report. **J Neurosurg** 53:707–709, 1980.
26. Steed DL, Webster MW, DeVries EJ, et al: Clinical observations on the effect of carotid artery occlusion on cerebral blood flow mapped by xenon computed tomography and its correlation with carotid artery back pressure. **J Vasc Surg** 11:38–44, 1990.
27. Tarr RW, Jungreis CA, Horton JA, et al: Complications of preoperative balloon test occlusion of the internal carotid arteries: Experience in 300 cases. **Skull Base Surg** 1:240–244, 1991.
28. Vishteh AG, Marciano FF, David CA, et al: Long-term graft patency rates and clinical outcomes after revascularization for symptomatic traumatic internal carotid artery dissection. **Neurosurgery** 43:761–768, 1998.
29. Winn HR, Richardson AE, Jane JA: Late morbidity and mortality of common carotid ligation for posterior communicating aneurysms. **J Neurosurg** 47:727–736, 1977.

CHAPTER

26

Selective Use of Extracranial–Intracranial Bypass as an Adjunct to Therapeutic Internal Carotid Artery Occlusion

BOB S. CARTER, M.D., PH.D, CHRISTOPHER S. OGILVY, M.D., CHRISTOPHER PUTMAN, M.D., AND ROBERT G. OJEMANN, M.D.

Therapeutic internal carotid artery (ICA) occlusion is an important strategy in the management of certain complex ICA aneurysms not amenable to direct surgical clipping and in the management of some skull base lesions. Proximal occlusion allows for reduction of blood flow through these complex lesions while preserving flow through important branch vessels and perforators. After therapeutic occlusion of the ICA, the patient is a risk for cerebral ischemia from the development of thromboembolus or decreased cerebral blood flow (CBF). In the former situation, clot propagation distal to the site of ICA occlusion may result in thromboembolism in the circle of Willis. The use of therapeutic permanent balloon occlusion (PBO) of the ICA allows for very distal ICA occlusion just before the origin of the opthalmic artery, thus markedly reducing the incidence of these embolic complications. This, coupled with the use of intensive care monitoring, periocclusion maintenance of blood pressure, and brief systemic anticoagulation has contributed to the significantly lower rates of ischemic complications reported in recent large case series of therapeutic PBO of the ICA artery (13).

Despite the reduction in thromboembolic complications with the use of endovascular balloon occlusion of the ICA, hemodynamic ischemia after ICA occlusion remains an important problem. Variability in cerebral collateralization is reflected in a varying ability to tolerate ICA occlusion without the development of stroke. Because of this, extracranial-intracranial (EC-IC) bypass is an important adjunct in the treatment of aneurysms that require occlusion of the ICA. The goal of the EC-IC bypass is to preserve adequate CBF to areas of brain that are at risk of decreased perfusion in the setting of ICA occlusion. Two strategies exist regarding the use of EC-IC bypass. Some experts prefer the use of EC-IC bypass as a prophylactic measure in each patient who requires therapeutic ICA occlusion (14). We contrast this to the alternative strategy of selective EC-IC bypass in which patients are tested for functional CBF reserve before any definitive treatment procedure. EC-IC bypass is considered for those patients in whom a poor functional reserve is demonstrated using balloon test occlusion (BTO) of the ICA. In this report, we review the treatment-related risks of each strategy.

RISK OF NEUROLOGICAL SEQUELAE AFTER THERAPEUTIC OCCLUSION OF THE INTERNAL CAROTID ARTERY

One important question is what percentage of all patients for whom therapeutic ICA occlusion is considered are at risk for neurological sequelae? Data from patients undergoing BTO and unselected patients undergoing PBO suggest that approximately 25% of unselected patients are at risk. DeVries (6) reported on a series of 136 patients who underwent BTO before management of skull base lesions. Eight percent of the patients failed the initial assessment that included neurological and electroencephalographic monitoring during test occlusion. Twelve percent of the remaining patients (11% of the total) were found to have inadequate CBF by xenon-computed tomography (CT) assessment. Thus, a total of 19% of all patients were found to have inadequate cerebral reserve to support ICA occlusion. The remainder of patients underwent ICA occlusion without sequelae. Similarly, Annon et al (1) reported that 20% of 40 patients studied failed BTO (assessed by neurological examination and xenon-CT). Linskey et al. (16) reported that 17% of 23 patients failed BTO coupled with xenon-CT blood flow analysis. HaceinBey et al (11) found that 25% (8 of 32 patients) could not tolerate BTO. This estimate correlates well with that of Linskey et al. (15), who summarized 254 cases from the literature and estimated an overall stroke risk rate of 25% in this group. Thus, when all patients are considered, approximately 20 to 25% of unselected patients would not tolerate ICA occlusion. It is important to develop a means for sensitively and specifically identifying these patients. Most studies that report on the sequelae of ICA occlusion have focused on immediately evident deficits. Roski et al. (26) also highlighted the fact that an additional 10 to 15% of patients may be at risk for late ischemic complications after ICA occlusion.

A SELECTIVE OR UNIVERSAL BYPASS STRATEGY?

The decision between a treatment strategy of offering all patients prophylactic bypass who are having therapeutic ICA occlusion and a strategy in which only those patients who are deemed at high risk of neurological sequelae are offered bypass depends on our ability to detect these patients. In practical terms, two questions must be answered in a decision analysis regarding the two strategies in question. 1) What is the likelihood of acute or delayed ischemic deficit after BTO and PBO using the best available adjunct methods to identify the 20 to 25% of patients who are candidates for therapeutic ICA occlusion and who are at risk for neurological sequelae? It is important to develop a means for sensitively and specifically identifying these patients. 2) What are the risks of performing an EC-IC bypass for the 75 to 80% of patients who do not require the bypass to tolerate the therapeutic ICA occlusion?

SENSITIVITY OF METHODS TO IDENTIFY PATIENTS AT RISK FOR NEUROLOGICAL SEQUELAE AFTER INTERNAL CAROTID ARTERY OCCLUSION

Several methods have been used to identify patients in whom the cerebrovascular reserve is insufficient to prevent symptomatic cerebral infarction after ICA PBO. The most common of these methods based on test occlusions of the ICA. During the period of occlusion, indirect and direct measures of CBF can be made by a variety of evaluations including clinical examination, ICA back pressure measurement, EEG analysis, transcranial Doppler studies, single-photon emission computed tomography (SPECT), positron emission tomography, and xenon-CT analysis. Measures of CBF are considered to be either qualitative, such as SPECT analysis, or quantitative, such as xenon-CT analysis. Although most authors agree that an ICA-occluded CBF study will enhance the sensitivity of detection of patients at risk for stroke, there remains debate regarding the most feasible technique.

There are pitfalls in analyzing the literature to estimate the false negative rate of BTO with or without adjunctive CBF analysis. One issue is that following PBO, neurological deficit may occur secondary to thromboembolus or hypoperfusion. However, the BTO only attempts to distinguish which patients are at risk for the latter complication. Thus, a 10% stroke rate following PBO may reflect both a 5% false negative BTO rate and a 5% incidence of embolic complications that could not be predicted with BTO. Furthermore, confounding factors can influence the neurological complication rate following PBO. If PBO is performed in the setting of ischemia (23) (vasospasm after ruptured ICA aneurysm) or subsequent cranial base surgery (24), the complication rate is higher than if PBO is performed as a final therapeutic maneuver for unruptured intracranial aneurysms. It is therefore important to carefully evaluate the management morbidity when attempting to compare protocols that involve the use of BTO followed by bypass and PBO and those protocols wherein BTO is eschewed in favor of a universal bypass strategy before PBO or surgical occlusion of the ICA.

Clinical Balloon Test Occlusion

The most widely accepted method of performing ICA test occlusion has been BTO. This strategy has the advantages of reproducibility and minimal invasiveness compared with the older techniques of digital compression and open surgical occlusion. In typical protocols, patients receive a baseline neurological examination. Transfemoral arteriography is performed with insertion of a double lumen catheter so as to permit simultaneous monitoring of the arterial waveform and monitor intraarterial pressures while the balloon is inflated. Balloon inflation continues until the arterial waveform is fully damped. A small amount of dye is infused to confirm the presence of a static contrast column. The test occlusion is maintained for 15 minutes with monitoring of the neurological status throughout. The risk of neurological deficit after balloon test occlusion has been estimated to be 0.4% in an analysis of 500 cases by Mathis et al. (19). The false negative rate of normotensive BTO (without adjuncts such as hypotensive challenge or CBF analysis) with subsequent PBO has been estimated to be in the 5 to 20% range (6, 10).

Clinical Ballon Test Occlusion with Hypotensive Challenge

Because of the unacceptably low sensitivity of normotensive clinical BTO, other authors have supplemented the standard BTO with hypotensive challenge (28). As performed in our institution, after standard BTO, an intravenous infusion of nitroprusside is used to reduce the systolic blood pressure to 70% of baseline. The balloon occlusion is maintained for an additional 15 minutes under this protocol for a total occlusion time of 30 minutes. Standard et al. (28), reported that during normotensive test occlusion, 9% of 47 patients had deficits, whereas 27% of the total patients showed deficits when a 20-minute hypotensive challenge was added to the regimen. The addition of the hypotensive challenge did not markedly alter the rate of test-associated complications, as only 1 of 47 patients experienced a transient neurological deficit. Despite the increased sensitivity of BTO with hypotensive challenge, Standard et al. (28) reported a false negative rate of 5%, with 1 of 19 patients who subsequently underwent permanent ICA occlusion experiencing stroke. Despite the conceptually attractive features of the hypotensive challenge, one report described the occurrence of hypoperfusion-related stroke in 2 of 13 patients who passed a hypotensive balloon test occlusion, yielding a false negative rate of 15% (5).

Although the clinical neurological examination is a valuable endpoint for determining tolerance of ICA occlusion during BTO, there remains a group of patients in whom subclinical ischemia may be present and who may be at risk for delayed ischemic deficits following PBO.

These patients may be near the threshold for maintaining cerebral function during the 30-minute BTO, yet after PBO, additional stressors such as profound intraoperative hypotension or intraoperative blood loss may cause the CBF to drop below this threshold and cause cerebral infarction. Because of this, there has been considerable interest in developing direct measures of CBF to visualize areas of the brain that are experiencing subclinical ischemia during BTO using SPECT or xenon-CT analysis.

Clinical Balloon Test Occlusion with 99m-hexamethylpropyleneamine oxime SPECT Cerebral Blood Flow Analysis

Qualitative CBF techniques, such as SPECT with 99-m hexamethylpropyleneamine oxime (HMPAO), can define a high-risk subgroup of patients for cerebral infarction following ICA occlusion based on visualized abnormalities of CBF during test occlusion (20, 25). ^{99m}Tc-HMPAO SPECT imaging involves the determination of a baseline study prior to BTO and an additional study after 20 minutes of BTO. Ten minutes after injection of 20 mCi of ^{99m}Tc-HMPAO, the presence of the tracer is detected with a SPECT camera. Because there is no generally accepted technique for quantitating rCBF in ml/100 g/min using ^{99m}Tc-HMPAO SPECT imaging, qualitative assessments of relative CBF have been used. In particular, a significant reduction of flow on the occluded versus the nonoccluded side has been used as an indicator for predicting patients who are at risk of stroke (20, 21, 25). It has been suggested that SPECT asymmetry analysis alone may have a high rate of false positive test results based on the fact that assymmetry of flow may develop not only because of differential decreases in CBF but also differential increases in CBF (29). Yonas et al. (30) used both qualitative and quantitative techniques to analyze data from 94 patients undergoing a vasodilatory challenge and showed that qualitative techniques had only a 50% positive predictive value for defining patients with compromised cerebrovascular reserves compared with quantitative CBF analysis.

Clinical Balloon Test Occlusion with Xenon-Enhanced Tomographic Cerebral Blood Flow Measurements

To reach the goal of a widely available method of quantitating CBF noninvasively, xenon-CT CBF imaging has been developed as an adjunct to clinical BTO (8). Xenon-CT CBF analysis involves CT imaging three 10-mm-thick levels of the brain spaced 20 mm apart following the inhalation of Xe133 tracer. Two baseline images are obtained at each level while the patient breathes room air. A 4 1/2-minute period of xenon inhalation follows, during which four CT scans are obtained at each of the three levels. A thermistor is used to detect end-tidal xenon concentration for the calculation of an arterial partial pressure of xenon curve. With this information in hand, the CBF is calculated for each CT voxel (1*1*10 mm). This quantitative flow of information is then displayed on the CT scanner console. Yonas et al. (29) have developed criteria for identification of patients at high risk as the development of asymmetrically reduced blood flow on the side of occlusion with development of CBF values below 30 ml/100 g/min.

Using quantitative CBF analysis with xenon-CT imaging and the criteria outline above for selecting patients likely to tolerate PBO, Linskey et al. (15), reporting on the large experience from the University of Pittsburgh, found a neurological deficit rate of 1 of 30 in their protocol for patients who passed both the BTO and xenon-CT CBF analysis. Five radiographic infarcts were detected among the 30 patients undergoing ICA occlusion: one confirmed by angiography as distal embolus, one associated intraoperative perforator sacrifice, and 3 of 30 felt possibly flow related. This low false negative rate has fueled efforts to make xenon-CT CBF analysis equipment more widely available.

The procedure-related risks of BTO coupled with xenon-CT have been reported in a series of 500 patients by Mathis et al. (19). They found that 3.2% of patients experienced procedure-related complications, including 1.6% asymptomatic complications (dissection, embolus, and pseudoaneurysm), 1.2% a transient neurological deficit, and 0.4% a permanent neurological deficit. Of note, logistic problems have been noted in performing CBF analysis with xenon-CT, especially the transportation of the patient from the site of BTO in the angiography suite to the CT scanner for xenon-CT analysis with an uninflated intracarotid balloon in place, and associated concern that a dissection could develop.

Clinical Balloon Test Occlusion:
Additional Adjunctive Studies under Evaluation

In addition to the aforementioend methodologies, transcranial Doppler sonography (9, 27), positron emission tomographic scanning (4), electroencephalographic and analysis (22) have also been used as adjuncts to the clinical examination during BTO. However, so far none of these evaluations have been reported to be superior to the studies discussed above.

Summary

Normotensive clinical BTO is accompanied by a high false negative rate in the 5 to 20% range for transient neurological symptoms and a permanent stroke morbidity in the 3 to 8% range (see *Table 26.1*). Supplementation of the clinical BTO with either hypotensive challenge or specific assessment of CBF can reduce the false negative rate for neurological symptoms to 5% or less (*Table 26.1*).

EC-IC BYPASS FOR ANEURYSM TREATMENT IN THE LITERATURE

Review of the major surgical series for EC-IC bypass performed for the treatment of aneurysms reveals a mortality rate of approximately 3% and a stroke rate ranging from 0 to 8% (3, 7, 11–14). When a selective bypass approach was used the percentage of patients undergoing bypass ranged from 5 to 30% (see *Table 26.2*). Drake et al. (7) performed selective EC-IC bypass in 21 of 72 (30%) patients with giant aneurysms proximal to the ICA bifurcation. Patients were chosen for bypass when BTO and xenon-CT suggested poor cerebrovascular reserve. There were no deaths in this series of patients. Several patients were reported to have transient neurological symptoms stated to have resolved with the use of hypertension and volume expansion. Anon et al. (1) reported on 40 patients with giant intracavernous aneurysms treated with a combination of BTO, EC-IC bypass (10%), and PBO. They reported three patients with transient neurological deficits, and one patient suffered a permanent hemiparesis. The permanent infarct was attributed to an embolus that occurred at the time of BTO. There were no deaths. Larson et al. (13) reported on a 15-year experience using PBO to treat ICA aneurysms in 58 patients. They reported three deaths (1 of 3 patients under going by-

TABLE 26.1
Series Using Balloon Test Occlusion before Therapeutic ICA Occlusion

Year	Author	No. Patients	Transient Neuro (%)	Permanent Neuro (%)	Mortality(%)	Other Compl (%)	Adjunct
1993	Awad (2)	12	16	8	8	1	Clinical exam
1993	Mathews (18)	12	0	0	0	n.s.	SPECT
1994	Drake (7)	56	10	0	0	n.s.	Xenon-CT
1994	Linskey (15)	30	7	3	0	n.s.	Xenon-CT
1995	Standard (28)	19	5.2	0	0	4	Hypotension
1995	Larson (13)	55	10	2	2	n.s.	SPECT
1997	Schneweis (27)	10	20	n.s.[a]	0	n.s.	TCD
1998	Dare (5)	20	15	5	0	n.s.	Hypotension

[a]n.s., not stated.

TABLE 26.2
Series Reporting EC-IC Bypass in the Treatment of Cerebral Aneurysms

Year Published	Author	Patients Bypassed	Percent Bypassed	ICA Occlusion Method	Adjunct to BTO	Transient Deficit	Permanent Deficit (%)	Mortality
1993	Mathews (18)	3	15	PBO	SPECT	0 of 3	0	0%
1994	Barnett (3)	7	n.s.[a]	PBO immed	None	1 of 7	0	0%
1994	Drake (7)	45	30	Selverstone (11), PBO (27), trapping (7)	Xenon-CT	n.s.	0	1 of 11-selverstone, 1 of 7 trapping, 0 of 27-PBO
1995	Larson (13)	3	5	PBO	Hypotension, SPECT	10%	5	1 of 3
1996	Lawton (14)	54	100	Trapping (51), PBO (3)	None	n.s.	8	2%
1997	Hacein-Bey (11)	8	25	PBO	Xenon-CT	n.s.	0	0%
1998	Jafar (12)	25	n.s.	n.s.	n.s.	n.s.	n.s.	1 of 25

[a]n.s., not stated.

pass with PBO and 2 of 55 patients undergoing PBO alone). Six patients had transient deficits (1 of 3 bypass patients and 5 of 55 PBO patients), and two patients had permanent deficits (2 of 55 PBO patients).

In the largest series wherein a universal bypass strategy was employed, Lawton et al. (14) reported a surgical mortality of 2%, cerebral infarcts in 5% and a worsened neurological deficit in 8%. Graft occlusions occurred in 5% of patients and caused stroke in 2% of patients. In general, for anterior circulation aneurysms that required EC-IC bypass, an attempt was made to trap these lesions with proximal clip ligation or proximal endovascular balloon occlusion used in those cases where trapping was not possible. This series highlights some of the additional complications that can be associated with a bypass, including epidural hematomas (8% of patients) and postoperative myocardial infarction (2% of patients) (14). Recent reports of therapeutic ICA occlusion supplemented with bypass are summarized in *Table 26.2*.

BENEFITS AND RISKS OF BYPASS STRATEGIES TO ALTER NATURAL HISTORY

The information provided above can allow us to make some estimates as to the expected outcome of two different management strategies: selective versus universal bypass. For this comparison, we have used the average values from the literature for the risk of stroke and death (see *Tables 26.1* and *26.2*). Though there is considerable variability in the data, stroke rates in the 0 to 8% range have been reported for patients undergoing therapeutic ICA occlusion with or without EC-IC bypass (*Tables 26.1* and *26.2*). The data suggest that the benefit provided by EC-IC bypass in preventing hypoperfusion-related infarcts is offset by procedure-related infarctions secondary to problems such as a graft thrombosis or embolization. Procedure-related mortality seems to be higher in patients undergoing EC-IC bypass (5 of 155 patients in *Table 26.2*) versus therapeutic ICA occlusion without bypass (2 of 214 patients in *Table 26.1*).

Because the overall stroke rate of both algorithms is similar, why do we favor selective EC-IC bypass? Usually only the most experienced surgeons have the low morbidity rate for EC-IC bypass reported in *Table 26.2*. With a selective bypass approach, the mortality is lower, and the risk of other postoperative complications (infection, epidural hematoma, deep venous thrombosis, and cardiopulmonary problems) is not present. Finally, in a population of 100 patients, a selective bypass approach may incur the cost of 20 to 25 craniotomies for bypass in those patients who fail test occlusion, whereas a universal bypass approach necessitates an extra 75 to 80 craniotomies in the population of patients who do not require bypass.

A PROPOSED ALGORITHM

In the above discussion, we have highlighted a set of expected outcomes using a selective EC-IC bypass approach in which CBF analysis identifies a group of "borderline" patients for whom clinical BTO is normal, yet CBF studies show some impairment of perfusion. We report on a modification on this strategy in which a selective bypass strategy is used for patients who clearly fail a clinical BTO with hypotensive challenge. Borderline patients are identified at the time of PBO using SPECT analysis and are managed with an aggressive regimen of hypervolemia, hypertension, anticoagulation, and slow mobilization during a period when the flow capacity of cerebral collaterals is expanded.

Our current protocol involves a clinical BTO in the neurointerventional suite. At 10 minutes after the initiation of BTO, the patient is injected with HMPAO for detection at a later time point with SPECT analysis. At 15 minutes after the initiation of BTO, an infusion of nitroprusside is used to reduce the SBP to 70% of its baseline value. The hypotensive portion of the BTO continues for 15 minutes for a total BTO time of 30 minutes. If the patient has tolerated BTO on clinical grounds, PBO is performed. Within 1 to 4 hours, SPECT detection of the HMPAO tracer is used to identify patients with borderline CBF. Although all patients undergo 48 hours of ICU management post-occlusion, the subset of "borderline" patients is selected for a several day course of hypervolemia with placement of a Swan-Ganz catheter to monitor volume status, anti-coagulation, and slow mobilization.

In our series of 48 patients treated with therapeutic ICA occlusion in the past 4 years, five patients (10%) failed the clinical portion of the BTO and underwent EC-IC bypass followed by successful ICA occlusion. Two of the patients with bypass experienced transient neurological deficit with documentation of radiographic infarct. Both infarcts were felt to be embolic. ICA occlusion without bypass was performed in 43 patients. There were two transient deficits (4%) and one permanent neurological deficit (2%) in this group. The overall management protocol had a 10% rate of radiological and a 2% rate of permanent neurological deficit. This compares favorably with the other studies outlined in *Table 26.2*.

In summary, we support an algorithm in which BTO is used to identify patients at high risk of post-PBO hypoperfusion stroke and to treat these patients with a prophylactic EC-IC bypass. These patients (approximately 10% of all patients tested) are then subjected to repeat BTO before PBO. "Borderline" patients who pass a clinical BTO with hypotensive challenge but show SPECT abnormalities do not undergo bypass, yet they are followed more closely in the postocclusion period to maximize medical management during a period when collateralization may be borderline. By focusing the use of prophylactic EC-IC bypass on the high risk group, the morbidity and mortality risk is avoided in patients who do not need this surgical procedure.

REFERENCES

1. Anon VV, Aymard A, Gobin Y, et al.: Balloon occlusion of the internal carotid artery in 40 cases of giant intracavernous aneurysm: Technical aspects, cerebral monitoring and results. **Neuroradiology** 34:245–251, 1991.
2. Awad I, Masaryk T, Magdinec M: Pathogenesis of subcortical hyperintense lesions on magnetic resonance imaging of the brain: Observations in patients undergoing controlled therapeutic internal carotid artery occlusion. **Stroke** 24:1339–1346, 1993.
3. Barnett D, Barrow D, Joseph G: Combined extracranial-intracranial bypass and intraoperative balloon occlusion for the treatment of intracavernous and proximal carotid artery aneurysms. **Neurosurgery** 35:92–98, 1994.
4. Brunberg J, Frey K, Horton J, et al: 15OH2O Positron emission tomography determination of cerebral blood flow during balloon test occlusion of the internal carotid artery. **Am J Neuroradiol** 15:725–732, 1994.
5. Dare A, Chaloupka J, Putman C, et al.: Failure of the hypotensive provocative test during temporary balloon test occlusion of the internal carotid artery to predict delayed hemodynamic ischemia after therapeutic carotid occlusion. **Surg Neurol** 50:147–155, 1998.
6. Devries E: A new method to predict safe resection of the internal carotid artery. **Laryngoscope** 100:85–88, 1990.
7. Drake C, Peerless S, Ferguson G: Hunterian proximal arterial occlusion for giant aneurysms of the carotid circulation. **J Neurosurg** 81:656–665, 1994.
8. Erba S, Horton J, Latchaw R, et al.: Balloon test occlusion of the internal carotid artery with stable xenon/CT cerebral blood flow imaging. **Am J Neuroradiol** 9:533–538, 1988.
9. Giller C, Mathews D, Walker B, et al.: Prediction of tolerance to carotid artery occlusion using transcranial Doppler ultrasound. **J Neurosurg** 81:15–19, 1994.
10. Gonzalez G, Moret J: Balloon occlusion of the icarotid artery prior to surgery for neck tumors. **Am J Neuroradiol** 11:649–652, 1990.
11. Hacein-Bey L, Connolly E, Duong H, et al.: Treatment of inoperable carotid aneurysms with endovascular carotid occlusion after EC-IC bypass surgery. **Neurosurgery** 41:1255–1234, 1997.
12. Jafar JJ, Huang PP: Surgical treatment of carotid cavernous aneurysms. **Neurosurg Clin N Am** 9:755–763, 1998.
13. Larson J: Treatment of aneurysms of the internal carotid artery by intravascular balloon occlusion: Long-term follow-up of 58 patients. **Neurosurgery** 36:26–30, 1995.
14. Lawton M, Hamilton M, Morcos J, et al.: Revascularization and aneurysm surgery: Current techniques, indications, and outcome.. **Neurosurgery** 38:83–94, 1996.
15. Linskey M, Jungreis C, Yonas H, et al.: Stroke risk after abrupt internal carotid artery sacrifice: Accuracy of preoperative assessment with balloon test occlusion and xenon-enhanced CT. **Am J Neuroradiol** 15:829–843, 1994.
16. Linskey M, Sekhar L, Horton J, et al.: Aneurysms of the internal carotid artery: A multidisciplinary approach to treatment. **J. Neurosurg** 75:525–534, 1991.
17. Lorberboym M, Pandit N, Machac J, et al.: Brain perfusion imaging during preoper-

ative temporary balloon occlusion of the internal carotid artery. **J. Nucl Med** 37:415–419, 1996.
18. Mathews D, Walker B, Purdy P, et al.: Brain blood flow SPECT in temporary balloon occlusion of carotid and intracerebral arteries. **J Nucl Med** 34:1239–1243, 1993.
19. Mathis J, Barr J, Jungreis C, et al.: Temporary balloon test occlusion of the internal carotid artery: Experience in 500 cases. **Am J Neuroradiol** 16:749–754, 1995.
20. Monsein L, Jeffrey P, vanHeerden B, et al.: Assessing adequacy of collateral circulation during balloon test occlusion of the internal carotid artery with 99mTc-HM-PAO SPECT. **Am J Neuroradiol** 12:1045–1051, 1991.
21. Moody E, Dawson R, Sandler M: 99mTc-HMPAO SPECT imaging in interventional neuroradiology: Validation of balloon test occlusion. **Am J Neuroradiol** 13:1043–1044, 1991.
22. Morioka T, Matsushima T, Fujii K, et al.: Balloon test occlusion of the internal carotid artery with monitoring of compressed spectral arrays (CSAs) of elecroencephalogram. **Acta Neurchir (Wein)** 101:29–34, 1989.
23. Nishioka H: Report on the cooperative study of intracranial aneurysms and subarachnoid hemorrhage. **J Neurosurg** 25:660–682, 1966.
24. Origtano T, Ossama A, Leonettie J, et al.: Vascular considerations and complications in cranial base surgery. **Neurosurgery** 35:351–363, 1994.
25. Peterman S, Taylor A, Hoffman J: Improved detection of cerebral hypoperfusion with internal carotid balloon test occlusion and 99mTc-HMPAO cerebral perfusion SPECT imaging. **Am J Neuroradiol** 13:1035–1041, 1991.
26. Roski R, Spetzler R, Nulsen F: Late complications of carotid ligation in the treatment of intracranial aneurysm. **J Neurosurg** 54:583–587, 1981.
27. Schnweis S, Urbach H, Solymosi L, et al.: Preoperative risk assessment for carotid occlusion by transcranial Doppler ultrasound. **J Neurol Neurosurg Psychiatry** 62:485–489, 1997.
28. Standard S, Ahuja A, Guterman L, et al.: Balloon test occlusion of the internal carotid artery with hypotensive challenge. **Am J Neuroradiol** 16:1453–1458, 1995.
29. Yonas H, Linskey M, Johnson D, et al.: Internal carotid balloon test occlusion does require quantitative CBF. **Am J Neuroradiol** 13:1147–1152, 1992.
30. Yonas H, Pindzola R, Meltzer C, et al.: Qualitative versus quantitative assessment of cerebrovascular reserves. **Neurosurgery** 42:1005–1010, 1998.

CHAPTER

27

Therapeutic Carotid Occlusion: Current Management Paradigms

SUNGHOON LEE, M.D., AND ISSAM A. AWAD, M.D., M.SC., F.A.C.S.

INTRODUCTION AND HISTORICAL OVERVIEW

Therapeutic carotid occlusion has become an accepted treatment strategy for the management of selected inoperable internal carotid aneurysms, the radical surgical management of base of skull and head and neck tumors, and in cases of impending carotid blowout from trauma, neoplasia, or other disease. Although its practice has had a long conceptual and experiential evolution, a critical evaluation of this therapeutic modality has only recently been elucidated.

Attempted therapeutic ligation of the carotid artery was documented as early as the 16th century for the surgical control of traumatic carotid rupture (52). In 1724, Johann J. Wepler accurately described the course of the internal carotid artery through the base of the skull to its position adjacent to the pituitary gland proposing its importance in carrying the "vital spirits" to the brain (4). John Abernethy (1764–1831) published his experience with a case of surgical ligation of the carotid artery in a patient who suffered a carotid laceration after an attack from an ox. Abernethy reported the death of this patient from ischemic complications related to the carotid ligation (2). In carefully documenting the associated stroke related to this case, Abernethy's case allowed a critical correlation of brain ischemia with carotid occlusive disease in addition to introducing carotid occlusion as a potentially useful but also a risky therapeutic intervention (4). The Abernethian approach to carotid ligation essentially followed previously articulated Hunterian principles of arterial ligation for peripheral aneurysms and consisted of direct surgical exposure and abrupt arterial occlusion. Cooper, in 1805 performed the first "elective" carotid occlusion for the treatment of a cervical carotid aneurysm. Although his first patient died, Cooper performed a successful ligation three years later (1808), which was published in 1836 (12).

After the work of Abernethy and Cooper, therapeutic carotid occlusion became popularized and gained a wider spectrum of applications and indications. Carotid occlusion was attempted in the treatment of seizures, trigeminal neuralgia, and psychosis, in addition to its application in the therapy of carotid rupture and aneurysms (51). The operative mortality of this era is best summarized by Pilz, who in 1868 reported a mortality rate of 43% in a patient population of 600 after therapeutic carotid ligations (49), suggesting a narrowing of its indications to include mainly the treatment of carotid aneurysms and carotid rupture. In the early twentieth century, the application of carotid occlusion remained a principal arm of therapy for the treatment of both extracranial and intracranial aneurysms. Harvey Cushing and Walter Dandy reported its application as a temporizing measure in the treatment of intracranial arteriovenous malformations (13, 14). The therapeutic efficacy and morbidity of carotid occlusion soon became a subject of ongoing debate in the neurosurgical community. Schorstein noted the high rates of morbidity and mortality of treating intracranial aneurysms with carotid occlusion, accurately noting the salient factors such as recent subarachnoid hemorrhage, severe anemia, and elevated intracranial pressures as the predictors of poor outcome (56).

In the modern era, the intracranial exposure of aneurysms and direct metal clip ligation as first described by Dandy (reported in ref. 66) have largely obviated the need for parent vessel sacrifice in the majority of circle of Willis aneurysms responsible for subarachnoid hemorrhage. Advances in microneurosurgery and cisternal dissection techniques popularized by Yasargil have greatly enhanced the safety and effectiveness of this direct therapeutic strategy for most intracranial aneurysms. However, in symptomatic aneurysms of the cavernous segment and in certain giant intracranial aneurysms where dysmorphic features preclude a direct reconstruction of the parent artery, carotid occlusion remains an accepted and efficacious therapeutic modality. Also, carotid occlusion has found an important role in the radical surgical management of skull base and head and neck neoplasms, allowing an oncologically meaningful resection in cases where the carotid cannot be preserved. Carotid ligation remains, as it has been for several centuries, a lifesaving intervention in cases of active or impending carotid blowout from trauma or other diseases.

The technical procedure of carotid occlusion has evolved markedly since the Hunterian-Abernethian abrupt ligation paradigm. In the second half of the twentieth century, there was a popular concept of gradual arterial occlusion using a variety of implanted devices (Saliba clamp, Crutchfield clamp, Selverstone clamp, etc.). Once implanted, these devices allowed gradual vessel occlusion, presumably allowing progressive maturation of collateral pathways. Equally important, these clamps allowed prompt reperfusion in the case of neurological symptoms. More recently, these have largely yielded to endovascular balloon occlusion, allowing temporary testing of tolerance to arterial occlusion while preserving the ability to deflate the balloon in case of acute ischemic symptoms. Adjuvant provocative testing and methods for assessment of cerebral blood flow have been advocated to enhance the sensitivity and specificity of balloon test occlusion. The role of adjuvant revascularization surgery to augment collateral reserves has been debated almost since the introduction of extracranial-intracranial (EC-IC) bypass surgery. Lastly, a variety of management adjuncts have been advocated, including periprocedure anticoagulation therapy, to prevent thromboembolism and hypervolemic hypertension to enhance hemodynamic reserves. We review these strategies within the context of current indications, contraindications, and potential complications of carotid occlusion and present a modern management paradigm aimed at minimizing morbidity and enhancing effectiveness of therapeutic carotid occlusion.

CURRENT INDICATIONS AND CONTRAINDICATIONS

Presently, there are four main indications for therapeutic carotid occlusion: the treatment of symptomatic cavernous segment aneurysms and those asymptomatic lesions with intradural extension or demonstrated expansion, the treatment of neoplastic processes involving the internal carotid artery, and the urgent or emergent treatment of carotid blowout syndrome (*Table 27.1*).

Prevailing strategies among head and neck surgeons for the treatment of neoplastic processes at the skull base have emphasized, first and foremost, an aggressive surgical resection (60). In light of such a treatment paradigm for base of skull tumors involving the carotid artery, the surgeon is confronted with several options. First, the option of carotid preserving resection should be considered, accepting the possibility of residual tumor adjacent to the carotid artery. The second option is the complete dissection of the tumor from the artery while maintaining its integrity. The third option of excising the artery with the tumor may be considered. The decision in relation to the preservation of the carotid artery is based on the malignancy of the tumor, the likelihood of a complete resection, and the hemodynamic reserve of the patient. In our institution, we have evolved the following algorithm. When the oncological goal is determined to be a total resec-

TABLE 27.1
Indications for Therapeutic Carotid Occlusion

Symptomatic intracavernous carotid aneurysm causing:
- Progressive ophthalmoplegia or visual loss
- Intractable ipsilateral facial or orbital pain
- Prior subarachnoid hemorrhage or epistaxis

Asymptomatic intracavernous carotid aneurysm with:
- Intradural extension at risk for future SAH
- Progressive radiographic enlargement of the aneurysm

Head and neck neoplasms with the involvement of the carotid artery where:
- Resection of the artery is deemed oncologically necessary
- Preservation of the artery is deemed technically impossible
- Carotid artery is considered to be at imminent risk of rupture

Carotid artery rupture as a result of:
- Neoplastic process
- Radiation therapy or radical neck flap failure
- Wound infection or pharyngocutaneous fistula
- Blunt or penetrating trauma with carotid artery disruption

tion including the resection of the carotid, it is reasonable to proceed with therapeutic carotid occlusion 4 to 6 weeks before the planned oncological resection in a patient who has passed provocative testing. In a patient who fails provocative testing with balloon test occlusion, it becomes prudent to reconsider the option of a carotid preserving procedure or consider a prophylactic revascularization before the occlusion.

Therapeutic carotid occlusion remains the principal modality of therapy for idiopathic intracavernous carotid aneurysms (40). Indications for the treatment of intracavernous carotid aneurysm are founded on the retrospective evaluations of its natural history. Asymptomatic intracavernous carotid aneurysms arising from the distal cavernous segment and extending intradurally into the subarachnoid space have been shown to have the potential for causing subarachnoid hemorrhage (39). Symptomatic intracavernous carotid aneurysms have been treated to halt their clinical progression. Accepted indications include progressive opthalmoplegia or visual loss, intractable ipsilateral facial or orbital pain, progressive radiographic enlargement of the aneurysm, and subarachnoid hemorrhage or epistaxis (40). Therapeutic endovascular carotid occlusion remains a reasonable option for the subset of patients meeting these treatment criteria with adequate hemodynamic reserves to tolerate ipsilateral carotid occlusion.

Carotid artery rupture is a dreaded complication in the management of head and neck tumors with an estimated rate of mortality of 40% and a rate of neurological morbidity of 25% (11). Its incidence has been estimated at a rate of 3 to 4% as a result of radical head and neck tumor resection. Radiation therapy, flap necrosis, wound infection, pharyngocutaneous fistula, and recurrent tumors have been shown to be significant associated risk factors in carotid artery rupture. Direct blunt and penetrating trauma can also cause carotid artery rupture (1, 10). Open surgical ligation of the carotid artery has been the traditional modality of treatment of carotid artery rupture. Recent applications of endovascular therapeutic carotid occlusion after balloon test occlusion have achieved marked improvements in the outcome. Citardi et al. (11) have reported a series of 12 patients treated with a current endovascular carotid occlusion paradigm without associated mortality or neurological sequelae. Endovascular carotid occlusion paradigm, with provocative testing, has become the standard of care in the treatment of carotid artery rupture.

Careful consideration of contraindications is prerequisite to proceeding with elective therapeutic carotid occlusion (*Table 27.2*). An absolute contraindication to therapeutic carotid occlusion is the presence of conditions that are certain to preclude adequate hemodynamic support for unilateral carotid occlusions. These clinical states include severe contralateral carotid occlusive disease, cardiogenic or hypovolemic shock, clinical or angiographic evidence of vasospasm, angiographic absence of circle of Willis collaterals, and the failure of provocative testing, with the development of focal neurological deficit or the evolution of major deficits on cerebral blood flow studies. Other relative contraindications include states that would prohibit periprocedural anticoagulation, such as recent subarachnoid hemorrhage, intracerebral hemorrhage, or recent surgery. Lastly, the presence of intracranial collateral pathway aneurysms is considered a relative contraindication because of the added hemodynamic stress and risk of aneurysm rupture.

Increased awareness of potential relative contraindications to therapeutic carotid occlusion can allow the development of specific strategies for risk management. Other relative contraindications include poor medical states, such as congestive heart failure or chronic renal failure, the presence of known vasculopathic risk factors such as smoking and diabetes, mild contralateral carotid stenosis, and the mild to moderate impaired collateral reserve on cerebral blood flow studies.

SPECTRUM OF POTENTIAL COMPLICATIONS

The modern era has been marked by a significant evolution in the understanding of the varied complications of therapeutic carotid occlusion. In the recent years, we have noted the distinction between hemo-

TABLE 27.2
Contraindications for Therapeutic Carotid Occlusion

Absolute contraindications
  Inadequate hemodynamic support for unilateral carotid occlusion:
    • Severe contralateral carotid occlusive disease
    • Cardiogenic or hypovolemic shock
    • Clinical or angiographic evidence of vasospasm or impending vasospasm
    • failure of provocative testing with:
      • The development of focal neurological deficit
      • Major deficits on CBF studies
  Conditions likely to require contralateral carotid occlusion:
    • Contralateral aneurysms or dolicoectasia of carotid artery
    • Contralateral neoplastic invasion or compression of carotid artery
Relative contraindications
  Clinical states likely to risk delayed hemorrhagic sequelae:
    • Intracranial collateral pathway aneurysms
  Poor general medical condition:
    • Congestive heart failure
    • Chronic renal failure
    • Respiratory failure
  Known advanced vasculopathic risk factors:
    • Heavy smoking, diabetes (?)
  Mild to moderate contralateral carotid stenosis (?)
  Mild to moderate compromise on CBF studies during test occlusion (?)
  Clinical states contraindicating anticoagulation therapy:
    • Recent subarachnoid hemorrhage with unsecured aneurysm
    • Recent intracerebral hemorrhage
    • Recent craniotomy, other surgery (?), or multiple trauma
  Family history of intracranial aneurysms (?)

dynamic and thromboembolic ischemic sequelae (*Figs. 27.1* and *27.2*) as potential complications of therapeutic carotid occlusion. We have learned to identify the subset of patients with unfavorable hemodynamic reserve with the advent of provocative test occlusion. Quantitative and qualitative measures of cerebral blood flow have increased the sensitivity of the selection of patients with marginal hemodynamic reserve. The care of these patients with subthreshold reserve has improved with the advances of bypass revascularization and cerebral blood flow enhancing critical care management.

The threat of thromboembolism has been recognized as a significant complication of carotid occlusion (16, 21, 30, 31, 37, 63). These can occur in the hours following carotid occlusion and despite apparent hemodynamic tolerance in the acute stage. Propagating thrombosis with devastating hemispheric infarction remains the most common cause of

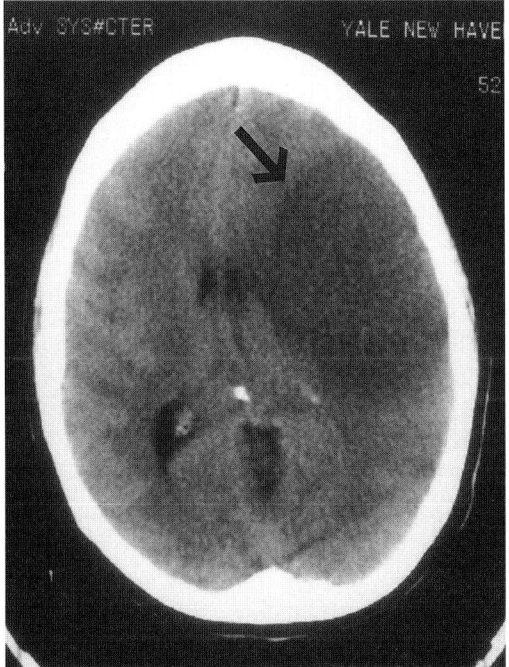

FIG. 27.1 CT scan of the brain with major arterial territory infarction, characteristic of embolism or propagating thrombosis.

death after carotid occlusion. Heros et al. reported the periprocedural use of full systemic anticoagulation to prevent embolic complications (30, 31). Heros also noted the potential increase in the thromboembolic risk in EC-IC revascularizations, postulating that new flow patterns induced by the revascularization could enhance the probability of thrombus propagation from either the aneurysm or the internal carotid artery (ICA) distal to the occlusion (30). Little et al. (41) have reported no instance of thromboembolic complications with 48 hours of systemic anticoagulation followed by prolonged course of antiplatelet therapy. In addition, endovascular carotid occlusion has further minimized the frequency of thromboembolic phenomena by decreasing the dead space in the carotid artery with a more distal anchorage of the balloon, closer to the level of pathology and to collateral pathways (16, 21, 63).

In addition to a further understanding of acute hemodynamic and thromboembolic sequelae, studies with long-term longitudinal follow-up have elucidated the phenomenon of delayed ischemia. The problem of delayed ischemia from carotid ligation was noted by Black and Ger-

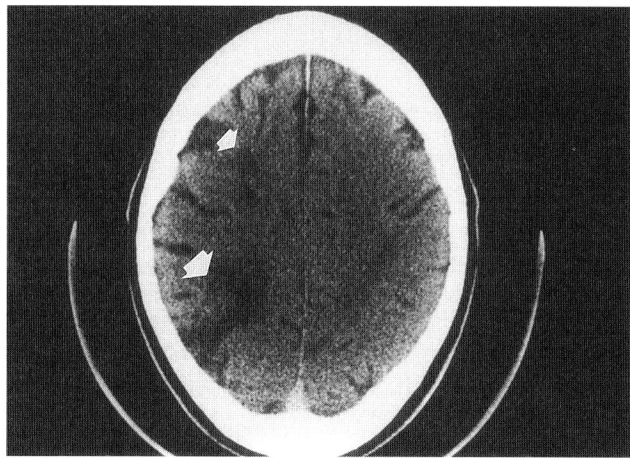

FIG. 27.2 CT scan of the brain with borderzone (watershed) infarction, characteristic of hemodynamic ischemia.

man, who estimated its incidence to be 6% (8). Roski et al. estimated the risk of delayed ischemic stroke at 7.5% (53). Other studies (43, 46) have also documented delayed hemiparesis with an incidence of 5 to 10%. More recently, magnetic resonance imaging has demonstrated delayed sequelae of subclinical ischemia after carotid occlusion. Awad et al. demonstrated the de novo appearance of subcortical hyperintense lesions on magnetic resonance images after therapeutic carotid occlusion (5) even in patients who tolerated acute occlusion and who were subjected to maximal prophylaxis against thromboembolism (*Fig. 27.3*). The authors proposed a potential mechanism of delayed collateral failure in these cases. Larson et al. (38) have also reported instances of delayed ischemic stroke that progressed despite anticoagulation and apparently involved watershed and borderzone brain territories. Prophylactic considerations for the prevention of delayed ischemia may include judicious blood pressure and volume management and avoidance of hypotension.

Several studies continue to demonstrate unacceptable ischemic complications from surgical or endovascular carotid occlusion in conjunction with skull base and head and neck neoplastic lesions. Brisman et al. reported that 4 of the 10 patients surgically managed for head and neck neoplasms with carotid occlusion suffered profound ischemic sequelae (9). Sen and Sekhar reported that 12 of 30 patients treated with carotid occlusion and revascularization procedures suffered ischemic sequelae (60). Some authors have suggested that such tumors per se de-

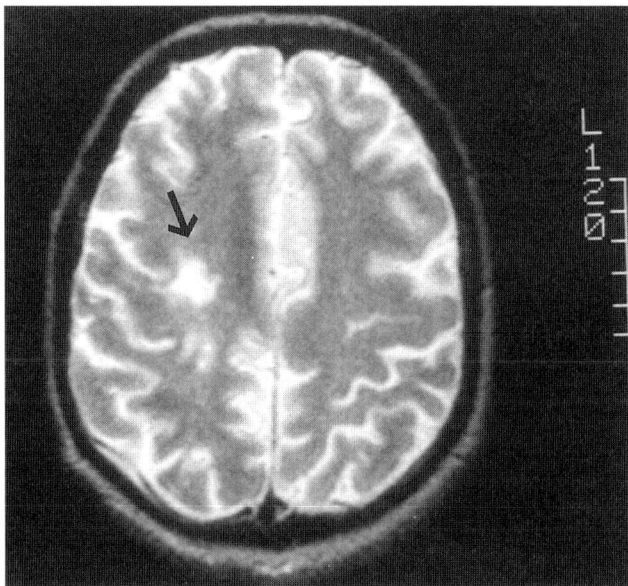

Fig. 27.3 Magnetic resonance image of the brain revealing subcortical white matter hyperintense lesion, which often develops (with or without minor ischemic symptoms) after carotid occlusion.

crease tolerance to carotid occlusion and have recommended aggressive adjuvant revascularization procedures. It is more likely, however, that complications are the result of suboptimal provocative testing, injudicious periprocedure management (anticoagulation, hemodynamic support, etc.), and early, major surgical intervention after carotid occlusion. The latter predisposes to hemodynamic stresses (blood loss, hypovolemia, anemia), hypercoagulability (or at least lack of anticoagulation or antiplatelet prophylaxis), and even mechanical manipulation of fresh thrombus in the occluded artery (surgical positioning and dissection). We have not encountered any higher prevalence of ischemic complications in our cases of head and neck neoplasia who were subjected to rigorous neurovascular protocol of carotid occlusion with all management adjuncts and with delay of major surgical procedures at least 4 weeks after carotid occlusion.

Delayed hemorrhagic complications from therapeutic carotid occlusion have been well documented. The potential for delayed hemorrhage from therapeutic carotid occlusion lies in the possibility of subarachnoid hemorrhage from the original aneurysm, the possible enlargement and rupture of another untreated aneurysm, or the de novo formation of a new aneurysm. Wright and Sweet reviewed a series of 112 patients treated with therapeutic carotid ligation and found 21 patients suffered delayed subarachnoid hemorrhage (69). German and Black reported similar rates (20%) of hemorrhagic complications from internal carotid ligation (24). Long-term follow-up study by Winn et al. (68) found delayed hemorrhages in 5 patients in a group of 37 patients treated with carotid ligation.

Although a large fraction of the patients with hemorrhagic complications likely suffered hemorrhages from the incomplete thrombosis of intradural aneurysms, other reports have confirmed enlargement and hemorrhage from untreated aneurysms, as well as the de novo formation of new aneurysms (*Fig. 27.4*). Miller et al. reported 4 cases of delayed hemorrhage from 72 patients whose aneurysms were treated by therapeutic carotid occlusion. Miller et al. noted that three of the four cases of subarachnoid hemorrhage were related to aneurysms that were previously undiagnosed. Dyste and Beck (18) and Fujiwara et al.

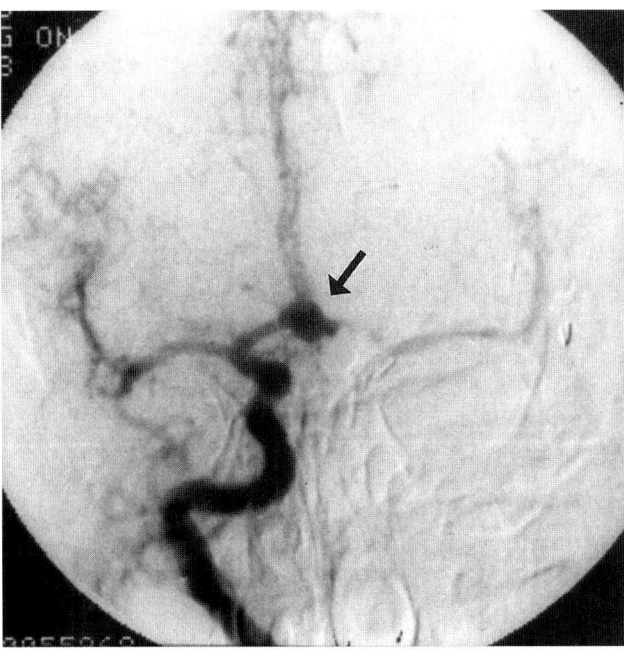

FIG. 27.4 Anterior communicating artery aneurysm presenting with subarachnoid hemorrhage 5 years after left internal carotid artery occlusion for giant aneurysm. The anterior communicating artery aneurysm was not present on angiogram at time of carotid occlusion.

(23) have also reported angiographically novel aneurysm formation after therapeutic carotid occlusion. Confirmed reports of growth and the increased risk of rupture in intracranial aneurysms contralateral to the side of occlusion after therapeutic occlusion have been published (6, 20). The mechanism of aneurysm growth and formation after carotid occlusion may be secondary to alterations in flow dynamics. This phenomenon has been compared with the increased incidence berry aneurysms in the patients with congenital hypoplasia of one carotid artery (40) and the association of aneurysms with hemodynamic stresses in arteriovenous malformations (23). It is possible that regular noninvasive surveillance with magnetic resonance imaging or computed tomography angiography might detect de novo aneurysms predisposing to hemorrhage, allowing prophylactic treatment of these lesions. Such surveillance might also identify progressive occlusive disease in the contralateral carotid or collateral arteries that might predispose to delayed ischemic sequelae.

ENDOVASCULAR OCCLUSION AND PROVOCATIVE TESTING

Before the advent of endovascular techniques of carotid occlusion, therapeutic approaches to carotid occlusion employed the application of various clamps such as those of Selverstone, Crutchfield, and Saliba. The outcomes reported from the wide application of occlusion clamps were varied. In the 1960s, Scott and Skwarok reported significant rates of mortality; 6% of the patients treated with clamp occlusion of the internal carotid artery and 11% of those treated with clamp occlusion of the common carotid artery suffered fatal complications (57). These authors also reported an overall significant morbidity in 22% and 11% of cases of internal and common carotid occlusions, respectively. Literature from this era also reported significant rates of delayed ischemic and hemorrhagic complications as noted previously (24, 51, 57).

A significant improvement in outcomes from therapeutic carotid occlusion has accompanied the advent of endovascular techniques. Endovascular detachable balloon technique has been noted to offer several advantages over conventional abrupt or gradual arterial ligation. A transfemoral arterial catheter approach allows the procedure to be performed in the awake patient under local anesthesia. Balloon test occlusion in the awake patient allows the close and continuous monitoring of the patient's neurological status while defining angiographic patterns of collateral supply of the territory of the occluded artery. This allows the dynamic definition of the patient's hemodynamic reserve before committing permanent arterial occlusion (32, 41, 44). If the patient develops a focal neurological deficit during the balloon test occlusion, the procedure can be aborted, and alternative treatment modalities such as EC-IC bypass surgery can be contemplated to enhance the patient's hemodynamic collateral reserves.

An important adjunct to balloon test occlusion is provocative hypotensive challenge. Typically, hypotension is induced after contrast stasis is noted after balloon inflation (*Fig. 27.5*). Upon reassessment of the patient's neurological examination after balloon inflation, and if the patient is found to have tolerated the balloon inflation without immediate flow-related neurological deficit, the hypotensive challenge can be initiated. Chemically induced hypotension is induced usually to 30 to 50% of the patient's baseline systolic blood pressure, whereas the patient is repeatedly examined for alterations in speech, motor loss, or sensory extinction (5, 15, 38). Although balloon test occlusion in the normotensive patient allows an assessment of immediate tolerance to hemodynamic ischemia, the addition of provocative hypotensive challenge may enhance the sensitivity to detect potential vulnerability to collateral failure.

Since its introduction in the mid-1970s, endovascular carotid occlusion has become the standard modality of therapy, gradually replacing

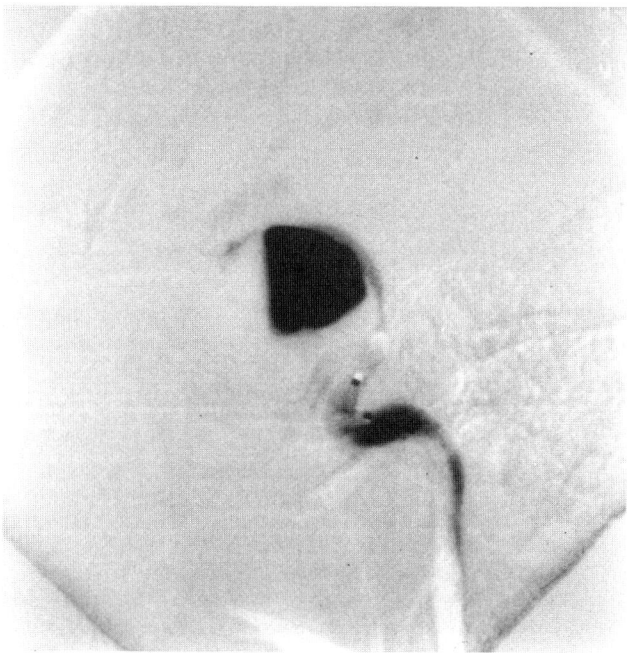

FIG. 27.5 Temporary internal carotid artery test occlusion with stasis of contrast agent in giant cavernous segment aneurysm.

abrupt surgical ligation and gradual arterial occlusion paradigms. Serbinenko reported in 1974 a series of 82 patients who had successful occlusions of the ICA with angiographically guided detachable balloons without discussion of related complications (61). Romodanov and Shcheglov (50) reported in 1981 the application of endovascular balloon occlusion, where they found a rate of mortality of 8.95% and a rate of morbidity of 4.48%. Later studies have cited rates of complications that are improved from these early reports. In 1984, Kupersmith et al. and Berenstein et al. reported the application of endovascular carotid occlusion without the occurrence of major morbidity (7, 37). Weil et al. (65) also reported favorable outcome, with a 4.7% rate of transient ischemia, 9.7% of permanent ischemia, and no instances of hemorrhage. In 1987, Fox et al. (22) reported a series of 68 patients with inoperable, infraclinoid aneurysms who were treated with proximal artery occlusion with detachable balloons. Although the authors reported only a single instance of serious morbidity in their series (permanent stroke) and no instances of mortality, they reported a rate of 13.2% of delayed ischemic complications. Those patients who have had partial or complete failures of provocative balloon test occlusion are identified as candidates for either aggressive post-procedural medical management (volume expansion and induced hypertension) or surgical revascularization.

Most recent clinical studies, with the benefit of long-term follow-up, have elucidated the delayed ischemic and hemorrhagic complications of endovascular carotid occlusion. Larson et al. (38) reported in 1995 the long-term evaluation of 58 patients with internal carotid aneurysms treated by intravascular balloon occlusion. The authors reported that 3% of their study population suffered permanent delayed ischemic sequelae between the 72 hours to 2-week period, whereas 10% suffered acute but transient ischemia that was reversed with volume expansion and anticoagulation. Larson et al. correctly suggested that endovascular occlusion and balloon test occlusion may not be protective against delayed thromboembolic or hemodynamic ischemia. Larson et al. (38) also noted the phenomenon of delayed hemorrhagic complication from carotid occlusion either from de novo aneurysm formation or from the enlargement and rupture of a previously noted aneurysm. The authors presented two patients in their series who presented with subarachnoid hemorrhage 2 and 4 years after their therapeutic occlusion.

ADJUNCTIVE ASSESSMENT OF CEREBRAL BLOOD FLOW

Although the clinical functional assessment of collateral reserve offered by balloon test occlusion has had a profound impact on decreasing acute hemodynamic ischemia, it has proven to have imperfect predictive value for subacute and delayed hemodynamic ischemia (5, 15). In the attempt to identify the subgroup of patients who pass the provocative balloon test occlusion but that are still "at risk" for subacute or delayed ischemia, indirect studies of cerebral blood flow (CBF) have become an important adjunct. Carotid stump pressures and ocular pneumoplethysmography have been used in the past but have been largely abandoned as they failed to relay information predictive of subsequent neurological compromise (35). The ocular pneumoplethysmography in particular has been questioned as it reflects only the distal pressures of the opthalmic artery (17).

Transcranial Doppler (TCD) ultrasound has also been useful as an adjunct to permanent balloon occlusion in predicting the risk for ischemia (19). The technique, as applied to therapeutic carotid occlusion, was introduced by Giller et al. in 1990 (25). The authors applied TCD measurements of the ipsilateral middle cerebral artery as a guide to a gradual carotid occlusion protocol (Crutchfield clamp) for the treatment of a giant intracavernous carotid aneurysm with supraclinoid extension. Applying the principle that TCD velocities are reflective of ipsilateral hemodynamically significant carotid artery stenosis (67), Giller et al. applied ipsilateral middle cerebral artery velocities as a gauge of evolving collateral formation with a gradual carotid occlusion. Eckert et al. (19) recently reported the application of TCD measurements (mean flow velocity and pulsatility index) in conjunction with permanent balloon occlusion of the internal carotid artery. In the retrospective analysis of 32 patients who underwent permanent balloon occlusion, the authors found that compromised TCD values noted at the time of the occlusion were predictive of delayed ischemic sequelae from hemodynamic compromise. Schneweis et al. (55) also reported a significant specificity in the relationship between compromised TCD velocities and the evolution of hemodynamic infarcts.

Over the past two decades, xenon-enhanced computed tomography (xenon-CT) has gained gradual acceptance for the accurate quantitative assessment of regional CBF (17, 72, 73, 75, 76). Its popularity in the neurosurgical community has been related to its ready accessibility and the relative ease of its interpretation as a consequence of its high resolution in conjunction with analogous CT images (17). The CBF values obtained from xenon-CT have been shown to correlate well with invasive laboratory measurements of CBF (27, 28). The xenon technology is easily assimilated into pre-existing CT scanners with relatively little expense (76). Furthermore, xenon-CT can be repeated in 20-minute intervals to reflect the possible changes in the cerebral hemodynamic state. Its application as an adjunct to endovascular carotid occlusion and provocative testing was introduced by deVries et al. (17). The authors showed that the combination of balloon test occlusion and xenon-CT allowed a greater accuracy in the prediction of ischemic risk, significantly increasing the safety of ICA occlusion and resection. Since its introduction, other studies have also included xenon-CT in the treatment protocol and have corroborated its contribution in assessing the hemodynamic reserve (33, 64, 73, 76).

However, the advantages of xenon-CT, in its high-resolution quantification of regional CBF and its efficacy in the identification of "at risk" brain territories in therapeutic carotid occlusion must be tempered by its disadvantages. Xenon as a gaseous element is associated with significant anesthetic properties that may affect level of consciousness and even induce apnea (76). It can result in severe effects on the sensorium, and studies may need to be aborted if the patient is intolerant to these effects. Xenon-CT assessment of CBF is also complicated by the phenomenon of "flow activation" that may result in artifactual signal and contaminated determination of CBF (76). Lastly, this technique requires that the patient be transported from the angiography table, with the temporary balloon occluded, for xenon-CT blood flow assessment. This necessitates close logistic coordination and may compromise hemodynamic and clinical monitoring during carotid test occlusion.

Single-photon emission computed tomographic (SPECT) brain imaging has also gained increasing acceptance in the differentiation of patients with poor hemodynamic reserve in the pre-procedural evaluation for therapeutic carotid occlusion (34, 36, 42, 47, 48). Since the early 1990s, SPECT has become established as a reliable measure of CBF and cerebral blood volume (54). Its usefulness as a predictor of hemodynamic outcome after therapeutic carotid occlusion has been examined in some detail. Komiyama et al. (36) reported that the application of SPECT studies of CBF, in conjunction with balloon test occlusion, may be potentially valuable in the prediction of hemodynamic outcome. Palestro et al. (48) examined 20 cases of SPECT performed during temporary balloon test occlusion and found that SPECT symmetry is correlated with favorable postocclusion outcome. Furthermore, the authors suggested that SPECT asymmetry might have significant predictive value of poor hemodynamic tolerance to carotid occlusion, thus serving as a foundation for alternative treatment modalities.

Unlike the xenon-CT, SPECT allows the assessment of CBF up to several hours after injection of the isotope. Patients are injected with the isotope ^{99m}Tc HMPAO at the time of the balloon test occlusion, and the imaging performed subsequently reflects the CBF at the time of the injection. This is related to the single pass uptake properties of the particular isotope, reflecting blood flow at the time of the injection and not at the time of imaging. SPECT also allows the direct visualization and relative quantification of "at risk" regions and vascular territories that may be more meaningful to the clinician than TCD values. Other advantages of SPECT include its ready availability at major medical institutions.

However, as with all adjunctive assessments of hemodynamic reserves, the sensitivity and specificity of SPECT at predicting ischemic sequelae are not absolute. Loberboym et al. (42) reported four cases of delayed clinical ischemia as a result of carotid occlusion in patients who had apparent SPECT symmetry. The study also noted, however, that the patients with SPECT asymmetry were directed toward alternative treatment strategies such as revascularization or carotid preservation with favorable surgical and neurological outcome. On the other hand, Monsein et al. (45) have reported a series in which a subgroup of patients with SPECT asymmetry suffered no ischemic sequelae after carotid occlusion. Our own experience has included three patients with severe SPECT asymmetry and early tolerance of carotid occlusion who subsequently developed delayed ischemia (41). We have also encountered at least four patients with mild-to-moderate SPECT asymmetry who tolerated acute carotid occlusion with hypotensive challenge. These cases received active hemodynamic support including hypertensive therapy, hypervolemia, and slow mobilization and did not develop subsequent clinically overt ischemia. We also encountered a case of SPECT asymmetry in association with catheter-induced brain embolism, who also tolerated carotid occlusion without further neurological sequelae.

In summary, adjunctive CBF assessment may define a subgroup of cases who exhibit serious compromise of collateral reserve (*Fig. 27.6*) and who are likely at high risk of subsequent ischemic complications. Other cases with less pronounced blood flow asymmetry (*Fig. 27.7*) may well tolerate carotid occlusion but are at moderate risk of delayed ischemia from collateral failure and could benefit from more judicious hemodynamic support during the periocclusion period.

THE DILEMMA OF PROPHYLACTIC BYPASS SURGERY

Prophylactic EC-IC bypass remains a point of controversy in whether it should play a major role in the management of therapeutic carotid occlusion. Recent literature has pointed to conflicting directions in regard to the benefit of prophylactic bypass. Notably, some authors have emphasized the value of prophylactic bypass in the select group of pa-

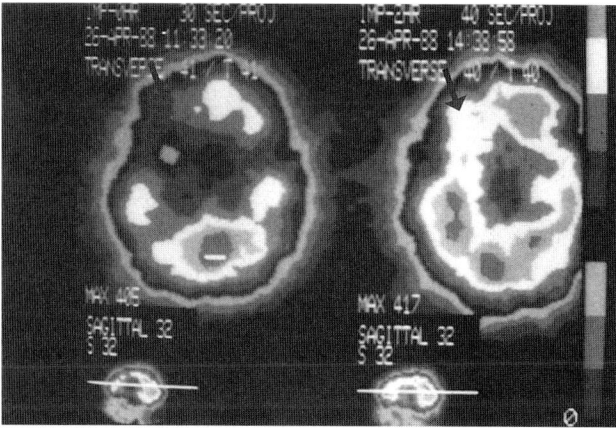

FIG. 27.6 SPECT scan showing major cerebral hypoperfusion ipsilateral to internal carotid artery occlusion. Such severe hypoperfusion is strongly predictive of subsequent cerebral infarction.

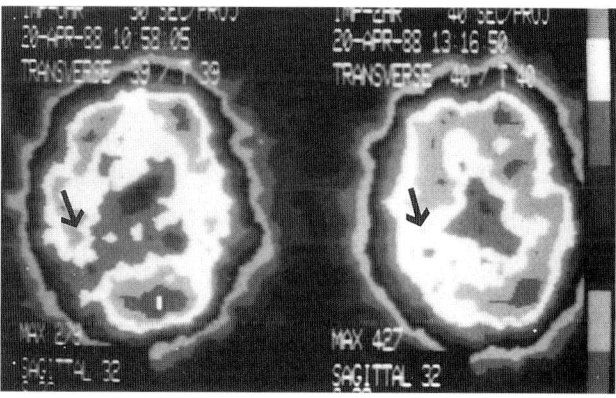

FIG. 27.7 SPECT scan showing mild cerebral hypoperfusion ipsilateral to internal carotid artery occlusion. Many such patients tolerate occlusion with judicious hemodynamic support and manifest no lasting neurological sequelae.

tients who have failed provocative testing. Hacein-Bey et al. (29) have reported their experience with the EC-IC bypass as an adjunct in therapeutic carotid occlusion for the treatment of inoperable internal carotid aneurysms. Their study population included patients who failed ICA balloon test occlusion or those that showed marked deficits in CBF (by xenon-133 washout technique), TCD readings, or carotid stump pressures. Excellent results are reported in this study with regard to the graft patency, aneurysm thrombosis, and symptomatic outcome without major irreversible morbidity. Other authors have also advocated treatment paradigms including EC-IC bypass for the "at-risk" patient population in trying to supplement the deficient hemodynamic reserve (58, 71, 74).

Although the concept of supplementing a deficient hemodynamic reserve has obvious intuitive and some experiential support, other studies have suggested still significant rates of thromboembolic complications. EC-IC graft thrombosis and the resultant embolic phenomenon from the thrombosed graft have been reported (62). The graft itself may alter hemodynamic patterns or may act as a direct channel of emboli from the stump of the occluded carotid artery to the middle cerebral artery territory. A review of cases collected from the neurovascular community reported a significant rate of embolic complications after prophylactic EC-IC bypass in conjunction with carotid occlusion (30). Recent series of the revascularization experience with carotid occlusion have estimated the prevalence of major associated morbidity to be from 10 to 30% (9, 59, 70). Brisman et al. evaluated a series of 17 patients who underwent a surgical management of head and neck tumors that involved the carotid artery at the skull base. Although their worst outcome is reported in the three patients without revascularization (two of whom passed balloon test occlusion), a significant rate of graft thrombosis and stroke were found (two of seven) in the patient group with revascularization. In a recent study, Abruzzo et al. reported that 8 of 15 patients subjected to prophylactic bypass before carotid occlusion suffered significant ischemic complications, despite patent bypass graft, whereas none of 17 patients undergoing therapeutic carotid occlusion after provocative testing and without prophylactic bypass suffered any neurological sequelae (3).

Other articles regarding the benefits of cerebral revascularizations have been reported in intracranial carotid to carotid bypass in the treatment of skull base lesions. Sen and Sekhar reported a series of 30 patients who underwent reconstructions of the internal carotid artery for the surgical management of lesions at the cranial base with a graft patency rate of 86% in a mean follow-up time of 18 months (60). The authors reported that only one of the four patients suffering a graft failure led to a massive stroke with ensuing death, whereas the other three remained asymptomatic. Furthermore, three of their patients suffered minor strokes as sequelae of the temporary ICA occlusion during the 2-hour operative revascularization period. These authors have recently abandoned this procedure (L Sekhar, unpublished comments, 1998) in favor of more conventional EC-IC bypass strategies, citing unacceptable complication rates.

Other arguments in favor of prophylactic bypass in every case of intended carotid sacrifice are often framed in emotional or anecdotal contexts, such as needing to preserve or restore two "God given" carotid circulations (T. Fukushima, unpublished comments, 1997). More objective rationale invokes the bypass as protecting against delayed ischemic and hemorrhagic complications of carotid occlusion, especially in young patients. There has been no scientific evidence whatsoever that bypass surgery protects in any way against such delayed sequelae. It may in fact provide an unjustified sense of security with less judicious surveillance for contralateral carotid occlusive disease or the genesis of intracranial berry aneurysms.

The major argument against prophylactic bypass surgery in every case with planned therapeutic carotid occlusion is that most patients in fact do tolerate therapeutic carotid occlusion without untoward sequelae (11, 26, 32, 38, 64). The arbitrary subjection of the whole universe of these cases to the risk and cost of major revascularization procedure can hardly be defensible. Most complications of carotid occlusion may be preventable by judicious provocative testing and adjunctive management protocols, and yet many of these complications are not necessarily preventable by prophylactic bypass surgery.

Cerebral revascularization remains an essential adjunct to therapeutic carotid occlusion in a select subgroup of cases. These include patients where a deficient hemodynamic reserve is noted by a failure of provocative test occlusion (overt acute symptoms or major cerebral blood flow compromise). In such instances, provocative testing is repeated after revascularization and before carotid sacrifice (*Fig. 27.8*). Verification of bypass patency is mandatory, and time may be allowed for the bypass to mature and provide sufficient collateral reserve. Unexpected intraoperative carotid sacrifice in cases (vascular or neoplastic) without preoperative tests of tolerance might also benefit from acute revascularization to enhance hemodynamic reserve. Cases with significant contralateral occlusive disease, or pathology that might dictate subsequent contralateral carotid sacrifice, require every effort at carotid preservation or prophylactic revascularization in conjunction with carotid occlusion.

PRACTICAL MANAGEMENT PROTOCOL

Risk Management: Pre-procedural Considerations

Before the permanent occlusion of the carotid artery, careful considerations are given to minimize post-procedural risk of ischemia (*Fig. 27.9*). Initially, a noninvasive examination of the cerebrovascular

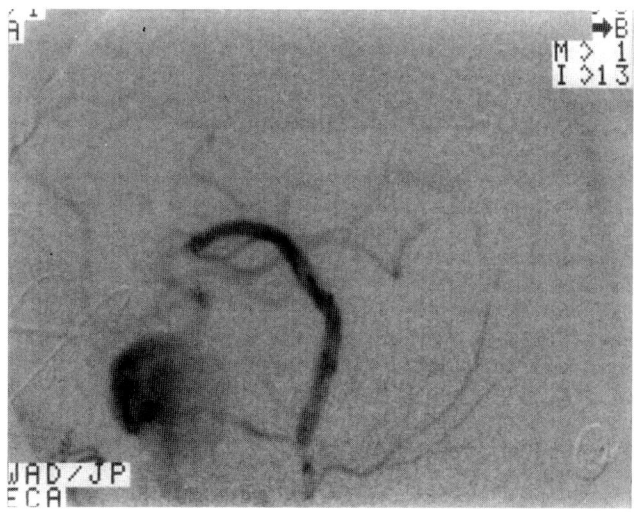

FIG. 27.8 Patient with symptomatic cavernous segment giant aneurysm developed dense hemiparesis and aphasia during test occlusion. She underwent short vein EC-IC bypass (postprocedure angiogram shown) and subsequently tolerated therapeutic carotid occlusion.

anatomy is specified for each patient. Magnetic resonance angiography or duplex Doppler carotid ultrasound may reveal a compromised patency of the contralateral carotid artery, making impossible the treatment option of ipsilateral carotid occlusion. In these instances, invasive catheter angiography can be prevented or other treatment modalities can be considered, including possible enhancement of the contralateral vascular supply with an endarterectomy procedure. These noninvasive examinations provide valuable pre-procedural risk evaluation, and they have become a part of the standard pre-procedural workup. Other standard laboratory evaluations and standard chest x-ray and electrocardiogram are obtained pre-procedurally to minimize post-procedural risks such as dye-related exacerbation of chronic renal failure or cardiogenic failure that may increase risks of hypotension and cerebral ischemia.

The central venous catheter, and in selected instances the Swan-Ganz catheter (advanced over a guidewire even in the anticoagulated patient), can be an important adjunct in the post-procedural critical care management to optimize fluid status and to enhance the hemodynamic reserve. Placement of such catheters after carotid occlusion often requires reversal of anticoagulation at a time when it may be most needed. We have made it standard practice at our

THERAPEUTIC CAROTID OCCLUSION MANAGEMENT PROTOCOL

Noninvasive Neurovascular Assessment
MR Angiogram, Carotid ultrasound

⇩

Central Venous Access and Arterial Line

⇩

Periprocedural Anticoagulation
Prevention of Thromboembolic Ischemia.
Aiming for PTT of 60–80 seconds.

⇩

Provocative Testing: Balloon Test Occlusion
Careful neurological monitoring for 15 to 30-minute period.
Adjunctive hypotensive challenge
CBF Studies (SPECT vs. xenon CT vs. TCD)

 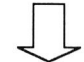 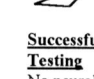

Failure of Provocative Testing
Neurological symptoms **or**
Major asymmetry on CBF studies

Partial Failure of Provocative Testing
No neurological symptoms **and**
Mild to moderate asymmetry on CBF studies **or**
Impaired angiographic collaterals

Successful Provocative Testing
No neurological symptoms **and**
No asymmetry on CBF studies

Abort Procedure
1) Consider carotid bypass surgery for the enhancement of hemodynamic reserve.
2) Reconsider carotid preservation and alternative treatment modalities.

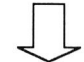

Aggressive Hemodynamic Support:
1) Volume and inotropic support.
2) Swan-Ganz catheter monitoring.
3) Continued systemic anticoagulation for 48 hours.
4) Slow mobilization

If subacute postprocedure symptoms   If no subacute symptoms

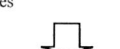

1) Maintain full systemic anticoagulation for 48 hours.
2) Rapid mobilization

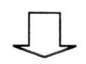

Delayed Management Paradigm
1) Delay elective surgical procedures for at least 4 weeks following therapeutic carotid occlusion (hypotension, dysautoregulation, anesthesia, positioning)
2) Maintain antiplatelet therapy
3) Avoid hypotension
4) Follow-up MRA surveillance contralateral ICA, de novo aneurysms

FIG. 27.9 Proposed management protocol for therapeutic carotid occlusion as currently implemented by the Yale Neurovascular Surgery Program. PTT, partial thromboplastin time.

institution to place a subclavian central line before embarking on potential carotid occlusion. In anticipation of the hypotensive challenge and the requirement for careful post-procedural blood pressure management, we have also made it standard practice to place a radial arterial line.

Balloon Test Occlusion and Adjunctive CBF Studies

Standard neuroangiographic techniques are applied to provide high-resolution digital subtraction imaging of the cervical and intracranial carotid circulation bilaterally. The balloon test occlusion is performed using commercially available nondetachable balloon catheters. The balloon is inflated to the minimal volume required to obtain a complete arrest of the anterograde blood flow.

Before the inflation of the balloon, the patients receive a bolus of 3000 U of intravenous heparin and are subsequently started on weight-based maintenance heparin with activated coagulation time controls. Maintenance heparin therapy is continued in the periprocedural period for a total of 48 hours, aiming for full systemic anticoagulation with partial thromboplastin time of 60 to 80 seconds. The rationale for the standardization of periprocedural anticoagulation in therapeutic carotid occlusion is inspired by the effective prophylaxis against thromboembolic ischemia documented by previous reports (30, 31, 41). We have not encountered any instances of major territorial arterial infarction (thromboembolic propagation) in more than one hundred consecutive carotid occlusions with periprocedure anticoagulation. Such enthusiasm for full anticoagulation must be tempered in special situations of continued vulnerablilty to hemorrhage, i. e., carotid blowout, multiple trauma, etc.

After the inflation of the test balloon, serial neurological examinations are performed every 2 to 3 minutes for 15 to 30 minutes. If the patient develops gross neurological deficit such as dense hemiparesis or aphasia, the balloon is deflated, and the planned carotid occlusion is aborted. If no neurologic symptoms develop during the balloon test occlusion, a chemically induced hypotension is initiated to further challenge the hemodynamic reserve. Infusion of intravenous sodium nitroprusside allows a controlled titration of the systolic blood pressure to a level that is at least 20% below the patient's baseline systolic blood pressure. Serial neurological examinations are continued at every 2 to 3-minute interval during the hypotensive challenge. The patient is immediately returned to normotensive systolic blood pressure if new neurological symptoms develop.

During the hypotensive challenge, the patient is injected with ^{99m}Tc HMPAO. Although ^{99m}Tc HMPAO SPECT images are obtained after the balloon test occlusion, the images are reflective of the regional CBF at the time of the provocative testing. As discussed previously, ^{99m}Tc SPECT provides a reliable prediction of post-procedural hemodynamic ischemia (36, 47, 48). We have applied qualitative ^{99m}Tc HMPAO SPECT in our carotid occlusion paradigm because of its excellent track record in the literature and its ready availability in our institution. However, other institutions have also reported excellent outcome with the adjunctive applications of xenon-CT and transcranial Dopplers in the assessment of cerebral blood flow (19, 73, 76).

Provocative Testing and Risk Assessment

Based on the results of the provocative balloon test occlusion and ^{99m}Tc HMPAO SPECT, each patient can be determined to be at "high risk," "moderate risk," or "low risk" of facing hemodynamic ischemic sequelae. Those patients who are determined to be in the "high risk" category are identified by the occurrence of neurological symptoms during balloon test occlusion or by the appearance of major asymmetry on SPECT. In this subset of patients, we have aborted the planned permanent balloon occlusion. In light of their poor hemodynamic reserves, consideration must be given to alternative modalities of therapy, such as a subtotal resection of a skull base tumor with preservation of the carotid artery. Furthermore, with the recent improvements in the technical aspects of carotid revascularization, the consideration must be given to prophylactic carotid bypass surgery to enhance the hemodynamic reserve before therapeutic occlusion. We have found the utility in repeating provocative testing after a successful prophylactic carotid bypass to assess the radiographic and hemodynamic enhancement from the revascularization. If the patient is able to pass provocative testing with a patent bypass graft, it is reasonable to proceed with carotid occlusion.

The patients who are determined to be at "moderate risk" develop no neurological symptoms at the time of the balloon test occlusion but are identified by a mild to moderate asymmetry on the SPECT. We have found that this subset of patients can also evolve post-procedural neurological sequelae despite normal clinical examination during provocative testing. However, with the application of aggressive, medical, hemodynamic support, this subset of patients is usually left with no permanent clinical sequelae. These patients are post-procedurally managed in the intensive critical care setting with frequent neurological monitoring. We have pursued aggressive volume and ionotropic support guided by central hemodynamic monitoring with the Swan-Ganz catheter. Typically, for the first 48 hours after the procedure, the pulmonary capillary wedge pressures are maintained at a moderately hypervolemic range to titrate the maximum cardiac output at the peak of the Starling curve. The patient's systolic blood pressure is maintained at 20% above the baseline, if necessary, with the institution of ionotropic agents. Systemic anticoagulation is maintained for the first 48 hours to prevent thromboembolic complications. After the first 48 hours, the hemodynamic support is weaned gradually, and the patient is mobilized in a slow and deliberate fashion with a close monitoring of the patient's neurological status.

The "low risk" group is determined by the absence of neurological symptoms during provocative testing and the absence of asymmetry on ^{99m}Tc SPECT. Although the potential for hemodynamic ischemia in this subset of patients is "low," reports of post-procedural hemodynamic strokes have been reported (15). Typically with patients in the "low risk" group, we have guided our volume resuscitation with central venous pressures and have instituted ionotropic support in the rare instances of appearance of neurological symptoms. These patients are otherwise rapidly mobilized within 48 hours of carotid occlusion. Full systemic anticoagulation is pursued for the first 48 hours, followed by aspirin therapy.

Delayed Management Paradigm

The proposed delayed management paradigm is aimed at the prevention of known mechanisms of delayed sequelae. Reports of delayed ischemia have been shown to be generated from both hemodynamic and thromboembolic sources (5, 8, 38, 53). In the prevention of delayed hemodynamic ischemia, we have made it standard practice to delay elective surgical procedures for 4 to 6 weeks after the carotid occlusion. The added hemodynamic risks associated with intraoperative anesthesia and positioning are avoided until the complete maturation of the cerebrovascular collaterals to the hemisphere ipsilateral to the occlusion. Furthermore, we emphasize caution against overjudicious hypertension management that may occur in the primary-care setting. It may be useful to withhold some antihypertensive agents for a few weeks after carotid occlusion. As prophylaxis from delayed thromboembolic sequelae, we routinely institute antiplatelet therapy with aspirin. Lastly, we recommend follow-up surveillance magnetic resonance angiographies for the assessment of the contralateral ICA as well as for the prophylactic screening for de novo intracranial aneurysms.

CONCLUSIONS

Therapeutic carotid occlusion remains a rational therapeutic approach for several clinical conditions facing the neurosurgeon. With its theoretical and technical evolutions, the neurovascular community is able to define indications and contraindications of therapeutic carotid occlusion and implement rational strategies of risk management to minimize its complications. A critical step in the progress of therapeutic carotid occlusion has been the advent of endovascular techniques of carotid occlusion and the implementation of rigorous provocative testing. Other adjunctive strategies including CBF studies, periprocedural anticoagulation, neurocritical care management, and post-procedural delay of elective surgical procedures have significantly decreased the morbidity and mortality associated with therapeutic carotid occlusion. Surgical progress in bypass revascularization of the carotid artery has allowed therapeutic options for patients with limited hemodynamic reserves. However, current evidence fails to present a good rationale for the indiscriminate application of bypass revascularization in every case of planned carotid sacrifice.

Future advances in outcome from therapeutic carotid occlusion will depend on the continued critical analysis of failures and morbidity related to this procedure. Management strategies of therapeutic carotid occlusion will need to maintain flexibility to accommodate future advances. It would be reasonable to expect that we will progress toward more sensitive and specific methods of provocative testing, including possible computer modeling of the cerebral circulation and more predictive imaging studies of flow, metabolism, and collateral reserves. Continued technical advances in cerebral revascularization will allow safer integration into the comprehensive management paradigm. Lastly, a higher level of awareness may result in better expectant and preventive strategies against delayed complications of carotid occlusion.

REFERENCES

1. Abad C, Diluch A, Espino JC: Isolated blunt trauma of the common carotid artery. **J Cardiovasc Surg** 34:507–509, 1993.
2. Abernethy J: In Rees LA (ed): *Surgical Observations*. London, 1804.
3. Abruzzo T, Miller DS, Owens RC, Dawson GJ, Shengelaia GG, Barrow DL: Prevention of cerebral ischemia after endovascular carotid sacrifice: The value of STA MCA bypass. ASITN/AANS/CNS Proceedings of the first joint meeting, Orlando, FL, February 1–4, 1998.
4. Awad IA: History of neurovascular surgery: II. Occlusive disease, cerebral hemorrhage, and vascular malformations. In: Greenblatt SH (ed): *A History of Neurosurgery*. Park Ridge, IL, AANS Publishers, 1997, pp 271–287.
5. Awad IA, Masaryk T, Magdinec M: Pathogenesis of subcortical hyperintense lesions on

magnetic resonance imaging of the brain: Observations in patients undergoing controlled therapeutic internal carotid artery occlusion. **Stroke** 24:1339–1346, 1993.
6. Batjer H, Mickey B, Samson D: Enlargement and rupture of distal basilar artery aneurysm after iatrogenic carotid occlusion. **Neurosurgery** 20:624–628, 1987.
7. Berenstein A, Ransohoff J, Kupersmith M, Flamm E, Graeb D: Transvascular treatment of giant aneurysms of the cavernous carotid and vertebral arteries: Functional investigation and embolization. **Surg Neurol** 21:3–12, 1984.
8. Black S, German WJ: The treatment of internal carotid artery aneurysm by proximal artery ligation. **J Neurosurg** 10:590–601, 1953.
9. Brisman MH, Sen C, Catalano P: Results of surgery for head and neck tumors that involve the carotid artery at the skull base. **J Neurosurg** 86:787–792, 1997.
10. Bula W, Loes DJ: Trauma to the cerebrovascular system. **Neuroimag Clin N Am** 4:753–772, 1994.
11. Citardi MJ, Chaloupka JC, Son YH, Ariyan S, Sasaki CT: Management of carotid artery rupture by monitored endovascular therapeutic occlusion (1988–1994). **Laryngoscope** 105:1086–1092, 1995.
12. Cooper A: Account of the first successful operation, performed on the common carotid artery, for aneurysm, in the year 1808: With the post-mortem examination in 1821. **Guys Hosp Rep** 1:53–58, 1836.
13. Cushing H, Bailey P: *Tumours Arising from the Blood-Vessels of the Brain: Angiomatous Malformations and Hemangioblastomas.* London, Balliere, Tindall, and Cox, 1928.
14. Dandy W: Arteriovenous aneurysms of the brain. **Arch Surg** 17:190–243, 1928.
15. Dare AO, Chaloupka JC, Putman CM, Fayad PB, Awad IA: Failure of the hypotensive provocative test during temporary balloon test occlusion of the internal carotid artery to predict delayed hemodynamic ischemia after therapeutic carotid occlusion. **Surg Neurol** 50:147–155, 1998; Discussion 155–156.
16. Debrun G: Balloon catheter techniques in neuroradiology, in *Interventional Radiology.* Philadelphia, WB Saunders, 1982, pp 707–730.
17. de Vries EJ, Sekhar LN, Horton JA, et al.: A new method to predict safe resection of the internal carotid artery. **Laryngoscope** 100:85–88, 1990.
18. Dyste GN, Beck DW: De novo aneurysm formation following carotid ligation: Case report and review of the literature. **Neurosurgery** 24:88–92, 1989.
19. Eckert B, Thie A, Carvajal M, Groden C, Zeumer H: Predicting hemodynamic ischemia by transcranial Doppler monitoring during therapeutic balloon occlusion of the internal carotid artery. **Am J Neuroradiol** 19:577–582, 1998.
20. Faria MA Jr, Fleischer AS, Spector RH: Bilateral giant intracavernous carotid aneurysms treated by bilateral carotid ligation. **Surg Neurol** 14:207–210, 1980.
21. Formanek G, Frech R, Amplatz K: Arterial thrombus formation during clinical percutaneous catheterization. **Circulation** 41:833–839, 1973.
22. Fox AJ, Vinuela F, Pelz DM, et al.: Use of detachable balloons for proximal artery occlusion in the treatment of unclippable cerebral aneurysms. **J Neurosurg** 66:40–46, 1987.
23. Fujiwara S, Fujii K, Fukui M: De novo aneurysm formation and aneurysm growth following therapeutic carotid occlusion for intracranial internal carotid artery (ICA) aneurysms. **Acta Neurochir (Wien)** 120:20–25, 1993.
24. German W, Black SPW: Cervical ligation for internal carotid artery aneurysms: An extended follow-up. **J Neurosurg** 23:572–577, 1965.
25. Giller CA, Steig P, Batjer HH, Samson D, Purdy P: Transcranial Doppler ultrasound as a guide to graded therapeutic occlusion of the carotid artery. **Neurosurgery** 26:307–311, 1990.

26. Graves VB, Perl J II, Strother CM, Wallace RC, Kesava PP, Masaryk TJ: Endovascular occlusion of the carotid or vertebral artery with temporary proximal flow arrest and microcoils: Clinical results. **Am J Neuroradiol** 18:1201–1206, 1997.
27. Gur D, Good WF, Wolfson SK Jr, Yonas H, Shabason L: In vivo mapping of local cerebral blood flow by xenon-enhanced computed tomography. **Science** 215:1267–1268, 1982.
28. Gur D, Wolfson SK Jr, Yonas H, et al.: Progress in cerebrovascular disease: Local cerebral blood flow by xenon enhanced CT. **Stroke** 13:750–758, 1982.
29. Hacein-Bey L, Connolly ES Jr, Duong H, et al.: Treatment of inoperable carotid aneurysms with endovascular carotid occlusion after extracranial-intracranial bypass surgery. **Neurosurgery** 41:1225–1231, 1997; Discussion 1231–1234.
30. Heros RC: Thromboembolic complications after combined internal carotid ligation and extra- to intracranial bypass. **Surg Neurol** 21:75–79, 1984.
31. Heros RC, Nelson PB, Ojemann RG, Crowell RM, DeBrun G: Large and giant paraclinoid aneurysms: Surgical techniques, complications, and results. **Neurosurgery** 12:153–163, 1983.
32. Higashida RT, Halbach VV, Dowd C, et al.: Endovascular detachable balloon embolization therapy of cavernous carotid artery aneurysms: Results in 87 cases. **J Neurosurg** 72:857–863, 1990.
33. Johnson DW, Stringer WA, Marks MP, Yonas H, Good WF, Gur D: Stable xenon CT cerebral blood flow imaging: Rationale for and role in clinical decision making. **Am J Neuroradiol** 12:201–213, 1991.
34. Keller E, Ries F, Urbach H, et al.: Endovascular balloon occlusion test of the internal carotid artery with increased hemodynamic monitoring for determination of circulatory reserve before planned carotid occlusion. **Rofo Fortschr Geb Rontgenstr Neuen Bildgeb Verfahr** 164:324–330, 1996.
35. Kelly JJ, Callow AD, O'Donnell TF, et al.: Failure of carotid stump pressures: Its incidence as a predictor for a temporary shunt during carotid endarterectomy. **Arch Surg** 114:1361–1366, 1979.
36. Komiyama M, Khosla VK, Tamura K, Nagata Y, Baba M: A provocative internal carotid artery balloon occlusion test with 99mTc- HM-PAO CBF mapping: Report of three cases. **Neurol Med Chir (Tokyo)** 32:747–752, 1992.
37. Kupersmith MJ, Berenstein A, Choi IS, Ransohoff J, Flamm ES: Percutaneous transvascular treatment of giant carotid aneurysms: Neuro- ophthalmologic findings. **Neurology** 34:328–335, 1984.
38. Larson JJ, Tew JM Jr, Tomsick TA, van Loveren HR: Treatment of aneurysms of the internal carotid artery by intravascular balloon occlusion: Long-term follow-up of 58 patients. **Neurosurgery** 36:26–30, 1995; Discussion 30.
39. Linskey ME, Sekhar LN, Hirsch WL Jr, Yonas H, Horton JA: Aneurysms of the intracavernous carotid artery: Natural history and indications for treatment. **Neurosurgery** 26:933–937, 1990; Discussion 937–938.
40. Linskey ME, Sekhar LN, Horton JA, Hirsch WL Jr, Yonas H: Aneurysms of the intracavernous carotid artery: A multidisciplinary approach to treatment. **J Neurosurg** 75:525–534, 1991.
41. Little JR, Rosenfeld JV, Awad IA: Internal carotid artery occlusion for cavernous segment aneurysm. **Neurosurgery** 25:398–404, 1989.
42. Lorberboym M, Pandit N, Machac J, et al.: Brain perfusion imaging during preoperative temporary balloon occlusion of the internal carotid artery (see comments). **J Nucl Med** 37:415–419, 1996.
43. Love J, Dart LH: Results of carotid ligation with particular reference to intracranial aneurysms. **J Neurosurg** 27:89–93, 1967.

44. Mathis JM, Barr JD, Jungreis CA, et al.: Temporary balloon test occlusion of the internal carotid artery: Experience in 500 cases. **Am J Neuroradiol** 16:749–754, 1995.
45. Monsein LH, Jeffery PJ, van Heerden BB, et al.: Assessing adequacy of collateral circulation during balloon test occlusion of the internal carotid artery with 99mTc-HMPAO SPECT (see comments). **Am J Neuroradiol** 12:1045–1051, 1991.
46. Oldershaw J, Voris HC: Internal carotid artery ligation: A follow-up study. **Neurology** 1966:937–938, 1966.
47. Palestro CJ: Temporary balloon occlusion, SPECT and carotid artery sacrifice (editorial; comment). **J Nucl Med** 37:419–420, 1996.
48. Palestro CJ, Sen C, Muzinic M, Afriyie M, Goldsmith SJ: Assessing collateral cerebral perfusion with technetium-99m-HMPAO SPECT during temporary internal carotid artery occlusion (see comments). **J Nucl Med** 34:1235–1238, 1993.
49. Pilz C: Zur Ligatur der Arteria carotis communis, nebst einer Statistik dieser Operation. **Arch Klin Chir** 9:257–445, 1868.
50. Romodonov A, Shcheglov VI: Intravascular occlusion of saccular aneurysms of cerebral arteries by means of a detachable balloon catheter. **Adv Tech Neurosurg** 9:25–49, 1982.
51. Roski RA, Spetzler RF: Carotid ligation, in Rengachary Wa. (ed): *Neurosurgery*. New York, McGraw-Hill, 1996, vol 2, pp 2333–2340.
52. Roski R, Spetzler RF: Carotid ligation in the treatment of cerebral aneurysms, in Hopkins L, Long DM (eds): *Clinical Management of Intracranial Aneurysms*. New York, Raven Press, 1982, pp 11–19.
53. Roski R, Spetzler RF, Nulsen FE: Late complications of carotid ligation in the treatment of intracranial anuerysms. **J Neurosurg** 54:583–587, 1981.
54. Sabatini U, Bossavy JP, Celsis P, et al.: Cerebral blood volume, endarterectomy and SPECT. **Rev Neurol (Paris)** 147:158–161, 1991.
55. Schneweis S, Urbach H, Solymosi L, Ries F: Preoperative risk assessment for carotid occlusion by transcranial Doppler ultrasound. **J Neurol Neurosurg Psychiatry** 62:485–489, 1997.
56. Schorstein J: Carotid ligation in saccular intracranial aneurysms. **Br J Surg** 28:50–70, 1940.
57. Scott M, Skwarok E: The treatment of cerebral aneurysms by ligation of the common carotid artery. **Surg Gynecol Obstet** 113:54–61, 1961.
58. Sekhar LN, Patel SJ: Permanent occlusion of the internal carotid artery during skull-base and vascular surgery: Is it really safe? (editorial; see comments). **Am J Otol** 14:421–422, 1993.
59. Sen C, Segal D: Is carotid artery reconstruction mandatory? **Clin Neurosurg** 42:135–153, 1995.
60. Sen C, Sekhar LN: Direct vein graft reconstruction of the cavernous, petrous, and upper cervical internal carotid artery: Lessons learned from 30 cases. **Neurosurgery** 30:732–742, 1992; Discussion 742–743.
61. Serbinenko FA: Balloon catheterization and occlusion of major cerebral vessels. **J Neurosurg** 41:125–145, 1974.
62. Takeuchi S, Tanaka R, Koike T, et al.: Frequent TIA in the territory fed by the anastomosed STA after combined therapeutic ICA occlusion and extracranial-intracranial bypass: Case report. **Acta Neurochir (Wien)** 133:206–210, 1995.
63. Tomsick TA, Tew JM Jr, Lukin RR, Johnson JK: Balloon catheters for aneurysms and fistulae. **Clin Neurosurg** 31:135–164, 1983.
64. Vazquez Anon V, Aymard A, Gobin YP, et al.: Balloon occlusion of the internal carotid

artery in 40 cases of giant intracavernous aneurysm: Technical aspects, cerebral monitoring, and results. **Neuroradiology** 34:245–251, 1992.
65. Weil SM, van Loveren HR, Tomsick TA, Quallen BL, Tew JM Jr: Management of inoperable cerebral aneurysms by the navigational balloon technique. **Neurosurgery** 21:296–302, 1987.
66. Weir B, Macdonald RL: Intracranial aneurysms and subarachnoid hemorrhage: An overview, in Rengachary Wa (ed): *Neurosurgery.* New York, McGraw-Hill, 1996, vol 2, pp 2191–2213.
67. Wilterdink JL, Feldmann E, Furie KL, Bragoni M, Benavides JG: Transcranial Doppler ultrasound battery reliably identifies severe internal carotid artery stenosis (see comments). **Stroke** 28:133–136, 1997.
68. Winn H, Richardson AE, Jane JA: Late morbidity and mortality of common carotid artery ligation for posterior communicating artery aneurysms. **J Neurosurg** 47:727–736, 1977.
69. Wright R, Sweet WH: Carotid or vertebral occlusion in the treatment of intracranial aneurysms: Value of early and late readings of carotid and retinal pressures. **Clin Neurosurg** 9:163–192, 1963.
70. Wright JG, Nicholson R, Schuller DE, Smead WL: Resection of the internal carotid artery and replacement with greater saphenous vein: A safe procedure for en bloc cancer resections with carotid involvement. **J Vasc Surg** 23:775–780, 1996; Discussion 781–782.
71. Yonas H: Predictability of extracranial/intracranial bypass function: A retrospective study of patients with occlusive cerebrovascular disease (letter; comment). **Neurosurgery** 41:1447–1448, 1997.
72. Yonas H: Use of xenon and ultrafast CT to measure cerebral blood flow (letter; comment). **Am J Neuroradiol** 15:794–795, 1994.
73. Yonas H, Jungreis C: Xenon CT cerebral blood flow: Past, present, and future (letter; comment). **Am J Neuroradiol** 16:219–220, 1995.
74. Yonas H, Kaufmann A: Combined extracranial-intracranial bypass and intraoperative balloon occlusion for the treatment of intracavernous and proximal carotid artery aneurysms (letter; comment). **Neurosurgery** 36:1234, 1995.
75. Yonas H, Linskey M, Johnson DW, et al.: Internal carotid balloon test occlusion does require quantitative CBF (letter; comment). **Am J Neuroradiol** 13:1147–1152, 1992.
76. Yonas H, Pindzola RP, Johnson DW: Xenon/computed tomography cerebral blood flow and its use in clinical management. **Neurosurg Clin N Am** 7:605–616, 1996.

CHAPTER

28

Therapeutic Carotid Occlusion: Indications and Potential Complications

DANIEL L. BARROW, M.D., C. MICHAEL CAWLEY, M.D.

Notwithstanding the remarkable technical and scientific developments in the treatment of disorders affecting the internal carotid artery (ICA), therapeutic carotid occlusion has remained a viable and durable method for treating selected disorders. Advances in microsurgical techniques and endovascular therapy have significantly reduced the indications for therapeutic carotid occlusion. Simultaneously, its role has been somewhat enhanced by the advent of extracranial–intracranial (EC–IC) bypass procedures to augment collateral blood flow, relatively reliable methods for determining one's ability to tolerate permanent carotid occlusion and endovascular methods for performing minimally invasive therapeutic carotid occlusion.

HISTORICAL PERSPECTIVES

The earliest indication for therapeutic carotid ligation was to control severe hemorrhage from the cervical carotid, usually as a consequence of penetrating trauma or erosion of the vessel by an adjacent neoplastic process. One of the earliest reports of carotid ligation was by Paré, who in 1585 treated a patient with life-threatening hemorrhage from a stab wound to the neck incurred during a duel (42). In 1785, John Hunter ligated the carotid artery of a stag belonging to King George III (25). Hunter observed that the stag's antler became cold and stopped growing after a few days but noted that the antler was warm and resumed growth a week later. After ordering the stag to be killed, Hunter identified enlargement of collateral vessels above and below the ligature and hypothesized that "under the stimulus of necessity," small tributary arteries will assume the function of the larger parent artery. He later used this technique to save the leg of a coachman with a popliteal aneurysm by ligating the popliteal artery. In 1792, Lynn reported the use of common carotid ligation to control hemorrhage encountered during the removal of a neck tumor (42).

In 1805, Sir Astley Cooper was the first to "electively" occlude the common carotid artery to treat an extracranial ICA aneurysm (8). The patient later died from respiratory compromise after developing a suppurative infection. In 1808, Cooper successfully repeated the operation for a similar patient (9). Sir Victor Horsley ligated the right common carotid artery to treat a right ICA aneurysm in a patient undergoing surgery for a lesion presumed to be a middle fossa tumor (4). The patient was alive and well 5 years later.

The first planned surgical carotid occlusion for an intracranial aneurysm diagnosed preoperatively was performed by Birley and Trotter in 1924 (5). In 1926, George Gray Tuner ligated the ICA of a patient who had been diagnosed with a cavernous segment carotid aneurysm on the basis of intracavernous cranial nerve involvement. Nattrass (32) reported this case in 1928.

The technique of carotid ligation was popular in the 19th century not only for the treatment of aneurysms but also for treating diverse conditions including epilepsy, trigeminal neuralgia, and "psychosis." By 1868, Pilz had amassed 586 cases of common carotid ligation with an operative mortality rate of 38.5% and a central nervous system morbidity rate of 32% (38). In 1900, Siegrist reported a significant difference among mortality rates depending on the indications for therapy (47). He found a mortality rate of 8.8% for ligations performed for pulsating exophthalmos (carotid cavernous fistula) and mortality rates of 28.3% and 50.8% for ligations performed during operations for tumor and for hemorrhage, respectively.

Several theories were advanced in those early days to explain the neurological complications resulting from carotid ligation. These theories included failure of the systemic circulation, raised intracranial pressure after subarachnoid hemorrhage, and thrombosis and subsequent embolism from the site of ligation. Perhaps the most widely accepted theory was (and is) a failure of collateral circulation to compensate for ligation of the carotid artery. As early as 1868, Pilz had emphasized the importance of sufficient collateralization of the circle of Willis to ensure the safety of carotid ligation (38).

In 1914, Matas advocated preoperative testing of the collateral cerebral circulation. This preoperative evaluation, which now bears his name, involved the use of digital compression of the carotid artery in the neck while examining the patient's neurological status (30). Dandy also advocated preoperative testing of the collateral circulation and claimed that such an evaluation allowed him to achieve relatively lower morbidity and mortality statistics (mortality rate, less than 4%; immediate complication rate, less than 4%; delayed complication rate, less than

2%) for 105 patients undergoing ligation or partial occlusion (10). In 1936, Dandy performed the first "trapping" procedure for an ICA aneurysm. This procedure involved ligation of the ICA in the patient's neck and intracranially. After performing two more of these procedures, Dandy reported all three cases in 1939.

The report by Schorstein in 1940, in which he reviewed 60 cases of intracranial aneurysms treated by carotid ligation, outlines several important clinical factors regarding the use of carotid ligation that are still applicable today (44). The operative mortality and morbidity were each 13.3% in these 60 cases. In this analysis, Schorstein noted that the complications from ICA ligation were more common in cases with severe anemia from previous hemorrhage. He hypothesized that severe anemia, the mass effect of a giant aneurysm, or intracranial hypertension led to poor cerebral perfusion. Schorstein observed superior results in patients with infraclinoid as opposed to supraclinoid aneurysms, and he noted a higher mortality rate in patients who had suffered a recent subarachnoid hemorrhage compared with patients having remote hemorrhage. Because the results were an improvement over the natural history of ruptured intracranial aneurysms, carotid ligation remained a major method of treatment for intracranial aneurysms for many years.

CURRENT INDICATIONS

Vascular

Carotid artery occlusion remains an important therapeutic option in the management of selected carotid artery aneurysms. Currently, therapeutic carotid occlusion is used most commonly to manage symptomatic cavernous segment aneurysms. A variety of therapeutic options are available for managing cavernous carotid aneurysms (8). Reconstructive options include surgical exposure of the cavernous segment for direct clip ligation and endovascular coil obliteration of the aneurysm with preservation of the parent vessel. A direct surgical approach to cavernous segment aneurysms is a formidable procedure associated with significant morbidity to the intracavernous cranial nerves. Unfortunately, many aneurysms of the cavernous segment of the carotid artery are associated with wide necks and are not readily amenable to endovascular coiling with current technology. Therefore, therapeutic carotid ligation remains a mainstay among the available therapeutic options.

Carotid occlusion for cavernous aneurysms can be performed by proximal surgical or endovascular common or ICA occlusion alone, surgical or endovascular ICA occlusion with an EC–IC bypass utilizing the superficial temporal artery, or a saphanous vein graft between a variety of donor and recipient sites or surgical or endovascular trapping with or without an EC–IC bypass (*Fig. 28.1*).

The majority of large or giant supraclinoid aneurysm are able to be managed by direct surgical clip ligation using a variety of adjuncts in-

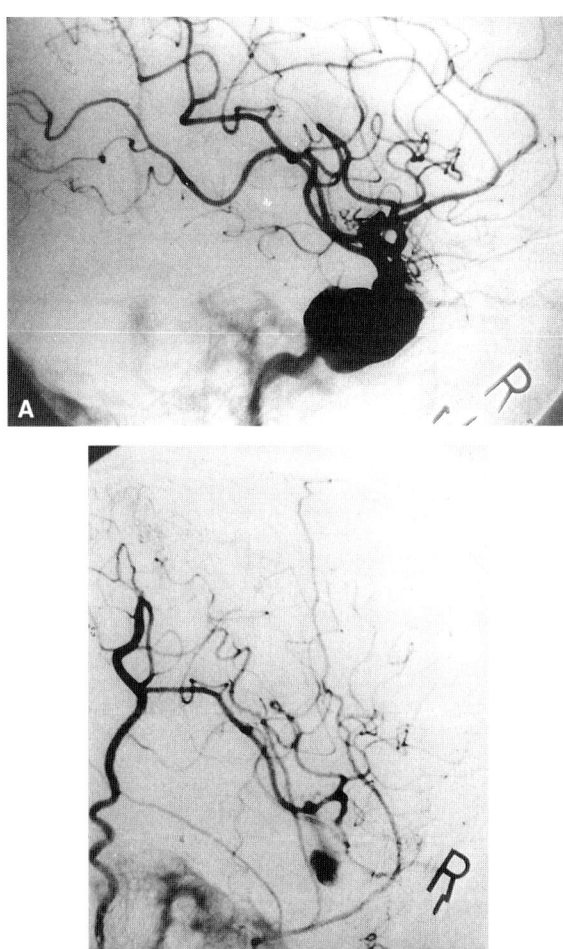

FIG. 28.1 (*A*) Lateral right carotid angiogram demonstrating a large intracavernous aneurysm that presented with retro-orbital pain and ophthalmoparesis. (*B*) Postoperative right external carotid angiogram revealing a patent superficial temporal artery to middle cerebral artery bypass filling the entire middle cerebral circulation after endovascular carotid sacrifice. Note that the bypass actually fills a portion of the aneurysm in a retrograde fashion.

cluding temporary occlusion, cerebral protection, aneurysm deflation, and preclipping aneurysmorrhaphy. However, some large and giant supraclinoid carotid aneurysms are simply not amenable to direct clip ligation or endovascular coiling because of extension of the neck into the cavernous sinus (*Fig. 28.2*), dense calcification of the neck (*Fig. 28.3*), large size of the neck, intraluminal thrombus, or other physical factors

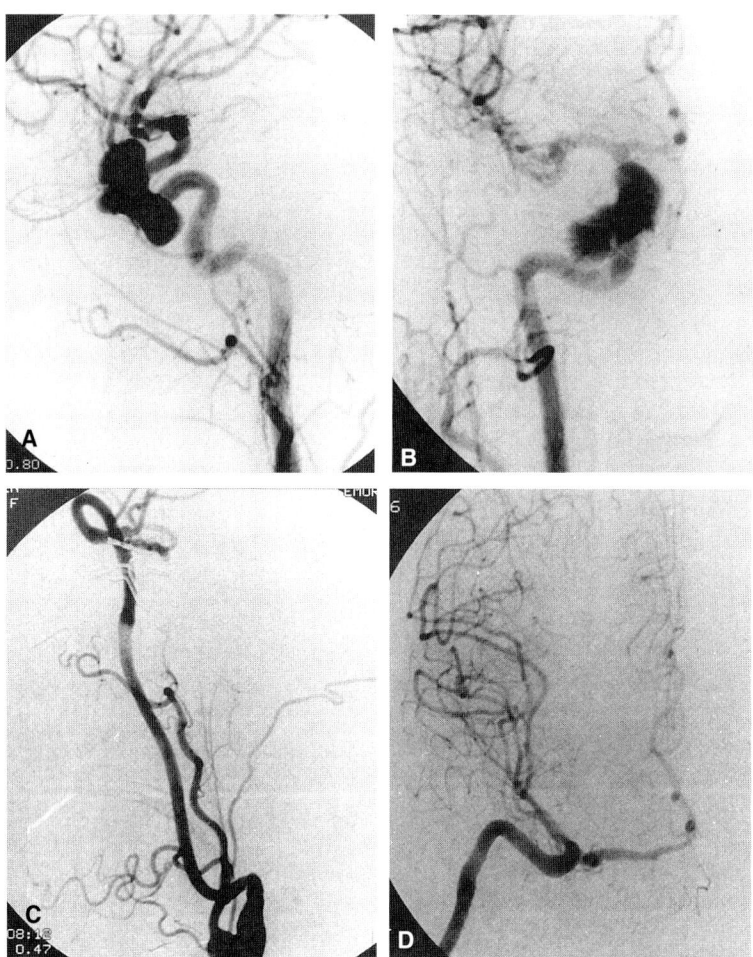

FIG. 28.2 (*A*) Lateral and (*B*) anteroposterior carotid angiograms showing a proximal carotid aneurysm involving the cavernous and clinoidal segments with supraclinoid extension into the subarachnoid space. (*C* and *D*) Follow-up angiogram after surgical trapping of the ICA and placement of a long saphenous vein graft between the cervical ICA and the middle cerebral artery.

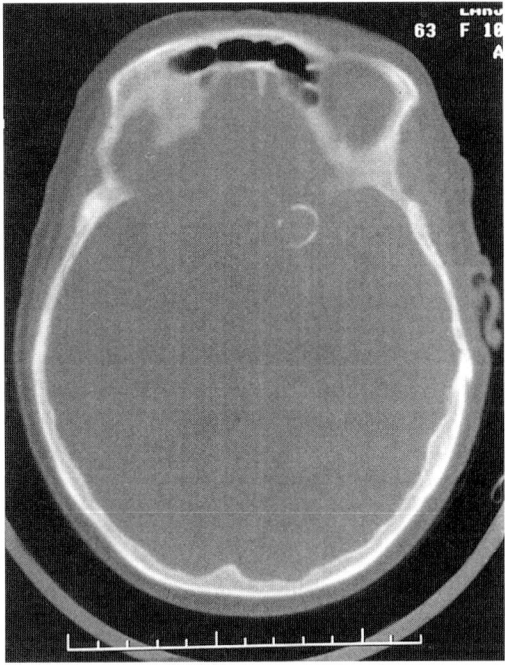

FIG. 28.3 Axial CT demonstrating dense calcification of the neck of a large ophthalmic segment ICA aneurysm that was unable to be clipped and required carotid sacrifice with an EC–IC bypass graft.

that preclude obliteration of the sac with preservation of the parent vessel. As with cavernous aneurysms, therapeutic options include a variety of methods for therapeutic carotid occlusion by endovascular or surgical means with or without augmentation of collateral circulation through an EC–IC bypass.

Therapeutic carotid occlusion is infrequently indicated in the treatment of certain carotid cavernous fistulae. The overwhelming majority of carotid cavernous fistulae are readily managed by modern endovascular techniques (21). Direct, high-flow fistulae are usually treated by endovascular detachable balloon or coil occlusion of the fistula, and indirect fistulae can usually be treated with minimal morbidity by transvenous endovascular approaches. There remain, however, some carotid cavernous fistulae that are unable to be obliterated by endovascular methods with maintenance of patency of the parent vessel. Occasionally, these lesions are best treated by therapeutic carotid sacrifice by endovascular methods. If a carotid cavernous fistula is to be treated by carotid sacrifice, it is essential that the carotid artery and the precise site of the fistula be completely obliterated by the endovascular device. Proximal occlusion of the parent vessel alone will allow the fistula to continue to fill by retrograde flow, resulting in a "cerebrovascular steal" with high risk of cerebral ischemia (3).

Therapeutic carotid occlusion is occasionally indicated for a variety of unusual aneurysms such as high cervical or petrous segment aneurysms that are difficult to access surgically. Extracranial carotid aneurysms are most often pseudoaneurysms that are the result of spontaneous traumatic carotid dissection (*Fig. 28.4*). Although therapeutic carotid occlusion remains a viable treatment option for selected lesions, the development of endovascular stents has reduced the need for carotid sacrifice due to extracranial carotid pseudoaneurysms (2). The carotid artery may also be injured as a result of either blunt or penetrating trauma. Some traumatic intracranial injuries result in pseudoaneurysm formation or irreparable disruption of the artery that requires carotid sacrifice to eliminate a potential source of hemorrhage or thromboembolism (*Fig. 28.5*).

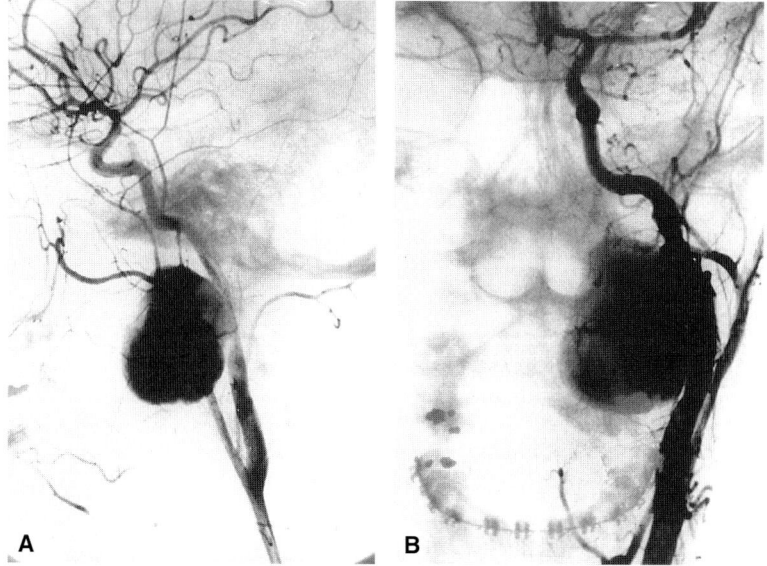

FIG. 28.4 (A) Lateral and (B) anteroposterior carotid angiogram revealing a large traumatic cervical carotid pseudoaneurysm that was treated by endovascular carotid sacrifice without a bypass after successful balloon test occlusion.

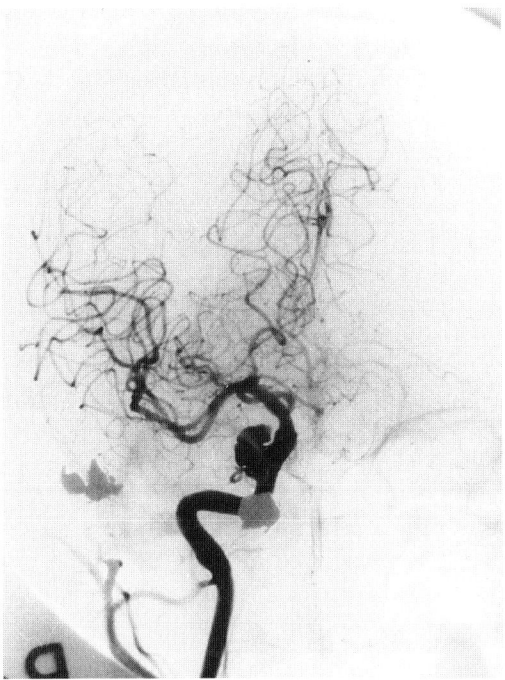

FIG. 28.5 Anteroposterior carotid angiogram showing a traumatic intracranial pseudoaneurysm resulting from a gunshot wound to the head that was treated by carotid occlusion.

Neoplasms

The advent and further development of skull-base techniques have resulted in a more aggressive surgical approach to a variety of neoplasms involving the cranial base. In selected cases, planned therapeutic sacrifice of the ICA serves as an adjunct to the aggressive removal of the tumor. In other cases, ICA resection may not contribute to a better patient outcome at all. Indeed, long-term control or cure of a slowly growing tumor is not worth a disabling or fatal stroke (46).

Most tumors involving the ICA do so through a slowly progressive process of displacement, encasement, and finally constriction. Early ischemic symptoms are more likely due to coexistent atherosclerosis than frank neoplastic arterial involvement. Malignant tumors that do invade the vessel wall include metastatic carcinoma (especially squamous cell), nasopharyngeal carcinoma, adenoid cystic carcinoma, and rhabdomyosarcoma in the cervical region. The petrous and intracavernous segments of the ICA may also be invaded by osteosarcomas, plasmacytomas, chondrosarcomas, and chordomas. Malignant processes do not usually involve the supraclinoid ICA. Benign neoplasms involving the ICA include carotid body tumors, paragangliomas, and nerve sheath tumors in the cervical region; more distal segments may be encased by glomus jugulare tumors, meningiomas, epidermoids, nerve sheath tumors, pituitary adenomas, and cavernous sinus hemangiomas.

The extent to which a given process involves the ICA determines whether the artery may be saved. Sekhar et al. described several factors that are unfavorable to ICA preservation, which include previous surgery and/or radiation therapy that might lead to scarring and weakening of the vessel wall, a firm tumor texture, and ICA neoplastic encasement and narrowing seen on magnetic resonance imaging or angiography (46). However, in his large series, Sekhar was unable to dissect the artery free of the tumor in only 7% of the cases of cervical/petrous ICA neoplastic involvement and in 26% of the cases of intracavernous/supraclinoid involvement. Despite the fact that in most cases the ICA may be dissected free, if a planned curative or aggressive procedure involves any exposure of risk to the ICA, pretreatment evaluation of the risk of ICA occlusion is wise. Appropriate flow augmentation procedures may be either planned as needed or performed prophylactically.

COMPLICATIONS

Ischemic

The most common and feared complication of therapeutic carotid occlusion is cerebral ischemia. Cerebral ischemia may result from hypoperfusion due to inadequate collateral circulation for sustaining the hemisphere ipsilateral to the occluded carotid. Additionally, embolic complications from propagating thrombus within the occluded artery may result in cerebral ischemia and infarction. Another potential mechanism for postocclusion ischemia is endovascular device emboli if carotid occlusion is accomplished through the use of endovascular balloons or coils.

Either common or internal carotid occlusion will result in a significant drop in the distal ICA pressure that is maintained well into the intracranial circulation. The risk of ischemic infarction due to hemodynamic insufficiency after carotid ligation is related to the adequacy of collateral circulation to the ipsilateral carotid circulation. In various reported series, morbidity of carotid sacrifice ranged from 0 to 46%, and mortality ranged from 0 to 29% (14–17, 22–24, 28, 31, 33, 36, 40, 43, 48, 51–53). In their 1961 review of 909 patients undergoing carotid occlusion from various series, Scott and Skwansk reported an operative mortality ranging from 0 to 18% (45). Given the high incidence of ischemic complications after carotid sacrifice in unselected populations, a variety of tests have been performed to select patients who can tolerate carotid occlusion.

Many authors have advocated gradual occlusion of the carotid with a Selverstone or Crutchfield clamp to allow the development of collateral circulation. Landolt and Millikan (26) as well as Nishioka (35) have demonstrated that there is no difference in morbidity from acute versus gradual carotid occlusion.

Propogation of thrombus up the occluded carotid and subsequent embolization is another potential source of ischemia after carotid sacrifice. Brackett (6) suggested that this is a much less common cause of ischemia than hypoperfusion.

The risk of ischemic complications after carotid sacrifice for tumor resection seems to be higher than the risk for carotid occlusion for aneurysms (37). This may be related to the subsequent manipulation and brain retraction required for tumor removal.

Inadequate Protection of Intracranial Aneurysms

The rationale for treatment of cavernous and supraclinoid carotid aneurysms by carotid ligation is based on the presumption that sacrifice of the carotid artery will produce a drop in blood pressure distal to the ligation to potentiate thrombosis and minimize the risk of aneurysm growth and rupture. The immediate and late alterations in ICA pressure, angiographic appearance of aneurysms, and blood flow changes within the carotid artery have all been studied extensively. Despite the documented reduction in pressure and flow distal to a carotid occlusion, the effects are sometimes inadequate to prevent continued filling of the aneurysm through collateral and retrograde blood flow. This may result in delayed enlargement of the aneurysm with associated symptoms of mass affect or rupture of those sacs that lie within the subarachnoid space.

In addition to cerebral ischemia, aneurysmal rebleeding is the most common complication of carotid sacrifice for the treatment of aneurysms. Kak and colleagues (23) reviewed the incidence of early aneurysmal rebleeding after carotid ligation in the major series reported from 1953 to 1973. In their review of 1298 patients, 57 suffered early rebleeding for an incidence of 4.4%.

Long-term Consequences of Carotid Occlusion

Late complications after therapeutic carotid sacrifice include delayed aneurysmal enlargement and rebleeding or delayed ischemic complications. Tomsick et al. reported on delayed complications of endovascular balloon occlusion of the ICA for aneurysms in 62 of their own patients, and reviewed the incidence of delayed complications in several reported series (54). They found that the incidence of delayed infarction was 0.8 per 100 patient-years of follow-up at 0.5, 2, 2.5, and 5 years posttreatment (mean, 2.5 years). Three of their four infarctions occurred in patients treated for clinoidal or ophthalmic segment aneurysms wherein the aneurysm neck was not trapped. The incidence for extradural ICA aneurysms was one per 371.5 patient-years, or 0.3 per 100 patient-years of follow-up. This incidence was similar to the 0.9 infarcts per 100 patient-years of follow-up in 258 patients reviewed from the literature (54).

In addition to the well-documented delayed ischemic complications of carotid occlusion, other sequelae have been reported. After occlusion of an ICA flow increases in the contralateral carotid. Winn et al. reported an increased incidence of hypertension after common carotid ligation in the treatment of intracranial aneurysms (55). Alterations in intracranial hemodynamics may result in the development of *de novo* aneurysms. Subarachnoid hemorrhage occurring from previously unrecognized contralateral aneurysms has been reported. Hassler (19) and Hashimoto et al. (18) demonstrated in an experimental model that ligation of the carotid artery can lead to contralateral aneurysm formation. In their analysis of 62 patients treated with balloon ICA occlusion, Tomsick et al. documented the incidence of subarachnoid hemorrhage due to *de novo* aneurysms to be 0.4 per 100 patient-years of follow-up (54). The incidence identified from their review of 510 patients from the literature was 0.4 per 100 patient-years of follow-up. In our own experience, we have seen patients who have developed *de novo* aneurysms of the anterior communicating artery after therapeutic carotid ligation for an ICA aneurysm.

CONTRAINDICATIONS

Absolute

The contraindications to therapeutic carotid ligation all represent situations in which collateral blood flow to the ipsilateral cerebral hemisphere may be severely impaired. The contraindications to the use of carotid ligation include: 1) severe hypovolemia; 2) a poor Hunt and Hess grade after subarachnoid hemorrhage; 3) presence of a recent Fisher Grade III subarachnoid hemorrhage; 4) cerebral vasospasm suspected clinically or noted on arteriogram or by transcranial Doppler; 5) presence of an intracerebral hematoma; 6) inability to tolerate carotid occlusion as documented by a Matas test or balloon test occlusion, and 7) significant drop of cerebral blood flow during balloon test occlusion measured by zenon-enhanced computed tomographic (CT) scan, positron emission tomographic (PET) scan or technetium-99-HMPAO single photon emission computed tomographic (SPECT) scan.

Relative contraindications to therapeutic carotid occlusion include: 1) presence of a contralateral ICA aneurysm or anterior communicating aneurysm filling from the contralateral carotid circulation, and 2) presence of contralateral significant atherosclerotic carotid disease. As mentioned previously, if a contralateral ICA aneurysm or an anterior communicating aneurysm exists, increased flow through the contralateral carotid artery after carotid ligation may increase the likelihood of subsequent aneurysm rupture. The presence of significant contralateral atherosclerotic stenosis of the carotid artery may increase the risk of ischemic complications due to inadequate collateral flow.

METHODS TO REDUCE COMPLICATIONS OF THERAPEUTIC CAROTID OCCLUSION

Ischemic

A variety of methods have been proposed to prospectively determine an individual patient's ability to tolerate therapeutic carotid sacrifice. As mentioned previously, the Matas test was one of the earliest methods used to select patients who could tolerate carotid occlusion (30). This technique involves the manual compression of the carotid artery in the neck for 10–15 minutes while examining the patient to determine whether ischemic symptoms develop. Miller et al. established comprehensive guidelines for selecting patients who could safely tolerate carotid occlusion by measuring zenon cerebral blood flow, electroencephalography, and distal ICA pressure (31). According to these authors, carotid ligation is safe if: 1) cerebral blood flow is greater than 40 ml/min per 100 g during carotid clamping; 2) cerebral blood flow during carotid clamping ranges from 20 to 40 ml/min per 100 g, provided that the reduction from the control flow is less than 25%; and 3) cerebral blood flow ranges from 20 to 40 ml/min per 100 g with up to a 35% reduction in flow from the control level, provided that the distal ICA pressure is greater than 60 mm Hg in normotensive patients. Carotid ligation is always considered to be unsafe if the cerebral blood flow during carotid occlusion is less than 28 ml/min per 100 g.

Subsequently, a number of innovative methods have been tested in an attempt to develop a reliable method for selecting patients who will tolerate therapeutic carotid occlusion. Currently, the majority of these methods involve a clinical neurological examination during temporary nondetachable endovascular balloon occlusion of the ICA. Development of an ischemic neurological deficit during test occlusion is associated with an unacceptably high risk of permanent ischemic complications after permanent carotid occlusion and represents a contraindication to carotid occlusion without augmentation of cerebral blood flow through the use of an EC–IC bypass. In addition to the balloon test occlusion, several methods for measuring cerebral blood flow have been used to enhance the reliability of test occlusion (12, 13, 41). Cerebral blood flow can be qualitatively evaluated with technetium-99-HMPAO SPECT scans (29). Quantitative cerebral blood flow can be measured by PET or zenon-enhanced CT scans (7). Extensive experience with all of these methods demonstrates their usefulness in assisting with the prediction of patients who are able to tolerate carotid occlusion without hemodynamic ischemic complications. However, no test is currently available that will reliably predict all hemodynamic ischemic complications.

The development of techniques for performing EC–IC bypasses provides an opportunity to augment collateral blood flow and markedly reduce the likelihood of ischemic complications after therapeutic carotid sacrifice (7, 11, 20, 22, 23, 49, 50, 52, 56). Options for EC–IC bypass include relatively low-flow bypasses such as a superficial temporal artery to middle cerebral artery bypass or a variety of high-flow grafts, including saphenous vein grafts from the cervical internal or external carotid artery to the middle cerebral or supraclinoid ICAs. Short vein bypass grafts from the petrous carotid to the supraclinoid carotid have also been used for high-flow augmentation of collateral circulation when occluding the cavernous segment of the ICA (49).

Although the utility of EC–IC bypass in augmenting cerebral blood flow and reducing the risk of ischemic complications from therapeutic carotid occlusion is undeniable, significant controversy exists regarding patient selection. There is virtually no disagreement that patients who develop an ischemic deficit during balloon test occlusion require an EC–IC bypass if therapeutic carotid occlusion is performed. Most surgeons agree that in this situation a high-flow bypass using a vein graft will be required to supply the necessary collateral flow to adequately minimize the risk of a hemodynamic complication. Likewise, patients who tolerate balloon test occlusion of the carotid artery but demonstrate significant reductions in blood flow in the ipsilateral hemisphere by zenon-enhanced CT, PET, or SPECT scans are at significant risk of an ischemic complication if an EC–IC bypass is not used to augment collateral circulation. Significant controversy exists over the necessity of an EC–IC bypass in patients who have minimal or moderate reductions in blood flow during balloon test occlusion. Many surgeons advocate the use of EC–IC bypass in younger patients, regardless of the results of balloon test occlusion, because of the concern of long-term complications in this population with significant life expectancy. Some highly experienced surgeons advocate the use of an EC–IC bypass in virtually all patients considered for therapeutic carotid occlusion, citing the relatively high incidence of delayed complications of carotid sacrifice (27).

After carotid sacrifice, use of hyperdynamic therapy to optimize the patient's fluid status, cardiac output, and blood pressure will reduce the incidence of ischemic complication in the early postocclusion period (39). It is imperative that hypovolemia and hypotension be avoided to minimize the risk of an ischemic complication after carotid sacrifice (16).

Ischemic complications resulting from thromboembolism can theoretically be reduced by the use of anticoagulation after therapeutic carotid sacrifice. Furthermore, occlusion of the carotid artery near the site of the aneurysm will theoretically reduce the dead space within the vessel and potentially minimize the column of propagating thrombus. The use of anticoagulants is relatively straightforward if endovascular techniques are used for carotid sacrifice. Furthermore, endovascular occlusion of the carotid can usually be performed high in the vessel near the site of the lesion to minimize dead space. Surgical or endovascular trapping of the diseased segment of the vessel will also theoretically minimize the risk of thromboembolic complications. This may be accomplished by endovascular techniques by placing the occluding balloon across the neck of the aneurysm or by placing endovascular devices proximal and distal to the aneurysm. Surgical trapping is accomplished by ligating the ICA in the cervical region and intracranially. For cavernous segment aneurysms, the intracranial ligation is usually performed below the ophthalmic artery.

To minimize the risk of device embolization, most interventional neuroradiologists use a second back-up balloon placed within the ICA proximal to the initial occluding balloon (*Fig. 28.6*). This dampens the residual pulsatile effect and markedly diminishes the risk of the initial balloon deflating and embolizing into the intracranial circulation.

Inadequate Protection

If an intracranial aneurysm continues to fill by retrograde flow after proximal carotid occlusion, the risk of further growth or subsequent hemorrhage can be eliminated by a trapping procedure performed by intracranial occlusion of the vessel distal to the lesion.

Theoretically, the placement of an EC–IC bypass to augment collateral flow will minimize the risk of enlargement of contralateral carotid aneurysms or the development of *de novo* aneurysms on the contralateral carotid or anterior communicating artery circulations.

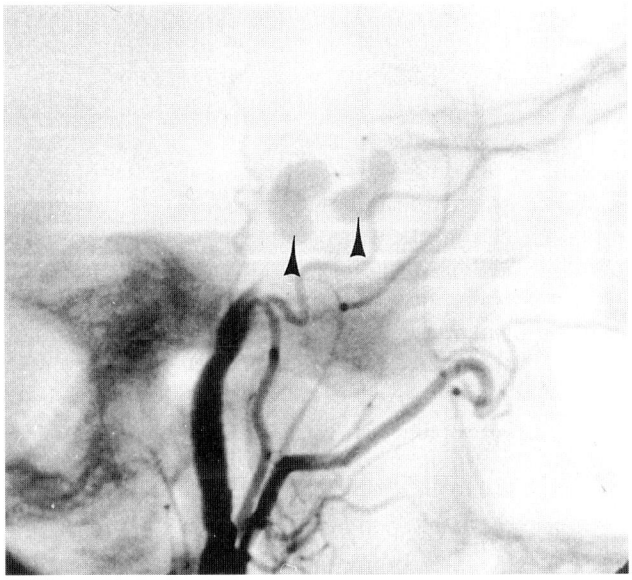

FIG. 28.6 Lateral carotid angiogram performed after endovascular balloon occlusion of the ICA. Arrows point to the primary and back-up balloons.

CONCLUSIONS

Despite the dramatic improvement in management of patients with intracranial aneurysms, including improved neurosurgical techniques and development of endovascular options, therapeutic carotid occlusion remains an important option in the treatment of selected carotid aneurysms, particularly those involving the cavernous segment of the ICA. Therapeutic carotid sacrifice is also a useful adjunct for skull-base surgeons in their attempt to extirpate neoplastic lesions involving the carotid artery. Through the judicious use of adjuncts, including preoperative testing of collateral circulation, EC–IC bypass procedures, anticoagulation, and appropriate perioperative medical therapy, therapeutic carotid sacrifice will remain an important adjunct in the management of selected patients in the future.

REFERENCES

1. Barrow DL, Alleyne CH Jr: Aneurysms of the intracavernous carotid artery, in Tindall GT, Cooper PR, Barrow DL (eds): *The Practice of Neurosurgery*. Baltimore, Williams & Wilkins, 1996, pp 2013–2023.
2. Barrow DL, Clare CE, Fazel I: Penetrating vascular injuries of the head and neck, in

Aarabi B, Kaufman HK (eds): *Missile Wounds of the Head and Neck,* Volume II. Park Ridge, Ill., American Association of Neurological Surgeons, pp 315–342, 1999.
3. Barrow DL, Fleischer AS, Hoffman JC: Complications of detachable balloon catheter technique in the treatment of traumatic intracranial arteriovenous fistulae. **J Neurosurg** 56:396–403, 1982.
4. Beadles CF: Aneurysms of the larger cerebral arteries. **Brain** 20:285–336, 1907.
5. Birley JL, Trotter W: Traumatic aneurysm of the intracranial portion of the internal carotid artery. **Brain** 51:184–208, 1928.
6. Brackett CE Jr: The complications of carotid artery ligation in the neck. **J Neurosurg** 10:91–106, 1953.
7. Brunberg JA, Frey KA, Horton JA, Deveikis JR, Ross DA, Koeppe RA: [0] H$_2$O positron emission tomography determination of cerebral blood flow during balloon test occlusion of the internal carotid artery. **Am J Neuroradiol** 15:725–732s, 1994.
8. Cooper A: A case of aneurysm of the carotid artery. **Med-Chir Trans** 1:1–10, 1809.
9. Cooper A: A second case of carotid aneurysm. **Med-Chir Trans** 222–223, 1809.
10. Dandy WE: Intracranial arterial aneurysms. Ithaca, Comstock, 1944.
11. Diaz FG, Ausman JI, Pearce JE: Ischemic complications after combined internal carotid artery occlusion and extracranial-intracranial anastomosis. **Neurosurgery** 10:563–570, 1982.
12. Eckard DA, Purdy PD, Bonte FJ: Temporary balloon occlusion of the carotid artery combined with brain flow imaging as a test to predict tolerance prior to permanent carotid sacrifice. **Am J Neuroradiol** 13:1565–1569, 1992.
13. Erba SM, Horton JA, Latchaw RE, et al: Balloon test occlusion of the internal carotid artery with stable Xenon/CT cerebral blood flow imaging. **Am J Neuroradiol** 9:533–538, 1988.
14. Galbraith JG, Clark RM: Role of carotid ligation in the management of intracranial carotid aneurysms. **Clin Neurosurg** 21:171–181, 1974.
15. German WJ, Black SPW: Cervical ligation for internal carotid aneurysms: An extended follow-up. **J Neurosurg** 23:572–577, 1965.
16. Giannotta SL, McGillicuddy JE, Kindt GW: Gradual carotid artery occlusion in the treatment of inaccessible internal carotid artery aneurysms. **Neurosurgery** 5:417–421, 1979.
17. Gurdjian ES, Linder DW, Thomas LM: Experiences with ligation of the common carotid artery for treatment of aneurysms of the internal carotid artery. **J Neurosurg** 23:311–318, 1975.
18. Hashimoto N, Handa H, Hazama F: Experimentally induced cerebral aneurysms in rats. **Surg Neurol** 10:3–8, 1978.
19. Hassler O: Experimental carotid ligation followed by aneurysmal formation and other morphological changes in the circle of Willis. **J Neurosurg** 20:1–7, 1963.
20. Ito Z: Long radial artery grafting, in Ito Z: *Microneurosurgery of Cerebral Aneurysms.* Amsterdam/Niigata, Elsevier/Nishimura, 1985, pp 270–279.
21. Jensen ME, Dion JE: Carotid cavernous sinus fistulae, in Tindall GT, Cooper PR, Barrow DL (eds): *The Practice of Neurosurgery,* Baltimore, Williams & Wilkins, 1996, pp 2241–2260.
22. Jha AN, Butler P, Lye RH, Fawcitt RA: Carotid ligation: What happens in the long term? **J Neurol Neurosurg Psychiatry** 49:893–898, 1986.
23. Kak VK, Taylor AR, Gordon DS: Proximal carotid ligation for internal carotid aneurysms: A long-term follow-up study. **J Neurosurg** 39:503–513, 1973.
24. Kapp J, Neill WR, Salter JE, Barnes TY: Systemic heparin in the early management

of ruptured intracranial aneurysms: Review of 104 consecutive cases and comparison with concurrent controls. **Neurosurgery** 20:564–570, 1987.
25. Kobler J: The reluctant surgeon: A biography of John Hunter. New York, Doubleday, 1960.
26. Landolt AM, Millikan CH: Pathogenesis of cerebral infarction secondary to mechanical carotid artery occlusion. **Stroke** 1:52–62, 1970.
27. Lawton NT, Hamilton MG, Morcos JJ, Spetzler RF: Revascularization and aneurysm surgery: Current techniques, indications, and outcome. **Neurosurgery** 38:83–94, 1996.
28. Love JG, Dart LH: Results of carotid ligation with particular reference to intracranial aneurysms. **J Neurosurg** 27:89–93, 1967.
29. Manskin LH, Jeffrey PT, van Heerden BB, et al: Assessing adequacy of collateral circulation during balloon test occlusion of the internal carotid artery with 99mTc-HMPAO SPECT. **Am J Neuroradiol** 12:1045–1051, 1991.
30. Matas R: Testing the efficiency of the collateral circulation as a preliminary to the occlusion of the great surgical arteries. **JAMA** 63:1441–1447, 1914.
31. Miller JD, Jawad K, Jennett B: Safety of carotid ligation and the role in the management of intracranial aneurysms. **J Neurol Neurosurg Psychiatry** 40:64–72, 1977.
32. Nattrass FJ: Aneurysm of the carotid artery in the cavernous sinus: Recovery. **Edinb Med J** 35:30–32, 1928.
33. Neill CL, Hodges LR, Neill WR: Cerebral aneurysms treated by common carotid ligation. **J Neurol Neurosurg Psychiatry** 31:87, 1968 (abstr).
34. Deleted in proof.
35. Nishioka H: Results of the treatment of intracranial aneurysm by occlusion of the carotid artery in the neck. **J Neurosurg** 25:660–682, 1966.
36. Odom GL, Tindall GT: Carotid ligation in the treatment of certain intracranial aneurysms. **Clin Neurosurg** 15:101–116, 1968.
37. Origitano TC, Al-Mefty O, Leonetti JP, Demonte F, Reichman H: Vascular considerations and complications in cranial base surgery. **Neurosurgery** 35:351–363, 1994.
38. Pilz C: Sur Ligatur der Arteria Carotis communis, nebst einer Statistik dieser Operation. **Arch Klin Chir** 9:257–445, 1868.
39. Polin RS, Shaffrey ME, Jensen ME, et al: Medical management in the endovascular treatment of carotid-cavernous aneurysms. **J Neurosurg** 84:755–761, 1996.
40. Poppen JL, Fager CA: Intracranial aneurysms: Results of surgical treatment. **J Neurosurg** 17:283–296, 1960.
41. Raymonel J, Theron J: Intracavernous aneurysms: Treatment by proximal balloon occlusion of the internal carotid artery. **Am J Neuroradiol** 7:1087–1092, 1986.
42. Roski RA, Spetzler RF: Carotid ligation, in Wilkins RH, Rengachary SS (eds): **Neurosurgery.** New York, McGraw-Hill, 1996, pp 2333–2340.
43. Roski RA, Spetzler RF, Nulsen FE: Late complications of common carotid ligation in the treatment of intracranial aneurysms. **J Neurosurg** 54:583–587, 1981.
44. Schorstein J. Carotid ligation of saccular intracranial aneurysms. **Br J Surg** 28:50–70, 1940.
45. Scott M, Skwansk E: The treatment of cerebral aneurysms by ligation of the common carotid artery. **Surg Gynecol Obstet** 113:54–61, 1961.
46. Sekhar LN, Linskey ME, Snyderman CH: Surgical management of neoplastic involvement of the internal carotid artery, in Carter LP, Spetzler RF, Hamilton MG (eds). **Neurovascular Surgery,** New York, McGraw-Hill, 1995, pp 1263–1299.
47. Siegrist A. Die gafahren der Ligatur der grossen Halsschlagadern fur das Auge und

das Leben des Menschen. **Arch Ophthalmol** 50:511–646, 1900.
48. Somach FM, Shenkin HA: Angiographic end-results of carotid ligation in the treatment of carotid aneurysm. **J Neurosurg** 24:966–974, 1966.
49. Spetzler RF, Fukushima T, Martin N, Zabramski JM: Petrous carotid-to-intradural carotid saphenous vein graft for intracavernous giant aneurysm, tumor and occlusive cerebrovascular disease. **J Neurosurg** 73:496–501, 1990.
50. Spetzler RF, Schuster H, Roski RA: Elective extracranial-intracranial arterial bypass in the treatment of inoperable giant aneurysms of the internal carotid artery. **J Neurosurg** 53:22, 1980.
51. Swearingen B, Heros RC: Common carotid occlusion for unclippable carotid aneurysms: An old but still effective operation. **Neurosurgery** 21:288–295, 1987.
52. Tindall GT, Kapp J, Odom GI, Robinson SC: A combined technique for treating certain aneurysms of the anterior communicating artery. **J Neurosurg** 33:41–47, 1970.
53. Tindall GT, Odom GL, Dillon ML, et al: Direction of blood flow in the internal and external carotid arteries following occlusion of the ipsilateral common carotid artery. **J Neurosurg** 20:985–994, 1963.
54. Tomsick TA, Van Loveren H, Tew JM Jr, Larson J, Ernst R, Khoury J: Delayed complications of balloon occlusion of the internal carotid artery for unclippable aneurysm. **J Neurovascular Disease** 64–67, 1997.
55. Winn HR, Richardson AE, Jane JA: Late morbidity and mortality of common carotid ligation for posterior communicating aneurysms. **J Neurosurg** 47:727–736, 1997.
56. Yasargil MG: Microsurgery applied to neurosurgery. New York, Academic Press, 1969, pp 105–117.

CHAPTER

29

Honored Guest Presentation: Therapeutic Decisions in Facial Pain

JAMAL M. TAHA, M.D., AND JOHN M. TEW, JR., M.D.

Several disorders that cause facial pain can be successfully treated by neurosurgical procedures. It is important for the neurosurgeon to accurately diagnose the disorder and identify the best treatment for each disorder. In the absence of randomized prospective studies, standardized methods of reporting, and standardized outcome criteria, it is difficult to compare the results of various surgical procedures and the different reported series of the same surgical procedure. Nevertheless, several important observations emerge from reviews of the literature and personal experience. These observations can serve as general guidelines for treatment. In the context of facial pain, some of these observations are the following:

1. Accurate diagnosis is required.
2. The diagnosis of typical trigeminal neuralgia (TGN) is seldom difficult.
3. In general, the length of the list of the patient's symptoms is directly proportional to the likelihood of treatment failure.
4. Medical treatment should be explored before surgery is contemplated.
5. There is no successful surgical procedure for treatment of atypical facial pain.
6. It is more difficult to treat neuropathic than neuralgic pain.
7. Patients with dysesthetic pain seldom respond to ablative sur-gery.
8. There is no single superior treatment for facial pain. The treatment should be individualized. Patients should have access to a broad spectrum of treatment options.
9. The effectiveness of surgical treatment diminishes as facial pain becomes more chronic.

In this chapter, the authors review their observations, review the literature for the past 10 years, and search for treatment guidelines that may be accepted for current practice.

TRIGEMINAL NEURALGIA

For over 30 years, neurosurgeons have been searching for the best surgical treatment for TGN. The fact that this matter is still debated reflects our lack of clear understanding of the pathogenesis of this disorder and the lack of a curative procedure among all current surgical procedures. When recommending treatment for a patient with TGN, the surgeon must understand the risks and benefits of surgery as applied to that specific patient. The surgeon must also review current information and personal experience and ask two questions: "What would I want to have done if I were the patient?" and "What is the best treatment for this patient?"

Generalizations regarding treatment of TGN have been presented in the literature. Whereas some surgeons advocate one procedure for all patients, others select different surgical procedures for different patients. In the midst of this controversy, surgeons must not lose sight of the facts and observations pertaining to the treatment of TGN. Following are some of the authors' observations:

RECOGNIZE ATYPICAL TGN AND STATUS TRIGEMINUS

One must distinguish atypical TGN from atypical facial pain. In atypical TGN, patients report lancinating pain or brief episodes of sharp or burning pain that last seconds to minutes and are associated with milder constant aching pain.

Some patients experience status trigeminus or continuous repeated episodes of pain of TGN. These patients present fatigued, often dehydrated, and in constant severe pain. They frequently report simple continuous pain rather than the typical episodic pain. Such patients usually require an urgent surgical procedure.

THERE IS NO CURRENT CURE FOR TGN

All current surgical procedures for TGN are associated with risk of pain recurrence (39). After successful surgery, pain of TGN can progress to involve other trigeminal divisions or the contralateral side. In some patients, pain of TGN is difficult to treat, regardless of what treatment is given. Longstanding chronic TGN is more difficult to treat.

LONG-TERM PAIN RELIEF IS HIGHEST AFTER MICROVASCULAR DECOMPRESSION AND PERCUTANEOUS STEREOTACTIC RADIOFREQUENCY RHIZOTOMY

Among the current treatment options, microvascular decompression (MVD) and percutaneous stereotactic radiofrequency (PSR) rhizotomy have comparable rates of pain relief that are highest among the available

TABLE 29.1
Results of Microvascular Decompression in Series of Approximately
100 Patients or More over the Past 10 Years

Series	No. of Patients	No. of Follow-up years	Long-term Pain Relief (%)	Significant DE[a] (%)	Corneal Analgesia (%)	TG Motor Weakness (%)	CN Palsy (%)	PO Morbidity (%)	Severe PO Morbidity or Mortality (%)
Bederson 1989[b]	166	5.1	75	3	0	0	3	21	0
Sindou 1990 (35)	120	4.8	79						
Klun 1992[b]	178	5.2	88	0	0.6	0.6	0.6	NR	1.4
Cutbush 1994 (9)	109	4.8	76	0	0	0	7	NR	1.8
Mendoza 1995 (25)	133	5.4	71	0	0	0	1.5	11	2
Barker 1996 (2)	1204	10	64	1	0	0	2	19	1.1
Kondo 1997 (20)	281	12.6	87	NR	NR	NR	5.5	NR	NR
Lee 1997 (23)	146	7.2	84						
Pagura 1996 (27)	203	5	68	0.5	0	0	1	13	0.5
TOTAL	2540	~7	77	0.8	0.1	0.1	3	16	1

[a]DE, dysesthesia; CN, cranial nerve; PO, perioperative; NR, not reported.
[b]Cited in Reference 44.

options. In a review of series of approximately 100 patients or more published in the past 10 years (2, 9, 15, 20, 23, 25–27, 35, 44, 49), the rates of pain relief calculated were 77% in 7 years for MVD (*Table 29.1*) and 75% in 6 years for PSR rhizotomy (*Table 29.2*). The timing of pain recurrence is similar for MVD and radiofrequency rhizotomy. In the series of Barker et al. (2), pain recurrence occurred primarily in the first 2 years after MVD, and then dropped to 2% per year in years 3 to 5, 1% per year in years 6 to 10, and 0.7% per year thereafter. In the authors' series (38), pain recurrence after PSR rhizotomy occurred in 3% of patients per year through the first 5 years, 1.4% per year in years 6 to 10, and 0.75% thereafter.

Glycerol rhizotomy and radiosurgery have the highest rates of pain persistence or recurrence. Pain relief is calculated to be 55% in 3 years for glycerol rhizotomy (4, 6, 10, 13, 14, 17, 37, 44, 46) (*Table 29.3*). Initial results of 129 patients from three series demonstrate a pain relief rate of 55% in 1.5 years after radiosurgery (22, 29, 48). Balloon compression has a recurrence rate that is higher than that of MVD and PSR rhizotomy, but lower than that of glycerol rhizotomy and radiosurgery. Pain relief was calculated to be 75% in 3 years for balloon compression (1, 5, 44) (*Table 29.4*).

ALL PERCUTANEOUS PROCEDURES ARE ASSOCIATED WITH DYSESTHESIA

Glycerol rhizotomy is frequently reported to be the preferred percutaneous destructive procedure because of its rare association with dysesthesia. The authors' review of the literature does not support this hypothesis. In a review of the results of 1751 patients in 10 series, significant dysesthesias occurred in 4% of patients after glycerol rhizotomy (*Table 29.3*), in 7% of patients after PSR rhizotomy (*Table 29.2*), and in 6% of patients after balloon compression (*Table 29.4*). Some surgeons relate the high incidence of dysesthesia to poor technique, such as the injection of glycerol without cisternography or injection of large volumes of glycerol during glycerol rhizotomy (13), production of anesthesia and analgesia during PSR rhizotomy (39), and prolonged balloon inflation during balloon compression (5). Supporters of glycerol rhizotomy and balloon compression estimate a lower incidence of dysesthesia in technically adequate procedures (13). Supporters of PSR rhizotomy estimate rates of dysesthesia and pain recurrence that are comparable with those of glycerol rhizotomy and balloon compression if lesions created by PSR produced hypalgesia only (39).

Contrary to percutaneous destructive procedures, MVD rarely produces significant facial numbness or dysesthesia (*Table 29.1*). In the authors' experience, facial sensory loss and dysesthesia complicated cases

TABLE 29.2
Results of Percutaneous Stereotactic Radiofrequency Rhizotomy in Series of Approximately 100 Patients or More over the Past 10 Years

Series	No. of Patients	No. of Follow-up years	Long-term Pain Relief (%)	Significant DE[a] (%)	Corneal Analgesia (%)	TG Motor Weakness (%)	CN Palsy (%)	PO Morbidity (%)	Severe PO Morbidity or Mortality (%)
Fraioli 1989[b]	533	6.5	89	NR	3	3	0.2	0.2	0
Frank 1989[b]	700	>3	75	NR	1	8	0.1	0.1	0
Miserocchi 1989 (26)	111	1–7	80	6.3	2	NR	0	0	0
Broggi 1990[b]	1000	9	78	6.5	17	10	0.5	0.5	0
Sweet 1990[b]	702	5.5	63	9	9	65	0.4	0.5	0
Ischia 1990 (15)	124	3.7	67	6	2	3	4	NR	NR
Nugent 1991[b]	1070	9	73	6.5	3.5	26	0.2	0.5	0.2
Zakrzewska 1993 (49)	265	3.8	71	8	9	NR	NR	NR	0
Tew 1995 (44)	1200	9	79	4	6	16	1	1.3	0
TOTAL	5705	~6	75	6.6	6	19 tr	0.3	0.4	0.03

[a]DE, dysesthesia; CN, cranial nerve; PO, perioperative; NR, not reported; tr, transient.
[b]Cited in Reference 44.

TABLE 29.3
Results of Glycerol Rhizotomy in Series of Approximately 100 Patients of More over the Past 10 years

Series	No. of Patients	No. of Follow-up years	Long-term Pain Relief (%)	Significant DE[a] (%)	Corneal Analgesia (%)	TG Motor Weakness (%)	CN Palsy (%)	PO Morbidity (%)	Major PO Morbidity or Mortality (%)
Young 1988[b]	162	0.5–5.5	63	3	2	0	0	0.6	0
Waltz 1989 (46)	200		55	2	NR	NR	0	NR	NR
Fujimaki 1990[b]	122	4.5	22	13	0	0	0	0	0
Ischia 1990 (14)	112	3.5	73	3	8	0	0	0	0
De La Porte 1990 (10)	120		NR	0	2.5	0	NR	0	0
Steiger 1991 (37)	122	5	41	13	16	4	0	0	0.8
Cappabianca 1995 (6)	191	1–7	70	0	10	6	0	6	NR
Bergenheim 1991 (4)	99	1	64	7	5	0	0	0	0
Jho 1997 (17)	523	0.5–11	46	2	0	0	0	0	0
Hakanson 1998 (13)	100	5.4	57	0	0	0	0	0	0
Total	1751	~3	55	4	5	1	0	0.7	0.1

[a]DE, dysesthesia; CN, cranial nerve; PO, perioperative; NR, not reported.
[b]Cited in Reference 44.

TABLE 29.4
Results of Balloon Compression in Series of Approximately 100 Patients or More over the Past 10 Years

Series	No. of Patients	No. of Follow-up years	Long-term Pain Relief (%)	Significant DE[a] (%)	Corneal Analgesia (%)	TG Motor Weakness (%)	CN Palsy (%)	PO Morbidity (%)	Severe PO Morbidity or Mortality (%)
Fraioli 1989[b]	159	3.5	81	7.6	NR	3	0	0	0
Frank 1989[b]	212	<3	75	0	0	9	0.9	1.8	0
Lichtor 1990[b]	100	1–10	78	4	0	0	0	2	0
Lubato 1990[b]	144	0.5–4.5	83	3	0	12	2.8	4.8	0
Addenneibi 1997 (1)	200	4.2	68	10.6	3	7	0	NR	0.5
Brown 1997 (5)	140	2	68	6	0	0	0	5	0
Total	955	~3	76	6	0.6	5 p	0.6	2.7	0.08

[a]DE, dysesthesia; CN, cranial nerve; PO, perioperative; NR, not reported; p, permanent.
[b]Cited in Reference 44.

of venous compression or excessive manipulation of the trigeminal rootlets. The initial results of radiosurgery demonstrate a rare association with sensory loss and dysesthesia, despite the fact that the nerve is deliberately injured (48).

POSTOPERATIVE CORNEAL ANESTHESIA IN PATIENTS WITH V-1 PAIN IS HIGHEST AFTER PSR RHIZOTOMY

Among the percutaneous destructive procedures, PSR rhizotomy has the highest risk of postoperative loss of corneal sensations after surgery for V-1 pain (*Tables 29.2–29.4*). PSR rhizotomy differentially affects the small myelinated and unmyelinated fibers, which mediate the corneal reflex (44). In contrast, balloon compression differentially affects large myelinated fibers (5). Glycerol has neurolytic effects on both small and large myelinated fibers (13). In the authors' review of the literature, the corneal reflex was lost in 6% of PSR rhizotomies, in 5% of glycerol rhizotomies, and in 1% of balloon compressions (*Tables 29.2–29.4*). MVD and radiosurgery have been rarely associated with corneal anesthesia.

POSTOPERATIVE TRIGEMINAL MOTOR WEAKNESS IS HIGHEST AFTER BALLOON COMPRESSION

Balloon compression carries the highest risk of postoperative motor trigeminal weakness (*Tables 29.2–29.4*). In a review of the literature, trigeminal weakness occurred transiently in 19% of patients after PSR rhizotomy, infrequently (1%) after glycerol rhizotomy, and permanently in 5% after balloon compression (*Tables 29.2–29.4*). Trigeminal motor weakness occurred rarely after MVD and radiosurgery. Complications such as trismus, otalgia, and hyperacusis have not been thoroughly discussed in the literature and are likely underestimated.

PERIOPERATIVE MORBIDITY AND MORTALITY ARE HIGHER AFTER MVD THAN AFTER PERCUTANEOUS DESTRUCTIVE PROCEDURES

Literature review demonstrates that the perioperative mortality or serious morbidity (e.g., stroke, hemorrhage, venous sinus occlusion, myocardial infarction, hydrocephalus), permanent hearing loss or facial palsy, and minor perioperative complications (e.g., wound dehiscence or infection, cerebrospinal fluid leak, pseudomeningocele, bacterial and aseptic meningitis, pulmonary complications, ataxia) were higher after MVD than after percutaneous procedures. After MVD, serious morbidity or mortality occurred in 1%, permanent hearing loss occurred in 3%, and minor complications occurred in 16% (*Table 29.1*). The risks are higher for patients who have an ectatic and tortuous vertebrobasilar system arterial tree (24). These results do not compare favorably with rates of 0.07% serious morbidity and mortality, 0.5% serious hearing loss, and 1.3% minor complications for percutaneous procedures (*Tables 29.2–29.4*).

Conclusion

All available surgical procedures for TGN have advantages and disadvantages (*Table 29.5*). MVD is highly successful in treating pain of TGN with a relatively low risk of pain recurrence, dysesthesia, corneal analgesia, and trigeminal motor weakness; however, one should not overlook the perioperative risks associated with this surgery, especially in the elderly. MVD may be best suited for healthy patients, but it is not the best procedure for patients in poor medical condition. Because of the risk of hearing loss, MVD may not be suitable for patients who have contralateral hearing loss. MVD may also not be the best procedure for patients who have a large, ectatic, and tortuous vertebrobasilar arterial system because of increased perioperative morbidity.

Percutaneous destructive procedures are appropriate procedures for the elderly and for those in poor medical condition. Because of its low pain recurrence rate, PSR rhizotomy generally seems to be the most appropriate procedure. By avoiding dense lesions, adverse effects of dysesthesias are greatly reduced. PSR rhizotomy may not be the best procedure for patients with V-1 pain and patients with pain distributed over the three trigeminal divisions.

Because glycerol rhizotomy is associated with a high recurrence rate, the procedure likely requires repetition. Multiple glycerol injections are associated with a higher risk of failure and adverse effects. During glycerol rhizotomy, surgeons and patients should be ready to convert the procedure to PSR rhizotomy if cerebrospinal fluid flow is not obtained. Because of its low risk of trigeminal motor dysfunction, glycerol rhizotomy is particularly advantageous for patients with contralateral pain, trigeminal motor weakness, and temporomandibular joint dysfunction. Glycerol rhizotomy is also appropriate for patients who have pain over V-1 or the entire face and are not candidates for a posterior fossa procedure.

Balloon compression seems particularly advantageous for patients who have V-1 pain and are not good candidates for microvascular decompression. Alternative procedures for these patients include glycerol rhizotomy, peripheral nerve section, and radiosurgery.

Other surgical procedures have a role in the treatment of TGN. Peripheral nerve section is appropriate for elderly patients with V-1 pain or with bilateral facial pain. Radiosurgery has a role in the treatment of patients who cannot safely undergo surgical procedures, such as patients who are receiving anticoagulants.

TABLE 29.5
Comparison of Results of Various Surgical Treatments for Trigeminal Neuralgia

	Long-term Failure	Dysesthesia	Trigeminal Motor Dysfunction	Corneal Analgesia in V-1 Pain	PO Morbidity	Mortality/Severe Morbidity
MVD[a]	+	+	+	+	+++	+++
PSR	+	-++	++	+++	+	+
Glycerol	+++	++	+	++	+	+
Balloon	++	-++	+++	+	+	+
Rhizotomy	+	-++	+	+++	+++	+++
Neurectomy	++	-++	+	+	+	+
Radiosurgery	+++	+	+	+	+	+

[a]MVD, microvascular decompression; PO, perioperative; PSR, percutaneous stereotactic radiofrequency; +, among the least effective; ++, in between; +++, among the most effective.

In summary, the authors conclude that the discipline of treating TGN should be similar to disciplines of treating other disorders, such as aneurysms, tumors, and vascular malformations. The discipline entails a multimodality approach conducted by a team who can offer medical and surgical treatments directed to the needs of the individual patient.

RECURRENT TRIGEMINAL NEURALGIA

Controversy also exists regarding the treatment of persistent or recurrent TGN. All procedures that currently treat initial TGN can effectively treat recurrent pain. To help select the best treatment, the authors review the following facts and observations:

TGN FREQUENTLY RECURS IN OTHER TRIGEMINAL DIVISIONS

TGN frequently recurs in trigeminal divisions previously free of pain. This observation, which can follow all surgical procedures, may represent progression of the underlying disorder rather than recurrence.

REPEAT MVD IS FREQUENTLY UNSUCCESSFUL

A second MVD is performed in less than one-third of all posterior fossa explorations for pain recurring after a prior MVD; therefore, most patients undergoing a second posterior fossa surgery require trigemi-

TABLE 29.6
Results of Rhizotomy and Decompression of the Vagal and Glossopharyngeal Nerves

Series	Procedure	No. of Patients	No. of Follow-up Years	Pain-Free n	%
White 1966[b]	rhizotomy	129	55	~100	
Rushton 1981[b]	rhizotomy	129		110	92
Giorgi 1984[b]	rhizotomy	4	3–20	4	100
Wakiya et al. 1989 (45)	MVD[a]	16	0.08–4	14	88
Sindou et al. 1991 (36)	MVD	8	3.5	8	100
	rhizotomy	3	3.5	3	100
Resnick et al. 1995 (32)	MVD	40	2	30 (76)	
Taha and Tew 1995 (41)	rhizotomy	12	7	11	92

[a]MVD, microvascular decompression.
[b]Cited in Reference 42.

nal rhizotomy (7, 31, 47). Repeat MVD is associated with increased risk of cranial nerve palsy, perioperative morbidity, and dysesthesia (7, 31, 47). In the series of Barker et al.(6), the risk of disturbing facial numbness increased to 8% after repeat MVD. In our experience, better results can be achieved by using percutaneous techniques (39). In less than 1% of cases, patients with intractable TGN require complete section of the sensory and motor root to achieve pain relief.

REPEAT GLYCEROL RHIZOTOMY IS FREQUENTLY UNSUCCESSFUL

Repeat glycerol rhizotomy is associated with a higher risk of technical failure because the trigeminal cistern becomes less accessible after repeated glycerol injections (13, 30). There is no documentation that PSR rhizotomy and balloon compression are associated with greater technical failure when these procedures are repeated. All percutaneous procedures have a higher risk of sensory complications when repeated.

PERCUTANEOUS DESTRUCTIVE PROCEDURES ARE NOT INDICATED IN PATIENTS WITH ANALGESIA

All percutaneous destructive procedures fail to relieve recurrent trigeminal pain for patients who are analgesic in the painful division. Such patients may require posterior fossa exploration for MVD or intracranial trigeminal rhizotomy, radiosurgery, dorsal root entry zone (DREZ) surgery, or motor cortex stimulation.

Conclusion

Posterior fossa exploration for recurrent trigeminal pain following MVD is not suitable for the majority of patients because of a low success rate. Superior results can be achieved by percutaneous destructive procedures, especially PSR rhizotomy, with less risk of perioperative complications. Otherwise healthy patients with pain recurring after a prior percutaneous destructive procedure are best treated by MVD. A repeat percutaneous procedure or radiosurgery is considered for patients who are medically unhealthy. Patients who have recurrent TGN in an analgesic area rarely benefit from repeat destructive surgery, but may find relief through decompression or complete section of the sensory and motor root.

TRIGEMINAL NEURALGIA ASSOCIATED WITH MULTIPLE SCLEROSIS

Trigeminal neuralgia associated with multiple sclerosis (TGN-MS) is difficult to alleviate due to multiple factors. Following are some facts and observations:

MVD FAILS TO TREAT TGN-MS

Even the strongest advocates of MVD do not recommend this surgery for TGN-MS because of its high failure rate (33).

PERCUTANEOUS DESTRUCTIVE PROCEDURES CAN EFFECTIVELY TREAT TGN-MS, ALTHOUGH A HIGHER RECURRENCE RATE IS ANTICIPATED

All percutaneous destructive procedures have successfully relieved pain of TGN-MS, but with a higher recurrence rate than primary TGN. This is especially true for glycerol rhizotomy (13, 31). Denser levels of hypalgesia are needed to control pain of TGN-MS than in primary TGN.

TGN-MS FREQUENTLY INVOLVES MULTIPLE DIVISIONS OR OCCURS BILATERALLY

TGN-MS may recur in different trigeminal divisions or on the contralateral side of the face. Therefore, it is appropriate to recommend a destructive procedure, such as PSR rhizotomy, which is most selective in achieving hypalgesia.

Conclusion

Patients with TGN-MS are more difficult to treat than those with TGN. There is no role for MVD in such patients. PSR rhizotomy seems to be the most appropriate treatment for TGN-MS because it is the most selective destructive procedure in tailoring the quantity and location of sensory deficit. The initial results of radiosurgery for TGN-MS have not been encouraging, with less than 50% of patients achieving acceptable pain control. Other techniques, such as motor cortex stimulation and percutaneous trigeminal nucleotomy-tractotomy, deserve investigation for multiple recurrent pain.

SYMPTOMATIC TRIGEMINAL NEURALGIA ASSOCIATED WITH TUMOR

Although reports document that patients with TGN who harbor tumors, aneurysms, vascular malformations, or cysts (TGN-MASS) are young, have sensory deficits, and experience more atypical pain, the authors have observed patients with symptomatic lesions who have typical TGN. Similar observations have led others to advocate performing imaging studies on all patients with TGN (28).

TGN-MASS can be effectively treated by tumor excision and MVD when vascular compression is found (16, 28). In the series of Barker et al. (3), pain relief was achieved in 81% of patients over 10 years by using that approach. PSR rhizotomy has achieved similar results for patients who are not candidates for elective surgical removal of the lesion (7, 28). Initial results of radiosurgery indicate a high rate of pain relief after radiation of tumors (48). Anecdotal data indicate that pain relief may follow embolization of arteriovenous malformations and clipping of aneurysms (3). The literature contains insufficient information to allow the comparison of the different techniques in treatment of TGN-MASS.

Conclusion

In TGN-MASS, the authors recommend directing the treatment to the intracranial mass. Percutaneous destructive procedures can effectively control pain if surgery or radiosurgery to the tumor is not otherwise indicated.

TRIGEMINAL NEUROPATHIC PAIN

Patients who experience pain distributed in the trigeminal nerve may have the typical symptoms of TGN. The following concepts and observations should be remembered when assessing and treating these patients:

RECOGNIZE PATIENTS WITH NEUROMA

Patients who experience facial pain after trauma or facial surgery may harbor a neuroma. These patients usually describe constant, dull, and burning pain along the distribution of a branch of the trigeminal nerve. A Tinel's sign and temporary relief with a lidocaine block can establish the diagnosis. These patients can improve after peripheral neurectomy.

TREATMENT OF PATIENTS WITH DYSESTHESIA

Dysesthesia that develops after percutaneous destructive procedures is usually mild and temporary. There is no good treatment for patients with persistent dysesthesia. Destructive procedures are not recommended because they usually worsen the symptoms. MVD has generally not been successful. Techniques such as trigeminal stimulation, motor cortex stimulation, caudalis DREZ surgery, and PSR nucleotomy-tractotomy require further evaluation.

VAGOGLOSSOPHARYNGEAL NEURALGIA

Current neurosurgical procedures for treating vagoglossopharyngeal neuralgia include PSR rhizotomy, open intracranial rhizotomy, MVD, and, recently, PSR trigeminal nucleotomy-tractotomy. When recommending treatment, one must consider the following observations:

OPEN INTRACRANIAL RHIZOTOMY HAS THE HIGHEST RATE OF LONG-TERM PAIN RELIEF

After open rhizotomy of the glossopharyngeal and upper vagal rootlets, long-term pain relief is consistently achieved in more than 90% of patients (41, 42). MVD has inconsistently achieved high rates of pain relief. Some surgeons reported pain relief in more than 90% of patients after MVD (36, 45); Resnick et al. (32) reported a 76% pain relief in patients followed for more than 2 years.

PSR RHIZOTOMY CARRIES THE HIGHEST RISK OF POSTOPERATIVE DYSPHAGIA, VOCAL CORD PARALYSIS, AND IRRITATIVE COUGH

The authors have had difficulty achieving precise controlled coagulation of the glossopharyngeal and vagal nerves. Many series have reported dysphagia and vocal cord paralysis after PSR rhizotomy (42). The authors restrict the use of PSR rhizotomy to patients with glossopharyngeal neuralgia from cancer who already have developed vocal cord paralysis and swallowing difficulty.

Open rhizotomy has been associated with 10 to 20% risk of temporary swallowing problems (43). Many authors have decreased this risk by restricting vagal rhizotomy to the upper two or upper third of the vagal rootlets and preserving the upper large-diameter vagal rootlets (42). The authors have not encountered cases of postoperative permanent dysphagia or vocal cord paralysis after they used intraoperative monitoring of the false vocal cord to differentiate motor from sensory vagal rootlets (43).

MVD was introduced to minimize the risks associated with section of the upper vagal rootlets; however, dysphagia and vocal cord paralysis can develop from excessive manipulation of the lower cranial nerves. In the series of Resnick et al. (32), 10% of patients developed transient paresis of the cranial nerves IX and X, and 2% developed permanent moderate swallowing difficulty.

PERIOPERATIVE CARE

Patients with glossopharyngeal neuralgia may develop hemodynamic instability during intubation, during manipulation of the lower cranial nerves, and postoperatively secondary to hypersensitivity to the vagus nucleus, ephaptic transmission between cranial nerves IX and X or nuclei, and hypersensitivity of the carotid sinus reflex. Before laryngeal intubation, topical anesthesia to the oropharynx and intravenous atropine should be administered. Intraoperatively, the surgeon should avoid excessive manipulation of the lower cranial nerves to decrease risks of severe fluctuations of blood pressure and heart rate. Atropine should be administered before section of the vagal rootlets. Strict postoperative control of blood pressure is required to avoid hypertensive crisis. These risks should be taken seriously. In the series of Resnick et al. (32) of MVD, the mortality rate from hemodynamic instability was 5%.

OPEN RHIZOTOMY IS RECOMMENDED FOR PATIENTS WITH VAGOGLOSSOPHARYNGEAL SYNCOPE

Ten percent of patients with vagoglossopharyngeal neuralgia develop sudden excessive vagal outflow during an attack—resulting in bradycardia, heart arrhythmias, hypotension, syncope, seizure, or cardiac arrest—known as vagoglossopharyngeal syncope. Bradyarrythmia can be transiently blocked by atropine, whereas hypotension usually responds to local injection of lidocaine near the carotid bifurcation (42). Vagoglossopharyngeal syncope can be successfully treated with carbamazepine and with open rhizotomy (42). Data are insufficient to support the use of MVD or other surgical procedures for this disorder.

OPEN RHIZOTOMY IS CONTRAINDICATED IN BILATERAL GLOSSOPHARYNGEAL NEURALGIA

In the rare event of bilateral glossopharyngeal neuralgia, open rhizotomy carries a high risk of swallowing problems from sectioning both glossopharyngeal nerves (42). In bilateral glossopharyngeal neuralgia, MVD is likely the treatment of choice.

Conclusion

Open rhizotomy seems to have the highest rate of long-term pain relief. Risks of postoperative dysphagia and vocal cord paralysis are minimized by using intraoperative vagal monitoring. MVD has a low risk of permanent dysphagia and vocal cord paralysis and a lower rate of long-term pain relief. Open rhizotomy is the treatment of choice for patients who experience vagoglossopharyngeal syncope. MVD is the treatment of choice for patients who develop bilateral glossopharyngeal syncope. PSR rhizotomy should be restricted to patients with pain of cancer who already have swallowing problems and vocal cord paralysis. Percutaneous trigeminal nucleotomy-tractotomy requires further evaluation before recommending it as a treatment option (18).

CLUSTER HEADACHE

The surgical treatment of chronic cluster headache is difficult, but worthy of consideration after an appropriate medical therapy has been explored. Two systems are implicated in the pathogenesis of cluster headache: the trigeminovascular system and the nervus intermedius-superficial petrosal-sphenopalatine system. Surgery directed to one or both of these systems include percutaneous destructive procedures (PSR trigeminal rhizotomy, glycerol rhizotomy, balloon compression), open trigeminal rhizotomy, MVD of the trigeminal root, superficial petrosal neurectomy, section of the nervus intermedius, MVD of the nervus intermedius, and caudalis DREZ surgery. The authors review the following facts and observations:

SURGERY OF EITHER SYSTEM CAN BE SUCCESSFUL

In combined series (12, 19, 34, 40, 42), long-term pain control was achieved in 62% of 210 patients who underwent surgery of the trigeminovascular system (*Table 29.7*) and in 54% of 203 patients who under-

TABLE 29.7
Surgery of the Trigeminal System for Cluster Headache

Series	Surgery	No. of Follow-up Years	No. of Patients	Pain Control	Sensory Complications[a]
White 1969[c]	open rhizotomy	4–15	2	2	
Mazars[c]	open rhizotomy		31	28	
Stowell 1970[c]	open rhizotomy		5	5	
Maxwell 1982[c]	PSR[b] rhizotomy	0.5–5	8	5	1
Watson 1983[c]	PSR rhizotomy	0.9–3	13	10	1
	open rhizotomy	2–8	8	2	
	glycerol rhizotomy	1	1	0	
Waltz 1985[c]	glycerol rhizotomy		5	0	
Onofrio 1986[c]	PSR rhizotomy	0.9–3	21	12	3
	open rhizotomy	1–5	10	6	1
Wake 1987[c]	open rhizotomy	1–25	4	3	
Ekbom 1987[c]	glycerol rhizotomy	0.5–5	7	2	
Gybels 1988[c]	open rhizotomy		3	0	1
Sweet 1988[c]	PSR rhizotomy	1–20	20	12	1
Mathew 1990[c]	PSR rhizotomy	0.5–5	27	17	1
Hassenbusch 1990[c]	glycerol rhizotomy	1	8	5	
Morgalender 1990[c]	open rhizotomy	0.1–2	10	1	
Kirkpatrick 1993 (19)	open rhizotomy	5.6	14	12	3
Grigorian 1995 (12)	PSR rhizotomy		6	2	
Taha and Tew 1995 (40)	PSR rhizotomy	2–20	7	5	1

[a]Sensory complications include significant dysesthesia and keratitis.
[b]PSR, percutaneous stereotactic radiofrequency.
[c]Cited in Reference 42.

went surgery of the nervus intermedius-superficial petrosal-sphenopalatine system (Table 29.8). Results of small series of surgery on both systems suggest rates of pain control approximating 80% (42). Regardless of the surgery that is performed, good pain control rather than complete pain relief is expected.

GLYCEROL RHIZOTOMY AND MVD ARE THE LEAST EFFECTIVE PROCEDURES FOR THE TRIGEMINOVASCULAR SYSTEM

In a review of combined series, long-term pain control was achieved in 62% patients who underwent PSR trigeminal rhizotomy, in 68% of patients who underwent open trigeminal rhizotomy, and in only 33% of patients who underwent glycerol rhizotomy. Glycerol rhizotomy is not recommended for the treatment of cluster headache by some specialists (13). Limited experience with isolated MVD of the trigeminal rootlets has been disappointing (42).

In patients with cluster headache who undergo PSR rhizotomy, pain is best controlled when a dense sensory lesion is made in the V-1 and V-2 regions (42). Experience with glycerol rhizotomy has been similar

TABLE 29.8
Surgery of the Nervus Intermedius-Superficial Petrosal-Sphenopalatine System

Series[a]	Surgery	No. of Follow-up Years	No. of Patients	Pain Control
Gardner	petrosal neurectomy	0.3–2	12	6
Trowbridge	petrosal neurectomy	<1	4	3
Ponti	petrosal neurectomy	2–5	6	5
White 1969	petrosal neurectomy	1.5–14	9	3
Stowell 1970	petrosal neurectomy		21	18
Duran	petrosal neurectomy	0.5–2	6	4
Alvarez	petrosal neurectomy	0.6–12	9	4
Denecke	petrosal neurectomy	<1	3	3
Kunkel 1974	petrosal neurectomy	4	12	6
Watson 1983	petrosal neurectomy	1–5	4	1
Wake 1987	petrosal neurectomy	1–20	6	3
Gybels 1988	petrosal neurectomy		13	1
	section nervus intermedius		4	2
Sachs	section nervus intermedius	1–16	8	5
Morgalender 1990	section nervus intermedius	0.1–8	12	3
Roweed 1990	section nervus intermedius	0.4–2	8	6
Sanders 1997	PSR[b] sphenopalatine gangliolysis	1–6	66	37

[a]All series are cited in Reference 42.
[b]PSR, percutaneous stereotactic radiofrequency.

(42). Patients who undergo open trigeminal rhizotomy require section of the rostral part of the nerve for good pain control (19, 42). Major sensory loss is associated with increased risks of keratitis and dysesthesia that can be up to 12% (42). For this reason, balloon compression may be worth considering for the treatment of cluster headache; however, results have not been reported.

SURGERIES TO THE NERVUS INTERMEDIUS-SUPERFICIAL PETROSAL-SPHENOPALATINE SYSTEM SEEM EQUALLY EFFECTIVE

In combined series, long-term pain control was achieved in 54% of patients who underwent superficial petrosal neurectomy, in 50% of patients who underwent section of the nervus intermedius, and in 56% of patients who underwent percutaneous PSR sphenopalatine gangliolysis. Limited experience with isolated MVD of the nervus intermedius has been disappointing (43).

CLUSTER HEADACHE IS OCCASIONALLY ASSOCIATED WITH INTRACRANIAL PATHOLOGY

There are anecdotal reports of patients with chronic cluster headache who achieve pain relief after surgery for tentorial meningiomas, pituitary tumors, arteriovenous malformations, and aneurysms (42). These patients most likely experience referred pain along the ophthalmic or maxillary divisions that can mimic pain of chronic cluster headache.

INNOVATIVE TREATMENTS

There may be a role for newer surgical approaches for cluster headache. Initial results of radiosurgery have been encouraging, with pain controlled in 6 of 8 patients followed for 8 to 14 months (11). Recently, ultrasonic trigeminal nucleotomy-tractotomy achieved pain control in 11 of 12 patients (12). The authors, however, are aware of several patients who underwent caudalis DREZ surgery with only transient pain relief.

Conclusion

In cluster headache, pain can be controlled by surgery to either the trigeminal system or nervus intermedius-superficial petrosal-sphenopalatine system. With either approach, the pain is rarely cured. In the authors' experience, periorbital pain is best relieved by PSR trigeminal rhizotomy or open intracranial rhizotomy with section of the nervus intermedius if pain radiates to the temple-ear region. To avoid sensory loss, surgeons may combine MVD with section of the nervus intermedius with less successful results. Other approaches, such as balloon compression, radiosurgery, and trigeminal nucleotomy-tractotomy require further investigation.

SUMMARY

The authors recommend a multidisciplinary approach for the diagnosis and treatment of facial pain. With this approach, several experts can accurately diagnose various disorders of facial pain and offer appropriate treatment options, which should be tailored to the specific needs and general condition of the patient. For reporting and comparison, seek standardization of methods of analysis and outcomes criteria. Associate with a good secretary and nurse. For your patients' benefit, be an optimistic, caring, and attentive listener.

REFERENCES

1. Addennebi B, Mahfouf L, Nedjahi T: Long-term results of percutaneous compression of the gasserian ganglion in trigeminal neuralgia. **Stereotact Funct Neurosurg** 68:190–195, 1997.
2. Barker F, Jannetta P, Bissonette D, Larkins M, Jho HD: The long-term outcome of microvascular decompression for trigeminal neuralgia. **N Engl J Med** 334:1077–1083, 1996.
3. Barker FG II, Jannetta PJ, Babu RP, Pomonis S, Bissonette DJ, Jho HD: Long-term outcome after operation for trigeminal neuralgia in patients with posterior fossa tumors. **J Neurosurg** 84:818–825, 1996.
4. Bergenheim A, Hariz M, Laitinen L, Olivecrona M, Rabow L: Relation between sensory disturbance and outcome after retrogasserian glycerol rhizotomy. **Acta Neurochir (Wien)** 111:114–118, 1991.
5. Brown J, Gouda J: Percutaneous balloon compression of the trigeminal nerve. **Neurosurg Clin North Am** 8:53–62, 1997.
6. Cappabianca P, Spaziante R, Graziussi G, Taglialatela G, Peca C, De Divitiis E: Percutaneous retrogasserian glycerol rhizolysis for treatment of trigeminal neuralgia. Technique and results in 191 patients. **J Neurosurg Sci** 39:37–45, 1995.
7. Cheng T, Cascino T, Onofrio B: Comprehensive study of diagnosis and treatment of trigeminal neuralgia secondary to tumors. **Neurology** 43:2298–2302, 1993.
8. Cho DY, Chang C, Wang YC, Wang FH, Shen CC, Yang DY: Repeat operations in failed microvascular decompression for trigeminal neuralgia. **Neurosurgery** 35:665–670, 1994.
9. Cutbush K, Atkinson R: Treatment of trigeminal neuralgia by posterior fossa microvascular decompression. **Aust NZ J Surg** 64:173–176, 1994.
10. De La Porte C, Verlooy J, Veeckmans G, Parizel P, de Moor J, Selosse P: Consequences and complications of glycerol injection in the cavum of Meckel: A series of 120 consecutive injections. **Stereotact Funct Neurosurg** 54–55:73–75, 1990.
11. Ford R, Ford K, Swaid S, Jennelle R: Gamma knife treatment of refractory cluster headache. **Headache** 38:3–9, 1998.
12. Grigorian IUA, Ogleznev KIA, Roshchina NA: Surgical treatment of migrainous neuralgia. **Zh Vopr Neirokhir im N N Burdenko** 4:16–19, 1995.

13. Hakanson S, Linderoth B: Injection of glycerol into the gasserian cistern for treatment of trigeminal neuralgia, in Gildenberg P, Tasker R (eds): *Textbook of Stereotactic and Functional Neurosurgery*. New York, McGraw-Hill, 1998, pp.1697–1706.
14. Ischia S, Luzzani A, Polati E: Retrogasserian glycerol injection: A retrospective study of 112 patients. **Clin J Pain** 6:291–296, 1990.
15. Ischia S, Luzzani A, Polati E, Ischia A: Percutaneous controlled thermocoagulation in the treatment of trigeminal neuralgia. **Clin J Pain** 6:96–104, 1990.
16. Jamjoom A, Jamjoom Z, Al-Fehaily M, El-Watidy S, Al-Moallem M, Nain-Ur-Rahman: Trigeminal neuralgia related to cerebellopontine angle tumors. **Neurosurg Rev** 19:237–241, 1996.
17. Jho HD, Lunsford D: Percutaneous retrogasserian glycerol rhizotomy. **Neurosurg Clin North Am** 8:63–74, 1997.
18. Kanpolat Y, Savas A, Batay F, Sinav A: Computed tomography-guided trigeminal tractotomy-nucleotomy in the management of vagoglossopharyngeal and geniculate neuralgias. **Neurosurgery** 43:484–490, 1998.
19. Kirkpatrick P, O'Brien M, MacCabe J: Trigeminal nerve section for chronic migrainous neuralgia. **Br J Neurosurg** 7:483–490, 1993.
20. Kondo A: Follow-up results of microvascular decompression in trigeminal neuralgia and hemifacial spasm. **Neurosurgery** 40:46–51, 1997.
21. Kondziolka D, Lunsford LD, Bissonette D: Long-term results after glycerol rhizotomy for multiple sclerosis-related trigeminal neuralgia. **Can J Neurol Sci** 21:137–140, 1994.
22. Kondziolka D, Lunsford D, Habeck M, Flickinger J: Gamma knife radiosurgery for trigeminal neuralgia. **Neurosurg Clin North Am** 8:79–85, 1997.
23. Lee KH, Chang JW, Park YG, Chung SS: Microvascular decompression and percutaneous rhizotomy in trigeminal neuralgia. **Stereotact Funct Neurosurg** 68:196–199, 1997.
24. Linskey M, Jho HD, Jannetta P: Microvascular decompression for trigeminal neuralgia caused by vertebrobasilar compression. **J Neurosurg** 81:1–9, 1994.
25. Mendoza N, Illingworth R: Trigeminal neuralgia treated by microvascular decompresssion: A long-term follow-up study. **Br J Neurosurg** 9:13–19, 1995.
26. Miserocchi G, Cabrini G, Motti ED, Granata G, Ferrari da Passano C: Percutaneous selective thermorhizotomy in the treatment of essential trigeminal neuralgia. **J Neurosurg Sci** 33:179–183, 1989.
27. Pagura J, Rabello J, De Lima W: Microvascular decompression for trigeminal neuralgia, in Gildenberg P, Tasker R (eds): *Textbook of Stereotactic and Functional Neurosurgery*. New York, McGraw-Hill, 1996, pp.1715–1721.
28. Puca A, Meglio M: Typical trigeminal neuralgia associated with posterior cranial fossa tumors. **Ital J Neurol Sci** 14:549–552, 1993.
29. Rand R: Leksell gamma knife treatment of tic douloureux. **Neurosurg Clin North Am** 8:75–78, 1997.
30. Rappaport Z, Gomori J: Recurrent trigeminal cistern glycerol injections for tic douloureux. **Acta Neurochir (Wien)** 90:31–34, 1988.
31. Rath S, Klein H, Richter H: Findings and long-term results of subsequent operations after failed microvascular decompression for trigeminal neuralgia. **Neurosurgery** 39:933–938, 1996.
32. Resnick D, Jannetta P, Bissonnette D, Jho HD, Lanzino G: Microvascular decompression for glossopharyngeal neuralgia. **Neurosurgery** 36:64–69, 1995.
33. Resnick D, Jannetta PJ, Lunsford LD, Bissonette DJ: Microvascular decompression for trigeminal neuralgia in patients with multiple sclerosis. **Surg Neurol** 46:358–361, 1996.

34. Sanders M, Zuurmond W: Efficacy of sphenopalatine ganglion blockade in 66 patients suffering from cluster headache: A 12- to 70-month follow-up evaluation. **J Neurosurg** 87:876–880, 1997.
35. Sindou M, Amrani F, Mertens P: Microsurgical vascular decompression in trigeminal neuralgia. Comparison of 2 technical modalities and physiopathologic deductions. A study of 120 cases. **Neurochirugie** 36:16–25, 1990.
36. Sindou M, Henry J, Blanchard P: Idiopathic neuralgia of the glossopharyngeal nerve. Study of a series of 14 cases and review of the literature. **Neurochirurgie** 37:18–25, 1991.
37. Steiger H: Prognostic factors in the treatment of trigeminal neuralgia. Analysis of a differential therapeutic approach. **Acta Neurochir (Wien)** 113:11–17, 1991.
38. Taha JM, Tew JM Jr: A prospective 15-year follow up of 154 consecutive patients with trigeminal neuralgia treated by percutaneous stereotactic radiofrequency thermal rhizotomy. **J Neurosurg** 83:989–993, 1995.
39. Taha JM, Tew JM Jr: Comparison of surgical treatments for trigeminal neuralgia: Reevaluation of radiofrequency rhizotomy. **Neurosurgery** 38:865–871, 1996.
40. Taha JM, Tew JM Jr: Long-term results of radiofrequency rhizotomy in the treatment of cluster headache. **Headache** 35:193–196, 1995.
41. Taha JM, Tew JM Jr: Long-term results of surgical treatment of idiopathic neuralgias of the glossopharyngeal and vagal nerves. **Neurosurgery** 36:926–931, 1995.
42. Taha JM, Tew JM Jr: Surgical management of glossopharyngeal and other uncommon facial neuralgias, in Tindall G, Cooper P, Barrow D (eds): *The Practice of Neurosurgery.* Baltimore, Williams & Wilkins, 1996, pp 3065–3080.
43. Taha JM, Tew JM Jr, Keith R, Payner TD: Intraoperative monitoring of the vagus nerve during intracranial glossopharyngeal and upper vagal rhizotomy: Technical note. **Neurosurgery** 35:775–777, 1994.
44. Tew JM Jr, Taha JM: Percutaneous rhizotomy in the treatment of intractable facial pain (trigeminal, glossopharyngeal, and vagal nerves), in Schmidek HH, Sweet WH (eds): *Operative Neurosurgical Techniques,* 3rd ed, Philadelphia: W.B. Saunders, 1995, pp 1469–1484.
45. Wakiya K, Fukushima T, Miyazaki S: Results of microvascular decompression in 16 cases of glossopharyngeal neuralgia. **Neurol Med Chir (Tokyo)** 29:1113–1118, 1989.
46. Waltz T, Dalessio D, Copeland B, Abbott G: Percutaneous injection of glycerol for the treatment of trigeminal neuralgia. **Clin J Pain** 5:195–198, 1989.
47. Yamaki T, Hashi K, Niwa J, et al: Results of reoperation for failed microvascular decompression. **Acta Neurochir (Wien)** 115:1–7, 1992
48. Young R, Vermeulen S, Grimm P, Blasko J, Posewitz A: Gamma knife radiosurgery for treatment of trigeminal neuralgia: Idiopathic and tumor related. **Neurology** 48:608–614, 1997.
49. Zakrzewska J, Thomas D: Patient's assessment of outcome after three surgical procedures in the management of trigeminal neuralgia. **Acta Neurochir (Wien)** 122:225–230, 1993.

IV

General Scientific Session IV

CHAPTER

30

Facial Pain Syndromes: Practical Considerations

KIM J. BURCHIEL, M.D., F.A.C.S.

The evaluation and treatment of facial pain is a common problem in neurosurgical practice. The history of the description of the various facial pain diagnoses as entities that we recognize today is fascinating, and for this background the reader is directed to the excellent review by Wilkins (6). Much has also been written of the taxonomy of this family of diagnoses (3, 4), and the neurosurgical treatment of facial pain (5). However, the goal of this chapter is not to be encyclopedic, but rather to share the author's view of the practical diagnosis and categorization of facial pain in the clinical setting. The chapter focuses or common clinical problems, exemplified by case studies. The author also presents a scheme for characterization of facial pain that is based partly on tradition, and partly on experience, and comments on the specific diagnosis of trigeminal neuralgia.

DIFFERENTIAL DIAGNOSIS OF FACIAL PAIN

Table 30.1 shows a broad overview of the diagnostic categories of facial pain. The most familiar of these is trigeminal neuralgia, or tic douloreux, which in its most common form is idiopathic. Trigeminal neuralgia can also be secondary to structural pathology, such as a tumor or aneurysm, or it can be the result of multiple sclerosis (so-called symptomatic trigeminal neuralgia). Atypical trigeminal neuralgia may be idiopathic or secondary and is characterized by constant facial pain combined with the more typical episodic pains of more typical trigeminal neuralgia. Trigeminal neuropathic pain has also been called posttraumatic trigeminal neuralgia, to denote its origin from facial trauma or prior orofacial surgery. By this categorization, atypical facial pain is diagnostically distinct from trigeminal neuropathic pain and implies a primarily psychogenic origin for the facial pain (4).

Because many other conditions include an important element of craniofacial pain, the evaluation of a patient with facial pain should al-

TABLE 30.1
Differential Diagnosis of Facial Pain

Trigeminal neuralgia (tic douloureux)
  Secondary trigeminal neuralgia
  Multiple sclerosis
Atypical trigeminal neuralgia
Trigeminal neuropathic pain
Atypical facial pain
Other cranial neuralgias
Temporomandibular joint disorders and dental pain
Headache syndromes

ways include include consideration of other related disorders. For example, other cranial neuralgias, discussed below, can manifest historical or clinical features that can be confused with trigeminal neuralgia. One should also not forget that the most common cause of orofacial pain is odontogenic pain. Thus, disorders of the teeth and temporomandibular joint should be added to the diagnostic possibilities. Lastly, headache syndromes are vastly more common than the rarities that neurosurgeons deal with. Unusual migrainous variants can easily be confused with atypical craniofacial neuralgias.

CLINICAL DIAGNOSIS OF FACIAL PAIN

The diagnosis of facial pain is almost entirely from the patient's history. The location and description of the pain, its temporal features, pain-free intervals (if any), pain trigger zones, and response to medication are perhaps the most important elements. The patient's past medical history may also give some clues to the diagnosis as well as help the neurosurgeon recommend the most appropriate therapy. Conversely, when the patient is impaired mentally or does not speak the neurosurgeon's primary language, the diagnosis of facial pain can be extraordinarily difficult and fraught with many unpredictable pitfalls.

The patient's physical examination, including detailed neurological evaluation, is likewise important in forming a differential diagnosis and treatment plan. For example, any clinically detectable facial numbness or cranial nerve palsy would necessitate reconsideration of the diagnosis of idiopathic trigeminal neuralgia. Review of all relevant imaging studies, including computed tomographic (CT) and magnetic resonance imaging (MRI) scans, is essential. For patients with suspected trigeminal neuralgia, at least one CT or MRI is required to rule out otherwise occult structural pathology.

What follows are descriptions of the most common facial pain diagnoses and a brief case study to highlight the characteristic features of each condition.

Trigeminal Neuralgia

Table 30.2 describes a history of typical trigeminal neuralgia. Pains are strictly unilateral, are within one or more of the divisions of the trigeminal nerve, and are episodic, lasting for seconds to 1 to 2 minutes. The pains are usually described as "electrical," or "shock-like." Minor pains or premonitory sensations can be described as "sparkles," or tingling paresthesias. They give the impression of traveling or lancinating within a given division or from one division to another. The pains more commonly occur in the third, or mandibular, division (V3), less commonly in the second (maxillary) division [V2], or the first (opthalmic) division (VI). There is frequently a peritoral trigger area, in which light tactile stimulation can trigger a typical bout of neuralgia. There is no clinically detectable sensory loss to tactile, thermal, or pinprick sensation. A history of pain-free intervals that can last for months or even many years is usually reported. Pain-free intervals are particularly common in patients in whom the pain developed in middle age, or younger. When a patient in the seventh or eighth decade develops trigeminal neuralgia, these "pain holidays" may be short to nonexistent. CT and MRI studies are almost invariably normal, except in the 1 to 2% of patients who have secondary trigeminal neuralgia.

Perhaps the most important feature of a facial pain that labels it as trigeminal neuralgia is unequivocal improvement with an anticonvulsant such as carbamazepine, gabapentin, or phenytoin. One can virtually be assured of the diagnosis of trigeminal neuralgia in a patient whose facial pain disappears with carbamazepine treatment, irrespective of the other historical features of the syndrome.

TABLE 30.2
Characteristics of Trigeminal Neuralgia

Episodic, lancinating, "electrical" pains
Unilateral, trigeminal distribution
V3>V2/V1
Perioral trigger
No sensory loss
Pain-free intervals
Normal imaging
Response to carbamazepine/gabapentin

CASE HISTORY 1: TRIGEMINAL NEURALGIA

A 62-year-old woman complained of a 10-year history of episodic, "shock-like" pains in her right jaw, gums, and tongue. For the first 2 years of her syndrome the pains were intermittent and were felt to be dental in origin. She underwent several tooth extractions before the diagnosis of trigeminal neuralgia was entertained. The patient was placed on carbamazepine 200 mg bid, and her pains resolved completely. Over the previous 8 years, there had been several periods, one lasting for almost 2 years, when the patient's pains completely subsided, and she was able to temporarily cease taking the medication. More recently pains had returned consistently and had remained refractory to separate trials of carbamazepine 200 mg qid and gabapentin up to 1200 mg per day. At these medication levels the patient developed somnolence and ataxia. Her past history is otherwise unremarkable. Physical examination revealed normal cranial nerve function, including normal facial sensation, and staggering on tandem gait. An MRI of the head was normal for the patient's age.

Secondary Trigeminal Neuralgia

Most cases of trigeminal neuralgia are considered to be idiopathic, because no clear pathology or predisposing condition can be determined preoperatively. The current theories and controversies surrounding the etiology of this entity are discussed elsewhere.

Rarely in about 1 to 2% of cases, the cause of trigeminal neuralgia is somewhat more clear. *Table 30.3* lists the various conditions that can be associated with so-called secondary trigeminal neuralgia. From the neurosurgeon's standpoint, the two most important, and in fact most common, causes of secondary trigeminal neuralgia are tumors and vascular lesions such as aneurysms or arteriovenous malformations. It is for this reason that CT or MRI imaging of the head must be obtained

TABLE 30.3
Causes of Secondary Trigeminal Neuralgia

Tumors
Vascular lesions
Granulomatous conditions, (sarcoid)
Syringobulbia
Paget's syndrome or acromegaly
Amyloidosis
Toxins
Dejerine-Sottas disease
Chiari malformation

at some point in all patients, and it is mandatory before surgical intervention for patients with trigeminal neuralgia.

There are two features of secondary trigeminal neuralgia that must be kept in mind. First, clinically detectable facial sensory loss is common in these cases. Second, atypical trigeminal neuralgia, with varying degrees of constant burning or aching background pain, is common. Patients manifesting either or both of these features have a much higher likelihood of harboring a structural abnormality or a condition that predisposes them to trigeminal neuropathy.

Atypical Trigeminal Neuralgia

Although the terms idiopathic or secondary trigeminal neuralgia denote the putative origin of the syndrome of trigeminal neuralgia, known or unknown, atypical trigeminal neuralgia is strictly a clinical distinction. It is based solely on how the patient describes the pain.

Whereas patients with classic trigeminal neuralgia have little in the way of background pain between the discrete bouts of neuralgia, patients with constant underlying pain, with more typical pains superimposed, are described as having atypical trigeminal neuralgia. *Table 30.4* lists the features of this syndrome. The background pains are often described as "aching" or "burning" in nature. As noted above, facial sensory loss on neurological examination and structural pathology on imaging are both more common than in the more typical syndrome. The response to carbamazepine may be partial, in that lancinating pains may disappear, leaving the background discomfort unrelieved.

Although at any point the syndrome of atypical trigeminal neuralgia may be a useful distinction, the differences between it and typical trigeminal neuralgia may actually be more quantitative than qualitative. After severe bouts of neuralgia, many patients with otherwise typical pains experience lingering background pain, which may last for hours. Furthermore, many patients with atypical pains give a prior history of exclusively episodic pains early in the course of their disorder. It is only over time that the more constant pains become a prominent aspect of their disorder. This concept will be discussed at the conclusion of this chapter.

TABLE 30.4
Characteristics of Atypical Trigeminal Neuralgia

Unilateral episodic pain superimposed on some degree of lingering background pain
Detectable sensory loss more common
Structural pathology (tumors) more common
Response to carbamazepine may be limited to episodic pain
Pain may have history of more typical trigeminal neuralgia pain early in course

CASE STUDY 2: ATYPICAL TRIGEMINAL NEURALGIA

A 55-year-old man gave a history of 8 years of episodic stabbing pains in his left cheek and forehead. These pains had always been associated with some degree of underlying pain in the same distribution, which he described as a "strong ache," but over the previous few yeas the constant pain had become almost as troublesome as the severe episodic stabbing pains. Although the episodic pains responded reliably to carbamazepine 400 mg tid, the constant pains remained refractory. The patient's past history was significant for non-insulin-dependent diabetes mellitus and hypertension. Physical examination revealed only a mild sensory loss to pinprick in the left V2 distribution, as well as "soreness" to touch in the left cheek. MRI showed a dolichocephalic basilar artery traversing the left cerebellopontine angle.

Trigeminal Neuropathic Pain

Table 30.5 lists the clinical characteristics of patients with trigeminal neuropathic pain (1). Patients who have experienced facial trauma, orofacial surgery, or sometimes complicated or difficult dental extractions can develop chronic pain in a trigeminal division or nerve distribution. This is termed trigeminal neuropathic pain, to identify it with other so-called neuropathic pains that can result from deafferenting injury to the peripheral or central nervous system (1).

The pain is described as having both episodic and constant components, although constant pain dominates. The pain is characterized as "burning" or "aching," and the area of pain may manifest allodynia, i.e., painful perceived sensation from what would be considered an innocuous stimulus. There may also be a Tinel's sign over the putative area of nerve injury.

In general, these pains have a poor response to medication, although recent experience with gabapentin has been more positive. As with

TABLE 30.5
Characteristics of Trigeminal Neuropathic Pain

History of facial trauma
History if difficult or complicated dental extraction, or sinus surgery
Pain in a branch or nerve distribution
Pain episodic and constant (dominates) components
Pain often described as aching or burning
May have facial allodynia, Tinel's sign
Poor response to medications
May respond to local anesthetic block, sympathetic block

other pains related to nerve injuries, local anesthetic block of the damaged nerve may temporarily alleviate the pain. In some cases, sympathetic blockade at the level of the stellate ganglion will also yield transient improvement.

CASE HISTORY 3: TRIGEMINAL NEUROPATHIC PAIN

A 45-year-old man had a history of an on-the-job injury in which he was struck with a metal rod under the left eye. He developed a hematoma and bruising at and below the inferior orbital rim but did not seek immediate medical attention. Since the injury, the patient has had unremitting aching pain in the right cheek and upper teeth, as well as episodic "shocks" in the same distribution. He had no improvement with either carbamazepine or gabapentin. The patient's past history was unremarkable. Physical examination showed a Tinel's sign under the left eye with radiation into the left upper lip and upper teeth. Sensory testing showed loss of pinprick sensation in the infraorbital nerve distribution. The patient had normal dentition and no dental tenderness. MRI scan was normal, and a review of old sinus x-rays revealed on old orbital rim fracture.

Atypical Facial Pain

Although atypical facial pain has little in common with trigeminal neuralgia or its variants, it is an entity that must be recognized to eliminate the possibility of inappropriate surgery.

Table 30.6 lists the characteristic features of atypical facial pain. Atypical facial pain is primarily a psychogenic pain syndrome, and it fits most closely what the American Psychiatric Association terms Psychogenic Pain Disorder. Pain can be bilateral and may include areas outside the trigeminal distribution. There is no response to carbamazepine, but some relief may be obtained with tricyclic antidepressants. The syndrome can cluster with other disorders such as fi-

TABLE 30.6
Characteristic of Atypical Facial Pain

Almost no common features with trigeminal neuralgia
Nonanatomic sensorimotor findings
Pain can be bilateral, and outside trigeminal distribution
No response to carbamazepine, gabapentin
May respond to tricyclic antidepressants
Diagnostic clusters (fibromyalgia, chronic fatigue syndrome)
Depression
American Psychiatric Association: Psychogenic Pain Disorder

bromyalgia, chronic fatigue syndrome, interstitial cystitis, and other controversial diagnoses that may be typified by a dearth of substantiating objective evidence. Patients are frequently clinically depressed. Psychological testing reveals corroboration of depression as well as strong evidence of somatization.

CASE HISTORY 4: ATYPICAL FACIAL PAIN

A 52-year-old woman complained of a constant burning pain in her right scalp to the occiput, V1 through V3 on the right, the left V3 distribution, and her entire tongue. The pain did not respond to carbamazepine or gabapentin. The pain was modestly improved by amitriptyline 100 mg at bedtime. Past medical history was remarkable for a diagnosis of fibromyalgia. The patient was seeing a counselor for "depression." Examination revealed diffuse, bilateral facial and somatic sensory loss, "give-away" weakness on motor testing, and nearly continuous pain behavior during the interview and examination. The patient was tearful at several points during the examination. Imaging studies, including head CT and MRI, as well as multiple x-rays of the sinuses, skull, c-spine, and L-spine, were unremarkable. Psychological testing demonstrated a conversion V (high hysteria and hypochondriasis scores) pattern on the Minnesota Multiphasic Personality Inventory, as well as depression on several indices.

Other Cranial Neuralgias

Other neuralgias of the head and face can mimic certain aspects of trigeminal neuralgia (*Table 30.7*). Postherpetic neuralgia always follows an acute herpetic outbreak (shingles), usually in the opthalmic division. Geniculate neuralgia is usually described as a stabbing pain deep in the ear, but these pains can radiate to the pinna, and region around the temporomandibular joint. Likewise, whereas glossopharyngeal neuralgia is usually described as stabbing pain in the tonsillar, lingual, or retropharyngeal area, complaints of pains in the third division, or anterior tongue, can create some diagnostic confusion with trigeminal neuralgia.

Occipital neuralgia, by definition, affects the occipital nerve distribution, which should remain posterior to the opthalmic division, suboccipital and peri-aural. However, occasionally, patients with atypical forms of trigeminal neuralgia can have pains in both the trigeminal and occipital nerve distributions. Appropriate treatment of the trigeminal neuralgia can alleviate the pains in the occipital nerve territory.

Rare conditions such as Raeder's paratrigeminal neuralgia, and sphenopalatine neuralgia are also of note, if only to show that other

TABLE 30.7
Other Cranial Neuralgias

Postherpetic neuralgia
Geniculate neuralgia
Glossopharyngeal neuralgia
Occipital neuralgia
Sphenopalatine neuralgia
Raeder's paratrigeminal neuralgia

syndromes exist that may fit the patient's description of the pain more closely than a more familiar diagnosis. The author's experience is that these rare diagnoses frequently remain dubious and virtually never lead to a surgical solution to the pain.

CAN ALL FACIAL PAIN BE CHARACTERIZED BY DISCRETE DIAGNOSES?

Certainly, classic trigeminal neuralgia is a highly recognizable objective diagnosis. This is significant, since it is the most medically and surgically tractable facial pain condition. As we move away from this diagnosis, the chances of improvement with surgery diminish dramatically. The conceptualization of the various types of trigeminal neuralgias as discrete entities (*Fig. 30.1*) is clinically very useful but should not be considered rigid or inviolate. Are the other diagnoses of atypical trigeminal neuralgia, trigeminal neuropathic pain, and atypical facial pain completely discrete clinical conditions? Experience indicates that rather than discrete entities, these conditions form a continuum, with intermediate forms of the conditions at each diagnostic interface (*Fig. 30.2*).

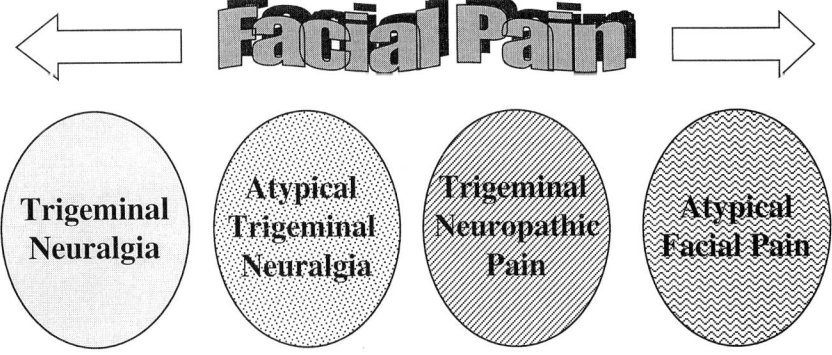

FIG. 30.1 Facial pain as a discrete diagnosis?

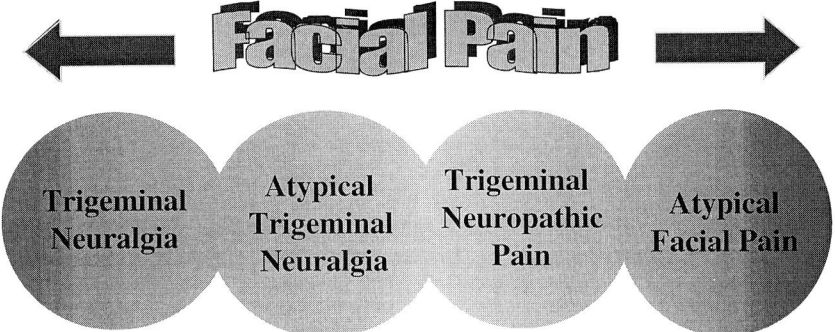

FIG. 30.2 Facial pain as a continuum of diagnoses.

Facial pain could then be considered a spectrum of conditions, rather than a collection of independent diagnoses.

FINAL COMMENTS

As more experience with trigeminal neuralgia is gained, a number of conclusions may be suggested:

1. Trigeminal neuralgia is a progressive disorder that worsens over a patient's lifetime. It never spontaneously regresses. Attacks become more frequent and severe, pain-free intervals disappear, and the pains become more refractory to medication.
2. Despite the fact that initially approximately 70% of patients will be rendered pain-free with medication alone, over time the majority of patients with trigeminal neuralgia will require surgical intervention.
3. Diagnostic distinctions of facial pain are useful but not inviolate. Facial pain is a continuum.
4. Surgical outcome is best with typical trigeminal neuralgia.
5. The pains of atypical trigeminal neuralgia and trigeminal neuropathic pain are also treatable, but the outcome is less predictable.
6. The cause of trigeminal neuralgia is still controversial.
7. The mechanism of the pains of trigeminal neuralgia is unknown. Further research is needed to clarify the fundamental nature of the disorder.
8. Trigeminal neuralgia remains an exception to the general intractability of most chronic pain states to surgical therapy.

REFERENCES

1. Burchiel KJ: Trigeminal neuropathic pain. **Acta Neurochir** 58:145–149, 1993.
2. Burchiel KJ: Neurovascular compression and trigeminal neuralgia. *APS Journal* 2(4):234–236, 1993.
3. Burchiel KJ: Treatment of facial pain, in, Gildenberg PL, Tasker RR (eds): *Textbook of Stereotactic and Functional Neurosurgery.* New York, McGraw-Hill, 1998, pp 1723–1728.
4. Burchiel KJ, Burgess J: Facial and cranial pain, in North R (ed): *Neurosurgical Management of Pain.* New York, Springer-Verlag, 1994, pp. 83–99.
5. Burchiel KJ, Moore KR: Neurosurgical treatment of pain: Trigeminal neuralgia, in Wilden JN, and Swash M (eds): *Outcomes in Neurological and Neurosurgical Disorders.* Cambridge, Cambridge University Press, 1998, pp 507–532.
6. Wilkins RH: Historical overview of surgical techniques for trigeminal neuralgia, in, Burchiel KJ (ed): *Techniques in Neurosurgery: Trigeminal Neuralgia.* Philadelphia, Lippincott-Williams & Wilkins, 1999, pp. 202–217.

CHAPTER

31

Contemporary Medical Management of Facial Pain

OREN SAGHER, M.D.

> Doctors pour drugs, of which they know little, for diseases of which they know less, into patients—of whom they know nothing.
> —*Voltaire*

INTRODUCTION AND HISTORY

Facial pain is an extremely vexing problem, with a wide spectrum of etiologies. Although neurosurgeons commonly associate facial pain with trigeminal neuralgia, the latter diagnosis comprises only a minority of patients with facial pain (22). Still, the history of facial pain treatment parallels that of the specific pain syndrome we now recognizes as trigeminal neuralgia.

The treatment of facial pain has historically ranged from the strange to the bizarre. Treatments such as blood-letting, purging, ingestion of wine, application of steam to the abdomen, irradiation, and appendectomy have all been reported (16). Medical treatments have included hemlock, vitamins, iron carbonate, and inhalational agents (6). Poor understanding of the various causes of facial pain syndromes as well as their natural history has contributed to the development of such improbable treatments.

Perhaps the most important observation regarding facial pain treatment was made by Armand Trousseau in 1853, who noted that facial pain tended to be paroxysmal (20). Although he was referring specifically to trigeminal neuralgia, his eponym for the disorder—neuralgia epileptiform—eventually led to the use of anticonvulsants in the treatment of facial pain. Indeed, these medications continue to be the most successful in the treatment of a variety of facial pain syndromes.

Despite the similarities that exist in the medical treatment of trigeminal neuralgia and other types of facial pain, it is important that the subtleties of pain characteristics are recognized and that underlying causes are thoroughly differentiated before initiation of treatment.

ETIOLOGIES OF FACIAL PAIN

The causes of facial pain are myriad but can be roughly classified into several categories (*Table 31.1*). Although many types of facial pain fall outside the expertise or practice of neurosurgery, it is nevertheless important for the neurosurgeon to consider the differential diagnosis before embarking on medical or surgical therapy.

The diversity of possible causes of facial pain represents the first (and sometimes most difficult) hurdle to treatment. When an anatomical cause can be found, as is the case in cancer of the head and neck, efforts can focus on treatment of the lesion or on palliative treatment. However, when no such lesion is apparent, the neurosurgeon must rely on other, indirect, diagnostic clues. Such factors as distribution of pain, pain triggers, and quality of pain provide important information on the origin of the pain as well as the most appropriate treatment. *Table 31.2* summarizes some of the salient features of commonly encountered facial pain syndromes.

GENERAL PRINCIPLES OF MEDICAL TREATMENT

The initial treatment of most facial pain syndromes is usually medical. Treatment, however, must be diagnosis-driven. Therefore, pain

TABLE 31.1
Facial Pain Etiologies

Cause	Examples
Neural	Trigeminal neuralgia
	Postherpetic neuralgia
	Trigeminal neuropathic pain
	Glossopharyngeal neuralgia
	Sphenopalatine neuralgia
	Geniculate neuralgia (Ramsay Hunt)
Dental/Periodontal	Dentinal, pulpal, or periodontal pain
	Temporomandibular disorders
Sinuses and Aerodigestive Tract	Sinusitis
	Head and neck cancer
Ocular	Tolosa-Hunt Syndrome
	Optic neuritis
	Iritis
	Glaucoma
Vascular	Giant cell arteritis
	Migraine
	Cluster headache (?)
Psychological	Psychogenic facial pain
	Atypical facial pain (?)

TABLE 31.2
Diagnostic Clues in Facial Pain

Diagnosis	Pain Character	Pain Distribution	Pain Triggers	Other Clues
Trigeminal neuralgia	Paroxysmal, lancinating	Trigeminal only V2 most frequent	Touch, chewing, talking, etc.	
Glossopharyngeal neuralgia	Paroxysmal, lancinating	Ear, throat	Swallowing	
Trigeminal neuropathic pain	Constant, burning, dull-throbbing	Trigeminal only	None	History of trigeminal nerve injury
Postherpetic neuralgia	Constant, crawling. May have paroxysmal component	Trigeminal only, V1 most frequent	Touch	History of herpes, zoster, ophthalmicus
Anesthesia dolorosa	Constant, burning, itching in an insensate region	Trigeminal only	None	History of trigeminal nerve lesion
Malignancy	Constant, but may have paroxysmal component	In area of neoplasm or referable to nerve compression	Possible of trigeminal nerve involved	Head/neck neoplasm
Atypical facial pain	Constant	Non-anatomic, often bilateral	None	Prominent psychiatric component

due to a head or neck neoplasm may be best treated by treatment of the lesion. Similarly, psychogenic pain is best addressed by treatment of the underlying psychiatric condition.

Medical treatment of facial pain is guided by the characteristics of the pain as much as it is by the underlying diagnosis. The primary differentiation that must be made is between nociceptive pain and neuropathic pain. Nociceptive pain is caused by normal and appropriate neuronal activity in the setting of local tissue damage. The primary example of nociceptive facial pain is that caused by head and neck cancer. Nociceptive pain is typically constant and aching, although it may sometimes also have a paroxysmal component. Nociceptive pain is usually best treated by the use of opioid medications, although one should consider treatment of the offending neoplasm as the first option.

Neuropathic pain is thought to result from abnormal and inappropriate neuronal activity and may occur in the absence of any anatomical lesion. Neuropathic pain frequently follows injury to the nervous system and is thought to involve aberrant regeneration or conduction. Neuropathic pain may be either paroxysmal or constant and is described frequently as electrical, burning, itching, or crawling. Neuropathic pain is thought to be relatively opioid-insensitive and treatment usually focuses on reducing abnormal neuronal activity through the use of anticonvulsants or psychotropic medications, such as the tricyclic antidepressants.

In addition to the important distinction between nociceptive and neuropathic pain, the differentiation between paroxysmal and constant pain also plays a key role in medical treatment. Paroxysmal pain, commonly seen in neuralgias, is thought to represent abnormal sensitization of the nerve that leads to attacks of lancinating pain in the distribution of the affected nerve. Constant neuropathic pain, on the other hand, is thought to occur in the setting of damage to the nerve or central nervous system. In the latter case, the pain is thought to result from an abnormal balance of inputs in neuromodulatory circuits. A general rule of thumb is that paroxysmal neuropathic pain is often best treated with anticonvulsants, whereas constant pain may respond better to the psychotropic medications, in particular, tricyclic antidepressants. The distinction between the two types of neuropathic pain is very useful when deciding on treatment options for facial pain. However, it is likely that this type of distinction represents a vast oversimplification of the differential causes of neuropathic pain.

The character of the pain, as well as its presumed cause, therefore guides the medical treatment of facial pain. *Figure 31.1* summarizes the general principles that guide the choice of medical therapy. In the next section, we will discuss the specific classes of medications used for treatment of the various facial pain syndromes.

MEDICATIONS USED IN TREATMENT OF FACIAL PAIN

Anticonvulsants

Following Trousseau's observation that trigeminal neuralgia resembled the epilepsies in the paraoxysmal presentation, a number of anticonvulsants have been effectively used in its treatment. Potassium bromide was first used successfully in the treatment of trigeminal neuralgia (23). In 1942, Bergouignan described the use of phenytoin for the treatment of trigeminal neuralgia (1). However, it was the development of a new anticonvulsant in 1961 that revolutionized the treatment of facial pain (2). Later known as carbamazepine, this medication still constitutes the mainstay of medical therapy in many facial pain syndromes. Other anticonsulvants have been subsequently developed and tested in the treatment of facial pain. Among these, only baclofen has

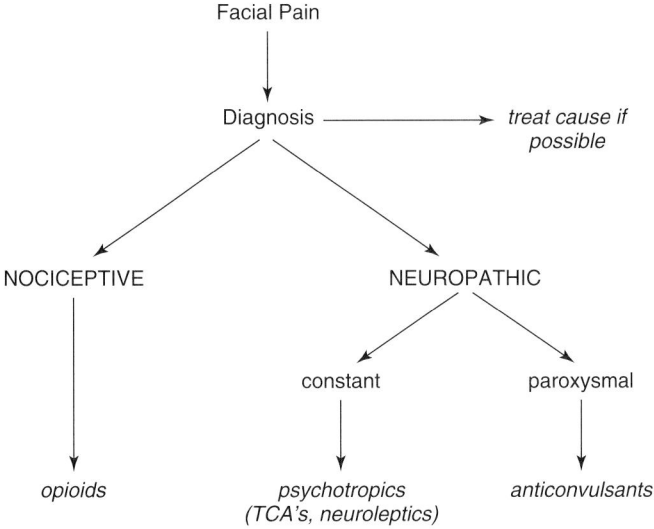

FIG. 31.1 General guidelines in the medical management of facial pain.

remained a first-line therapy in trigeminal neuralgia, although more recently there have been anecdotal reports detailing treatment with gabapentin for trigeminal neuralgia and other facial pain syndromes. *Table 31.3* outlines the typical anticonvulsant medications used in the treatment of facial pain.

The mode of action of anticonvulsants in the treatment of facial pain is not entirely clear. However, animal studies have indicated that both carbamazepine and baclofen act to enhance inhibitory neuronal activity in the trigeminal nucleus oralis (19). As it seems that this sensory nucleus plays an important role in trigeminal neuralgia, it is likely that the action of anticonvulsants at the level of the brainstem sensory nuclei is at least partially responsible for their beneficial effects.

In addition to their important therapeutic role in trigeminal neuralgia, anticonvulsants are used to treat other paroxysmal facial pain syndromes, such as trigeminal neuropathic pain, malignant facial pain, and postherpetic neuralgia.

Antidepressants

The antidepressants have found a prominent role in the treatment of neuropathic pain of a variety of causes. Although the precise mecha-

TABLE 31.3
Anticonvulsants Used in Facial Pain

Anticonvulsant	Class	Typical Dosage	Side Effects
Carbamazepine[a]	Tricyclic imipramine	200 to 1,000 mg/day	Dizziness, diplopia, rash, bone marrow suppression
Dilantin[a]	Hydantoin	300–500 mg/day	Lethargy, ataxia, rash, Stevens-Johnson (rare)
Baclofen[a]	GABA analogue	30–60 mg/day	Lethargy, ataxia, nausea
Clonazepam	Benzodiazepine	1–8 mg/day	Lethargy, fatigue, rash, thrombocytopenia
Valproic acid	Short-chain branched fatty acid	600 mg/day	Irritability, gastric irritation, alopecia, weight gain

[a]Considered first-line medications in facial pain.

nism by which they relieve pain is unclear, it is thought to involve alterations in monoamine levels in the central nervous system (17). In particular, elevations in brain/cerebrospinal fluid levels of serotine (5-hycroxytryptamine), norepinephrine, and dopamine are thought to be important. Inasmuch as the monomaines are believed to play a prominent role in chronic neuropathic pain, it is no surprise that these medications prove useful.

In addition to their independent analgesic effects, these agents probably also have a beneficial effect through their antidepressant effects. Because chronic pain is often compounded by a depressive component, these medications may work, in part by improving mood. Finally, they may benefit pain partially through their sedative activity by improving sleep.

The beneficial alteration of monoamine neurotransmitters is sometimes accompanied by anticholinergic and psychomimetic effects. It is an unfortunate reality that efficacy and side effects go hand-in-hand with antidepressants; the most consistently effective antidepressants are among the most poorly tolerated. Nevertheless, these drugs remain extremely useful in the treatment of constant, neuropathic pain. *Table 31.4* outlines some of the antidepressants commonly used in facial pain.

Neuroleptics

Neuroleptics are a class of psychotropic medications traditionally used for their antipsychotic effects. Like the antidepressants, neuroleptics modify neurotransmitter levels in the central nervous system.

Table 31.4
Antidepressants Used in Facial Pain[a]

Class	Examples	Typical Dose (mg/day)	5-HT[b] Effect	NE[b] Effect	Anti-cholinergic Effect	Sedation
Tricyclic	Amitriptyline	10–150	High	Mild	High	Moderate
	Desipramine	75–100	Mild	High	Minimal	None
	Doxepin	30–200	Mild	Minimal	Moderate	High
	Imipramine	20–150	Moderate	High	Mild	Minimal
	Nortriptyline	50–150	Mild	Moderate	Mild	Minimal
MAOI	Phenelzine	45–75	Minimal	Minimal	Minimal	None

[a]Adapted from Ref. 15.
[b]5-HT, 5-hydroxytryptamine; NE, norepinephrine.

Their mode of action is similarly nebulous, but it is thought to be related to a combination of direct neurotransmitter effects, antipsychotic activity, and sedative effects (3, 13). Unlike the antidepressants, however, they work predominantly to alter dopaminergic transmission and have little effect on the other monoamines.

Neuroleptics play a role in the treatment of facial pain under several special circumstances. The phenothiazine, fluphenazine, has been reported to be effective in treating the "crawling" pain of postherpetic neuralgia (8, 14). Neuroleptics may also be used as adjuncts to narcotic analgesia in malignant facial pain. In addition, neuroleptics may also be helpful in the treatment of the psychotic features that may accompany severe or psychogenic facial pain.

OPIOIDS

Nociceptive facial pain, such as that seen with malignancy, is usually treated with opioid medications. In cases wherein treatment of the offending lesion with surgery, radiation therapy, or chemotherapy is not possible, opioids should be routinely and liberally used. In these cases, the guidelines developed by the World Health Organization and the Agency for Health Care Policy and Research are relevant and useful (9, 21). In situations when adequate systemic opioids result in unacceptable sedation, opioids may be delivered intrathecally or intraventricularly (4, 10).

The use of chronic opioids for treatment of facial pain *not* related to malignancies is fraught with difficulties. First, many non-malignant facial pain syndromes are neuropathic or neuralgic and, therefore, respond poorly to opioid analgesics. Second, the treatment of facial pain with a prominent psychiatric component with opioids (such as may be the case in atypical facial pain) is usually counterproductive. Finally, the issue of opioid tolerance plagues most long-term administrations of these medications.

Other Medications Used in Facial Pain

LOCAL ANESTHETICS

Local anesthetics, such as lidocaine, have a minor role in the treatment of facial pain. They have been reported to be useful in temporarily halting paroxysms of trigeminal neuralgia (18). Mexiletine, an orally available anesthetic related to lidocaine, may be tried in cases of lidocaine-sensitive pain. Tocainide, another orally available anesthetic, has been reported to be effective in the treatment of trigeminal neuralgia but was associated with serious hematological complications (12).

CAPSAICIN

The neurotoxin, capsaicin, is primarily used in the treatment of painful neuropathies (such as diabetic neuropathy). Its mechanism of action is presumed to be related to a depletion of substance P in the dorsal horn. Capsaicin is used primarily in the treatment of postherpetic neuralgia, although there have been few reports of its use in the treatment of other types of facial pain (5, 7, 11).

SALICYLATES

Salicylates may have a role in the treatment of facial pain with an inflammatory component. Disorders of the temporomandibular joint, for example, may be treated with salicylates. Topical salicylates may also be used in neuropathic pain syndromes such as postherpetic neuralgia.

CONCLUSIONS

Neurosurgeons are frequently called upon to diagnose and treat facial pain. Although surgical options for specific facial pain syndromes are quite attractive, it is crucial that neurosurgeons be familiar with the myriad facial pain syndromes that do not respond to surgery. Moreover, it is important to arrive at a rational treatment regimen that addresses not only the cause of pain, but the character of the pain as well. A better appreciation of the neuroanatomical and chemical changes that occur in chronic pain has allowed us to rationalize our medical treatment of different pain syndromes. As our understanding of the pathophysiology of facial pain improves, so will our ability to hone our treatment, both medical and surgical.

REFERENCES

1. Bergouignan M: Cures hereuses de neuralgie faciales essentielles par le diphenylhydantoinate de soude. **Rev Laryngol Otol Rhinol** 63:34–41, 1942.
2. Blom S: Tic doulourex treated with a new anticonvulsant. **Arch Neurol** 9:285–290, 1962.
3. Bodnar RJ, Nicotera N: Neuroleptic and analgesic interactions upon pain and activity measures. **Pharmacol Biochem Behav** 16:411–416, 1982.
4. Donnadieu S, Nguyen S, Bertrand J, Dru M, Laccourreye O, Laccourreye H: Evaluation and treatment of chronic pain after cervicofacial cancer surgery. **Ann Oto-Laryng Chir Cervico-Faciale** 109:211–214, 1992.
5. Epstein JB, Marcoe JH: Topical application of capsaicin for treatment of oral neuropathic pain and trigeminal neuralgia. **Oral Surg Oral Med Oral Pathol** 77:135–140, 1994.
6. Fromm GH, Sessle BJ: Trigeminal Neuralgia: *Current Concepts Regarding Pathogenesis and Treatment* Boston, Butterworth-Heinemann, 1991.
7. Hersh EV, Pertes RA, Ochs HA: Topical capsaicin-pharmacology and potential role in the treatment of temporomandibular pain. **J Clin Dentistry** 5:54–59, 1994.
8. Hurtig HI: Fluphenazine and postherapetic neuralgia. **JAMA** 263:2750, 1990.
9. Jacox AK, Carr DB, Payne R: Agency for Health Care Policy and Research. Management of cancer pain. Clinical practice guideline no. 9. 1994 1994. Report No.: AHCPR publication no. 94-0592.
10. Karavelis A, Foroglou G, Selviaridis P, Fountzilas G: Intraventricular administration of morphine for control of intractable cancer pain in 90 patients. **Neurosurgery** 39:57–61, 1996.
11. Lincoff NS, Rath PP, Hirano M: The treatment of periocular and facial pain with topical capsaicin. **Neuro-Ophthalmol** 18:17–20, 1998.
12. Lindstrom P, Lindblom U: The analgesic effect of tocainide in trigeminal neuralgia. **Pain** 28:45–50, 1987.
13. Merskey H: Pharmacological approaches other than opioids in chronic non-cancer pain management. **Acta Anaesth Scand** 41:187–190, 1997.
14. Milligan NS, Nash TP: Treatment of post-herpetic neuralgia. A review of 77 consecutive cases. **Pain** 23:381–386, 1985.
15. Monks R: Psychotropic drugs, in: Bonica J, Loeser JD, Chapman CR, Fordyce WE (eds). *The Management of Pain,* 2nd ed, Vol. 2, Philadelphia, Lea & Febiger, 1990, pp. 1676–1689.
16. Penman J: Trigeminal neuralgia, in Vinken PJ, Bruyn GW (eds), *Handbook of Clinical Neurology.* Amsterdam, Elsevier Science, 1968, pp. 296–325.
17. Richelson E, Nelson A: Antagonism by antidepressants of neurotransmitter receptors of normal human brain in vitro. **J Pharmacol Exp Therap** 230:94–102, 1984.
18. Spaziante R, Cappabianca P, Saini M, de Divitiis E: Topical opthalmic treatment for trigeminal neuralgia. **J Neurosurg** 82:993–997, 1995.
19. Terrence CF, Sax M, Fromm GH, Chang CH, Yoo CS: Effect of baclofen enantiomorphs on the spinal trigeminal nucleus and steric similarities of carbamazepine. **Pharmacology** 27:85–94, 1983.
20. Troussea A. De la neuralgie epileptiforme. **Arch Gen Med** 1:33–44, 1853.
21. World Health Organization: Cancer pain relief and palliative care. 1990. Report No.: 804.
22. Yoshimasu F, Kurland LT, Elveback LR: Tic douloureux in Rochester, Minnesota, 1945–1969. **Neurology.** 22:952–956, 1972.
23. Zakrzewska JM: *Trigeminal Neuralgia.* Vol. 28, London, W. B. Saunders, 1995. in Warlow CP, van Gijn (eds), *Major Problems in Neurology.*

CHAPTER

32

Percutaneous Treatment of Trigeminal Neuralgia: Advances and Problems

JEFFREY A. BROWN, M.D.

ETIOLOGY

Love et al. (18) studied biopsy fragments of trigeminal roots at the time of microvascular decompression (MVD). For a number of years Sweet has urged neurosurgeons to do just that. Their examination revealed a zone of chronic demyelination in the proximal (centrally myelinated) part of the root, near its junction with peripheral nerve. The zone of demyelination contained closely packed axons. There was no intervening glial cytoplasm. Also present were small numbers of thinly myelinated axons. In some cases a single thin myelin sheath encircled several adjacent axons that were still in close apposition (18). These data are the most convincing available that trigeminal neuralgia is a consequence of proximal demyelination. Yet, when closely evaluated over several years, patients with detectable sensory loss after MVD did just as well as patients without sensory injury, indicating that root injury is not the cause of pain relief after MVD (2). What, then, is the status of percutaneous techniques for the treatment of classic trigeminal neuralgia?

THERMAL RHIZOTOMY

The most comprehensive recent review of thermal rhizotomy was a study of the treatment of 500 patients with trigeminal neuralgia who underwent radiofrequency rhizotomy at the University of Cincinnati Medical Center between 1981 and 1986. Their results are compared with literature reports of 6205 patients who underwent radiofrequency rhizotomy, 1217 patients who had glycerol rhizotomy, 759 patients who had balloon compression, 1417 patients with MVD, and 250 patients who underwent partial trigeminal rhizotomy. MVD had the lowest rate of technical success. RF rhizotomy and MVD had the highest rates of initial pain relief and the lowest rates of pain recurrence. Glycerol rhizotomy had the highest rate of pain recurrence. Balloon compression had the highest rate of trigeminal motor dysfunction. Balloon compression and MVD had the lowest rates of corneal anesthesia or keratitis. MVD had the lowest rates of facial numbness and dysesthesia. The incidence of dysesthetic pain was similar in ablative procedures. Permanent cranial nerve deficit (other than Vth) occurred most commonly after intracranial surgery, which also had the highest rates of intracranial hemorrhage, infarction, and other perioperative morbidity and mortality. The authors concluded that thermal rhizotomy is the procedure of choice for most patients undergoing first surgical treatments, and they recommended MVD for healthy patients who have isolated pain in the ophthalmic trigeminal division or in all three trigeminal divisions and for patients who do not wish to have a sensory deficit (25).

Taha et al. (26) also reviewed Tew's results in 154 consecutive patients with trigeminal neuralgia treated by thermal rhizotomy and prospectively followed the group for 15 years. Ninety-nine percent of the patients obtained initial pain relief after one procedure. Dysesthesia occurred in 23%: in 7% with mild initial hypalgesia; in 15% with dense hypalgesia; and in 36% with analgesia. Dysesthesia was mild and did not require treatment in most patients. The corneal reflex was absent or depressed in 18% of patients, and keratitis developed in three patients. In 14% of patients there was trigeminal motor weakness; the paresis resolved within 1 year in 86% of these patients. The authors estimated using Kaplan-Meier analysis that the 14-year recurrence rate was 25% in the total group, 60% in patients with mild hypalgesia, 25% in those with dense hypalgesia, and 20% in those with analgesia. Timing of pain recurrence varied according to the degree of sensory loss. All pain recurrences in patients with mild hypalgesia occurred within 4 years after surgery; 10% more of patients with dense hypalgesia had pain recurrences within the first 10 years compared with patients with analgesia. The median pain-free survival rate was 32 months for patients with mild hypalgesia and more than 15 years for patients with either analgesia or dense hypalgesia. Of the 100 patients followed for 15 years after one or two procedures, 95% rated the procedure excellent or good. The authors concluded that dense hypalgesia in the painful trigger zone, rather than analgesia, should be the goal in thermal rhizotomy (25–26).

A number of extensive series have recently been published that retrospectively analyze the results of various treatment methods. A large Korean study concluded that thermal rhizotomy had a lower dysesthesia rate than glycerol rhyzolysis and recommended it as the treatment of choice, but the study did not use other percutaneous approaches. The investigators analyzed 417 patients with trigeminal neuralgia who underwent MVD (n = 146), thermal rhizotomy (n = 235), or glycerol rhizotomy (n = 36) over a 25-year period. MVD and thermal rhizotomy had the highest rates of initial pain relief (glycerol rhizotomy had only an 82% initial success compared with 97% for MVD and 93% for thermal rhizotomy). Thermal rhizotomy had a 5.1% and glycerol a 3.3% incidence of facial dysesthesia. MVD had the lowest incidence (0.3%) (16).

At the University of Genoa in Italy, a method for performing trigeminal thermorhizotomy, guided by trigeminal nerve-evoked potentials (TNEPs), was used in 30 patients. TNEPS are produced by stimulation of the supraorbital, infraorbital, and mental nerves and are recorded from electrodes at both the scalp and trigeminal nerve. A cannula is modified to produce a concentric bipolar electrode that is suitable for both recording and lesion making. Baseline scalp TNEPs are first obtained from the derivation of the cervical vertex to C-7 to ensure that all stimulating electrodes are correctly placed. TNEPs from the trigeminal electrode after stimulation of the peripheral nerve trunks are obtained to ascertain the electrode's position relative to the root bundles. The trigeminal electrode position is ascertained by recording the root activity evoked by stimulation of cutaneous trigger points or of the most painful areas. The position relative to the motor root is learned by stimulating the nerve through the electrode and observing the masseter muscle responses. TNEPs are evaluated before and after each lesion. Thermal lesions are made until the scalp-recorded wave W2 decreases its amplitude by 20 to 50% of the original value or until it is delayed by 0.30 ms. The authors believe that the procedure has the potential for precise monitoring of both the position of the trigeminal electrode within the nerve and the extent of the lesion (14).

BALLOON COMPRESSION

New Zealand white rabbits were used to determine whether changes in the Vth cranial nerve sensory root after compression were associated with loss of a specific subclass of Vth cranial nerve ganglion cells, the disappearance of a distinct subset of primary afferent terminals in Vth cranial nerve nucleus caudalis, and/or injury to a specific axonal fiber type. There was no significant difference in the size of surviving ganglion cells after Vth cranial nerve compression, as measured 2 to 3 months after injury ($P > 0.5$, n = 4). Densitometric analysis of the nerves of rabbits that survived more than 2 months after compression showed no significant difference in the immunoreactivity of substance P and calcitonin gene-reactive protein between compressed and control sides ($P > 0.1$, n = 4). Fink-Heimer staining of the Vth cranial nerve subnucleus caudalis showed that transganglionic degeneration was most dense in the deeper layers, which are the sites of termination of large myelinated fibers. Ultrastructural evaluation of the type of myelinated axons injured by Vth cranial nerve compression in rabbits killed 7, 14, 37, and 270 days after injury was studied, and morphometric analysis was performed. The frequency distribution of axon diameters was significantly different for injured and control areas. The injured areas had higher ratios of small-diameter (<3 μ) to large-diameter axons compared with the control distribution. Balloon compression thus causes loss of fibers from the Vth cranial nerve sensory root and extensive transganglionic degeneration in the Vth cranial nerve brainstem complex. Cell size measurements and immunocytochemical data suggest that there is no specific loss of small ganglion cells or fine-caliber primary afferents. These experiments suggest that balloon compression relieves trigeminal pain by injuring the myelinated axons involved in the sensory trigger to the pain (4).

An interesting related study of remyelination of demyelinated CNS axons was done at Yale University. The authors examined the issue of restoration by cell transplantation of the conduction properties of demyelinated axons in the adult CNS. The dorsal columns of the adult rat spinal cord were demyelinated by x-irradiation and intraspinal injections of ethidium bromide. Cell suspensions of cultured astrocytes and Schwann cells derived from neonatal rats transfected with the (beta-galactosidase) reporter gene were injected into the glial-free lesion site. After 3 to 4 weeks the investigators found that nearly all of the demyelinated axons were remyelinated by the transplanted Schwann cells. The dorsal columns were removed and maintained in an in vitro recording chamber. Axons remyelinated by transplantation of cultured Schwann cells exhibited restoration of conduction through the lesion, with reestablishment of normal conduction velocity. The axons remyelinated after transplantation showed enhanced impulse recovery to paired-pulse stimulation and greater frequency-following capability as compared with both demyelinated and control axons. Functional repair of demyelinated axons in the adult CNS by transplantation of cultured myelin-forming cells from the peripheral nervous system in combination with astrocytes is thus possible. This study is of interest for the potential treatment of trigeminal root injury by ablative techniques such as balloon compression or glycerol rhyzolysis when demyelination has occurred (8).

In San Sebastian, Spain, the macroscopic changes that take place on the gasserian ganglion and the surrounding structures were studied on 20 trigeminal nerves of 10 fresh adult cadavers. There was compression on the ganglion and on the trigeminal nerve, and there were changes in the position of the trigeminal root, with shortening of its cisternal segment. When the balloon was inflated to capacity (0.75–1.0 ml), dural stretching in an area of 15 x 10 mm took place. This stretching of the dura extended from the lateral wall of the cavernous sinus to the level of the porus trigemini. The authors never found a rupture or tear on the dura or the trigeminal nerve fibers. When a pear shape is not obtained and the nerve is not compressed, it is because the balloon is positioned lateral to the porous trigeminous beneath the temporal lobe rather than because of a dural rupture (28).

One hundred and eighty three patients with classic symptoms of unilateral trigeminal neuralgia underwent 236 percutaneous compressions between 1983 and 1987 at The Medical College of Ohio. The patients' mean age was 64 years (range, 27–95 years). First division pain was present in 37%; 30% had had previous destructive procedure and 7% had multiple sclerosis. None of the patients had an associated tumor. All were treated initially with carbamazepine, and some with dilantin, baclofen, or gabapentin. The indications for surgery were similar to those for other percutaneous procedures for the treatment of trigeminal neuralgia.

The mean follow-up period was 55 months (range, 2–156 months); 93% were initially relieved of their pain, and 61% had detectable numbness postoperatively. This was mild in 80%, moderate in 14%, and severe in 6% (data are available only for the first 142 patients). Nineteen percent had minor ipsilateral masseter weakness that resolved in one year or less. Anesthesia dolorosa did not occur in any patient, and the corneal reflex was lost in only one patient.

The overall recurrence rate was 25%. Sixty eight percent of patients with a recurrence had a repeat balloon compression, which provided relief in 68% of the total. Thirty-seven percent of patients had involvement of the first division either alone or in combination with other sensory divisions. Pain relief without recurrence was achieved in 69% of these patients. This rate was higher than the success rate (62%) without first division pain after first balloon compression (3).

At The University of Algiers in Algeria, 150 patients with trigeminal neuralgia were treated by balloon compression during the past 8 years. The technique used is the original one described by Mullan wherein the balloon is inflated for 6 minutes with 0.7 ml of contrast medium. Over a follow-up period ranging from 6 months to 8 years with an average of 4 years, 69% remained pain-free. Postoperative complications included dysesthesias in 11%, hypesthesia in 93%, hypo-acousia and otalgia in 1%, and masticatory weakness in 1%. The recurrence rate was 30%. According to the authors, the main advantages of the procedure are a low incidence of severe dysesthesias, rare corneal complications, and a short hospital stay. They see the use of a general anesthetic as a disadvantage (1).

Percutaneous compression of the trigeminal ganglion for trigeminal neuralgia was performed over 5 years in Marseille in 70 patients. Ninety-eight percent of the patients were initially relieved of their pain. There were 14 recurrences (21%); 9 of these 14 patients underwent a second compression with 8 having excellent results. The follow-up examination at a mean of 1.25 years showed that 89% of patients were free of pain. There was hypesthesia in 14%; loss of the corneal reflex without keratitis in 11%; and dysesthesias without anesthesia dolorosa in 11%. The authors believe that this technique should be the first operation considered for trigeminal neuralgia for aged and for poorly cooperative patients, especially when V1 or V1-V2 pain is present, for symptomatic neuralgia (especially multiple sclerosis), or after recurrences after other procedures (22).

GLYCEROL RHYZOLYSIS

A series of 191 patients treated at The University of Naples in Italy between 1983 and 1990 using glycerol rhyzolysis was recently published. Technical failures occurred in 6% of the patients because of failure to penetrate the foramen ovale. In an additional 9% of patients, cerebrospinal fluid could not be obtained from the trigeminal cistern. Complete relief of pain was achieved in 93% of patients; in 65% pain relief was immediate; in 28% relief occurred within 1 week; and the operation was unsuccessful in 7%. There was no postoperative sensory loss in 17% of patients. Mild hypesthesia was present in 46%; the sensory loss was confined to the affected divisions in 24% and extended beyond the involved divisions in 23%. Moderate hypesthesia occurred in 32% of patients; this was restricted to the target divisions in 19% and exceeded them in 14%. Anesthesia dolorosa did not occur. Complications were as follows: herpetic eruptions in 33% of patients; minor dysesthesia in 18%; impairment of the corneal reflex in 10%, the first branch being the target of the treatment in 58% of these patients; 6% masseter/pterygoid weakness; and aseptic meningitis in 1%. Follow-up ranged from 1 to 7 years. A recurrence was observed 23% of patients. In 8% a partial relapse occurred, which was well controlled by drug therapy; in 15% another ablative procedures was required. The mean time until recurrence was 31 months. The overall recurrence rate in the series at the end of the follow-up period was 23% (6).

Kumar et al. (12), in New Delhi, prospectively investigated the blink reflex in 28 patients before and after glycerol rhizolysis. In 54% of the patients, there were varying degrees of sensory loss in the trigeminal nerve distribution before glycerol injection was done. After glycerol injection 18 patients had graded sensory loss. Before glycerol the blink reflex showed abnormal R1 wave in 57% patients, whereas direct and consensual R2 waves were abnormal in 43 and 48%, respectively. Postinjection R1 wave was abnormal in 64% patients, direct R2 waves were abnormal in 33% patients. Thus, clinical findings of sensory loss correlated well with pre- and postinjection blink reflex abnormality. Postoperatively R1 latencies deteriorated in 7% of patients and consensual R2 latency improved in 10%, suggesting improved function on the contralateral side after relief of pain by glycerol rhizotomy (12).

RADIOSURGERY

A laboratory study of the resistance of cranial nerves to radiation-induced injury noted that the trigeminal nerve is much more resistant than the optic nerve. No sign of neuropathy was seen in patients for whom the cranial nerves of the cavernous sinus received radiation doses of between 5 and 30 Gy (15).

Young et al. (29) reported their results on treatment by gamma knife radiosurgery of 60 patients with classic trigeminal neuralgia who did not have a response to pharmacological treatment, including 22 who had undergone some form of surgical treatment. A radiosurgical maximum dose of 70 Gy was delivered to the trigeminal nerve root adjacent to the pons through a 4-mm collimator helmet in 51 patients. Stereotactic magnetic resonance imaging localized the root. A third party not involved in the patients' clinical care accomplished follow-up assessment of pain relief. Within a latency period of 1 day to 4 months after treatment, 75% were pain-free. An additional 14% experienced reduced pain from 50 to 90%. At a mean of 16 months (range, 6–36 months) after treatment, 80% remained pain-free or had marked pain reduction. All 26 patients with classic symptoms of trigeminal neuralgia with no atypical features who had no prior surgery had complete or nearly complete pain relief, and none of these patients had recurrent pain. Nine patients with trigeminal neuralgia from tumors received standard radiosurgical treatment directed at their tumors, and 89% had pain relief. Of the total of 60 patients treated for trigeminal neuralgia, 82% had complete or nearly complete relief of pain at last follow-up. Only one patient with preexisting facial sensory loss due to a tumor had a mild increase in facial numbness. No other patient experienced either loss of facial sensation or any other complication (29). At The University of Pittsburgh 51 patients who had typical trigeminal neuralgia were treated by gamma knife. In all cases, a 4-mm isocenter was targeted at the proximal nerve at the root entry zone. The target dose varied from 60 to 90 Gy. Eighty-six percent of the patients had undergone prior surgery. The mean follow-up after radiosurgery was 10 months (range, 2–29 months). The initial response rate was 86%. At the last follow-up, 37% had excellent control (pain-free), 41% had good control (50–90% relief), and 21% did not respond to treatment. No patient developed further sensory loss or deafferentation pain. A maximum radiosurgery dose more than or equal to 70 Gy was associated with a significantly greater chance for complete pain relief (10).

A multi-institutional study was conducted that reviewed 55 patients at five centers; 32 patients had undergone prior surgery. The mean number of procedures that had been performed was 3 (range, 1–7). The target dose of the radiosurgery used in the current study varied from 60 to 90 Gy. The median follow-up period after radiosurgery was 18 months (range, 11–36 months). Fifty-eight percent of the patients were pain-free postoperatively, 36% had 50–90% pain relief, and 6% failed to benefit. The median time to pain relief was 1 month (range, 1 day-7 months). Recurrence occurred in 6% (at 5, 7, and 10 months). At 2 years 54% of the patients were pain-free, and 88% had 50 to 100% relief. A maximum radiosurgical dose of 70 Gy or greater was associated with a significantly greater chance of complete pain relief (72% versus 9%, $P = 0.0003$). Six percent of the patients developed increased facial paresthesia after radiosurgery, which resolved totally in one case and improved in another. No patient developed other deficits or deafferentation pain. The proximal trigeminal nerve and root entry zone, which is well defined on magnetic resonance imaging, is thought to be the appropriate target for radiosurgery (11).

MEDICAL TREATMENT

The Oxford Pain Relief Unit designed a study to determine effectiveness and adverse effects of anticonvulsant drugs in pain management. They performed a systematic review of randomized controlled trials of anticonvulsants for acute, chronic, or cancer pain identified through Medline, hand searching, searching reference lists, and contacting investigators. Twenty reports, of four anticonvulsants, were eligible. The only placebo-controlled study in acute pain found no analgesic effect of sodium valproate. Anticonvulsants were found to be effective for trigeminal neuralgia, diabetic neuropathy, and for migraine prophylaxis. Minor adverse effects occurred as often as benefit (20). Delcker et al. (7) studied the side effects of carbamazepine when initiated (7). Many patients recently have been treated with gabapentin before being referred for surgical intervention, but there are no controlled studies showing its effectiveness. Indeed the only study available is a report of two cases using gabapentin for idiopathic trigeminal neuralgia (24).

Lamotrigine was used in a double-blind placebo controlled crossover trial in 14 patients with refractory trigeminal neuralgia. Patients continued to take a steady dose of carbamazepine or phenytoin throughout the trial over a 31-day period. Each arm of the trial lasted 2 weeks, with an intervening 3-day washout period. The maintenance dose of lamotrigine was 400 mg. Lamotrigine was superior to placebo ($P = 0.011$), based on analysis of a composite efficacy index that compared the numbers of patients assigned to greater efficacy on lamotrigine with those assigned greater efficacy on placebo. Efficacy for one treatment over another was determined according to a hierarchy of: 1) use of escape medication, 2) total pain scores, or 3) global evaluations. Eleven of the 13 patients eligible for inclusion in the composite efficacy index showed better efficacy on lamotrigine compared with placebo. Global evaluations further suggested that patients did better on lamotrigine than placebo ($P = 0.025$). The adverse reactions with both lamotrigine and placebo were predominantly dose-dependent effects on the central nervous system. A 14th patient withdrew from the study because of severe pain during the placebo arm of the trial. Lamotrigine seems to have antineuralgic properties (20). At The University of Genoa another study on this drug in 15 patients was performed. Patients with trigeminal neuralgia secondary to multiple sclerosis were included. They detected pain relief proportional to daily dosage and to drug plasma levels. Eleven of the patients affected by the "essential" form of neuralgia showed complete pain relief on reaching their maximum daily dosage. All patients affected by the symptomatic form had complete relief at the end of the follow-up period 3 to 8 months after the end of the study (19).

TRIGEMINAL NEUROPATHY

Twenty patients with deafferentation pain were treated by chronic stimulation of the motor cortex by Nguyen et al. (21) in France. The central fissure was localized using stereotactic magnetic resonance imaging. The motor cortex was mapped using intra-operative somatosensory-evoked potentials. Seven patients with trigeminal neuropathic pain had pain relief varying between 40 and 100%. Ten patients had central pain from central nervous system lesions. Long-lasting pain control (pain relief > 40%) was obtained in half of the patients. One patient with pain from peripheral nerve injury obtained more than 80% pain relief. Two patients had pain from spinal cord lesions. One did not respond to treatment, but the other obtained an excellent long-term result. The location of the effective stimulation plots corresponded with the somatotopic maps of the primary motor cortex. One patient developed a small extradural hematoma, which resolved spontaneously. None of the patients developed seizure activity. This study confirms the potential value of motor cortex stimulation for treating certain forms of intractable pain, especially patients with trigeminal neuropathic pain (21). Sixty-eight patients with chronic pain syndromes who underwent deep brain stimulation (DBS) were prospectively studied over 15 years. Electrodes for DBS were implanted within the periventricular gray matter, specific sensory thalamic nuclei, or the internal capsule. Each patient was followed on a 6-month basis and evaluated with a modified visual analog scale. Follow-up periods ranged from 6 months to 15 years, with a mean follow-up of 6 years. The mean age of the 54 men and 14 women in the study was 51.3 years. Indications for DBS included 43 patients with failed back syndrome, 6 with peripheral neuropathy or radiculopathy, 5 with thalamic pain, 4 with trigeminal neuropathy, 3 with traumatic spinal cord lesions, 2 with causalgia, 1 with phantom limb pain, and 1 with carcinoma pain. Effective pain control was achieved in 62% of patients. Patients with failed back syndrome, trigeminal neuropathy, and peripheral neuropathy fared well with DBS, whereas those with thalamic pain, spinal cord injury, and postherpetic neuralgia did not (13).

At The University of Toronto, Ontario, Canada, Taub et al. (27) used an implanted system for chronic electrical stimulation of the gasserian ganglion in 34 patients for relief of chronic medically intractable facial pain. The pathogenesis of the pain was peripheral damage to the trigeminal nerve in 22 (65%), central (stroke) damage in 7 (21%), postherpetic neuralgia in 4 (12%), and unclassifiable cause in 1 (3%). All patients received a trial of transcutaneous stimulation (Stage 1). Successful trials in 56% were followed by implantation of a permanent system (Stage 2). Trial and postimplantation stimulation were deemed successful when there was a reduction of pain by at least 50% whenever the stimulator was on. Success rates varied from 71% for central pain to 23% for peripheral pain and none for postherpetic neuralgia. The median follow-up duration in successful cases was 22.5 months. Infections occurred in seven patients, all of whom had undergone permanent implantation. Infections were more frequent when the stimulating electrode from Stage 1 was left in place for Stage 2 (6 [43%] of 14) than when completely new hardware was used and prophylactic antibiotic drugs were administered (1 [20%] of 5). Other complications included iatrogenic injury to the trigeminal nerve or ganglion in 9%, transient diplopia in 6%, increased pain in 6%, and various technical problems in 29%. Taub et al. (27) concluded that pain of central origin (stroke) is the type most likely to be relieved by this procedure. The risk of infection seems to be lower when completely new hardware is used for Stage 2 and prophylactic antibiotic drugs are administered.

Lee et al. (16) compared the effect of high thoracic epidural block with that of stellate ganglion block to relieve moderate-to-severe facial acute herpetic neuralgia. The authors compared the results of treating six patients with stellate ganglion blocks and seven patients using high thoracic epidural blocks. Six milliliters of 1% mepivacaine was given to each patient. Acute herpetic pain was evaluated before and up to 60 minutes after the blocks, using a visual analog scale (VAS) of pain. There was no significant difference in VAS pain scores between the groups before, or after, the blocks, but there were significant ($P < 0.05$) decreases in VAS pain scores for both groups between 10 and 60 minutes after the blocks. High thoracic epidural block was as effective as stellate ganglion block in relieving moderate-to-severe acute herpetic pain involving the trigeminal and cervical regions (16).

In a very preliminary case report, two patients with trigeminal and glossopharyngeal neuralgia, respectively, were treated with electrical stimulation of the motor cortex. Alleviation of pain occurred after activation of the flat quadripolar electrode placed epidurally on the precentral cortical area; relief lasted as long as the stimulator was "working." By changing the polarity of the electrodes, it was possible to induce tingling sensations and muscle activation not only contralaterally to the stimulated motor cortex, but also in the ipsilateral part of the face. No stimulator-independent pain reduction resulted from long-term use of the stimulation device. During a follow-up period of 18 months, a sufficient and relatively stable analgesic effect of electrostimulation was observed. One major complication of motor cortex stimulation during the follow-up period was a single generalized epileptic seizure in one patient (23). In a more detailed series, Nguyen et al. (21) treated seven patients with neuropathic facial pain using motor cortex stimulation, which relieved the pain in 40 to 100% of the patients.

PROBLEMS

The fundamental conceptual difficulty with the percutaneous treatment of trigeminal neuralgia is that though it involves a minimal access approach, it remains a destructive treatment. The ideal surgical solution to the pain of tic douloureux is an operation that is minimally invasive, cures all pain, and removes the cause of the disease. Though the percutaneous procedures are minimally invasive, there is an inherent recurrence risk present and the cause of trigeminal neuralgia is not eliminated. This section will discuss several areas in which problems still exist.

Selective Injury

The more difficult case is that with a first division trigger. Fortunately, this is rare, although one-third of patients have a component of pain radiating to the eye or forehead. First division treatment is possible using either glycerol, thermal rhizotomy, or balloon compression. Each technique has technical manipulations directed toward injury of the more superomedial first division fibers. Glycerol must be layered superiorly in the trigeminal cistern to achieve first division selective injury. Lesser volumes will injure the third division or the second and third divisions together. It is not usually possible to selectively injure the second division fibers with glycerol. The third division may be protected, though. Gamma knife injury is not selective of any division, but it does not appear to cause detectable numbness.

The electrode for thermal rhizotomy, if curved, must be angled superiorly and advanced farther than it is for a limited third division lesion. Histological studies of the fibers injured by heating do not show selectivity by fiber type. The neurosurgeon's concern is that excessive heating will injure the corneal reflex. If one uses the more slender cordotomy type electrode needle, it is possible to let the patient remain awake during the final stages of heating. The blink reflex can be repeatedly tested during heating with a light sponge. Should this response diminish, the heating can be stopped. Still, there is much room for experience and judgment. There are no exact rules and no precise temperatures or times that can guide the surgeon.

Similarly, the issues to be solved with glycerol remain. How much glycerol? More than 0.3 ml is discouraged by Linderoth and Hakanson (17) because of the risk of sensory deficit. How long should glycerol remain in contact with the nerve? Usually a 1-hour duration is recommended. Interestingly, these investigators were concerned that contact of short duration with the nerve can cause extensive and less well-controlled injury, whereas Sweet believed that contact with the first division of the nerve for longer than 12 minutes can cause corneal anesthesia. Other issues regarding glycerol include incomplete pain relief and cisternal adhesions that prevent adequate cisternography or third division selectivity. If adhesions prevent complete contrast drainage from the cistern, then the glycerol will not contact the inferior third-division fibers. The fibers will be selectively protected, not injured. The technique for glycerol, like that for others, has inherent subtleties in needle positioning. Fibers more directly in contact with the injected glycerol are injured preferentially. Placement of the needle tip in the superomedial cistern adjacent to first division fibers is suggested in the process of selectively injuring these fibers as well as glycerol layering. Glycerol is a mild demyelinating agent, selective for larger myelinated fibers, similar to the balloon. The hypertonicity of the glycerol is the likely agent of myelin injury (9). It induces a short episode of increased spontaneous axonal firing, a response specific to myelinated fibers (5).

The balloon is selective according to the site of the balloon tip. Fibers that are closer to it are compressed more. By manipulating the catheter tip to the lateral, middle, or medial porous sections, fiber divisions can be selected. The duration and pressure of compression need not vary; this simplifies the issue of judgment but sometimes prolongs the operation because of the need to adjust the angle of catheter entry and site of the catheter tip. Facial soft tissue anatomy varies, making entry site selection between 2 and 3 centimeters lateral to the edge of the lip, and at, above, or below the horizontal point from the edge of the lip, variable and subject to the surgeon's judgment. Because the balloon selectively preserves the small myelinated and unmyelinated fibers that mediate the corneal reflex, however, it may make treatment of first division pain safer—especially for neurosurgeons without lengthy experience in thermal rhizotomy.

Communication with older patients who are emerging from fast-acting barbiturates makes the decision to continue with heating often a difficult one. The advantage of allowing the patient to remain awake to assist in the evaluation of lesion density and location is not always evident. Success depends on the neurosurgeon's or anesthetist's expertise in the pharmacology of sedation. Airway protection may be an issue during the deeper moments of sedation.

Selective fiber injury is thus a function of the expertise and experience of the neurosurgeon performing the procedure. Third division selectivity is easiest in thermal rhizotomy and more difficult with glycerol injection. First division selection is more difficult with both glycerol injection and thermal rhizotomy, but is perhaps safer with balloon compression.

Multiple Division Pain

There are technical difficulties in treating multidivisional pain using each of the percutaneous options. This can prolong the operating time for selective thermal rhizotomy. Balloon compression can create a more diffuse injury with a single compression. It may be easier to perform balloon compression in such a situation than thermal rhizotomy. Glycerol can also injure multiple divisions by varying the volume instilled.

Anesthetic

In the traditional approach to thermal rhizotomy, it is the neurosurgeon who is responsible for directing the level of anesthetic sedation. Balloon compression differs in that it is the anesthesiologist who shares this responsibility. The problem for the neurosurgeon is that there is little opportunity to obtain the experience and judgment required to learn this "anesthetic" technique. Most studies evaluating the treatment outcome have used intravenous methohexital for sedation because it is rapidly metabolized and repeated infusions are easier without dose accumulation. Difficulty occurs when communication with the patient is unclear and lesion location/size cannot be accurately surmised.

The challenge in the neurosurgical treatment of facial pain is to develop a standardized anethesiology technique that maximizes pain control and minimizes cognitive effect after patients awaken. Most anesthesiologists are familiar with the use of propofol for short-acting anesthesia but not methohexitol. Future treatment regimens probably will move toward the effective use of intravenous propofol, and neurosurgeons must develop familiarity with it.

Anesthesia Dolorosa

Anesthesia dolorosa is the greatest challenge to ablative treatment of trigeminal pain. The overriding intent is to mimimize injury to the trigeminal nerve while maximizing pain relief. The objective is to perform selective divisional injury when possible with a goal of hypesthesia. Sometimes patients find the resultant degree of sensory loss bothersome. In most series this occurs less than 5% of the time, but treatment for it remains a problem.

Anesthesia dolorosa is a descriptive term for the extreme degree of neuropathic pain. Neuropathic pain comes from functional abnormality of the nervous system that leads to ongoing pain without an active tissue-damaging process to explain it. The experiential component to this definition is dysesthesia and hyperpathia. The odd feelings experienced are described as sensations of intermittent "worm crawling," constant burning, and hypersensitivity. The McGill pain questionnaire summarizes and categorizes these descriptions very well, is a helpful adjunct to the evaluation of difficult-to-describe pain syndromes, and provides a means of quantification and evaluation of treatment alternatives.

Neuropathic pain is often treated medically with amitriptyline and other antidepressants. Surgical treatment is problematic after the extent of injury becomes an issue. Deep brain stimulation has been used primarily in Canadian centers. Its effectiveness is limited and potential morbidity is significant. Recent experience with motor cortex stimulation by Nguyen et al. (21) suggested an effective surgical therapy with less invasiveness and consequent morbidity. An inhibitory motor pathway to the sensory system is the suggested mechanism for the effective relief of neuropathic pain (21).

NEUROPATHIC PAIN

The diagnosis of classic trigeminal neuralgia can be made in the "blink of an eye." For example, a 65-year-old female patient describes intermittent electric shock pains in the jaw and cheek triggered by light touch to her face, a cool breeze, chewing, or speaking. When the description becomes longer or more complex, the diagnosis may be less certain. There may be a greater component of neuropathic pain than simple tic douloureux. The treatment of such syndromes then becomes more complicated. Frequently there may be elements of both lancinating pain and neuropathic pain that must be addressed separately. Percutaneous treatment of tic douloureux can address only the lancinating component of the pain. It is possible that the neuropathic pain will resolve secondarily, but this issue has not been completely examined in research studies and reviews of treatment outcome. If severe, the neuropathic pain may be aggravated by percutaneous injury.

The term atypical facial pain is better thought of as a miscellaneous category for pain that is not well described or understood. The more severe descriptions of neuropathic pain have greater emotional components. Atypical facial pain is likely descriptive of the more severe secondary emotional elements of neuropathic pain that emerge after facial pain becomes chronic. It is best that the term be retired from use.

A number of advanced ablative techniques are available but are not well known or often practiced for the treatment of these patients. These techniques include medial thalamotomy, either radiosurgically or by stereotactic radiofrequency lesioning, and cingulotomy. The effectiveness of such therapy is usually 50% or less by whatever criteria are used to define outcome.

MEDICAL ISSUES

Anticoagulation

Patients with trigeminal neuralgia compose an aged population with medical elements to their health care. They may require anticoagulation for atrial fibrillation, coronary artery disease, or stroke prevention. The risk of discontinuing warfarin anticoagulation must be carefully assessed. There is a low risk of hemorrhage from these percutaneous procedures. The length of time that reversal is allowed and the risk of reversal are variable and best reviewed in conjunction with a cardiologist and hematologist. Patients with a high risk of stroke may not tolerate reversal for long, or heparin infusion must be initiated very soon after the procedure has been completed, usually by the next day.

Mass Lesions

Trigeminal neuralgia is rare but definitely caused by compressive masses. The decision to treat the tic pain is distinct from the decision to excise the mass inasmuch as decompression or percutaneous injury are both effective. Gamma knife treatment of a compressive lesion may alleviate tic pain without injuring the nerve.

Carotid Artery Puncture

Carotid puncture is a known complication of thermal rhizotomy that is performed with a sharp #22-gauge spinal needle. The hemorrhagic complications that have occurred during balloon compression when a sharp #14-gauge cannula was used have not been repeated after the instrumentation was redesigned to include only a blunt cannula. These complications are clearly a consequence of using sharp instrumentation and should be reducible by limiting the intracranial use of such instruments.

The central problem for percutaneous treatment of trigeminal neuralgia is for neurosurgeons to develop a technique for creating standardized, reproducible, selective injury to the trigeminal system. Selective injury would limit bothersome numbness yet cure the terrible pain of this peculiar disease, which has eluded our mastery across generations of careful attention from physicians since it was first described in the clear words of John Locke 300 years ago.

REFERENCES

1. Abdennebi B, Mahfouf L, Nedjahi T: Long-term results of percutaneous compression of the gasserian ganglion in trigeminal neuralgia. (Series of 200 patients). **Stereotact Funct Neurosurg** 68:190–195, 1997.
2. Bergenheim AT, Shamsgovara P, Ridderheim PA: Microvascular decompression for trigeminal neuralgia: No relation between sensory disturbance and outcome. **Stereotact Funct Neurosurg** 68:200–206, 1997.
3. Brown JA, Gouda JJ, Sangvai DG: Percutaneous balloon compression for trigeminal neuralgia: Results in 183 consecutive patients. **J Neurosurg** 88:417A, 1998 (abstr).
4. Brown JA, Hoeflinger B, Long PB, et al: Axon and ganglion cell injury in rabbits after percutaneous trigeminal balloon compression. **Neurosurgery** 38:993–1003, 1996.

5. Burchiel KJ, Russell LC: Blycerol neurolysis: Neurophysiological effects of topical glycerol application on rat saphenous nerve. **J Neurosurg** 63:784–788, 1985.
6. Cappabianca P, Spaziante R, Graziussi G, Taglialatela G, Peca C, De Divitiis E: Percutaneous retrogasserian glycerol rhizolysis for treatment of trigeminal neuralgia. Technique and results in 191 patients. **J Neurosurg Sci** 39:37–45, 1995.
7. Delcker A, Wilhelm H, Timmann D, Diener HC: Side effects from increased doses of carbamazepine on neuropsychological and posturographic parameters of humans. **Eur Neuropsychopharmacol** 7:213–218, 1997.
8. Honmou O, Felts PA, Waxman SG, Kocsis JD: Restoration of normal conduction properties in demyelinated spinal cord axons in the adult rat by transplantation of exogenous Schwann cells. **J Neurosci** 16:3199–3208, 1996.
9. King JS, Jewett DL, Sundberg HR: Differential blockade of cat dorsal root C-fibers by various chloride solutions. **J Neurosurg** 36:569–585, 1972.
10. Kondziolka D, Flickinger JC, Lunsford LD, Habeck M: Trigeminal neuralgia radiosurgery: The University of Pittsburgh experience. **Stereotact Funct Neurosurg** 66[Suppl 1]:343–348, 1996.
11. Kondziolka D, Lunsford LD, Flickinger JC, et al: Stereotactic radiosurgery for trigeminal neuralgia: A multiinstitutional study using the gamma unit. **J Neurosurg** 84:940–945, 1996.
12. Kumar R, Mahapatra AK, Dash HH: The blink reflex before and after percutaneous glycerol rhizotomy in patients with trigeminal neuralgia—A prospective study of 28 patients. **Acta Neurochir (Wien)** 137:85–88, 1995.
13. Kumar K, Toth C, Nath RK: Deep brain stimulation for intractable pain: A 15-year experience. **Neurosurgery** 40:736–46; 746–7 (discussion), 1997.
14. Leandri M, Gottlieb A: Trigeminal evoked potential-monitored thermorhizotomy: A novel approach for relief of trigeminal pain. **J Neurosurg** 84:929–939, 1996.
15. Leber KA, Berglof J, Pendl G: Dose-response tolerance of the visual pathways and cranial nerves of the cavernous sinus to stereotactic radiosurgery. **J Neurosurg** 88:43–50, 1998.
16. Lee KH, Chang JW, Park YG, Chung SS: Microvascular decompression and percutaneous rhizotomy in trigeminal neuralgia. **Stereotact Funct Neurosurg** 68:196–199, 1997.
17. Linderoth B, Hakanson S: Retrogasserian glycerol rhizolysis in trigeminal neuralgia, in Schmidek HH, Sweet WS (eds): Operative Neurosurgical Techniques: Indications, Methods and Results. Philadelphia, Saunders, 1995, pp 1523–1536.
18. Love S, Hilton DA, Coakham HB: Central demyelination of the Vth nerve root in trigeminal neuralgia associated with vascular compression. **Brain Pathol** 8:1–11; 11–2 (discussion), 1998.
19. Lunardi G, Leandri M, Albano C, et al: Clinical effectiveness of lamotrigine and plasma levels in essential and symptomatic trigeminal neuralgia [see comments]. **Neurology** 48:1714–1717, 1997.
20. McQuay H, Carroll D, Jadad AR, Wiffen P, Moore A: Anticonvulsant drugs for management of pain: A systematic review. **Rev BMJ** 311:1047–1052, 1995.
21. Nguyen JP, Keravel Y, Feve A, et al: Treatment of deafferentation pain by chronic stimulation of the motor cortex: Report of a series of 20 cases. **Acta Neurochir Suppl (Wien)** 68:54–60, 1997.
22. Peragut JC, Gondin-Oliveira J, Fabrizi A, et al: Microcompression of Gasser's ganglion. A treatment of essential facial neuralgia. Apropos of 70 cases. **Neurochirurgie** 37:111–114, 1991.
23. Rainov NG, Fels C, Heidecke V, Burkert W: Epidural electrical stimulation of the mo-

tor cortex in patients with facial neuralgia. **Clin Neurol Neurosurg** 99:205–209, 1997.
24. Sist T, Filadora V, Miner M, Lema M: Gabapentin for idiopathic trigeminal neuralgia: Report of two cases. **Neurology** 48:14–67, 1997.
25. Taha JM, Tew JM Jr: Comparison of surgical treatments for trigeminal neuralgia: Reevaluation of radiofrequency rhizotomy. **Neurosurgery** 38:865–871, 1996.
26. Taha JM, Tew JM Jr, Buncher CR: A prospective 15-year follow up of 154 consecutive patients with trigeminal neuralgia treated by percutaneous stereotactic radiofrequency thermal rhizotomy. **J Neurosurg** 83:989–993, 1995.
27. Taub E, Munz M, Tasker RR: Chronic electrical stimulation of the gasserian ganglion for the relief of pain in a series of 34 patients. **J Neurosurg** 86:197–202, 1997.
28. Urculo E, Martinez L, Arrazola M, Ramirez R: Macroscopic effects of percutaneous trigeminal ganglion compression (Mullan's technique): An anatomic study. **Neurosurgery** 36:776–779, 1995.
29. Young RF, Vermeulen SS, Grimm P, Blasko J, Posewitz A: Gamma knife radiosurgery for treatment of trigeminal neuralgia: Idiopathic and tumor related. **Neurology** 48:608–614, 1997.

CHAPTER

33

Neurovascular Decompression: The Procedure of Choice?

RONALD I. APFELBAUM, M.D.

Trigeminal neuralgia is one of the most painful afflictions known to humanity. Having observed the dreadful suffering its victims experience, it's not surprising that so many physicians have sought to understand the nature of trigeminal neuralgia and devise methods to control the pain. Thus, many diverse techniques have been advocated. Historically, however, effective relief that persisted has been achieved only by destructive lesions placed within the trigeminal system. Such lesions, which usually produce significant sensory loss, can be associated with very bothersome dysesthesia, anesthesia dolorosa, corneal anesthesia, and neuroparalytic keratitis. The latter can result in loss of vision, whereas patients who develop anesthesia dolorosa are in such misery that they are scarcely better than they were with trigeminal neuralgia, and with few treatment options available to them. As Taarnhøj (52) has so eloquently stated:

> Every neurosurgeon with a reasonable amount of experience in treating patients with trigeminal neuralgia by sacrificing the trigeminal nerve fibers has seen the misery that some of these patients are left in after such surgery; it does not help the patient (but it might help the neurosurgeon) to tell the patient that such misery is the price he has to pay. (52)

It is not surprising, therefore, that efforts have been directed toward developing less destructive techniques. Unfortunately, such techniques as Taarnhøj's middle fossa technique (53) and Shelden's compression technique (46), although initially embraced with great enthusiasm by the neurosurgical community, ultimately proved unsatisfactory owing to a high recurrence rate. With this disappointment not too distant in their professional memory, there was great skepticism expressed by most neurosurgeons when Dr. Peter Jannetta (22) proposed his concept of neurovascular compression as the origin of a number of syndromes affecting the lower cranial nerves and manifesting symptoms of hyperactive dysfunction. The most common of these conditions, of course, are trigeminal neuralgia and hemifacial spasm.

This chapter analyzes the basis of Jannetta's concepts, addresses criticisms that have been raised, and reviews the experience that has accumulated in the 30 years since the concept was first espoused. For the technique to be the "procedure of choice," it must be shown to be effective and to offer real advantages over the alternatives.

HISTORICAL PERSPECTIVES

Peter Jannetta was not the first to suggest that neurovascular compression might be the cause of trigeminal neuralgia and hemifacial spasm. In the early years of this century, the overwhelming favorite intracranial surgical procedure of choice for treating trigeminal neuralgia was the middle fossa approach with section of the preganglionic trigeminal rootlets. First advocated by Sir Victor Horsley and colleagues in 1891 (21), with modifications suggested by Hartley (20) in New York and Krause (33) in Germany in1892, it was popularized by Spiller and Frazier's (48) work in Philadelphia starting in 1901. Their initial complete section gave way to partial section as their experience and that of a number of other skilled surgeons, such as Stookey and Ransohoff (49) and Peet and Schneider (44) expanded.

In contradistinction, Walter Dandy (11, 12), at the Johns Hopkins Medical Center, advocated partial sectioning of the trigeminal nerve in the posterior fossa. Working in the days before the employment of the operating microscope, which offers magnified vision and improved illumination, Dandy's technique was considered by most neurosurgeons to be more risky than Frazier's (48). However, Dandy's was able to make unique observations relevant to the posterior fossa anatomy that those who operated by middle fossa approach could not make and that were denied by many until the operating microscope proved him correct. Thus, Dandy (10), in the course of this posterior fossa nerve sections, noted vascular loops impinging on the root entry zone of the trigeminal nerve. He published an illustrations (*Fig. 33.1*) of such a case and stated, "Since the writer has been dividing the sensory root by the cerebellar route, tumors and aneurysms have been found in 10% of the cases, over 500, and in almost every additional case, a large arterial branch of the anterior inferior artery lies upon or under the sensory root. In many instances the nerve is grooved or bent in an angle by the artery. This I believe is the cause of tic douloureux (13).

Dandy, however, appears never to have made the next logical step of proposing or attempting to move the vessel to decompress the nerve.

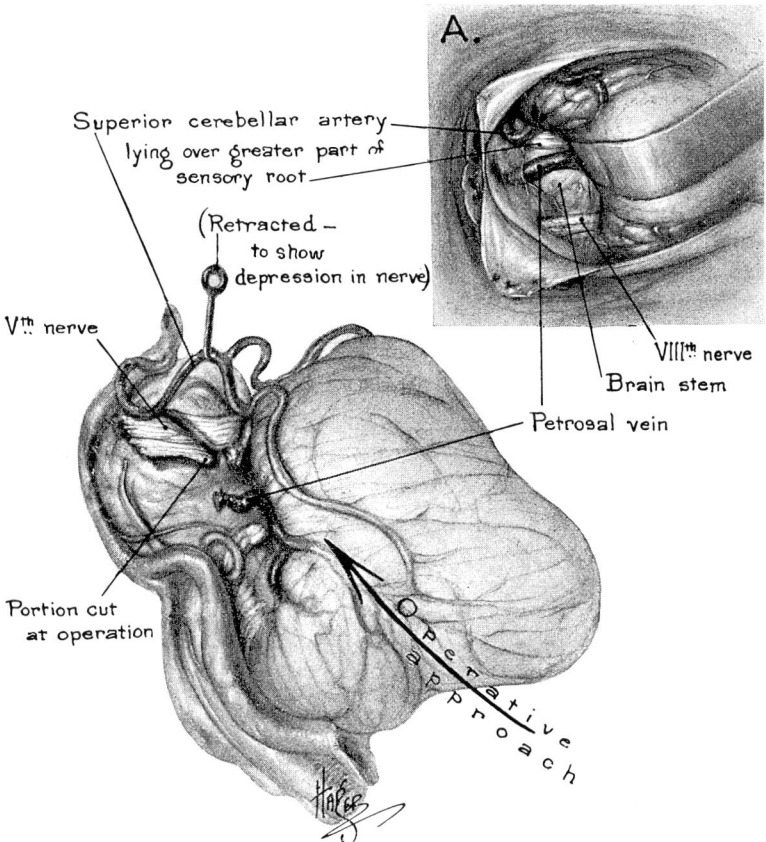

FIG. 33.1 Illustration from Ref. 13 demonstrating vascular compression of the trigeminal nerve adjacent to the brainstem. Although Dandy wrote that this usually was the "anterior inferior" artery, he correctly illustrated it as the superior cerebellar artery. (Reprinted with permission.)

Rather, he continued to sacrifice a portion of the nerve to treat the pain of trigeminal neuralgia.

Vascular impingement on the facial nerve causing hemifacial spasm was reported by Campbell and Keedy in 1974 (9) when they described two cases with aneurysmal compression. Gardner and Sava (17) also suggested a possible vascular origin. They treated hemifacial spasm and reported good success from manipulating the nerve gently in the region of the porus acousticus while forcefully irrigating it with a stream of Ringer's solution. In 7 of 19 patients so treated, a vascular loop compressing the nerve was found. However, the authors were not routinely inspecting the root exit zone of the nerve at the brainstem, rather they were operating at the porus acousticus. Again, no recommendation to decompress the nerve by moving the offending vascular structure and an incomplete understanding of the site of compression characterized these otherwise thoughtful pioneering reports.

It wasn't until Peter Jannetta (22), in 1967, became the first neurosurgeon to apply the surgical operating microscope to the posterior fossa exploration of these nerves that the concept of microvascular decompression began to develop. Jannetta noted the high incidence of vascular loops impinging on the cranial nerves of patients with these syndromes of hyperactive cranial nerve dysfunction and advocated moving these vessels and securing them with a nonabsorbable synthetic plastic sponge prothesis to avoid recompression of the nerve. The concept of microvascular decompression without any intentional trauma or disruption of the nerve was proposed and, indeed, vigorously advocated.

Jannetta reasoned that a group of clinical syndromes seemed to manifest signs of hyperactive dysfunction of a single cranial nerve. All of these syndromes exhibited brief, repetitive, paroxysmal events, the nature of which was determined by the type of cranial nerve involved. In the case of sensory nerves such as the fifth and ninth cranial nerves, patients had paroxysms of very intense electric shock-like pain confined to the distribution of the nerve. That is, they had trigeminal neuralgia or tic douloreux if the fifth nerve was involved and glossopharyngeal neuralgia if the ninth never was involved. In the case of a motor nerve such as the facial or seventh nerve, patients had paroxysms of uncontrolled brief, repetitive, painless twitching of the face; that is, hemifacial spasm. Jannetta has also suggested that a similar situation might effect the eighth nerve and produce Ménière's syndrome and disabling positional vertigo.

Jannetta and colleagues (23–26) published extensively on their experience with microvascular decompression and all of the related syndromes, and they suggested additional areas for further research. Although most neurosurgeons were initially (not inappropriately) skeptical of microvascular decompression, given the past history of nondestructive techniques, the growing experience of many has helped to validate Jannetta's observations and data. Still, some remain unconvinced and have raised a number of arguments that must be addressed.

PATHOPHYSIOLOGY

The pathophysiology of trigeminal neuralgia and hemifacial spasm (i.e., the abnormal or altered physiological events that lead to the clinical manifestations of these syndromes) remains elusive. This has led some to question the whole concept vascular compression. However, certain clues from previous research can be assembled into a plausible theory that fits all known observations.

W. James Gardner (15) devoted much thought to the problem of trigeminal neuralgia and summarized his views in the lead chapter of volume 15 of this publication (16). Gardner noted the following observations, which may be components of a unified theory. He summarized a workshop devoted to anatomical and etiological aspects of trigeminal neuralgia, which was printed as a supplement to the January 1967 issue of the *Journal of Neurosurgery,* as follows: "Demyelination of axons occurs with aging (Kerr [27], Moses [41]) and is more severe in patients with trigeminal neuralgia (Beaver [5], Kerr [29]). In the cat and monkey myelin changes are prominent at the junction of the glial and neurilemmal portions of the root, which suggests increased vulnerability at that point (37). The changes in the axons in trigeminal neuralgia suggest that in addition to aging there may be a compressive factor (28, 29).

The electrical transmission of a nerve impulse at a false synapse (ephapse) has been postulated, but, of course, this is difficult to establish clinically. However, laboratory demonstration of nerve cross-stimulation is well established using divided nerve preparations. This was examined further by Granit and Leksel (18) in 1944, who showed that mildly compressive lesions that did not block nerve conduction could also result in ephaptic conduction (short-circuiting or cross-stimulation). Gardner notes that List and Williams in 1957 (35) "proposed the concept that the paroxysm of tic douloureux represents a pathological, multineuronal reflex in the trigeminal system of the brain stem. The mechanism operates as follows. The tactile or proprioceptive stimulus evokes a pathologically increased delayed response in a hyperritable trigeminal nucleus; from there efferent (antidromic) impulses are conducted back to the periphery where they reverberate and re-excite the central trigeminal connections. This process of self-exciting, repetitive after-discharge, then continues until the firing neurons become refractory. This theory supposes a peripheral reverberating circuit between antidromic and orthodromic impulses together with a hyperirritability of the trigeminal nucleus; it fails to take into account the factor of cross stimulation at the nerve root level." Further observations by Kugelberg and Lindbolm (34) led them to conclude that a simple interaction or short-circuiting between touch and pain fibers could produce the initial jab of pain in trigeminal neuralgia.

Calvin et al. (8) proposed a persuasive neurophysiological theory for the pain mechanism of tic doulourex. The full discussion of this theory is beyond the scope of this chapter, but it is described in detail in chapter 39 of volume 24 of this publication (36). In essence, however, the authors argue that trigeminal neuralgic pain could be explained by combining the dorsal root reflex with impulses "reflected backwards from sites where the duration of the propagating impulse lengthens enough to re-excite a region to the rear where refractoriness is terminating." They noted that "whenever a sudden change occurs along the length of an axon that broadens or delays impulses (axon enlargement or change in myelination) . . . one has the possibility of reflections of the propagated impulse. Besides reflections, demyelinated regions can exhibit postpriming repetitive firing: following a short chain of impulses the site may initiate a train of impulses sometimes lasting several minutes." They suggest that the trigger of the pain of trigeminal neuralgia is carried by large myelinated afferents, but that these might be involved in setting up a reverberating circuit in the smaller Aδ or C fibers, which "would result in a high frequency burst of impulses arriving at the central axon terminals."

Calvin et al.'s (8) theory, combined with the prior cited observations can account for the clinical features of trigeminal neuralgia: spontaneous pain, pain triggered by non-noxious stimuli (which are not always in the same division or region as the pain), increased frequency with aging, and frequent lack of sensory loss. The paroxysmal, lancinating nature of the pain, the duration of the attacks, and the pain-free intervals can all be accounted for. In addition, the theory predicts the temporary pain relief afforded by peripheral deinnervation procedures that interrupt the initiating impulse and by minor trauma to the ganglion that would alter the timing of reflected impulses. The drugs that best help trigeminal neuralgia, carbamazepine and diphenylhydantoin, reduce presynaptic depolarization in the trigeminal system and would therefore (according to this theory) help alter such reverberating circuits as a mechanism of affording relief.

A significant reflectance site for such a reverberating circuit would be at the area of focal compression and/or demyelination at the root entry zone produced by a vascular compressive loop, neoplasm, or area of demyelination associated with multiple sclerosis (MS). It is notable that all patients having MS with trigeminal neuralgia who have been studied at autopsy have plaques in the nerve at the root entry zone, that is, at the junction between central and peripheral myelin.

Removal of the vascular compression by microvascular decompression can be expected to promptly reverse the pathophysiology, as has been demonstrated in experimental mild compression. Failure to resolve the intraneural abnormal circuits, as might occur in some patients (especially after longer periods of compression), could explain failures of such treatment. Duration of symptoms before surgery is, indeed, the only factor we have been able to correlate with failure to respond to MVD microvascular decompression (3). This correlation has also been validated by the analyses of Bederson and Wilson (6) and Barker et al. (4). One could postulate that with long or severe enough compression, axonal disruption would also occur, resulting in interruption of the abnormal circuitry and clinical periods of remission until adjacent fibers were sufficiently involved for the pain to recur.

The theory, therefore, accounts for all of the clinical features of trigeminal neuralgia and offers a plausible rationale for treatment. Undoubtedly, the real situation is more complex than has been so far elucidated. Lack of a complete understanding, however, should not restrict treatment for trigeminal neuralgia any more than it does elsewhere in medicine.

Much has been made of the frequency of vascular compression in patients both with and without trigeminal neuralgia (1, 40). In addition, the type of compression (i.e., arterial versus venous) has been questioned. The presence of vascular contact in the absence of symptoms should not be taken as a negative finding with regard to the hypothesis, because not only vascular contact but specific internal neural derangements sufficient to allow the abnormal circuitry to develop must occur. Duration of compression, therefore, may be important and there may be additional, as yet undefined, cofactors necessary for such pathophysiology.

How vessels come to be in contact with and, ultimately, compress nerves is also speculative, but because many vessels contacting the trigeminal nerve are clearly elongated and tortuous, such elongation seems likely to be a factor. With aging there is stretching of all body tissues—we invariably get wrinkles and sags. Vessels, too, elongate—both arteries and veins. The truth of the latter statement is clearly evident when one compares the torturous veins on the dorsum of an elderly patient's hands with those of his or her younger relatives. Because the origin and termination of vessels is relatively constant, elongation results in increased tortuosity. In some patients such tortuous vessels will come in contact with nerves, often, in the case of trigeminal neuralgia, getting caught in the axilla of the nerve where it joins the brainstem at an oblique angle. So trapped, further elongation must result in increased neural compression, and at the very site where the central myelin changes to peripheral; i.e., the root entry zone (Obersteiner-Redlick zone).

The questions as to whether compression adequate to cause these problems must be pulsatile has also been raised, largely in the context of suggesting the veins are not an adequate etiological explanation for neurovascular compression. On the one hand, no evidence exists that pulsatile compression is required—indeed, in animal experiments it is not—and on the other hand, these syndromes can be seen when tumors are present as the sole source of root entry zone compression. In this case the brain pulsating against the nerve may be the pulsatile source, if that indeed is required. Veins connecting to the cerebral venous sinuses, however, can pulsate, because no valves are present between them and the heart. This will vary with intrathoracic pressure, the patient's position, and intracranial pressure. Such pulsation is often observed when patients are operated on in the sitting position. This, too, appears to be a moot point from the standpoint of outcomes, at least in the analysis of our results.

One must also address the question of whether every patient in these clinical syndromes has root entry zone compression. In the case of hemifacial spasm, this seems to be the case in most clinical series in which careful neurosurgical inspection of the facial nerve is done by a surgeon who is educated and experienced in exposing the area properly. Interestingly, hemifacial spasm is not recognized as a symptom of intrinsic neural disease such as MS, and it is not likely to be mistakenly misdiagnosed.

Negative explorations do occur in patients undergoing surgery for trigeminal neuralgia. The reasons for this are probably multiple. First is the accuracy of the diagnosis. I have seen quite a few patients diagnosed with trigeminal neuralgia who clearly do not have the syndrome. A number of these patients have had various operations for trigeminal neuralgia, including microvascular decompression and, of course, are not relieved of their pain. With a very consistent clinical picture from patient to patient, trigeminal neuralgia should be easy to diagnose accurately. Variations in the pain quality, duration, or location should immediately alert the physician to question the diagnosis, as should failure to respond to adequate doses of carbamazepine or diphenylhydantoin. I have found that inquiring as to the patient's behavior during the attacks is helpful when assessing a patient who is a vague historian. Tic patients instantly stop what they are doing, freeze, and may cry out or grimace. They may bring their hand up near their face to guard it but rarely touch the area. In contrast, patients with other types of pain tend to pace about, throw themselves on the floor or bed, rub the area, or apply hot or cold poultices.

Certainly, there also is an experience factor that separates surgeons. Most who have followed their patients carefully note an increased incidence in the finding of vascular compression as their operative experience increases. Walter Dandy himself revised his estimation of the incidence of compressing vascular loops as his series grew. I have been able to demonstrate large, convincing vascular loops when assisting other capable surgeons who pronounced a negative exploration. This may reflect inexperience on their part with fully defining the root entry zone, thereby only inspecting the nerve distal to that region, or failure to recognize a vessel behind dense arachnoid or one obscured by the nerve Fig. 33.2). My point is that the technique must be learned by observing experienced surgeons and by operating under their tutelage. One cannot simply assume that prior operative experience, including experience with other posterior fossa surgical techniques, is adequate training for these procedures. All operations have their subtleties and nuances, and attention to these can make the difference between success and failure.

These explanations notwithstanding, there still seem to be instances of negative exploration; the reason for many if not all of these may be found in the well-documented observation that trigeminal neuralgia might be the symptomatic manifestation of MS. Estimates of 1–3% of trigeminal neuralgia patients who are affected with MS exist, but the actual incidence is not truly known. As noted before, all MS patients with trigeminal neuralgia who have been studied have shown demyelinating plaques in the centrally myelinated portion of the trigeminal nerve adjacent to the root entry zone. Many also have plaques elsewhere in the central nervous system, including the brainstem portion of the trigeminal system. How often trigeminal neuralgia is the initial presenting symptoms of MS is unknown. Neither is it clear whether focal trigeminal nerve demyelination can occur and provoke trigeminal neuralgia as the only symptom of MS or other diseases of myelin. The low incidence of truly negative explorations, however, is quite consistent with the incidence of known demyelinating conditions affecting the trigeminal nerve and therefore may explain many such cases. The few not so explained remain a puzzle but are rare enough not to negate the overwhelmingly positive correlation that exists.

RESULTS

Multiple surgeons have reported their experience with microvascular decompression. It seems worthwhile to analyze the larger series to reflect the results of the surgeons with the most experience and, presumably the greatest interest in the problem. Unfortunately, most of the reported series are small or of short-term follow-up.

Jannetta followed his patients carefully and used annual question-

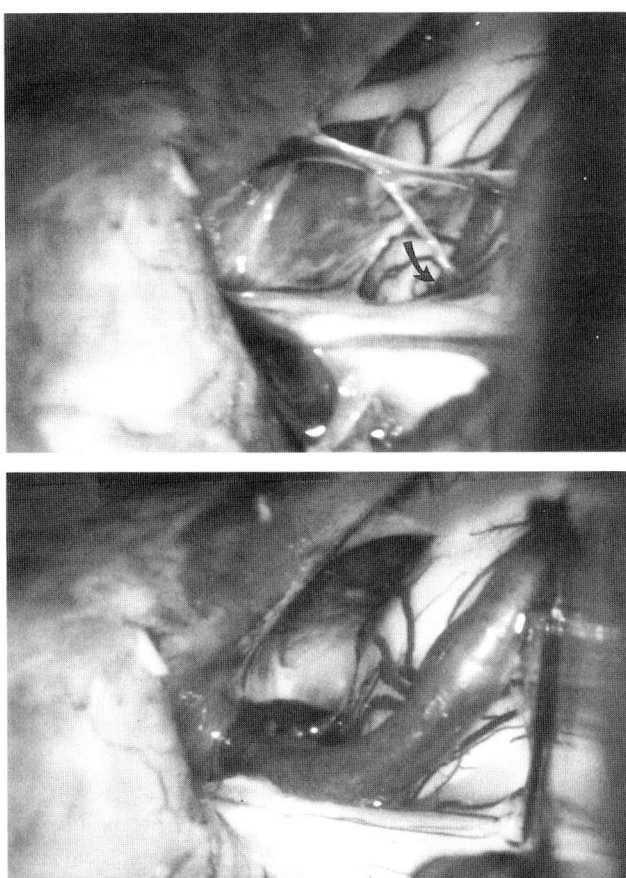

FIG. 33.2 (A) Operative findings in a patient with trigeminal neuralgia caused by compression of the trigeminal nerve by an elongated loop of the superior cerebellar artery. Note that the compression is immediately adjacent to the brainstem and that the only initial clue to this is the presence of the compressing vessel (superior cerebellar artery) emerging from behind the nerve at the brainstem (*arrow*). (B) The remainder of the vessel was hidden behind the nerve until elevated. Failure to fully visualize the most medial 2 to 3 millimeters of the nerve would fail to reveal the vessel and could lead the surgeon to the false conclusion of a "negative exploration."

naires to assess long-term outcome, recurrences, and further treatment for trigeminal neuralgia. The results of this landmark study were published in the *New England Journal of Medicine* in 1996 (4) and are detailed in *Tables 33.1–33.3*). The investigators had 1185 patients whom they operated on over a 20-year period for typical trigeminal neuralgia.

Patients whose symptoms were due to known MS, tumors, aneurysms, or arteriovenous malformations were excluded in the study, as were patients who were operated on with atypical trigeminal neuralgia. In *Table 33.1* some of the demographics of this group are tabulated. Patients ranged in age from 5 to 87 with a median age of 57 years. Sixty percent were female, and 61% had symptoms on the right side of the face. Bilateral trigeminal neuralgia was operated on in 19 patients (2%). At the initial surgical procedure (Table 33.1), vascular compression was most often caused by the superior cerebellar artery, with 10% being due to the anterior inferior cerebellar artery, and 4% other named arteries. Veins contributed to the compression in 68% of patients and were the only vessel in 13%. Serious complications (*Table 33.2*) include two operative deaths (a 69-year-old and a 79-year-old patient), both from cerebral infarction, with no deaths since 1980 (773 consecutive patients). Six patients developed cerebral infarction and two developed supratentorial hematomas. Seven of these patients were reoperated on and all resolved without sequelae. Other significant complications were rare, with 1.1% severe ipsilateral hearing loss (3% initially, 1% since using brainstem auditory-evoked response monitoring), 0.9% facial weakness (12 patients; transient in 10) and 1.2% extraocular muscle palsy (transient in 13 of 15).

TABLE 33.1
Microvascular Decompression for Trigeminal Neuralgia: Jannetta's Series[a]

Patients (n = 1145)	Operations (n = 1204)
Age: 5–87 yr; median 57 yr	Division Involved (%)
	V1 (3)
Gender (%)	V2 (18)
Female (60)	V3 (15)
Male (40)	V1, V2 (17)
Side of pain	V2, V3 (36)
Right (61)	V1, V2, V3 (12)
Left (37)	
Both (2)	
Cause of compression (%)	
SCA[b] (75)	Veins (68)
AICA (10)	Veins only (13)
PICA (1)	
Vertebral artery (2)	
Basilar artery (1)	
Unspecified small artery (15)	

[a]Adapted from Ref. 4.
[b]SCA, superior cerebellar artery; AICA, anterior inferior cerebellar artery; PICA, posterior inferior cerebellar artery.

TABLE 33.2
Complications in 1204 Microvascular Decompression Operations Jannetta's Series[a]

Major
    Deaths (2)
    Brainstem infarction (1)
    Cerebellar hemorrhage or edema (4)
    Supratentorial hematoma (2)
Cranial nerves:
    Facial paresis
        Transient (10)
        Mild (1)
        Severe (1)
    Ipsilateral hearing loss
        Mild (1)
        Severe (1)
    Extraocular muscle palsy
        4th nerve, transient (11)
        Permanent (2)
        6th nerve, transient (2)
    Severe facial numbness (22)
Other:
    Cerebrospinal fluid leak (20)
    Pseudomeningocele (4)
    Bacterial meningitis (5)

[a]Adapted from Ref. 4.

Outcomes are as follows (*Table 33.3*): Patients were considered to have excellent results with full relief and good results with partial relief. Initially 80% of patients had complete relief and 16% partial relief, with 2% not responding to treatment. At one year, 75% of the patients had excellent results, 9% had good results, and with a second operation for some patients with recurrence, these numbers rose to 80% excellent and 8% good. A 10 years the singly operated patients had a 64% excellent and 4% good outcome, with 70% excellent and 4% good if patients who had a second operation are included. Recurrences tended to occur early. They were less than 2% per year at 5 years and less than 1% per year after 10 years.

Thirty-four percent of patients with recurrent pain were controlled medically, 20% underwent an ablative procedure, 22% received both, and 24% and did not get further treatment. Analysis of these data by a proportional-hazards analysis suggests that the predictors of recurrence were female gender, preoperative symptoms greater than 8 years, venous compression, and lack of immediate postoperative relief.

I recently reviewed my experience with the various surgical procedures for treating trigeminal neuralgia (*Table 33.4*) during a 20-year

TABLE 33.3
Results of 1204 Microvascular Decompression Operations: Jannetta's Series[a]

	Excellent (%)	Partial (Good) (%)	Failure (%)
Initial	82	16	2
At 1 yr			
After first operation	75	9	16
After second operation	80	8	12
At 10 yrs			
After first operation	64	4	32
After second operation	70	4	26

[a]Adapted from Ref. 4.

interval using questionnaires to ascertain the follow-up status of the patients. During this period 702 patients were treated for trigeminal neuralgia, 406 by microvascular decompression, 20 by posterior fossa partial trigeminal root section, and 352 by percutaneous trigeminal neurolytic procedures. One hundred twenty-five of the latter had radiofrequency lesioning procedures and 243 had glycerol chemoneurolytic procedures. Some patients had multiple types of procedures. The average elapsed time since surgery was 13.9 years, with confirmed follow-up at an average of 6.9 years, and a minimum of 2 years postoperative follow-up required for inclusion in the study. In patients undergoing microvascular decompression (Table 33.5), the average age was 55.1 years (range, 18–83 years), 64% female, and 60% had pain on the right side. Vascular compression (*Table 33.5*) was due to arterial channels, either alone or in conjunction with veins or arteriovenous malformations in 83%, with 80% of these caused by the superior cerebellar artery, 85% due to the anterior inferior cerebellar artery, and 10% caused by both. Thirteen percent of the vascular compression was solely venous, 3% due to tumors, and 1.2% were negative explorations (five patients).

Major complications (*Table 33.6*) include five deaths (1.2%). These were due to cerebellar hemorrhagic infarction in three patients and supratentorial stroke in two patients. Five patients survived serious neurological compromise (3 with cerebellar infarction, 1 with supratentorial stroke, and 1 with brainstem stroke) but were left with neurological impairments. Cranial nerve palsies included 3.4% fourth nerve, 0.5% sixth nerve, and 0.5% seventh nerve, and 3.5% eighth nerve dysfunction. All of the patients with oculomotor, and 5 of 6 with facial nerve, palsies fully recovered, but 9 of 14 patients with eighth nerve dysfunctions remained affected (2 mild, 7 severe).

TABLE 33.4
Author's 20-Year Surgical Experience Treating Trigeminal Neuralgia[a]

MVD[b] procedures (406)
PFN section (20)
PTN procedures (352)
  RFL (125)
  GLY (243)
Average elapsed time since surgery: 167 mo (13.9 yr)

[a]n = 702 patients; some patients had multiple procedures.
[b]MVD, microvascular decompression; PFN, posterior fossa partial trigeminal nerve section; PTN, percutaneous trigeminal neurolysis; RFL, radiofrequency lesioning; GLY, glycerol chemoneurolysis.

This series, although only about one-third the size of Jannetta's is comparable in demographics and in surgical findings. Our fatality rate was higher, however, owing to cerebellar hemorrhagic infarction in three patients who died despite prompt attempts to remove the hem-

TABLE 33.5
Author's Experience with Microvascular Decompression for Trigeminal Neuralgia

Patients (n = 406)	Operations
Age: 18–83 yr; average 55.1 yr	Division Involved (%)
	V1 (1.5)
Gender (%)	V2 (21)
Female (64)	V3 (27)
Male (36)	V1, V2 (13)
Side of pain (%)	V1, V2, V3 (9)
Right (60)	
Left (40)	
Operative findings (%)	
Arterial channels (alone, w/veins, or w/AVMs) (83)	
SCA (67)	
AICA (7)	
Both (8)	
Basilar (1.5)	
Unnamed (0.25)	
Veins (alone or w/AVM (13)	
Tumors (5 w/arterial compression) (3)	
Negative exploration (1)	

[a]AVM, arteriovenous malformations; SCA, superior cerebellar artery; AICA, anterior inferior cerebellar artery.

TABLE 33.6
Author's Experience with Complications Using Microvascular Decompression for Trigeminal Neuralgia[a]

Major
  Death (5)
  Cerebellar hemorrhagic infarctions (6, 3 fatal)
  Supratentorial stroke (3, 2 fatal)
  Brainstem stroke (1)
Cranial nerve deficits
  Fourth nerve palsy (14)
  Sixth nerve palsy (2)
  Seventh nerve palsy
    Mild (0)
    Moderate (1)
    Severe (5, 1 permanent)
  Eighth nerve dysfunction
    Mild (5, 2 permanent)
    Severe (9, 7 permanent)

[a] n = 406 patients.

orrhage and infarcted tissue. Three other patients were saved by similar surgery for the same complication.

The outcomes, too, are comparable (*Table 33.7*). Excellent and complete initial pain relief was achieved in 91% of our patients and reduced pain in 6%. These results were correlated with my operative findings (*Table 33.8*). I prospectively graded the degree of vascular compromise as definite if the vessel clearly compressed or distorted the nerve and questionable if the vessel was only slightly touching the nerve. There was a trend toward less complete pain relief in the latter group, but this was not statistically significant because the numbers in these groups were small. In contrast with the results of Jannetta's series, no differences were seen when veins were the sole source of definite compression as compared with arteries.

On long-term follow-up, excellent pain relief, defined as pain-free or occasional mild pain not requiring medication, was achieved in 66% of

TABLE 33.7
Author's Results of Using Microvascular Decompression for Trigeminal Neuralgia[a]

	Excellent (%)	Partial (Good) (%)	Failure (%)
Initial	91	6	2
Follow-up	66	15	19

[a] Minimum, 2 yr of follow-up; average; 6.9 yr.

TABLE 33.8
Results According to Type of Compression Observed[a]

		Initial (%)			Long-term (%)		
	No.	Pain Relieved	Reduced Pain	Pain Unchanged	Excellent	Good	Failure
All patients	406	91.3	6	1.5	65.5	15.4	19.0
Definite arteries	319	93.4	5.3	1.2	66.3	15.3	18.5
Veins only	51	94	6	0	70.8	12.5	16.7
Questionable arteries and veins	20	85	15	0	31.6	31.6	36.8

[a] n = 406 patients.

patients. Fair relief, defined as pain that had recurred but was controlled medically, was noted in 15% of patients. Failure, that is, severe pain not medically controlled, was noted in 19%. It should be noted all of these patients were in severe pain and refractory to medication before surgery. As such, the patients in the "fair" group were generally happy with the result and considered it a good outcome. The same degree of patient satisfaction has been noted by Jannetta and others who have surveyed their patients. Questionable vascular compression patients as defined above seemed to have less durable results, with more patients achieving incomplete pain relief. The numbers in these groups are so small, however, that the failure rates fail to achieve statistical significance ($P > 0.05$ by Fisher exact 1-tailed test). The results of these two studies and several other reports with at least 70 patients are tabulated in *Table 33.9*. Not all of the authors presented the data in the same way, so they cannot all be completely compared. The similarities and long-term outcome, however, are strikingly similar.

COMPARISON WITH ALTERNATIVE PROCEDURES

Radiofrequency Lesioning

The alternative surgical approaches most used are percutaneous trigeminal neuroltyic techniques which can be accomplished in several ways. The technique that Sweet and Wepsic (51) introduced that used radiofrequency generated thermal energy to damage the preganglionic trigeminal rootlets in Meckel's cave has been adopted by many.

The end point of such lesioning was initially analgesia in the desired division. Touch sensation could often be preserved in "some or all of the trigeminal nerve rendered analgesic" (51). Nugent and Berry (43) also reported pain relief "usually with preservation of touch sensation in the face." Precise control of the extent of such a lesion is not always possi-

TABLE 33.9
Outcomes of Microvascular Decompression for Trigeminal Neuralgia

Series	No. of Patients	Average yrs of Follow-up	Initial Results (%)			Complications (%)		Long-Term Results (%)		
			Excellent	Good	Failure	Fatalities	Other Serious	Excellent	Good	Poor
Barker et al. (4)	1185	6.2	82	16	2	0.2	0.7	70	4	26
Apfelbaum (3)	406	6.9	91	6	1.5	1.2	1.5	66	15	19
Piatt and Wilkins (45)	103	4				1	3	72	5	23
Bederson and Wilson (6)	166	5.1				0	~1	75	7	18
Kondo (31)										
Series 1	127	12.6		93[a]	7					10.2[b]
Series 2	154	7.0		97[a]	3					6.5[b]
Taarnhøj (52)	86	5.8			5.8	1.2		80		12.8
Kolluri and Heros (30)	72	5	96		4	0	0	78	3	19

[a]Good to excellent.
[b]Recurrences.

ble, however, as Sweet has described: "Our biggest disappointments have been in patients in whom successful heatings were developing a gradually increasing zone of pure analgesia in the second and possibly a little loss in the first division; however the very next increment of heat, perhaps only five degrees centigrade hotter, would abruptly yield complete anesthesia and analgesia throughout both of these areas."

Abnormal unpleasant sensations of itching, burning, or crawling can accompany sensory loss and are increasingly frequent with more dense sensory loss. When severe, these sensations are as distressing to the patient as their original pain, since they can be present continuously as a severe burning discomfort (anesthesia dolorosa or analgesia dolorosa) and be intractable to treatment.

Loss of feeling in the first trigeminal division makes the cornea insensate and leaves the patient at risk for corneal ulceration and neuroparalytic keratitis, which can lead to loss of vision. Tew and Keller's (55) report of their first 400 cases typifies these complications. Although most patients were relieved of their pain, 19% reported bothersome paresthesias, 0.3% were classified as anesthesia dolorosa, and 20% developed corneal ulceration.

With the introduction of less destructive procedures, such as glycerol chemoneurolysis, described by Håkason (19) in 1981, it became clear that dense analgesia was not required for good pain relief. Radiofrequency lesioning advocates modified their technique to attempt to produce only hypesthesia of varying degrees and in so doing have reduced somewhat the rate of these disturbing complications. Taha and Tew (54) however, when reporting on 500 patients with a modified electrode and the end point of "dense hypalgesia," still note essentially the same incidence of anesthesia dolorosa (0.2% versus the previously reported 0.3%), although these figures are significantly less than Taha and Tew's estimated incidence of 1.5% anesthesia dolorosa in seven published series (54). Results in a number of large series are tabulated in *Table 33.10*.

Sweet (50) compiled an analysis of complications of various treatments of trigeminal neuralgia. He noted other complications of radiofrequency lesioning, which are infrequent but include oculomotor palsy in up to 6.5% of patients and trigeminal motor deficit in 25–40% of patients. Fortunately, almost all of these have been temporary. Sweet, however, reported 24 cases of bacterial meningitis, 1 of which was fatal, and several intracranial abscesses, 3 of which were fatal. He noted 6 cases of optic nerve lesions from misdirected needles, 20 intracranial hemorrhages with 2 deaths thought to be due to venous puncture, and 5 incidences of arterial puncture that resulted in 3

TABLE 33.10
Comparative Results of Radiofrequency Lesioning[a]

Series	No. of Patients	Average yr of Follow-up	Percentages (%)						
			Rcr	PR	MP	OP	CA	DY	AD
Siegfried (47)	1000	5–7	21	98	25	4	2.8	24	3
Tew (55), with curved electrode (54)	400 500	4 9	14 20	98 98	22 7	2 0	20 3	19 11	0.3 0.2
Moraci et al. (39)	568	2–10	16	96	11	0	0.6	21	0.3
Fraioli et al. (14)	527	5.8	10	98	3	0.2	3	15	1.5
Menzel et al. (38)	315	12	80	97	50			93	2
Sweet (51)	274	4	22	91	43	0	9	2	1
Apfelbaum (3)	109	8.8	19	92		0	1.2	26	2
Taha and Tew (54) (literature review)	6205	2–9	23	98	24		7	24	1.5

[a]Rcr, recurrences; PR, pain relief; MP, motor palsy; OP, oculomotor palsy; CA, corneal anesthesia; DY, dysesthesia, AD, anesthesia dolorosa.

deaths. Fifteen intracranial hematomas occurred, with 8 deaths. Inadvertent carotid punctures are usually innocuous, but in 2 cases hemiplegia with recovery and permanent infarction with deficit were noted.

These complications are noted not to imply that radiofrequency lesioning is very dangerous—it is not—but neither is it risk-free, and these risks must be considered when evaluating the various therapeutic options.

PERCUTANEOUS GLYCEROL CHEMONEUROLYSIS

Glycerol chemoneurolysis is the preferred percutaneous procedure of choice by many neurosurgeons. The advantages are ease of performance and removal of the need for patient cooperation and feedback for determining the end point of lesioning. As such, glycerol chemoneuroloysis can be performed with an anesthetized patient, improving patient comfort, at least compared with the awake lesioning techniques advocated by Nugent for maximal control of the lesion density. The technique can also be performed in patients who are not able to cooperate and make discriminative judgments. It is a much easier, easily learned, and less technically demanding procedure, and it does not require any special equipment, (2). Glycerol is also a relatively mild neurolytic agent, which has the advantage of less dense lesioning with usually only mild sensory loss, and rare oculomotor or dysesthetic sequelae. Of course, as a percutaneous technique glycerol chemoneurolysis has the same risks of meningitis and needle misdirection injury as any other like procedure.

TABLE 33.11
Author's Results with Percutaneous Trigeminal Neurolysis

	RFL[a] (%)	Gly[b] (%)	Results
Number of patients	109	227	
Number of procedures	118	352	
Initial Results			
Relieved	40 ⎫ 87	72 ⎫ 83	Excellent
Minimal pain, no medication	47 ⎭	11 ⎭	
Pain controlled w/medication	6	9	Fair
Pain not relieved	7	8	Good
Follow-up Results			
No recurrence	65 ⎫	46 ⎫	
Recurrent pain	⎬ 71	⎬ 52	Excellent
Mild pain, no medication	6 ⎭	6 ⎭	
Pain controlled w/medication	10	12	Fair
Severe pain; uncontrolled	19	36	Failure

[a] RFL, radiofrequency lesioning.
[b] Gly, glycerol injection.

The disadvantages of the technique are the need to prepare one's own sterile anhydrous glycerin (which most hospital pharmacies can easily do), and a somewhat higher recurrence rate. These are not thought by many to be significant disadvantages, as the procedure is well tolerated by patients and can be easily repeated.

Many authors have commented on the clear correlation between density of lesion and duration of relief of tic pain. A higher recurrence rate is to be expected with less dense lesions, but so are fewer denervation and dysesthetic complications, which increase with greater lesion density. Trading fewer of these very distressing complications and less numbness for the need for repeat procedures is very desirable to many patients.

As noted above we have used percutaneous techniques extensively in our practice as well as microvascular decompression. We initially used radiofrequency lesioning, adopting Nugent's cordotomy electrode technique. The tip can be bent at an angle to improve precision of placement within the appropriate trigeminal fibers, much like Tew's curved thermistor electrode. Our initial goal with radiofrequency lesioning was analgesia; that is, the inability to distinguish between the sharp versus dull end of a safety pin. This was commonly advocated as the appropriate end point at the time we were using radiofrequency lesioning. We changed to glycerol chemoneurolysis for the reasons already delineated in 1982 and have used it primarily since, reserving radiofrequency lesioning for the rare patient in whom we cannot cannulate the trigeminal cistern or in whom repeated glycerol injection fails to provide adequate relief.

As noted in *Table 33.11*, we have performed 118 radiofrequency lesions in 109 patients, and 352 glycerol injections in 227 patients. Initial pain relief, although while less than with our microvascular decompression experience, was good with both techniques, but more radiofrequency lesioning patients reported persistence of an aching facial pain after the procedure. Excellent relief was reported by 71% of radiofrequency lesioning patients, with a 19% failure rate. Ten percent had what we have defined earlier as a fair result; that is, pain control but requiring medication when they could not be controlled medically before the procedure. With glycerol more recurrences led to a 52% excellent, 12% fair, and 36% failure rate.

The average time to recurrence was 19 months, with a majority of patients treated by repeat procedures and attaining additional relief. Seventy-two percent of glycerol patients had at least 3 years of relief with one injection. Radiofrequency lesioning patients in our series averaged 1.15 procedures per patient, whereas glycerol injection patients averaged 1.53.

Complications included bacterial meningitis in two patients, aseptic meningitis in two, a transient sixth nerve palsy in one, and, most seriously, a temporal lobe hematoma with permanent neurological impairment in one radiofrequency lesioning patient. Sensory loss occurred in all radiofrequency lesioning patients and usually was moderate-to-severe. Two percent had anesthesia dolorosa and 26% had bothersome dysesthesia. Twenty percent developed corneal anesthesia and 2% developed keratitis. Glycerol patients usually had only mild sensory loss, with more severe sensory loss in only 20% of patients. One percent had corneal anesthesia and there was no keratitis. No glycerol patient developed anesthesia dolorosa, and only 0.5% complain of bothersome dysesthesia.

In summary, in our experience both procedures are quite safe and effective, but we feel that avoidance of significant sensory loss dysesthetic sequelae, and corneal anesthesia, as well as increased ease of performance and tolerability of the glycerol neurolysis technique far outweighs the somewhat longer duration of pain relief with radiofrequency lesioning. Treating recurrences is much easier than treating dysesthesia. Glycerol neurolysis, therefore, is our percutaneous procedure of choice.

An alternative technique is balloon microcompression, as described by Mullan and Lichtor (42). Because of the severe bradycardia the technique can produce, some advocate doing the procedure under general endotracheal anesthesia with an external cardiac pacemaker (7). In the absence of any significant advantage over glycerol chemoneurolysis, this seems unnecessarily complicated. The results seem comparable except for the significantly increased risk of motor root paralysis, which can last for a number of months.

Recently gamma knife irradiation of the trigeminal root has been proposed (32, 56). Despite enthusiastic promotion by gamma knife owners, information comparable to that reported for other procedures is lacking. Reports so far have considered 50 to 90% reduction of pain as good and 10 to 50% as fair. Even with these questionable definitions the results are barely comparable. No pathological data have been reported regarding the immediate and long-term effects of high-dose radiation (70–90 Gy) to the nerve adjacent to the brainstem, with so far unreported dosimetry involving the actual dose that the margin of the brainstem receives. Although certainly a suitable subject for research, this remains an experimental, expensive, and unproven technique at this time.

PROCEDURE OF CHOICE

The progress made in this century allows us to state unequivocally that trigeminal neuralgia is an eminently treatable condition. Often it can be controlled medically for significant periods of time. If medical treatment fails or is limited by significant side effects, good surgical options exist.

Patients must be fully informed of the options and must participate in the therapeutic decision process. Pain relief can be obtained by microvascular decompression or percutaneous trigeminal neurolysis (using whatever technique the surgeon is most comfortable with) in almost all patients. Neither is assuredly permanent, but most patients treated with microvascular decompression will be "cured," and most patients treated with percutaneous trigeminal neurolysis will obtain relief for a number of years and will easily tolerate repeat of the procedure if necessary.

How, then, can the surgeon recommend, and the patient decide on, one procedure over another? Clearly, there is no one correct answer for every patient. The key to this decision should involve consideration of the patient's age, associated illnesses, and assessment of the risks the patient is willing to assume. Age is a factor in two ways. First, younger patients have a better chance of tolerating an open procedure without complications. Second, they have a longer future life expectancy in which to deal with the deinnervation problems that can follow percutaneous lesioning. Being younger, they have a higher risk of recurrence from the palliative procedures and, although treatable, they will likely need more future treatments and thus will have increased cumulative effects with regard to deinnervation.

Older patients have increased risks of surgical complications, especially for an open procedure, and a shorter remaining life expectancy. Therefore, they likely will require fewer repetitions of percutaneous procedures with less cumulative deinnervation sequelae.

But what is the appropriate transition age between the "young" and "old" groups? In my experience most serious and life-threatening complications with microvascular decompression have occurred in patients older than 65 to 70 years of age. Although many patients in their 70s, and a few in their 80s, have tolerated the procedure well. I believe that the risks increase above the age of 65 to 70, and so advise patients. These numbers, of course, are not absolute and are adjusted for the patient's overall medical status.

Obviously, the presence of significant associated illness, such as chronic obstructive pulmonary disease, coronary artery disease, and diabetes mellitus (which increase the risks of a major surgical procedure), tip the balance in favor of percutaneous trigeminal neurolysis.

All procedures have their risk, however, small. Patients must be well and honestly informed so they can direct their treatment as to the type and degree of risk they are willing to assume. Some patients would rather take the risk of death with microvascular decompression (1% overall, but much lower for younger, low-risk patients) than have a lifetime of facial numbness and the chance of anesthesia dolorosa or corneal ulceration; others would not. My patients who have had a successful microvascular decompression are much happier than even those with a "good" percutaneous trigeminal neurolysis results. Both groups are pain-free, but the latter inquire whether "my face will always feel this way," even with mild numbness, not dysesthetic sequelae. Patients are bothered by the fact that their nose may run, or they may drool and not feel it, and they have a constant reminder of their problem and its eventual recurrence. How much worse is it for the patient with severe numbness or dysesthetic sequelae? These are quality-of-life issues, and for different individuals there are different choices.

I think there is great wisdom in the recommendations of Dr. C. Hunter Sheldon, who, in a discussion of trigeminal neuralgia in 1959, said, "In all likelihood the proper method would be to decide which operation you would prefer if you were the patient." There is no question that if I had trigeminal neuralgia I would prefer a microvascular decompression if I thought my condition was such that I'd likely tolerate the procedure.

I think there is little question for most "younger" patients and for some selected "older" patients that microvascular decompression clearly is their best option and is therefore the procedure of choice.

REFERENCES

1. Adams CBT, Chir M: Microvascular compression: An alternative view and hypothesis. **J Neurosurg** 57:1–12, 1989.
2. Apfelbaum RI: Glycerol trigeminal neurolysis, in Burchiel KJ (ed). *Techniques in Neurosurgery,* vol 5, Philadelphia, Lippincott Williams & Wilkins, 1999, pp. 225–231.
3. Apfelbaum RI: Surgery for tic dolourex, in Weiss M (ed). *Clinical Neurosurgery,* vol 31, Baltimore, Williams & Wilkins, 1983, pp. 351–358.
4. Barker FJ, Jannetta PJ, Bissonette DJ, Larkins MV, Joh HD: The long-term outcome of microvascular decompression for trigeminal neuralgia. **N Engl J Med** 334:1077–1983, 1996.
5. Beaver DL: Electron microscopy of the gasserian ganglion in trigeminal neuralgia. **J Neurosurg** 26:138–150, 1967.
6. Bederson JB, Wilson CB: Evaluation of microvascular decompression and partial sensory rhizotomy in 252 cases of trigeminal neuralgia. **J Neurosurg– 71:359–367, 1989.**
7. Brown JA, Preul MD: Trigeminal depressor response during percutaneous microcompression of the trigeminal ganglion for treigminal neuralgia. **J Neurosurg** 33:745–748, 1988.
8. Calvin WH, Loeser JD, Howe JF: A neurophysiologic theory for the pain mechanism of tic douloureux. **Pain** 3:147–154, 1977.
9. Campbell E, Keedy C: Hemifacial spasm. A note on the etiology in two cases. **J Neurosurg** 4:342–347, 1947.
10. Dandy WE: Concerning the cause of trigeminal neuralgia. **Am J Surg** 24:447–455, 1934.
11. Dandy WE. Section of the sensory root of the trigeminal nerve at the pons. **Bull Johns Hopkins Hosp** 36:105–106, 1925.
12. Dandy WE: The treatment of trigeminal neuralgia by the cerebellar route. **Ann Surg** 96:787–795, 1932.
13. Dandy WE: Trigeminal neuralgia and trigeminal tic douloureux, in Lewis D (ed). *Practice of Surgery.* vol XII, Hagerstown, W. F. Prior Co., 1932, pp. 177–200.
14. Fraioli B, Esposito V, Guidetti B, Cruccu G, Manfredi M: Treatment of trigeminal neuralgia by thermocoagulation, glycerolization, and percutaneous compressing of the gasserian ganglion and/or retrogasserian rootlets: Long-term results and therapeutic protocol. **Neurosurgery** 24:239–245, 1989.
15. Gardner WJ: Concerning the mechanism of trigeminal neuralgia and hemifacial spasm. **J Neurosurg** 19:947–958, 1962.
16. Gardner WJ: Trigeminal neuralgia, in : Ojemann RG (ed). *Clinical Neurosurgery,* vol 15, Baltimore, Williams & Wilkins, 1968, pp. 1–56.
17. Gardner WJ, Sava GA: Hemifacial spasm—A reversible pathophysiologic state. **J. Neurosurg** 19:240–247, 1962.
18. Granit R, Leksell L: Fibre interaction in injured or compressed region of nerve. **Brain** 67:125–140, 1944.
19. Håkason S: Trigeminal neuralgia treated by the injection of glycerol into the tregiminal cistern. **Neurosurgery** 9:638–646, 1981.
20. Hartley F: Intracranial neurectomy of the second and third divisions of the fifth nerve: A new method. **NY Med J** 55:317–319, 1892.
21. Horsley V, Taylor J, Colman WS: Remarks on the various surgical procedures devised for the relief or cure of trigeminal neuralgia (tic douloureux). **Br Med J** 2:1139–1143; 1191–1193; 1249–1252, 1891.
22. Jannetta PJ: Arterial compression of the trigeminal nerve at the pons in patients with trigeminal neuralgia. **J Neurosurg** 26:159–162, 1967.

23. Jannetta PJ: Microsurgical approach to the trigeminal nerve for tic douloureux, in: Krayenbuhl H, Maspes PE, Sweet WH, (eds). *Progress in Neurological Surgery,* vol 7, Basel, S. Karger 1976, pp 180–200.
24. Jannetta PJ: Neurovascular compression in cranial nerve and systemic disease. **Ann Surg** 192:518–525, 1980.
25. Jannetta PJ: Observations on the etiology of trigeminal neuralgia, hemifacial spasm, acoustic nerve dysfunction and glossopharyngeal neuralgia: Definitive microsurgical treatment and results in 117 patients. **Neurochirurgia (Stuttg)** 20:145–154, 1977.
26. Jannetta PJ, Abbasy M, Maroon JC, Ramos FM, Albin MS. Ethology and definitive microsurgical treatment of hemifacial spasm: Operative techniques and results in forty-seven patients. **J Neurosurg** 47:321–328, 1977.
27. Kerr FWL: Correlated light electron microscopic observations on the normal trigeminal ganglion and sensory root in man. **J Neurosurg** 26:132–137, 1967.
28. Kerr FWL: Evidence for a peripheral etiology of trigeminal neuralgia. **J Neurosurg** 26:168–174, 1967.
29. Kerr KWL: Pathology of trigeminal neuralgia: Light and electron microscopic observations. **J Neurosurg** 26:151–156, 1967.
30. Kolluri S, Heros RC: Microvascular decompression for trigeminal neuralgia. A five-year follow-up study. **Surg Neurol** 22:235–240, 1984.
31. Kondo A: Follow-up results of microvascular decompression in trigeminal neuralgia and hemifacial spasm. **Neurosurgery– 40:46–52, 1997.**
32. Kondziolka D, Lunsford LD, Flickinger JC, et al: Stereotactic radiosurgery for trigeminal neuralgia: a multiinstitutional study using the gamma unit. **J Neurosurg** 84:940–945, 1996.
33. Krause F. Resection des Trigeminus innerhalb der Schadelhohle. **Arch Klin Chir** 44:821–832, 1892.
34. Kugelberg E, Lindblom U: The mechanism of the pain in trigeminal neuralgia. **J Neurol Neurosurg Psychiatry** 22:36–43, 1959.
35. List CF, Williams JR: Pathogenesis of trigeminal neuralgia. A review. **Arch Neurol Psychiatry** 77;36–43, 1957.
36. Loeser JD, Calvin WH, Howe JF: Pathophysiology of trigeminal neuralgia, in Keener EB (ed). **Clinical Neurosurgery** vol 24, Baltimore, Williams & Wilkins, 1977, pp 527–537.
37. Maxwell DS: Fine structure of the normal trigeminal ganglion in the cat and monkey. **J Neurosurg** 26:127–131, 1967.
38. Menzel J, Piotrowski W, Penzholz H: Long-term results of gasserian ganglion electrocoagulation. **J Neurosurg** 42:140–143, 1975.
39. Moraci A. Buonaito C, Punzo A, Parlato C, Amalfi R: Trigeminal neuralgia treated by percutaneous thermocoagulation. Comparative analysis of percutaneous thermocoagulation and other surgical procedures. **Neurochirurgia (Stuttg)** 35(2):48–53, 1992.
40. Morley TP: Case against microvascular decompression in the treatment of tragemi-nal neuralgia. **Arch Neurol** 42:801–802, 1985.
41. Moses HL: Comparative fine structure of the trigeminal ganglia, including human autopsy studies. **J Neurosurg** 26:112–126, 1967.
42. Mullan S, Lichtor T: Percutaneous microcompression of the trigeminal ganglion for trigeminal neuralgia. **J Neurosurg** 59:1007–1012, 1983.
43. Nugent GR, Berry B: Trigeminal neuralgia treated by a differential percutaneous radiofrequency coagulation of the gasserian ganglion. **J Neurosurg** 40:517–523, 1974.

44. Peet MM, Schenider RC: Trigeminal neuralgia: A review of six hundred and eighty-nine cases with a follow-up study of sixty-five percent of the group. **J Neurosurg** 9:367–377, 1952.
45. Piatt JH, Wilkins RH: Treatment of tic douloureux and hemifacial spasm by posterior fossa exploration: therapeutic implications of various neurovascular relationships. **Neurosurgery** 14:462–471, 1984.
46. Sheldon CH: Compression procedure for trigeminal neuralgia. **J. Neurosurg** 25:374–381, 1966.
47. Siegfried J: Percutaneous controlled thermocoagulation of gasserian ganglion in trigeminal neuralgia. Experiences with 1000 cases, in Samii M, Jannetta PJ (eds). *The Cranial Nerves,* Berlin, Springer-Verlag, 1981, pp. 322–330.
48. Spiller WG, Frazier CH: The division of the sensory root of the trigeminus for relief of tic douloureux: An experimental, pathological and clinical study with a preliminary report of one surgically successful case. **Philad Med J** 8:1039–1049, 1901.
49. Stookey B, Ransohoff J: *Trigeminal Neuralgia. Its History and Treatment.* Springfield, IL, Charles C Thomas, 1959.
50. Sweet WH: Complications of treating trigeminal neuralgia: An analysis of the literature and response to questionnaire, in Rovit RL, Murali R (eds). *Trigeminal Neuralgia,* Baltimore, Williams & Wilkins, 1990, pp. 251–279.
51. Sweet WH, Wepsie JG: Controlled thermocoagulation of trigeminal ganglion and rootlets for differential destruction of pain fibers. **J Neurosurg** 40:143–156, 1974.
52. Taarnhøj P: Decompression of the posterior trigeminal root in trigeminal neuralgia. A 30-year follow-up review. **J. Neurosurg** 57:14–17, 1982.
53. Taarnhøj P: Decompression of the trigeminal root. **J Neurosurg** 11:299–305, 1954.
54. Taha JM, Tew JM: Comparison of surgical treatments for trigeminal neuralgia: Reevaluation of radiofrequency rhizotomy. **Neurosurgery** 38:864–871, 1996.
55. Tew JM, Keller JT: The treatment of trigeminal neuralgia by percutaneous radiofrequency technique, in Keener EB (ed). *Clinical Neurosurgery* vol 24 Baltimore, Williams & Wilkins, 1977, pp. 557–578.
56. Young RF, Vermeulen SS, Grimm P, Blasko J, Posewitz A: Gamma knife radiosurgery for treatment of trigeminal neuralgia: idopathic and tumor related. **Neurology** 48:608–614, 1997.

CHAPTER

34

Trigeminal Neuralgia: Vascular Compression Theory

ANDREW H. KAYE, M.D., M.B.B.S., F.R.A.C.S.

The concept of microvascular compression as a basis for a variety of clinical syndromes has been appropriately credited to Peter Jannetta and his pioneering work since the 1960s (12, 14). Walter Dandy, in 1934 (5), noted that in a substantial percentage of cases, trigeminal neuralgia was associated with compression of the Vth cranial nerve by tumor, aneurysm, or other vascular malformation or by an otherwise normal artery or vein. Vascular compression of the VIIth cranial nerve resulting in hemifacial spasm was described by Campbell and Keedy in 1947 (4). Gardner, in 1962, speculated that both trigeminal neuralgia and hemifacial spasm were "a reversible pathophysiologic state caused by a mild compression of the nerve root which permits transaxonal excitation while not interfering with axonal conduction" (7). Previously, Gardner and Miklos had reported on the response of trigeminal neuralgia to a vascular decompression in 1959 (8). However, it was Jannetta's use of the operating microscope in performing microvascular decompression, principally in patients with trigeminal neuralgia, but also for those with hemifacial spasm and glossopharyngeal neuralgia, that popularized the procedure for these conditions (12–15, 18).

It is particularly unfortunate that the debate concerning the vascular compression theory has not been without acrimony and rancor. We are all very much influenced by our teachers, particularly in neurosurgery, where concepts and clinical practice evolve from both an understanding of basic and applied neuroscience and the "art" of surgery. I have no special knowledge of the vascular compression syndromes, but I have had a considerable interest in the topic over 20 years. During that time, I have watched a debate that has "consumed" some of the giants of modern neurosurgery and neurosurgeons for whom I have had considerable respect.

During my initial neurosurgery training in Melbourne, Australia, the concept of the vascular compression syndrome was accepted without question, the procedure having been performed since 1973. Similar views were held by my teachers at the Cleveland Clinic in the early 1980s, although it is difficult to be sure how much this was influenced by William Gardner, who had played a major role in developing neurosurgery at the Clinic. It is fair to say that in Oxford in the early 1980s, the concept had met with some skepticism (1, 2). I should emphasize that I have considerable admiration for all the neurosurgeons involved in the debate. Nonetheless, as clinical scientists we have an obligation to both our patients and to neurosurgery to question and evaluate concepts and theories. We must do so without "fear or favor," and without intimidation.

Whatever the validity of the theory of microvascular compression, it is the procedure of choice that I have used since 1983 in the treatment of patients with trigeminal neuralgia and hemifacial spasm. However, over the last 20 years there have been a number of factors regarding the theory that have continued to perplex me. These include the following:

- What is the definition of compression, and what constitutes compression?
- Why are only certain cranial nerves affected?
- Why is compression evident in asymptomatic patients?
- Why are symptoms intermittent?
- Why are the symptoms nearly always unilateral, but it would seem that compression is often bilateral?
- Why are there recurrences after undergoing microvascular decompression?

WHAT IS COMPRESSION?

The fundamental basis of the theory is vascular compression at the root entry or exit zone, which is defined as a "junctional area between central and peripheral myelin," although there is no clear definition as to what constitutes compression (17). Whereas compression is self-evident if the nerve is grooved or distorted by a vessel, the initial concept of "pulsatile compression" is less easy to understand if compression by a small venule or arachnoid band is accepted as the cause (16). Some authorities have even proposed that failure to identify definite compression at operation can be due to the position of the head at surgery, or to the early division of arachnoid bands, which can alter the preoperative usual nerve–blood vessel relationship.

Obviously, different surgeons have different thresholds for accepting what constitutes compression and, in particular, what is pulsatile compression (10). In Jannetta's very large series of over 1200 patients operated on for trigeminal neuralgia, an "unnamed small artery or vein only" was found in 18.5% of cases (11). In my comparatively modest series of 302 patients, the nerve was grooved or distorted by an artery in 83% of cases (*Table 34.1*). In my series, 5% of cases showed no vessel to be in intimate association with the root entry zone. Table 1 shows the "offending" vessels and the percentage in which each was causing compression. The superior cerebellar artery was implicated in 75% of cases, and in 90% of these it was compressing or distorting the nerve. However, only 50% of small unnamed arteries and 42% of veins were thought to be causing compression.

The issue of "cause and effect" is not easily resolved by the surgical result. In 1952, Taarnhøj (27) noted that decompressing the gasserian ganglion without nerve section could successfully relieve trigeminal neuralgia. Of note, in my own series, excellent results as defined using Janetta's classification (11), were achieved 1 year after microvascular decompression in 87% of patients having obvious grooving or distortion of the nerve, compared with 78% in whom the findings were more subtle.

It would seem that there are two groups of neurosurgeons—those who believe there must be overt pulsatile compression that clearly distorts the nerve at the root entry zone, and the "minimalists," who believe that the compression can be subtle. For each group, there are some apparent contradictions of the theory, as detailed below. that are not easily explained.

TABLE 34.1
Vessels Compressing the Trigeminal Nerve in 302 Consecutive Operations on Patients with Typical Trigeminal Neuralgia

Vessel	n	%	No. of Distorting Nerve (%)
SCA[a]	227	75	206 (90)
AICA	30	10	10 (100)
PICA	1	0.33	0 (0)
Vertebral	1	0.33	1 (100)
Basilar	5	1.7	4 (80)
Unnamed small artery	32	10.5	16 (50)
Vein only	33	11	14 (42.4)
Vein and artery	159	52.6	—
No vessels	15	5	—

[a]SCA, superior cerebellar artery; AICA, anterior inferior cerebellar artery; PICA, posterior inferior cerebellar artery.

WHY ARE OTHER CRANIAL NERVES NOT AFFECTED?

Although much remains to be learned about the pathophysiology of the so-called "hyperactive cranial nerve syndromes," I have found no satisfactory explanation as to why other cranial nerves are not affected. In particular, one might expect to see spasm of the masseter and temporalis muscle with trigeminal neuralgia and of the stylopharyngeal muscle with glossopharyngeal neuralgia. I have never seen a case of neuralgia of nervus intermedius with hemifacial spasm. This is a very small nerve, and it would be expected to be easily distorted or compressed.

It is likely that there are other intrinsic factors within the root entry zone of the different cranial nerves or in the brainstem that make them resistant to the effects of pulsatile compression, but this is merely conjecture.

ASYMPTOMATIC COMPRESSION

Asymptomatic compression must occur in an extraordinarily large number of people. Of course, the number with asymptomatic compression would be proportional to the tolerance of defining what is "symptomatic" compression. For the "minimalists" who believe that symptomatic compression can be due to a venule, arachnoid band, or very small artery, there would have to be an explanation as to why a large percentage of the population had asymptomatic compression. For those who have a more strict definition of compression, and who believe that a compressive lesion has to cause grooving or distortion of the nerve, there is less need to explain this phenomenon. Of course, this does not exclude vascular compression as being part of the syndrome, but it adds to the view that there must be some as yet undiscovered factor that is necessary to produce the syndrome in addition to the compression (20). Although this may reside in the root entry zone, a more central basis is just as likely.

INTERMITTENT SYMPTOMS

A classic feature of trigeminal neuralgia involves remissions of pain that are frequent and may last for months or even years. Although this could be understood if the minimalist view of nerve compression is accepted, it is difficult to explain in those patients where there is evidence of considerable distortion of the nerve by a large vessel. The other "unidentified" factor needs to be invoked to explain this phenomenon.

UNILATERAL SYMPTOMS

Bilateral trigeminal neuralgia, hemifacial spasm, or glossopharyngeal neuralgia are uncommon. In accepting the vascular compression theory, the less stringent the requirement for a vessel to be the "cause" of trigeminal neuralgia, the more likely it would be that vessels are present bilaterally (and at multiple sites). The study by Hardy and Rhoton (9) investigating the relationship of the superior cerebellar artery and trigeminal nerve in cadavers has been used by proponents both for and against the microvascular compression theory, but as the authors themselves conclude, "any study of cadaver specimens must be of limited value in discussing the aetiology of pain producing conditions such as trigeminal neuralgia. . . ." Nevertheless, of the 50 nerves examined, 29 had a point of contact with a major artery between the pons and the point where the nerve passed beneath the tentorial attachment to enter Meckel's cave. In 10 of the 25 cadavers, there were vascular contacts with the trigeminal nerve on both sides.

FAILURE OF MICROVASCULAR DECOMPRESSION

The success or failure of microvascular decompression has been used by both the proponents of the concept and opponents to the theory to further their arguments. It is unfortunate that some have used the argument to attack other surgeons' technical expertise. In Jannetta's study of 1204 patients who underwent first microvascular decompression for typical trigeminal neuralgia at the Pennsylvania University Hospital (11), 75.2% of patients had an excellent result 1 year after microvascular decompression and 63.5% had an excellent result 10 years after the operation. A further 8.9% had a partial relief 1 year after and 3.5% 10 years after the procedure. A total of 132 patients (11%) were submitted to reoperation; 79.7% of patients had an excellent result at 1 year after microvascular decompression, and 69.6% had an excellent result 10 years after the procedure. These results are of considerable interest in considering the theory, as it would be expected that at least the 1-year results would have been much better if a microvascular compressive cause was the sole determinant of trigeminal neuralgia. There would be very few neurosurgeons or departments that would have had more experience in the use of microvascular decompression, yet at 1 year after surgery, 20% of patients still had some pain. Although in the honored guest lecture of 1996 (11), Jannetta provided an excellent analysis of his results, it would have been interesting for the outcomes relating to the severity of compression to have been analyzed in more detail. However, three of the four Cox proportional hazard models did identify venous compression as a significant predictor of long-term failure. As indicated previously, in a personal series of 225 patients followed for 5 years, the recurrence at 5 years was much higher in those patients in whom the nerve was neither grooved nor distorted by an artery.

Table 34.2 shows the results of my personal series, comparing outcome between those patients who had definite distortional compression of the nerve with those in whom either no vessel was found or the "offending" vessel was neither distorting nor grooving the nerve. Any vessel associated with the nerve was mobilized away from the nerve using a standard microsurgical technique, and then padded away from the nerve initially using Ivalon sponge and, over the past 5 years, Teflon pads. In those patients in whom no vessel was found, the nerve was rubbed vigorously.

Assessment of outcome in patients with trigeminal neuralgia is less objective than for hemifacial spasm, particularly in those patients in whom the relief is less than complete. The definition of the outcome results are as described by Janetta, with an excellent outcome being assigned if the patient was "free of lancinating pain, or at least 98% pain free, without medication for trigeminal neuralgia." A grade of "partial or good" relief was assigned if the trigeminal neuralgia symptoms were relieved in ". . . by 75% or greater. Intermittent treatment with low doses of medication for trigeminal neuralgia was considered compatible with partial success." A "poor or failure" outcome was assigned if ". . . more than 25% of preoperative symptoms were present without medication, or if chronic medication was resumed by any dose." The 5-year outcome results in my series are similar to those of Janetta, and better results were obtained where the nerve was noted to be distorted or grooved by a vessel. Statistical analysis using the Cochran Armitage test for trends shows significance at $p = 0.0051$ when comparing the results at 5 years for those patients with definite distortion or grooving of the nerve compared with those without a compressive lesion or with minimal compression. It could be argued that in those cases with more nerve compression, there was more manipulation of the nerve to obtain a satisfactory decompression,

TABLE 34.2
Five-year Results of a Consecutive Series of 225 Patients Treated for Trigeminal Neuralgia[a]

		Results					
		Excellent		Good		Poor	
	n	n	(%)	n	(%)	n	(%)
Vessel grooving or distorting nerve	187	155	(82.9)	10	(5.3)	22	(11.8)
No distortion/no vessel	38	24	(71)	3	(7.9)	11	(28.9)
Total		179	(79.6)	13	(5.8)	33.3	(14.7)

[a]Comparing patients in whom either no vessel was found or the vessel was considered not to be distorting or grooving the nerve. The Cochrane Armitage statistical test for trends shows significance at $p = 0.0051$.

but this is not necessarily so. In fact, there was often more manipulation of the nerve when no major compressive vessel was found, to be certain of the finding. In addition, Sindou (26) reported similar results in a technique he uses where there is no manipulation of the nerve.

The 1-year follow-up of patients following microvascular decompression is much harder to interpret in view of the known effect described by Taarnhøj of manipulation of the nerve, as at least some manipulation of the nerve is usually associated with the procedure and this manipulation will produce a temporary effect.

CONCLUSION

The vascular compression concept as a cause of a range of clinical syndromes as diverse as hemifacial spasm (4, 10, 14), trigeminal neuralgia, glossopharyngeal neuralgia, vertigo (19, 24, 25), tinnitus (23), and hypertension has rightly been subject to considerable debate as to its exact phathogenesis (1, 2, 22, 26) and the results of surgery compared with other techniques (3, 6). The relative role of vascular compression in each of these syndromes may vary and is still to be absolutely defined. However, what is clear is that, whatever the merits of the theory, the operation of microvascular decompression is successful in a large percentage of cases in relieving the disabling symptoms of trigeminal neuralgia (3, 11, 20, 21, 26, 27). In my opinion, it is the operation of choice in the vast majority of patients.

There are many mysteries in medicine, and these may be particularly hard to resolve in disease processes for which no definite pathophysiology has been defined. Hopefully, the revolution that has occurred in neurological imaging will help in the future to better elucidate the exact pathology that is the basis of trigeminal neuralgia. Until then, constructive enquiry and debate should be welcomed.

REFERENCES

1. Adams CBT: Microvascular compression: An alternative view and hypothesis. **J Neurosurg** 57:1–12, 1989.
2. Adams CBT: Trigeminal neuralgia: Pathogenesis and treatment. **Br J Neurosurg** 11:493–495, 1997.
3. Apfelbaum RI: A comparison of percutaneous radiofrequency trigeminal neurolysis and microvascular decompression of the trigeminal nerve for the treatment of tic douloureux. **Neurosurgery** 1:16–21, 1977.
4. Campbell E, Keedy C: Hemifacial spasm: A note on the etiology in two cases. **J Neurosurg** 4:342–347, 1947.
5. Dandy WE: Concerning the cause of trigeminal neuralgia. **Am J Surg** 24:447–455, 1934.
6. Ferguson GG, Brett DC, Peerless SI, Barr HWK, Girvin JP: Trigeminal neuralgia: A

comparison of the results of percutaneous rhizotomy and microvascular decompression. **J Can Sci Neurol** 8:207–214, 1981.
7. Gardner WJ: Concerning the mechanism of trigeminal neuralgia and hemifacial spasm. **J Neurosurg** 19:947–958, 1962.
8. Gardner WJ, Miklos MV: Response of trigeminal neuralgia to decompression of sensory root. **JAMA** 170:1773–1776, 1959.
9. Hardy DG, Roton AL: Microsurgical relationship of the superior cerebellar artery and the trigeminal nerve. **J Neurosurg** 49:669–678, 1978.
10. Hunn MK, Eldridge PR, Miles JB, West B: Persistent facial pain following microvascular decompression of the trigeminal nerve. **Br J Neurosurg** 12:23–28, 1998.
11. Jannetta PJ: Outcome after microvascular decompression for trigeminal neuralgia, hemifacial spasm, tinnitus, disabling positional vertigo and glossopharyngeal neuralgia. **Clin Neurosurg** 44:331–381, 1996.
12. Jannetta PJ: Arterial compression of the trigeminal nerve at the ons in patients with trigeminal neuralgia. **J Neurosurg** 26:159–162, 1967.
13. Jannetta PJ: Microsurgical approach to the trigeminal nerve for tic douloureux. **Prog Neurol Surg** 7:180–200, 1976.
14. Jannetta PJ: Observations on the etiology of trigeminal neuralgia, hemifacial spasm, acoustic nerve dysfunction and glossopharyngeal neuralgia: Definitive microsurgical treatment and results in 117 patients. **Neurochirurgie** 20:145–154, 1977.
15. Jannetta PJ: Microsurgery of cranial nerve cross-compression. **Clin Neurosurg** 26:607–615, 1979.
16. Jannetta PJ: Hemifacial spasm caused by a venule: Case report. **Neurosurgery** 49:669–678, 1978.
17. Jannetta PJ: Treatment of trigeminal neuralgia by micro-operative decompression in Youmans JR (ed): *Neurological Surgery*. Philadelphia, W.B. Saunders Co., 1982, ed 2, vol 6, pp 3589–3603.
18. Jannetta PJ, Abassy M, Maroon JC, Ramos FM, Albin MS: Etiology and definitive microsurgical treatment of hemifacial spasm. **J Neurosurg** 47:321–328, 1977.
19. Jannetta PJ, Moller MB, Moller AR: Disabling positional vertigo. **N Engl J Med** 310:1700–1705, 1984.
20. Lovely TJ: Efficacy and complications of microvascular decompression: A review. **Neurosurg Q** 8:92–106, 1998.
21. Lovely TJ, Jannetta PJ: Microvascular decompression for trigeminal neuralgia: Surgical technique and long-term results. **Neurosurg Clin N Am** 8:11–29, 1997.
22. Moller AR: The cranial nerve vascular compression syndrome: II—A review of pathophysiology. **Acta Neurochir (Wien)** 113:24–30, 1991.
23. Moller MB, Moller AR, Jannetta PJ, Jho HD: Vascular decompression surgery for severe tinnitus: Selection criteria and results. **Laryngoscope** 103:421–427, 1993.
24. Moller MB, Moller AR, Jannetta PJ, Jho HD, Sekhar LN: Microvascular decompression of the eighth nerve in patients with disabling positional vertigo selection criteria and operative results in 207 patients. **Acta Neurochir (Wien)** 125:75–82, 1993.
25. Moller MB, Moller AR, Jannetta PJ, Sekhar LN: Diagnosis and surgical treatment of disabling positional vertigo. **J Neurosurg** 64:21–28, 1986.
26. Sindou M, Mertens P: Microsurgical vascular decompression (MVD) in trigeminal and glosso-vago-pharyngeal neuralgia: A 20 year experience. **Acta Neurochir (Wien)** 58:168–170, 1993.
27. Taarnhøj P: Decompression of the trigeminal root and the posterior part of the ganglion as treatment in trigeminal neuralgia: Preliminary communication. **J Neurosurg** 9:288–290, 1952.

CHAPTER

35

Endoscopic Pituitary Surgery

CARL B. HEILMAN, M.D., WILLIAM A. SHUCART, M.D.,
ELIE E. REBEIZ, M.D., AND HARSHA GOPAL, M.D.

Endoscopic pituitary surgery is gaining in popularity as neurosurgeons become more familiar with endoscopic techniques (1–7). This chapter presents one method for the removal of pituitary adenomas, best termed the "endoscopic sphenoidotomy" approach. The endoscopic sphenoidotomy procedure is performed by working through one nostril without a septal dissection. This approach eliminates the need for postoperative nasal packing, eliminates the incidence of lip numbness and oronasal fistulas, and is less painful to the patient.

At New England Medical Center in Boston, the sublabial transseptal approach was used for resection of pituitary adenomas up until 1989. From 1989 to 1993 pituitary adenomas were removed by the transnasal transseptal approach to eliminate lip numbness and to decrease postoperative patient discomfort. In 1993 the authors began using the endoscope in addition to the microscope during pituitary tumor resection after a transnasal transseptal exposure. The endoscope was used to identify tumors superiorly and laterally within the sella beyond the visual field of the microscope. In May 1995 we began performing the endoscopic transnasal sphenoidotomy approach to the sella without a septal mucosal dissection. To date, we have used this approach on 34 lesions, 27 of which were pituitary adenomas (*Table 35.1*). This chapter summarizes our experience and current surgical technique.

TABLE 35.1
Endoscopic Sphenoidotomy Approach to the Sella[a]

Pituitary adenomas
  Nonsecretors (17)
  Acromegalics (7)
  Cushing's (3)
Sellar lesions other than adenoma (7)

[a]Study of 34 patients conducted May 1995 to August 1998.

ANATOMY

All surgeons who perform transsphenoidal pituitary surgery are familiar with the anatomy of the nasal septum, vomer, rostrum of the sphenoid sinus, sphenoid sinus septations, sella floor, carotid arteries, and cavernous sinuses. The anatomy of the superior nasal turbinate and sphenoid sinus ostium must also be understood to safely perform the endoscopic sphenoidotomy approach. The sphenoid sinus ostium is located above the floor of the sphenoid sinus. This ostium is just above the midpoint between the sphenoid sinus floor and the planum sphenoidale. When viewed from within the nasal cavity, the sphenoid sinus ostium is located in the lateral aspect of the posterior nasal cavity just above the inferior margin of the superior turbinate. It is often initially obscured by nasal mucosal tissue. Gentle lateral retraction of the superior turbinate usually brings it into view.

SURGICAL TECHNIQUE

The endoscopic sphenoidotomy technique is performed by using 0- and 30-degree rigid rod endoscopes. A 70-degree endoscope is necessary only on rare occasions. Instruments are passed beside the endoscope and not through a working channel. A 0-degree Storz or Aesculap endoscope connected to a three-chip camera and light source are ideal. The Endoscrub device (Xomed-Treace) can be used to keep the tip of the endoscope clean of blood. C-arm fluoroscopy is used as an added safety measure. Lateral fluoroscopy of the head is used intermittently to check the superior and inferior extent of the sphenoidotomy and to confirm the location of instruments in the suprasellar space during the removal of macroadenomas. In recurrent adenomas or selected cases with abnormal sphenoid sinus septations, we have used the Radionics frameless stereotactic navigational device (Optical Tracking System, Radionics, Burlington, MA) for intraoperative guidance as an additional safety measure.

The endoscopic sphenoidotomy technique is performed by holding the endoscope in the left hand while supporting it superiorly against the soft tissue of the nares. Instruments are then inserted under the endoscope. Learning to work with the endoscope and instruments, one above another, provides the surgeon with a significant amount of working space. If the surgeon tries to use the endoscope and an instrument side-by-side, the working space is diminished, the scope and instrument interfere with one another, and the procedure is difficult.

A number of instruments are available in the ENT–Functional Endoscopic Sinus Surgery (FESS) catalogs that have indwelling suction ports. Microdissectors, pituitary rongeurs, and curettes all can be purchased with attached indwelling suction ports to allow the surgeon to suction and dissect with the dominant hand while holding the endoscope with the nondominant hand. Endoscope holding devices attached to the operating room table can sometimes be used to free up both hands to allow the surgeon to suction and dissect simultaneously. However, downward drift of the endoscope because of the weight of the attached camera is a common problem.

The patient is positioned supine in three-point Mayfield pin fixation with the head elevated above the heart and turned to the patient's right. The surgeon then stands next to the patient's right arm and has direct visual access up the nose to the sella.

The periumbilical region is prepped and draped for a fat graft to pack the sella if intraoperative cerebrospinal fluid leak occurs. Cotton patties soaked in cocaine are placed in the right nostril for vasoconstriction. While vasoconstriction is occurring, the endoscope equipment is set up. If frameless stereotactic navigation is used, the patient's head position is registered by sequentially touching the scalp and facial fiducial markers. The nasal region is prepped and draped in the usual fashion. The endoscope is placed into the right nasal opening, and the anterior aspect of the inferior turbinate is identified. The middle turbinate is then identified, and a Penfield 1 dissector is used to gently move the middle turbinate laterally away from the nasal septum. The endoscope is then advanced between the middle turbinate and the nasal septum until the anterior aspect of the superior turbinate is identified. The superior turbinate is gently compressed laterally until the sphenoid sinus ostium is identified (*Fig. 35.1*). If the sphenoid sinus ostium cannot be identified, lateral C-arm fluoroscopy is used to help determine its location. If the ostium still cannot be identified directly, a small dissector or suction catheter can usually be gently pushed through the mucosa in the region of the sphenoid sinus ostium into the sphenoid sinus to make an ostium. A small curette is used to widen the natural sphenoid sinus ostium in a downward and medial direction toward the vomer or rostrum of the sphenoid.

The sphenoidotomy is widened until the right sphenoid sinus cavity is visualized (*Fig. 35.2*). A dissector is then used to dissect through the right septal mucosa and posterior vomer into the submucosal plane of the contralateral nasal cavity. This opening is made at the junction of the posterior aspect of the vomer with the rostrum of the sphenoid sinus and is the only difficult aspect of the exposure. Once the septal bone has been detached from the anterior aspect of the sphenoid sinus rostrum, the mucosa of the contralateral nasal cavity is dissected off of the

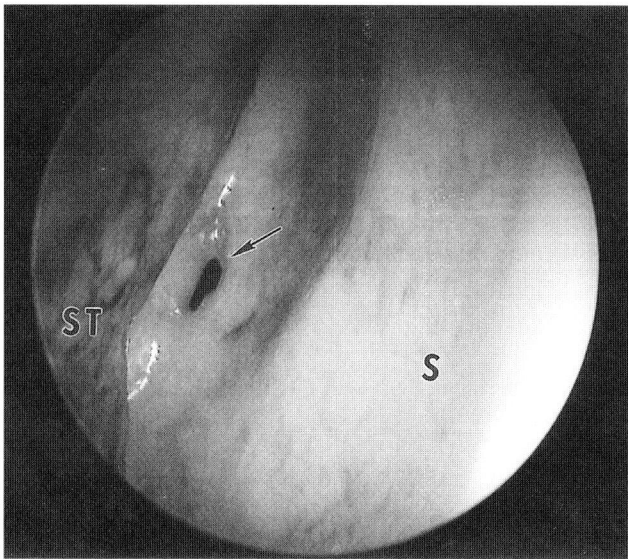

FIG. 35.1 The endoscopic view of a right sphenoid ostium (*arrow*). The nasal septum is on the right (*S*). The superior turbinate (*ST*) is to the left of the ostium.

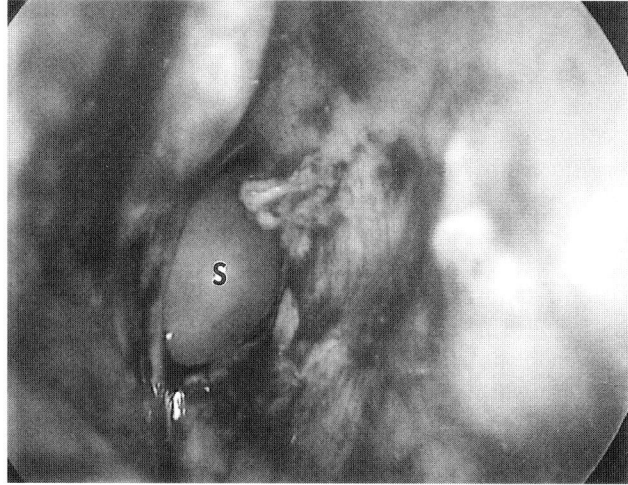

FIG. 35.2 The sphenoid ostium has been widened in a downward and medial direction. A view is obtained into the sphenoid sinus (*S*).

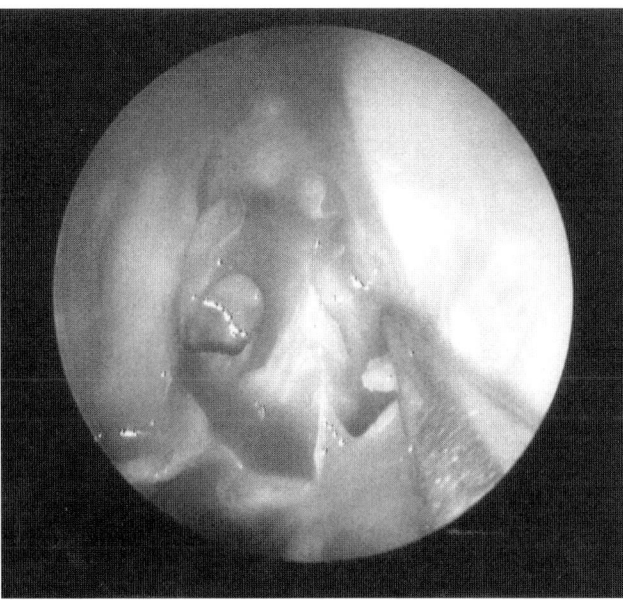

FIG. 35.3 The posterior aspect of the nasal septum has been separated from the rostrum of the sphenoid sinus. The suction tip is in the contralateral sphenoid sinus ostium. The bone exposed must be removed for exposure of the sella. (Reprinted from Ref. 3 with permission.)

anterior aspect of the left sphenoid sinus until the contralateral sphenoid sinus ostium is identified (*Fig. 35.3*). The exposure of the sphenoid sinus is thus midline, with visualization present from sphenoid ostium to ostium. The rostrum of the sphenoid is then removed using a pituitary forceps, small curettes, or, occasionally, a small osteotome.

The sphenoid sinus is inspected with the endoscope. The sphenoid sinus septum is removed using a pituitary rongeur. The carotid and optic nerve impressions are identified if visible, and the sellar outline is determined (*Fig. 35.4*). A pediatric Hardy nasal speculum is inserted into the right nasal cavity. An adult speculum usually takes up too much space for this approach. The pediatric speculum reaches just past the anterior half of the middle turbinate and holds it laterally, away from the nasal septum, providing a wider working space. The surgery can be performed without a nasal speculum, but we have found that the speculum adds no discomfort to the patient and makes the introduction of instruments during surgery much easier.

The sphenoid septum is removed back to the floor of the sella. The floor of the sella is opened with a small curette, a Penfield 4 dissector,

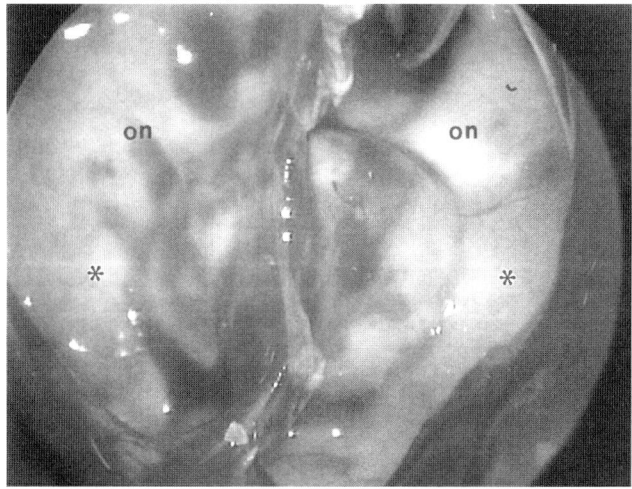

FIG. 35.4 Endoscopic view within the sphenoid sinus showing the impression of the sella into the sphenoid sinus. The sphenoid sinus septum has been partially removed. The impression of the optic nerves (*on*) and internal carotid arteries (*) can be seen. (Reprinted from Ref. 3 with permission.)

or, if thick, an osteotome or drill is required. The opening is widened using a kerrison punch until there is wide exposure of the anterior aspect of the sella. A standard transsphenoidal bipolar forceps is used to coagulate the dura. The dura is opened in a cruciate fashion using a bayonet #11 blade.

The tumor can usually be removed by working solely with the endoscope. A self-retaining retractor can hold the endoscope so two instruments can be introduced below it. However, even the best self-retaining retractors tend to drift a little with the weight of the endoscope and camera. If the tumor is vascular or troublesome bleeding occurs from the edges of the dural opening, the intraoperative microscope can be brought into use and the tumor resected in the usual microsurgical fashion.

The tumor is removed using ring curettes, suction, and pituitary rongeurs. In large tumors the lateral aspect of the tumor is removed first, leaving the central portion to the end. Air introduced by a lumbar spinal catheter can be used during removal of a macroadenoma to cap the top of the tumor as seen by lateral C-arm fluoroscopy. Alternatively frameless stereotactic navigation can be used with light-emitting diodes attached to ring curettes or dissecting forceps. Once the majority of the tumor has been removed, the endoscope is advanced into the sella for direct inspection. Additional tumor is often visible along the lateral aspects of the sella and superiorly, and is removed under endoscopic vision.

In microadenomas wherein CSF is not seen at surgery, the tumor cavity is filled with Gelfoam or Surgicel and no abdominal fat is used. The sellar floor is not reconstructed. In macroadenoma surgery without CSF leak, the sella is packed with a small abdominal fat graft. In cases when CSF is seen during surgery, the sella and sphenoid sinus are packed with abdominal fat, anterior rectus fascia, Gelfoam, and fibrin glue. The sphenoid sinus mucosa must be removed as much as possible when packed with fat. A postoperative spinal drain is used on occasion, depending on the size of the CSF leak, the adequacy of packing, and the healing capabilities of the patient.

The endoscope is removed and anesthesia reversed. No nasal packing is needed. Patients are observed in the hospital overnight. If there is no evidence of CSF leak or polyuria, the patient is discharged home on postoperative day 1 or 2 (*Table 35.2*).

RESULTS

Nine of 11 patients with visual loss due to optic chiasm compression showed improvement in their visual fields. Five of the seven patients with acromegaly had normalization of growth hormone levels postoperatively. Only one of the three patients with Cushing's disease returned to normal. Two patients with Cushing's disease showed persistently abnormal adrenocorticotropic hormone and cortisol levels. Both of these patients had had prior transsphenoidal surgery by the sublabial transseptal approach years before the current procedure. Their persistent Cushing's disease was thought to be secondary to microscopic residual disease in the cavernous sinus. One of these patients has had an adrenalectomy.

TABLE 35.2
Hospital Stay after Endoscopic Sphenoidotomy for Pituitary Adenoma[a]

No. of Patients	Postoperative Discharge Day
8	1
9	2
5	3
3	4
1	5
1	12

[a]n = 27 patients.

Eight patients were discharged home the morning after surgery. Nine patients went home on postoperative day 2. Complications included the following: two patients with postoperative CSF leaks, both requiring repeat endoscopic packing of the sella and sphenoid sinus (three other intraoperative CSF leaks seen); one patient developed permanent diabetes insipidus and two others had transient diabetes insipidus; and one patient had an abdominal fat graft harvest site hemotoma. There were no cases of lip numbness, oronasal fistula, denture problems or eating discomfort, visual deterioration, septal perforation, or nasal deformity in the immediate postoperative period. In addition, there were no cranial nerve injuries, carotid injuries, or deaths.

The two Cushing's disease patients who had had prior sublabial transseptal approaches commented that the endoscopic sphenoidotomy approach was less painful and made for an easier recovery than the transseptal approach.

In summary, the endoscopic sphenoidotomy approach to pituitary adenomas is an excellent surgical technique. It provides the surgeon with an almost identical exposure of the sella as provided by the sublabial transseptal approach. If necessary, the microscope can still be used through this exposure. The endoscopic sphenoidotomy approach has become our procedure of choice for sellar lesions.

REFERENCES

1. Cappabianca P, Alfieri A, de Divitiis E: Endoscopic endonasal transsphenoidal approach to the sella: Towards functional endoscopic pituitary surgery (FEPS). **Minim Invasive Neurosurg** 41:66–73, 1998.
2. Carrau RL, Jho HD, Ko Y: Transnasal-transsphenoidal endoscopic surgery of the pituitary gland. **Laryngoscope** 106:914–918, 1996.
3. Heilman CB, Shucart WA, Rebeiz EE: Endoscopic sphenoidotomy approach to the sella. **Neurosurgery** 41:602–607, 1997.
4. Jho HD, Carrau RL: Endoscopic endonasal transsphenoidal surgery: Experience with 50 patients. **J Neurosurg** 87:44–51, 1997.
5. Jho HD, Carrau RL, Ko Y, Daly Ma: Endoscopic pituitary surgery: An early experience. **Surg Neurol** 47:213–223, 1997.
6. Sethi DS, Pillay PK: Endoscopic management of lesions of the sella turcica. **J Laryngol Otol** 109:956–962, 1995.
7. Yaniv E, Rappaport ZH: Endoscopic transseptal transsphenoidal surgery for pituitary tumors. **Neurosurgery** 40:944–946, 1997.

CHAPTER

36

Endoscopic-assisted Tumor and Neurovascular Procedures

CHARLES TEO, M.B.B.S., F.R.A.C.S.

Endoscopic-assisted microneurosurgery is the use of a rigid endoscope, in the evaluation and treatment of pathology, that is approached through a standard microsurgical technique. The aim of the endoscope is to minimize retraction, decrease complications that may occur because of limited visualization and evaluate effectiveness of the procedure, e.g., the completeness of tumor removal or the patency of perforators around in aneurysm. These benefits are difficult to assess objectively, especially when the evaluator is also an advocate of the technique. Furthermore, benefits, such as enhanced surgeon's confidence, improved resident teaching, and shortened operative time, are difficult to accurately measure. This chapter aims to objectively evaluate the usefulness of the endoscope when used as an adjunct to standard microsurgical techniques.

MATERIALS AND METHODS

The charts of the last 100 patients who underwent endoscopic-assisted microsurgery were evaluated. The patients were gathered from the Arkansas Children's Hospital, the University of Arkansas for Medical Science Medical Center, and the John McLellan Veteran's Hospital in Little Rock, Arkansas. Information gathered from the charts addressed operative time, technique used, benefits or otherwise from the endoscope, and any complications that would not have occurred without the endoscope. Examples of objective evidence of benefit included the following:

- definition of tumor boundaries that could not be elucidated with the microscope and that resulted in expeditious tumor removal
- a more limited approach because the endoscope revealed pathology that would normally have required a bigger craniotomy
- discovery of residual tumor that could not be seen with the microscope alone

- identification of perforators or improved definition or aneurysm anatomy
- identification of occluded perforators or "unclipped" aneurysm after application of the clip
- ability to perform a definitive procedure e.g., an endoscopic third ventriculosotmy instead of a shunt.

The mean age of patients was 22 years with a range from 2 weeks to 72 years of age. The patients included 58 males and 42 females. In all cases, standard microsurgical techniques were used, and the rigid endoscope was introduced in one of the following ways:

Ipsilateral

The endoscope is introduced through the craniotomy either under microscope control or free-hand while watching the screen. This is the least invasive and most used method. The obvious advantage is that further dissection is not necessary, and therefore, there is virtually no chance of added morbidity. The major disadvantage is the clutter of instruments in an already crowded corridor. The ipsilateral method is ideal for tumor and neurovascular procedures, for which the surgeon needs added visualization of structures that are hidden from the microscope, e.g., perforators behind an aneurysm or a tumor in the apex of the internal acoustic meatus.

Contralateral

The endoscope is introduced through a contralateral burr hole or craniotomy, attached to a self-retaining retractor, and left in position while the pathology is approached through a separate opening using standard microsurgical techniques. Contralateral is the least used method and clearly the most invasive. It requires another opening, and unfortunately the patient becomes vulnerable to all the risks inherent to creating another opening e.g., neurovascular damage, seizures, postoperative hematoma, and infection. The advantages of the contralateral method include a unique perspective on the pathology and no cluttering of instruments. Ideal situations for use of this method would include giant aneurysms where an ipsilateral approach would not offer any benefit because the size of the dome would prevent visualization around it.

Transventricular

The endoscope is introduced into the ventricle through a separate burr hole. This transventricular method offers visualization of the intraventricular component of the pathology. Other advantages of this method include the ability to address any intraventricular pathology such as hydrocephalus. The disadvantage is the added morbidity of another burr hole and ventricular puncture. Invariably, patients that may benefit from this technique would have required a ventricular puncture anyway. Typical examples are the patient with a suprasellar tumor and secondary hydrocephalus or the patient with a basilar tip aneurysm that had ruptured into the third ventricle with secondary hydrocephalus. In both examples, the scope introduced into the third ventricle can add a unique perspective to the case and yet has not increased the morbidity of the procedure.

TRANSSPHENOIDAL

The endoscope is introduced through the nose, and access to the sphenoid sinus is made by expanding the sphenoid ostium. The transsphenoidal endoscopic method is ideal for large pituitary tumors that have suprasellar and infrasellar extension. These tumors sometimes need a combined approach and the endoscope may help in two ways. First, an initial endoscopic approach may obviate the need for a craniotomy if the entire tumor can be removed from below, and second, if a craniotomy is required in the future, the scope can be left in position to aid in visualization, illumination, and irrigation.

RESULTS

A retrospective analysis was performed on the last 100 consecutive cases where the endoscope was used during a standard microsurgical procedure. An independent assessor then reviewed their charts and completed a questionnaire (Table 36.1). Table 36.2 lists the pathological process that were seen. There were 70 tumors, 42 were found in adults and 28 in pediatric patients. Most of the tumors were skull based, but there were also pineal and intraventricular lesions. The other 30 patients had aneurysms, 23 in the anterior circulation and 7 in the posterior circulation. A rigid scope was used in 88 patients and a flexible fiber-optic scope in 12 patients. Scope introduction was ipsilateral in 85 patients, transventricular in 10, and transsphenoidal in 5; the contralateral approach was never used. The scope proved to be a definite benefit in 70% of cases. In another 15 cases, the scope was thought to be of some subjective benefit; the scope could be a good teaching aid or possibly save operative time. Although the scope caused no disadvantages there was no objective proof of benefit in the remaining patients. The overall complication rate in this series was 12%, which

TABLE 36.1
Questionnaire for Objectively Assessing Efficacy of Endoscopic-assisted Surgery

Patients name _____	Medical record number _____
Diagnosis _____	
Start time _____	Finish time _____
Craniotomy _____	Type _____
Type of scope _____	Method of introduction _____
(i = ipsilateral, c = contralateral, t = tranventricular, s = transsphenoidal)	
Reason for endoscope _____	Beneficial Yes ___ No ___
If yes, why? _____	If no, why? _____
Added benefit (e.g., good teaching aid) ___	
Complications _____	Complications of endoscope ___

included temporary cranial nerve dysfunction, meningitis, and panhypopituitarism. However, the use of the scope could only be definitely implicated in two of those cases. The first was a cerebrospinal fluid leak after a combined approach to a pituitary tumor, which could have occurred anyway. The second complication was an asymptomatic frontal contusion from a transventricular approach.

The following cases illustrate cases in which the scope was objectively beneficial.

Case 1

The patient was a 5-year-old female with a recurrent craniopharyngioma. The tumor extended into the third ventricle and had a satellite lesion within the lateral ventricle. There was secondary hydrocephalus.

Treatment of the patient began with a right frontal burr hole, placement of a peelaway sheath, and insertion of a rigid 4mm, 30-angled scope for removal of the metastatic, intraventricular lesion. The scope was then removed, and the peelaway sheath was left to maintain access to the ventricle. The patient was then repositioned to allow a stan-

TABLE 36.2
Pathology in Patients in whom Endoscopic-assisted Microneurosurgery was Used

Pathology	No. of Patients
Tumors	
Adult	42
Pediatric	28
Aneurysms	
Anterior circulation	23
Posterior circulation	7

dard pterional cranitomy. The scope was then repositioned in the ventricle and gave the surgeon an excellent view of the intraventricular component of the tumor. The tumor was removed in the usual microsurgical fashion with excellent illumination from within the third ventricle, easier determination of the tumor-hypothalamic plane, and reassurance that the tumor was completely removed from the ventricle. Apart from diabetes insipidus, no other complications occurred, and the patient was discharged within a week of the surgery.

Case 2

An 11-year-old male patient was referred to our service with a partially resected chordoma of the lower clivus, which had shown aggressive biological activity by regrowing within 6 weeks of the initial resection. The patient underwent a transcondylar approach to the tumor, with preservation of the anterior half of the occipital condyle. Unfortunately, this did not enable complete visualization of the tumor, which meant either complete removal of the condyle or an incomplete resection. A rigid 30-degree angled scope was introduced ipsilaterally, which gave excellent visualization of the rest of the tumor (*Fig. 36.1*) and allowed complete macroscopic clearance. The child did extremely well postoperatively, without complication and with a stable atlantooccipital joint. Approximately 1 year after proton-beam irradiation, he is tumor-free with full range of movement of his neck.

Case 3

A 54-year-old woman presented with a cerebellopontine angle meningioma. It was causing increasing dysesthesia and pain. Magnetic resonance imaging demonstrated that the tumor was mostly in the posterior fossa, but there was a tail of enhancement extending through the tentorial incisura and into the middle cranial fossa.

The patient underwent a standard retrosigmoid craniectomy, with preparation for a petrosal approach for removal of the supratentorial component if necessary. Once the cerebellopontine angle portion was removed, a rigid scope was introduced ipsilaterally, but which the tail of tumor could be seen and removed. The patient did not need a more extensive cranitomy and the postoperative magnetic resonance imaging showed no residual tumor. Her postoperative course was uneventful and she remains tumor-free.

DISCUSSION

The endoscope has many different applications. Pure endoscopic surgery describes surgery that is performed through working channels,

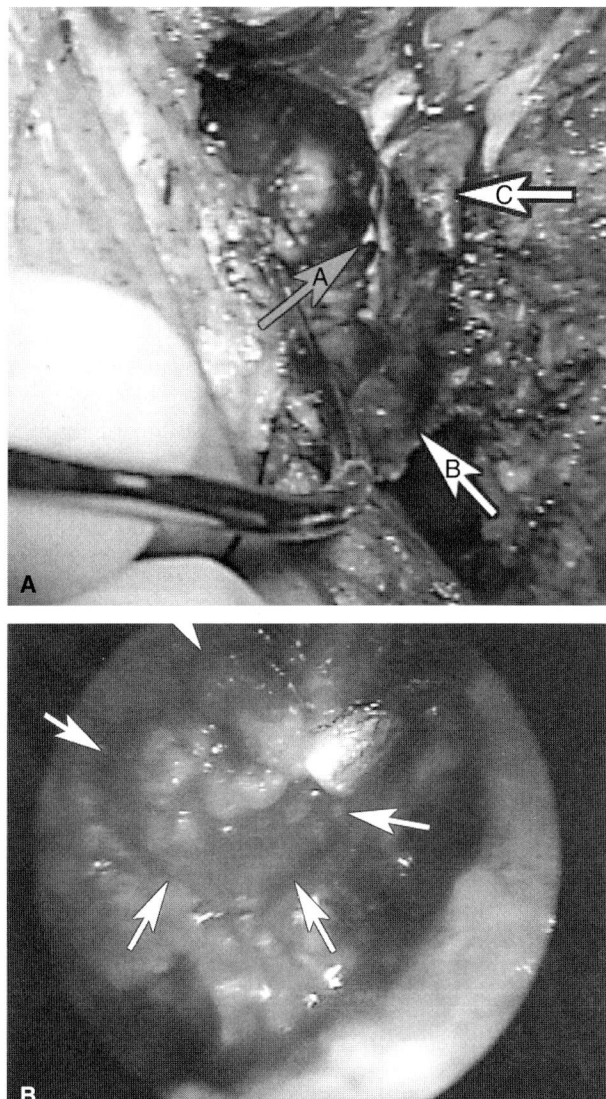

FIG. 36.1 (*A*) View through the microscope of apparent complete removal of a chordoma through a right transcondylar approach. *Arrow A*, area examined with endoscope; *Arrow B*, vertebral artery; *Arrow C*, anterior half of occipital condyle. (*B*) Residual tumor in the clivus area seen through a 30° angled rigid endoscope. The ultrasonic aspirator is seen in the *right upper corner*.

such as bronchoscopy and cystoscopy. Pure endoscopic surgery can perform, most intraventricular procedures. However, there are many limitations, not the least of which is the selection of instrumentation. Tools are small, clumsy, and fragile. Endoscopic guided surgery is surgery performed under endoscopic visualization only, such as laparoscopic and arthroscopic surgery. The endoscope provides the only means of visualization, and instruments are passed down separate portals. Examples, of neurosurgical endoscopy are endoscopic transsphenoidal surgery, laparoscopic anterior spinal surgery, and thoracoscopic sympathectomy. The obvious advantage of this technique is the freedom to use instruments that are not limited in their size and do not have to be flexible.

Endoscopic assisted microneurosurgery is the marriage of the microscope and the endoscope. The microscope has many positive features; the magnification is variable, the view is stereoscopic, and it does not get in the way of the instruments. However, the microscope cannot look around corners, and illumination is diminished by the size and depth of the incision. The endoscope, on the other hand, "takes" light to the pathology, is not effected by the size or depth of the incision, and can look around corners. It seems only natural to combine the two tools. The advantages are that one is not dependent on a single source for one's image, there is no restriction on instrumentation, and the anatomical information is doubled.

A few important safety rules should be followed when endoscopic-assisted microneurosurgery is performed. The scope should be placed into the field under direct vision, either with the naked eye or the microscope. Placing the scope under control of its own image can cause damage to structures that are not in the field of view. Once the scope is in a good position, it should be fixed with a flexible and lockable device so that the surgeon can operate with both hands. The precaution becomes even more important when the transventricular or contralateral routes are used.

This series demonstrates the subjective (85%) and objective (70%) benefits gained by adopting endoscopic-assisted microsurgery. Although the literature is sparse, the concept is not new (1–10). With endoscopy, tumors can be resected more completely with less morbidity, their borders can be defined more accurately, and their degree of resection can be assessed more precisely (*Fig. 36.2*). Aneurysm anatomy can be more readily clarified (*Fig. 36.3*), and once clipped, the integrity of perforators can be determined confidently (*Fig. 36.4*). Furthermore, endoscopy appears to be a very effective teaching aid, which gives residents a new perspective on anatomy. Most microsurgical procedures

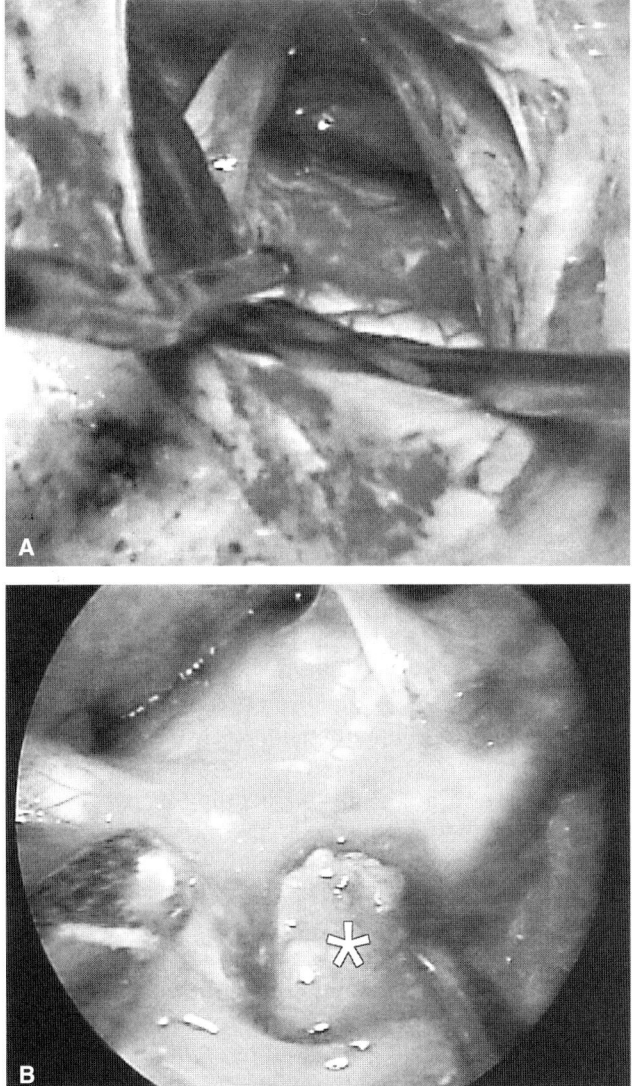

FIG. 36.2 (A) Apparent complete removal of a posterior fossa ependymoma as seen through the microscope. (B) A 30° angled endoscope clearly reveals residual tumor (*) in the foramen of Luschka.

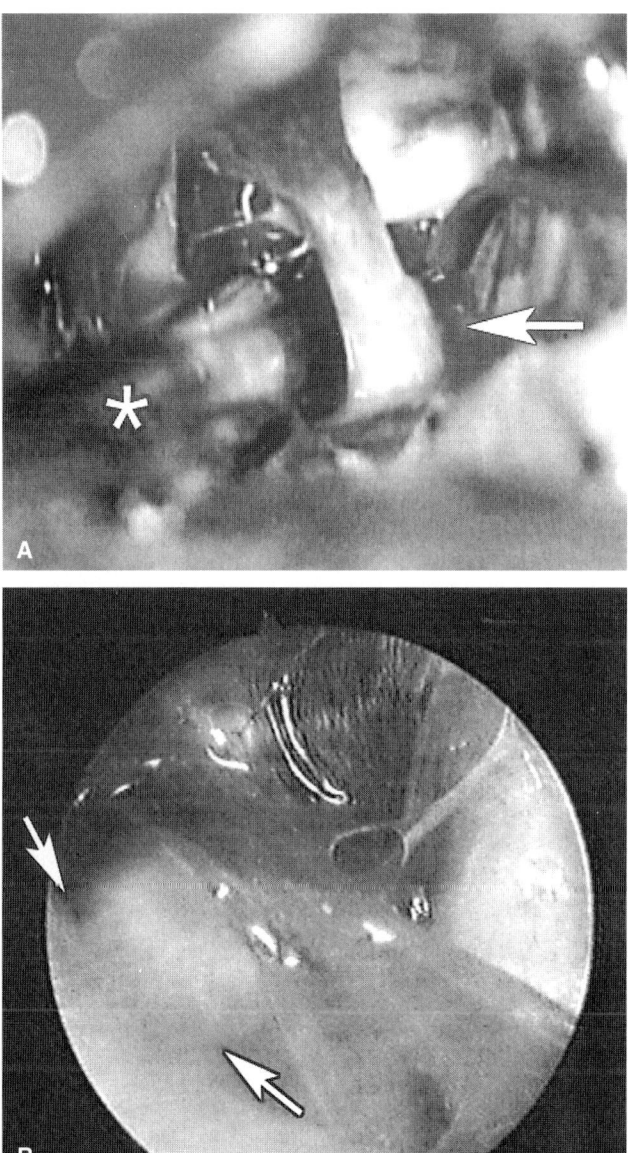

FIG. 36.3 (*A*) This right-sided anterior choroidal artery aneurysm is directly "beneath" the internal carotid artery and hidden from the microscope. *Arrow* points to unseen aneurysm; * indicates the endoscope. (*B*) View of the aneurysm neck through the endoscope (*) placed through the optico-carotid window.

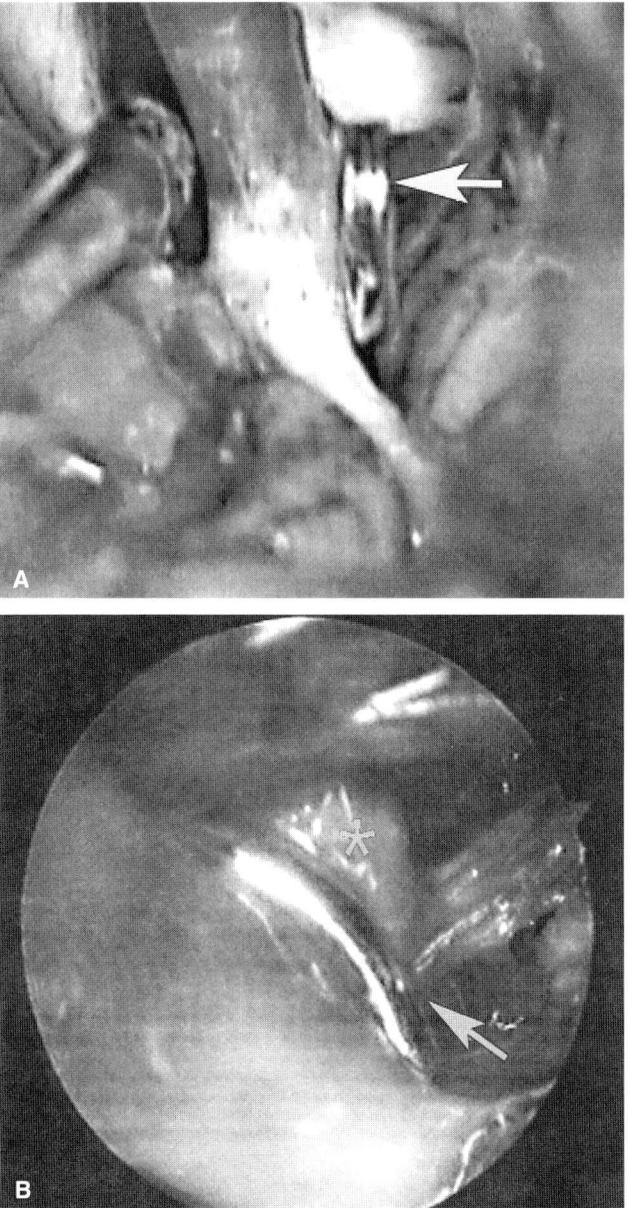

FIG. 36.4 (A) The aneurysm seen in Fig. 36.3B is now clipped. (B) The endoscope reveals a perforator caught in the aneurysm clip. *Arrow* points to the clipped perforator; * indicates the aneurysm.

will be enhanced with endoscopy, and the most common method will be the introduction of a rigid 30°-angled scope through the craniotomy itself and immobilization of the scope with a rigid holder.

CONCLUSION

Applications for neuroendoscopy are rapidly expanding. Initially the importance of endoscopy in the management of intraventricular pathology placed the pediatric neurosurgeon at the helm. Endoscopic-assisted microneurosurgery, as it applies to pathology in the subarachnoid space, should have particular interest to the adult neurosurgeon. The microscope will never replace the headlight and loupes, nor will the endoscope ever replace the microscope. It will simply move us one step closer in our perpetual quest for minimally invasive and maximally effective surgery, with the ultimate goal of providing better care for our patients.

REFERENCES

1. Apuzzo MLJ, Heifetz MD, Weiss MH, Kurze T: Neurosurgical endoscopy using the side-viewing telescope: Technical note. **J Neurosurg** 46:398–400, 1977.
2. Cohen AR, Perneczky A, Rodziewicz GS, Gingold SI: Endoscope-assisted craniotomy: Approach to the rostral brain stem. **Neurosurgery** 36:1128–1129, 1995.
3. Fries G, Perneczky A: Endoscope-assisted brain surgery: Part 2—Analysis of 380 procedures. **Neurosurgery** 42:226–232, 1998.
4. Fries G, Reisch R: Biportal neuroendoscopic microsurgical approaches to the subarachnoid cisterns: A cadaver study. **Minim Invasive Neurosurg** 39:99–104, 1996.
5. Fukushima T: Endoscopy of Meckel's cave, cisterna magna and cerebellopontine angle: Technical note. **J. Neurosurg** 48:302–306, 1978.
6. Grotenhuis JA: Endoscope-assisted craniotomy, in *Techniques in Neurosurgery*. Philadelphia, Lippincott-Raven Publishers, 1996, pp 201–212.
7. Perneczky A, Fries G: Endoscope-assisted brain surgery: Part 1—Evolution, basic concept, and current technique. **Neurosurgery** 42:219–225, 1998.
8. Prott W: Cisternoscopy-endoscopy of the cerebellopontine angle. **Acta Neurochir (Wein)** 31:105–113, 1974.
9. Teo C: Endoscopic neurosurgery, in Andrews R (ed): *Intraoperative Neuroprotection*. Baltimore, Williams and Wilkins, 1996, pp 423–443.
10. Teo C. Neuroendoscopy: Current application and future directions. *Surgical Technology International*. San Francisco, Universal Medical Press, 1997, 327–333.

CHAPTER

37

Endoscopic Spine Surgery

CURTIS A. DICKMAN, M.D., PAUL W. DETWEILER, M.S., M.D.,
AND RANDALL W. PORTER, M.D.

The recent trend toward minimally invasive surgery of the spine has been facilitated by a number of factors, including rapid improvements in video-assisted endoscopic technology, patients' desire to limit their postoperative pain and the time needed to recover, and the current emphasis on delivering cost-effective care (5, 6, 10, 18, 19, 27, 29, 31, 32). Modern endoscopic equipment has been applied primarily to facilitate surgery of the thoracic and lumbar spine and paravertebral structures. Endoscopic spinal procedures include thoracoscopy, retroperitoneal endoscopy, laparoscopy, percutaneous lumbar foramenoscopy and discectomy, and microsurgical endoscopic discectomy (*Table 37.1*). Our experience at the Barrow Neurological Institute has been predominantly focused on thoracoscopy and laparoscopy, which are endoscopic techniques for accessing the thoracic and lumbar spine anteriorly. These two methods are the topic of this chapter. Common applications for these approaches include thoracic discectomy and vertebrectomy (6, 11, 12, 26, 27), thoracic sympathectomy (1, 4, 5, 13, 20, 21, 25, 28, 30), and lumbar interbody fusion (7, 8). This technology can be used to resect intrathoracic nerve sheath tumors (*Fig. 37.1*) (9) and is also being applied to correct spinal deformities in patients with kyphosis and scoliosis (*Table 37.2*) (10, 11).

ANESTHESIA FOR THORACOSCOPY

The anesthetic considerations for thoracoscopic spine surgery are similar to those for an open procedure. The patient's cardiopulmonary status should be carefully evaluated preoperatively. Pulmonary function tests and arterial blood gas analysis are evaluated in patients who smoke cigarettes and in those with lung disease, chronic obstructive pulmonary disease, or morbid obesity. A chest radiograph is routinely obtained.

Thoracoscopic procedures require general endotracheal anesthesia. Use of a double-lumen endotracheal tube facilitates single-lung

TABLE 37.1
Comparison of Endoscopic Approaches to the Thoracic and Lumbar Spine[a]

Endoscopic Approach	Approach Replaced	Levels Accessed	Working Space Created By	Technical Difficulty[b]	Indications
Posterolateral endoscopic lumbar microdiscectomy and foramenoscopy	Open far-lateral lumbar discectomy and facetectomy	L1–L2 through L5–S1	Cannula with saline irrigation	+++[b]	Far-lateral disc herniation or foraminal disc herniation (limited)
Posterior microsurgical endoscopic discectomy	Open midline posterior lumbar microdiscectomy	L1–L2 through L5–S1	Cannula/dilator and tissue sheath	+	Contained or free-fragment disc herniation (identical to open microdiscectomy). Lumbar stenosis or lateral recess stenosis.
Laparoscopic approaches	Laparotomy for anterior lumbar approaches	L4–L5 and L5–S1	CO_2 insufflation or gasless techniques	++	L4–L5 or L5–S1 degenerative instability or foraminal stenosis. Congenital spondylolisthesis (Grade I or II).
Endoscopic retroperitoneal approaches	Open retroperitoneal approach	L1–L4	Balloon dilators, CO_2 insufflation, and fan retractors	+++	L1–L4 vertebral body or disc space pathology requiring an anterolateral interbody fusion, biopsy, or corpectomy
Thoracoscopy	Thoracotomy	T1–T12	Single-lung ventilation with ipsilateral pneumothorax and atelectasis. Creates empty space in hemithorax.	+++	Sympathectomy, anterior release of thoracic spinal deformity, resection of herniated thoracic discs, resection of intrathoracic nerve sheath tumors, corpectomy and thoracic vertebral, reconstruction, biopsy of thoracic vertebral lesions

[a] Reprinted from Dickman CA: Guest Editor Commentary. **Techniques in Neurosurgery** 3(4):336–337, 1997 with permission.
[b] +, relatively easy; ++, moderately difficult; +++, requires extensive training and practice.

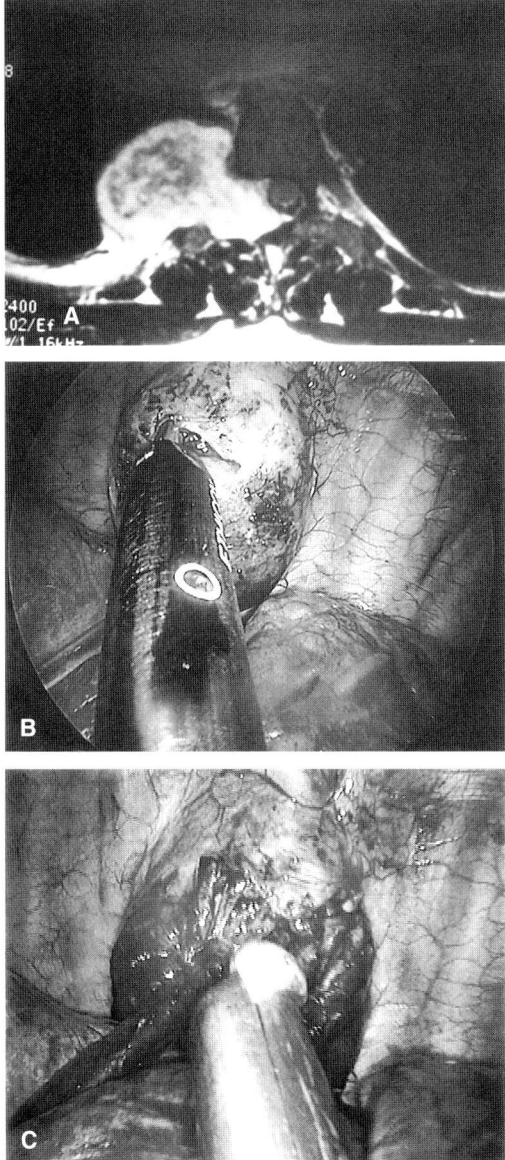

FIG. 37.1 (*A*) Axial T1-weighted magnetic resonance image with intravenous contrast demonstrating an intraspinal–extraspinal right-sided T5–T6 ganglioneurofibroma. (*B*) Thoracoscopic view of the ganglioneurofibroma. The tumor capsule is opened with electrocauterization. (*C*) The tumor is resected with a thoracoscopic pituitary rongeur.

TABLE 37.2
Barrow Neurological Institute Experience with 146 Thoracoscopic Spinal Surgeries: 1993–1998

Procedures	n
Discectomy	41
Sympathectomy	92
Biopsy	1
Nerve Sheath Tumor Resection	3
Spinal Deformity Correction[a]	2
Corpectomy	7

[a]For kyphosis or scoliosis.

ventilation on the nonoperative side. The selection of the side from which to approach the spine depends on the site of the pathology. Single-lung ventilation of the dependent lung is performed (called the down-side lung), while ventilation is blocked ipsilateral to the operative side, which allows the lung to collapse. The endotracheal tube can be placed under direct visualization or with the assistance of a fiberoptic bronchoscope. The distal endotracheal tube and balloon cuff are placed in the proximal left mainstem bronchus. A second cuff is inflated in the trachea. The bronchus on the operative side is obstructed, leading to slow collapse of the lung on that side. Several options for single-lung ventilation are available for pediatric patients, including a double-lumen endotracheal tube or a single-lumen endotracheal tube with an obstructive device (bronchial blocker) in the bronchus of the lung on the operative side.

A tidal volume of 10 to 15 ml/kg and inspired oxygen content of 100% are appropriate for a patient with no cardiorespiratory disease. Respiratory rate is adjusted to titrate the end-tidal partial pressure of carbon dioxide between 35 and 40 mm Hg. If oxygen saturation decreases during the procedure, auscultation over the inflated lung should be performed to verify that the endotracheal tube is placed appropriately. Bronchoscopy can be used as an adjunct if the placement of the endotracheal tube is in question. Alternatively, 5 to 10 mm Hg of continuous positive airway pressure can be added to the ventilated lung opposite the operative side. When pediatric patients are ventilated with a single-lumen endotracheal tube, the tube can be moved back into the trachea and the uninflated lung ventilated until the respiratory status is stabilized. To minimize postoperative atelectasis, the deflated lung is reinflated intraoperatively for 5 to 10 minutes for every hour of operating time.

A chest tube is placed at the end of the procedure to drain any fluid or blood collecting in the chest. In the case of thoracoscopic sympathectomy, both chest tubes are removed during a positive pressure breath while the patient is still under anesthesia in the operating room. In the case of discectomy or corpectomy, chest tubes are usually left in place for 24 hours after surgery. A chest radiograph always is obtained in the recovery room to verify full inflation of the lungs and to rule out or investigate a residual pneumothorax. Aggressive pulmonary care, which may include bronchodilators, deep suctioning, and deep coughing, is initiated if the patient has a significant history of respiratory difficulties.

THORACOSCOPIC SYMPATHECTOMY

Thoracic sympathectomy has become widely accepted as a permanent cure for intractable palmar and axillary hyperhidrosis (1, 4, 5, 13, 21, 25). Hyperhidrosis can have debilitating effects on social, interpersonal, recreational, and work activities. Axillary hyperhidrosis causes malodor and stains and destroys clothing. Palmar hyperhidrosis produces excessive sweating of the palms and can cause individuals to avoid shaking hands, to drop objects, and to destroy computer keyboards, among other problems. Students often destroy test paper from the perspiration. The excess sweating is produced by palmar, plantar, and axillary eccrine glands innervated by sympathetic fibers. The prevalence of hyperhidrosis is approximately 0.6 to 1.0% (13). About 25% of the cases are familial. Entities that can mimic hyperhidrosis include lymphoma, thyrotoxicosis, pheochromocytoma, carcinoid tumor, diabetes, hypothalamic pituitary dysfunction, and hypoglycemia and should be excluded preoperatively (14, 15).

Thoracic sympathectomy has also been used to treat causalgia, Raynaud's disease, essential hypertension, bronchial asthma, peptic ulcer, angina pectoris, and hyperthyroidism (1, 4, 5, 13, 20, 21, 23, 25, 28, 30). The efficacy of this procedure for treating hyperhidrosis has been established, and its success rate is 95 to 100% (1, 4, 5, 13, 14, 21, 25). Typically, the procedure is considered after medical treatment has failed. Some of these therapies may include topical antiperspirants, astringents, powders, biofeedback, botulinum toxin injections, and anticholinergics (4, 14, 20, 28). Available medical treatments work only temporarily and do not cure the hyperhidrosis. In comparison, surgical sympathectomy cures hyperhidrosis permanently. Less commonly, the procedure is used in select cases of causalgia and Raynaud's disease if patients have responded to sympathetic blocks. It is used rarely to treat other disease entities (1, 20, 21, 25, 28, 30).

Multiple open approaches have been described but are associated with significant rates of morbidity and mortality (14, 28). These approaches include the posterior midline, posterior paravertebral, anterior supraclavicular, axillary transthoracic, and axillary extrathoracic approach (8, 14, 25). The thoracoscopic approach is efficacious but, more importantly, results in better visualization of the sympathetic chain with less injury to the soft tissue of the thoracic wall than the open approaches (1, 13, 21, 23, 25). Consequently, hospitalization is briefer compared with that for an open approach. The potential complications of thoracoscopic sympathectomy are listed in *Table 37.3*. Most complications are rare (less than 1% risk). However, a compensatory increase in sweating elsewhere on the patient's body (i.e., trunk and legs) has been reported in 30 to 50% of patients (1, 4–6, 13–15, 17–21, 23, 25, 27, 28, 30).

The extent of resection or ablation of the sympathetic chain is variable. Typically, the second and third sympathetic ganglia are resected for palmar hyperhidrosis, and the fourth and fifth ganglia are also resected if axillary hyperhidrosis is present (1, 4, 5, 13–15, 20, 21, 25, 28, 30). Treatment failures are extremely rare (less than 1% in most series). Failures have been ascribed to insufficient resection of the sympathetic chain or inability to recognize the existence of the nerve of Kuntz (13, 25). Failure can be avoided by monitoring the palmar temperature intraoperatively. If the temperature rises more than 1°C, an adequate sympathectomy has been achieved.

Surgical Technique

The patient is positioned supine on the operating room table, and general endotracheal anesthesia is instituted. A double-lumen endo-

TABLE 37.3
Potential Complications of Thoracic Sympathectomy

Horner's syndrome (< 1%)
Compensatory sweating (30–50%)
Gustatory sweating (< 1%)
Vascular injury
Pneumothorax
Hemothorax
Intercostal neuralgia
Bradycardia
Phrenic nerve injury
Wound infection
Axillary anesthesia
Atelectasis
Subcutaneous emphysema

tracheal tube is used. The patient is rolled into the lateral decubitus position, and the upside arm is elevated above the chest. With the ipsilateral elbow flexed 90°, the forearm is secured to a padded instrument stand. This maneuver is performed to move the scapula out of the operative field. A generous sterile preparation is performed to facilitate conversion to an open procedure if necessary. Fortunately, we have never had to convert a thoracoscopic sympathectomy to an open thoracotomy. The patient is secured to the operating room table with tape. The table is placed in reverse Trendelenburg and rotated 40° anteriorly. This position allows gravity to retract the lung, which usually falls away from the upper thoracic spine without inserting a lung retractor.

The endoscopic portal is placed along the posterior axillary line between the fourth and fifth ribs. One or two working portals are placed along the anterior axillary line in the third and fifth intercostal spaces under direct visualization with the endoscope. The apex of the lung is retracted away from the spine. Adhesions can easily be transected with endoscopic scissors (20). If severe adhesions are encountered, converting to an open procedure should be considered. The stellate ganglion, which is located over the head of the first rib, and the upper thoracic sympathetic chain are identified (*Fig. 37.2*). The chain is located just beneath the parietal pleura and courses superficial to the intercostal vessels over the heads of the ribs. The pleura is opened distal to the T3

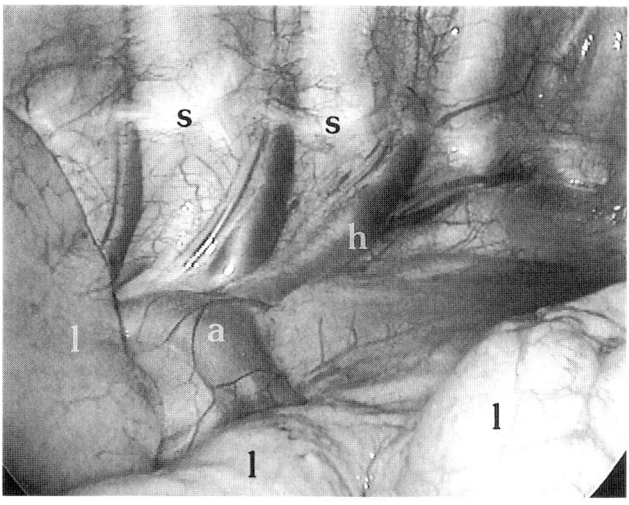

FIG. 37.2 Thoracoscopic view of the upper right sympathetic chain (S). *h*, highest intercostal vein; *a*, azygos vein; *l*, deflated lung.

or T4 ganglia and is advanced rostrally over the sympathetic chain just caudal to the inferior aspect of the stellate ganglion. If an accessory nerve of Kuntz is identified, it is exposed and excised. Starting below the T3 or T4 ganglion, the trunk is electrocoagulated and transected (*Fig. 37.3*). The upper sympathetic trunk is grasped and elevated to facilitate blunt and sharp dissection rostrally toward the stellate ganglion. The rami that communicate with each ganglion possess a rich vascular supply. Consequently, they are coagulated with bipolar cauterization before they are cut. Finally, the trunk is transected *below* the stellate ganglion and removed en bloc. The stellate ganglion is preserved to avoid Horner's sydrome.

The palmar skin temperature is monitored during the procedure. A unilateral increase of at least 1° to 3° is highly predictive of a successful clinical outcome (15). This effect is attributable to peripheral vasodilation and increased blood flow in the extremity. The increased blood flow is maximal immediately after the sympathectomy but decreases after 1 week. Failure to achieve this temperature increase should prompt a search for an aberrant accessory sympathetic trunk, such as the nerve of Kuntz (13). If an accessory trunk is not found, the inferior third of the stellate ganglion can be resected. This maneuver must be performed with great care because resection or manipulation of the stellate ganglion can produce a unilateral Horner's syndrome (13). An alternative technique for endoscopic sympathectomy involves transecting the sympathetic chain using cautery scissors and leaving the chain in situ (*Fig. 37.4*). This technique requires only two 5-mm portals. It can be performed rapidly with minimal blood loss and has become our technique of choice.

Clinical Results

We have performed 92 sympathectomies using video-assisted endoscopic treatment in 47 patients. Forty-five of the patients had bilateral sympathectomies for palmar and/or axillary hyperhidrosis. Two patients had unilateral sympathectomies for reflex sympathetic dystrophy. The endoscopic sympathectomies yielded a cure of palmar hyperhidrosis and axillary hyperhidrosis in 100% of the patients. All patients were relieved of their hyperhidrosis. We are in the process of comparing the clinical outcomes of patients treated with chain resection and those treated with in situ chain transection. No complications have been permanent. One pneumothorax occurred and was treated with chest-tube drainage. Two cases of transient postoperative intercostal neuralgia occurred and resolved. In comparison, the pain symptoms of both patients with reflex sympathetic dystrophy only margin-

534 CLINICAL NEUROSURGERY

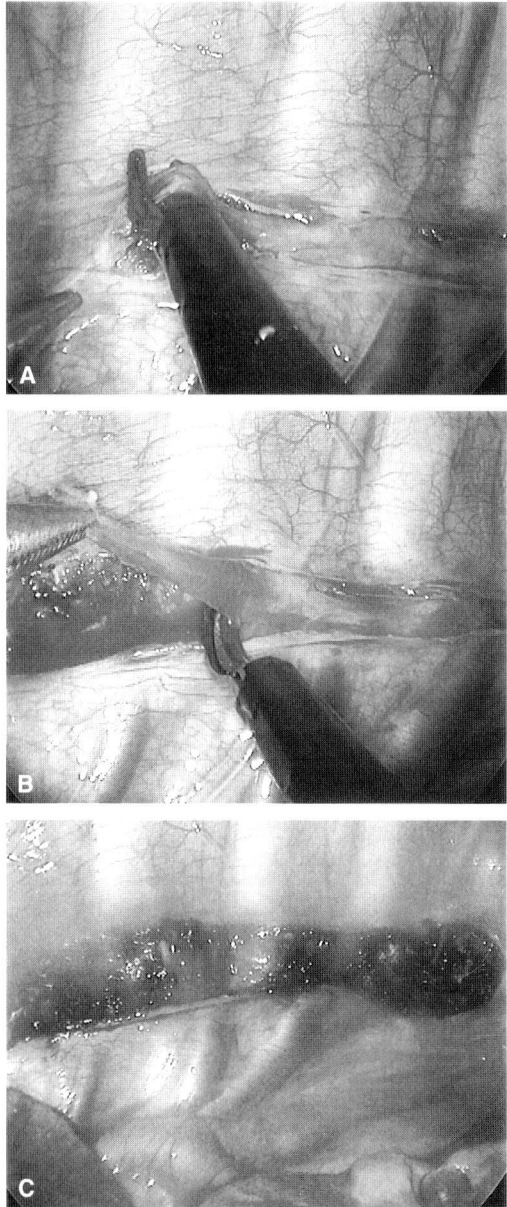

FIG. 37.3 (A) The pleura over the sympathetic chain has been opened, and the sympathetic chain is transected at T4. (B) The sympathetic chain is meticulously mobilized using scissors and electrocauterization. (C) Resection site after the sympathetic chain has been removed from T4 to the inferior stellate ganglion.

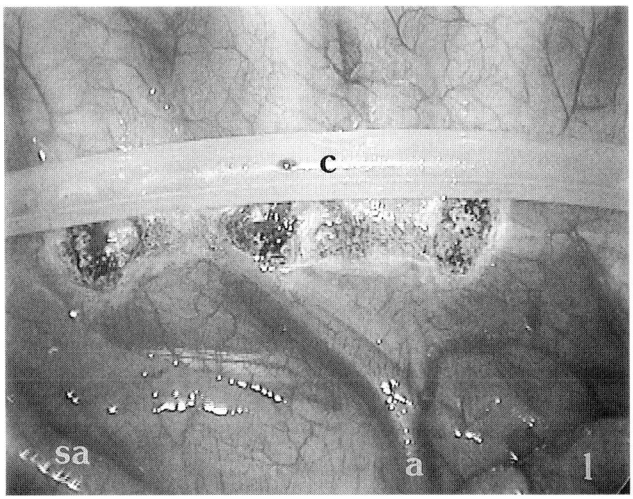

FIG. 37.4 Thoracoscopic sympathectomy of the left sympathetic chain at T2, T3, and T4. c, chest tube; a, azygos vein; l, deflated lung; sa, subclavian artery.

ally and temporarily improved, even though the sympathectomy was adequate.

THORACOSCOPIC DISCECTOMY

Classically, thoracic disc herniations manifest clinically with myelopathy and radiculopathy. Myelopathy is produced by compression of the spinal cord and is a compelling reason to pursue surgical decompression. Surgical intervention for the treatment of thoracic radiculopathy produced by compression of the thoracic root by a disc fragment depends on the length and degree of the patient's symptomatology.

Various posterior surgical approaches to the spine have been described, including the posterolateral, lateral, and transpedicular. Drawbacks of these approaches include iatrogenic spinal instability, partial visibility of midline structures, and increased postoperative pain due to extensive muscle transection (27). To optimize visibility of the anterior thecal sac and spinal cord, surgeons have adopted a transthoracic approach for midline, broad-based, and calcified disc herniations. The visibility of the ventral spinal cord is improved compared with that obtained with the posterior and posterolateral approaches. Thoracotomy is associated with morbidity, including atelectases and a significant degree of postoperative pain. Both of these drawbacks can be overcome by using a thoracoscopic approach, which provides a microsurgical view of the entire ventral surface of the spine and spinal cord. Compared with the posterolateral approaches through the thoracic spine, thoracoscopy provides better visualization and access to the ventral spine and spinal cord and facilitates a more complete resection of midline and calcified discs.

Surgical Technique

The patient is placed in a lateral decubitus position (*Fig. 37.5*). The side on which the patient is positioned is determined on the basis of the

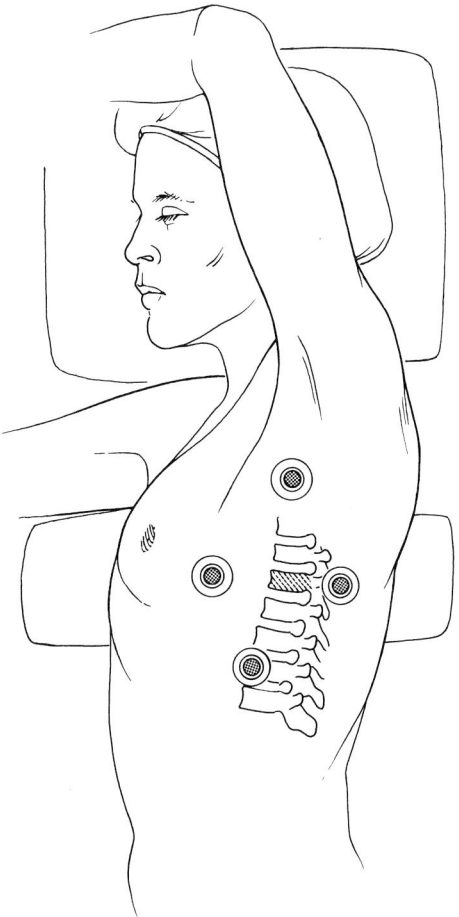

FIG. 37.5 Patients are positioned in the lateral decubitus position for either a thoracoscopic discectomy or corpectomy. The portals are placed circumferentially to surround the level of the pathology. Reprinted with permission from Barrow Neurological Institute.

side of surgical access. Single-lung ventilation is used, and the ventilated lung is positioned dependently. Before proceeding with a sterile preparation of the operative field, the level of surgery is localized using a fluoroscopic C-arm, and the skin is marked to assist with the placement of portals. The patient's skin is prepared using routine sterile technique. The portals are placed in a strategic fashion to encircle the level of pathology. This placement ensures optimal visualization and helps to prevent the working instruments from crossing over each other (referred to as fencing).

Once the endoscope has been inserted, the lung is mobilized from the surface of the spine and the ribs are counted rostrally to caudally until the disc space of interest is identified. The pleura over the adjacent rib head is cauterized to mark it, and the fluoroscopic C-arm is again used to verify that the localization is accurate. The ribs are counted using fluoroscopy, beginning caudally at the twelfth rib and counting rostrally.

A radiopaque object such as a curette or needle is placed in the disc space to confirm the localization. The parietal pleura is incised over the proximal disc space and rib and then mobilized laterally to expose the disc space, rib head, and the adjacent segmental arteries and veins. The segmental vessels are carefully mobilized, electrocoagulated, and occluded with hemoclips. Then, they are sharply transected and further mobilized. The importance of this step cannot be overemphasized, because these segmental vessels can bleed considerably. The neurovascular bundle (intercostal nerve and vessels) is also separated from the undersurface of the rib using subperiosteal dissection with curettes and periosteal elevators. Bleeding is controlled with bipolar cauterization. When the spine is approached from the patient's left side, the aorta can be mobilized if it obstructs access to the disc space of interest. Multiple segmental vessels are also isolated and transected above and below the disc space of interest, and the aorta is gently retracted laterally.

The proximal rib is transected 2 cm from the rib head and removed after the costotransverse and costovertebral ligaments have been detached with periosteal elevators and rib dissectors. The pedicle caudal to the disc space is identified, and the foraminal ligaments are cut from its superior edge. The epidural space is exposed by removing the pedicle with a Kerrison rongeur to facilitate the direct visualization of the anterolateral border of the spinal canal, ensuring that the surgeon remains oriented to the position of the spinal cord (*Fig. 37.6A*).

Using a pneumatic drill, a pyramidal-shaped cavity is produced in the dorsolateral vertebral bodies and disc space to provide an entryway to the herniated disc and epidural space (*Fig. 37.6B*). This maneuver

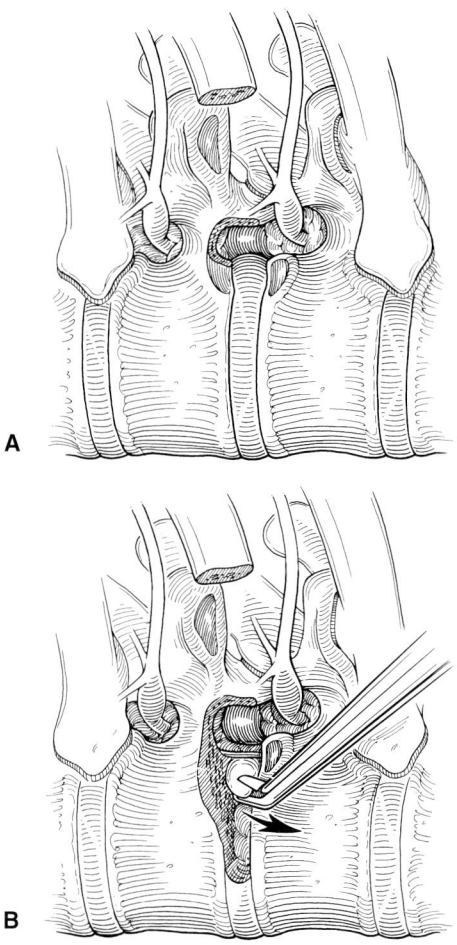

FIG. 37.6 (*A*) Spinal exposure for performing a thoracoscopic discectomy. The proximal rib and upper edge of the caudal pedicle have been removed to expose the ventrolateral dura. (*B*) A small cavity is made in the dorsal edge of the disc space. Disc material is removed using microsurgical tools. Reprinted with permission from Barrow Neurological Institute.

provides space for the surgeon to work and minimizes the placement of tools into the compromised epidural space. The cavity is large enough to facilitate safe decompression of the epidural space using microsurgical technique, but not large enough to produce spinal instability. After the spinal cord has been decompressed meticulously, the extent of the decompression can be verified using fluoroscopy.

Meticulous hemostasis is achieved with a variety of hemostatic agents and irrigation. One or two chest tubes are placed through the working portals under endoscopic guidance. The lung is reinflated and the chest tubes are left in place for approximately 24 hours (until their output is less than 100 ml/d). Chest radiographs are obtained in the recovery room to ensure that the lung is inflated completely.

Figure 37.7 is the thoracic computed tomographic scan of a middle-aged patient who became symptomatic with progressive myelopathy. The hyperdense mass in the ventral portion of the spinal canal represents a calcified herniated disc. A thoracoscopic surgical approach was used, and the disc space and associated rib were localized using intraoperative fluoroscopy (*Fig. 37.8A*). The intercostal artery and vein were then isolated, transected, and mobilized (*Fig. 37.8B*). The proximal rib head was removed, and a cavity was created by drilling the dorsal vertebral bodies above and below the disc space of interest (*Fig. 37.8C*). The disc was removed completely without sequelae. The patient was discharged from the hospital on the second day after surgery.

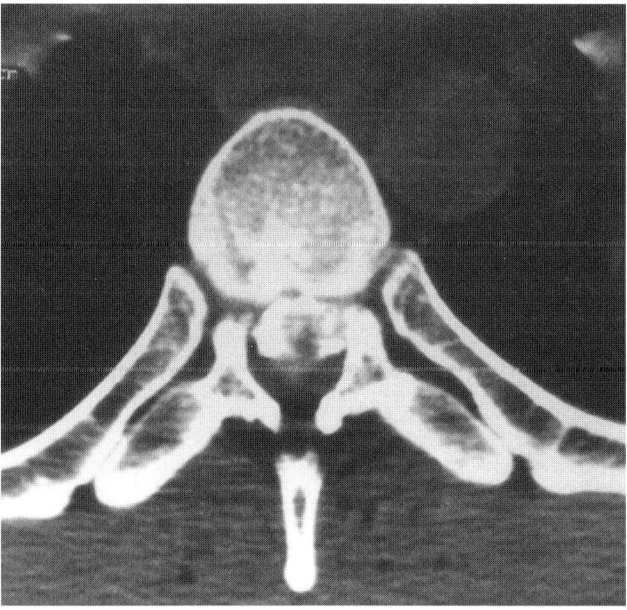

FIG. 37.7 Axial computed tomogram at T6–T7 demonstrating a large herniated midline (calcified) disc compressing the thecal sac and spinal cord.

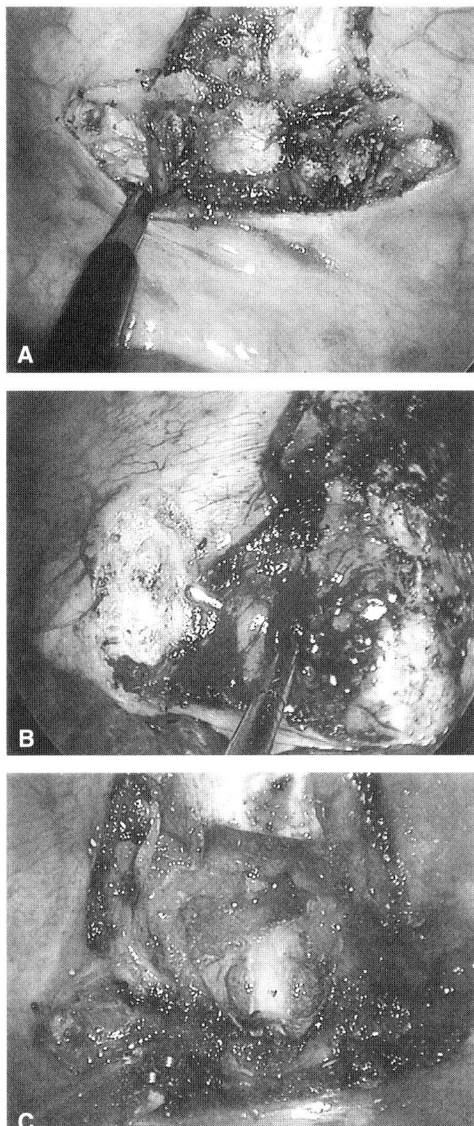

FIG. 37.8 (A) The calcified disc at T6–T7 was resected using a right thoracoscopic approach. The right T7 rib head and lateral aspect of the T6 and T7 vertebral bodies are exposed by coagulating and mobilizing the overlying pleura. (B) The segmental arterial-venous bundle at each level is mobilized as it courses from ventral to dorsal along the lateral midportion of the vertebral body. The vascular bundle is coagulated, clipped, and transected. (C) The head of the T7 rib has been removed. The inferior–posterior aspect of the T6 body and the superior–posterior aspect of the T7 body have been drilled away, providing excellent exposure of the T6–T7 disc.

Clinical Results

We reported the clinical results for thoracoscopic microdiscectomy in a collaborative publication (26). The results of applying this technique were excellent. We reviewed 55 consecutive patients who underwent video-assisted thoracoscopic discectomy. Sixty-five percent presented with myelopathic signs and symptoms due to spinal cord compression, whereas 35% had severe thoracic radiculopathy without myelopathy. The procedure was performed at one level in 43 patients, at two levels in 11 patients, and at three levels in one patient. The mean operative time was 3.5 hours (range, 80–542 min), and the mean blood loss was 327 ml (range, 124–1500 ml).

Clinical information was compared with that obtained from 18 patients treated with thoracotomy and from 15 patients treated with costotransversectomy for the same symptoms produced by a herniated thoracic disc. Compared with thoracotomy, thoracoscopy was associated with 1 hour less operative time and half the blood loss. Postoperatively, the length of chest tube drainage and utilization of narcotics were significantly less in the thoracoscopic group. Thoracotomy was also associated with a significantly greater incidence of intercostal neuralgia and postoperative atelectases. Compared with costotransversectomy, the endoscopic approach facilitated a more complete resection of calcified and midline thoracic discs, which was attributed to better visualization of the ventral surface of the dura.

Clinical outcomes in the thoracoscopic group were excellent: 60% of the myelopathic patients recovered neurologically. Among the 36 patients with myelopathy, 22 completely recovered neurologically, 5 improved functionally but had some residual myelopathic symptoms, and 9 stabilized. Among the 19 patients with isolated thoracic radiculopathy, 79% recovered completely (n = 15) and 21% improved moderately (n = 4). No patients had worsened radicular pain.

THORACOSCOPIC VERTEBRECTOMY

The surgical technique used to perform a thoracoscopic vertebrectomy is similar to that used for a thoracoscopic discectomy.

Surgical Technique

The positioning of the patient, anesthesia, and approach to the spine are the same as for thoracoscopic discectomy. After the disc space above and below the vertebral body of interest is localized, proximal rib heads are removed and saved for later fusion. As with the thoracoscopic discectomy, the pedicles serve as a key landmark. Pedicles are removed at both levels using a Kerrison rongeur. The dura is visualized and the dis-

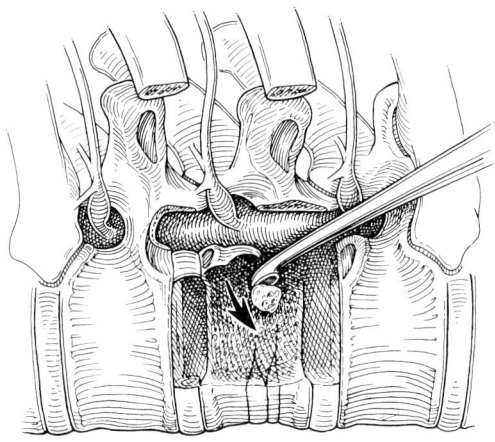

FIG. 37.9 The ventral spinal cord is decompressed by curetting the herniated disc material away from the dura. Reprinted with permission from Barrow Neurological Institute.

cectomy is performed at both levels. The vertebrectomy is performed using a variety of osteotomes, Leksell and Kerrison rongeurs, curettes, and high-speed drills. Compressive pathology, including the posterior cortex and posterior longitudinal ligament, is dissected away from the spinal cord into the defect created in the vertebral body (*Fig. 37.9*). Visualization and palpation of the contralateral pedicle ensure that the decompressive pathology has been completely removed (*Fig. 37.10*). Various options are available for vertebral reconstruction, including methylmethacrylate, allograft (*Fig. 37.11A*), or autograft utilizing the resected rib or iliac crest (*Fig. 37.11B*). Screw plate fixation can also be performed under endoscopic and fluoroscopic guidance.

Clinical Results

We previously reported our collaborative experience with 17 patients who underwent thoracoscopic vertebrectomy for a variety of pathologies (12). Thirteen patients had myelopathy and four had radiculopathy. The causes of the normal compression included tumors (n = 7), fractures (n = 6), infection (n = 3), and calcified herniated disc (n = 1). Lesions were approached from the right side in 15 patients and from the left side in two patients. The vertebral body was reconstructed with a bone graft in 9 patients and with methylmethacrylate in 5 patients. Internal fixation was performed in 14 cases. The mean length of surgery was 347 minutes, and operative blood loss averaged 1117 ml. The mean duration of chest tube drainage was 2.8 days. The duration of the intensive care unit and total hospital stay was 2.6 and 8.7 days, respectively.

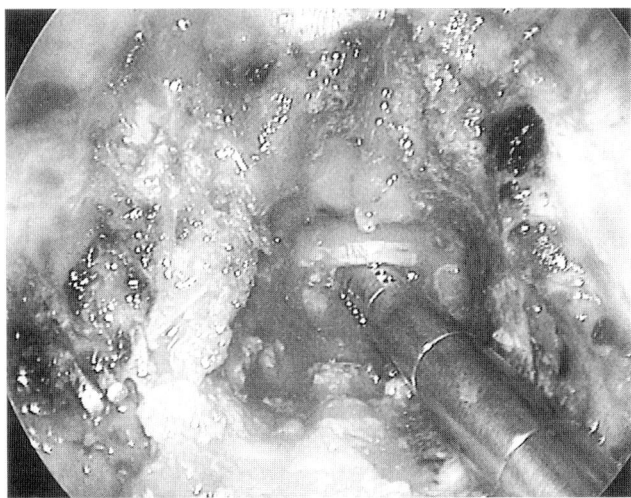

FIG. 37.10 The ventral thecal sac and spinal cord have been completely decompressed. The thoracoscopic irrigation/suction device touches the contralateral T6 pedicle without impinging upon the dura.

Complications included transient intercostal neuralgia (n = 2), pleural effusion (n = 1), and atelectasis and pneumonia (n = 1). No cases of neurological worsening complicated surgery. On follow-up there were no nonunions or instrumentation failures. No patients had persistent pain from spinal instability or neural compression.

This endoscopic cohort was compared with a matched cohort of patients who had undergone thoracotomy for vertebrectomy. The operative time and estimated blood loss were similar in the thoracoscopic vertebrectomy group when compared with the open thoracotomy group. Chest tube drainage was decreased by 1 day in the thoracoscopic vertebrectomy group. The most dramatic difference was seen in the narcotic pain utilization, length of stay in the intensive care unit and the length of hospital stay in patients treated endoscopically: All of these parameters were half that of the cohort undergoing thoracotomy.

LAPAROSCOPIC INTERBODY FUSION OF THE LUMBAR SPINE

Clinical application of the endoscope for surgery on the lumbar spine has gained popularity over the past decade (7, 8, 22, 29, 32). General surgeons and obstetricians have used the laparoscope to perform a variety of procedures, including hernia repairs, cholecystectomies, appendectomies, small and large bowel resections, ovarian resections and tubal ligations, and hysterectomies.

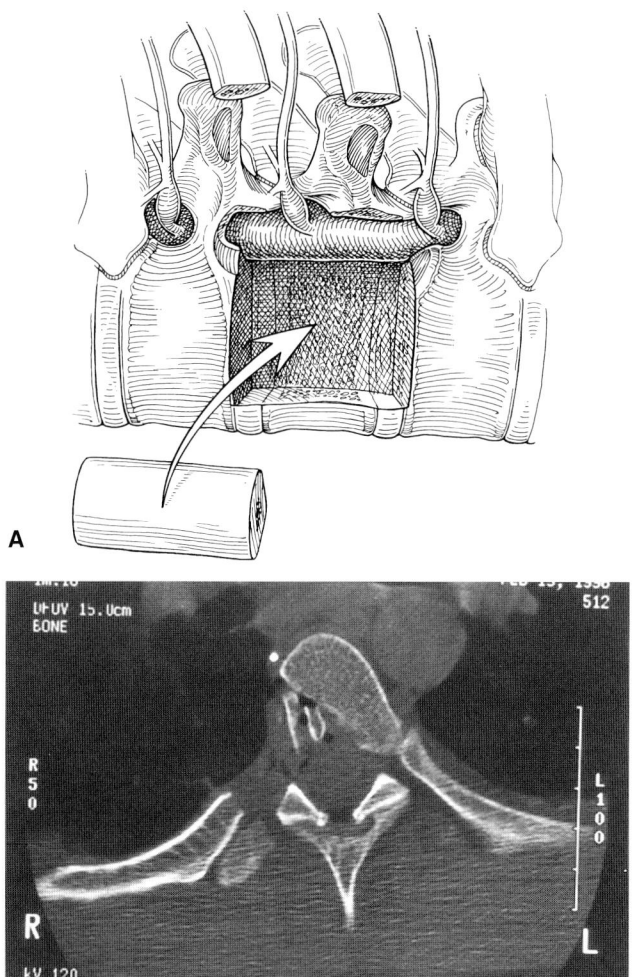

FIG. 37.11 (*A*) Cavity produced after removal of the vertebral body and cranial and caudal discs. The thecal sac has been completely decompressed. An allograft or autograft strut is used to create a fusion across the defect. (*B*) Postoperative axial computed tomogram demonstrating medial resection of the right T7 rib and the wedge-shaped ventral decompression of the T6 vertebral body, thecal sac, and spinal cord. Two strut grafts were fashioned from the resected portion of the rib. Reprinted with permission from Barrow Neurological Institute.

Compared with an open approach for lumbar interbody fusion, the benefits of laparoscopy include minimal incision of the tissue of the abdominal wall, less postoperative pain, and better cosmetic results. Although technically more difficult than an open procedure, the skills required to operate based on three-dimensional images projected on a television screen can be mastered by spine surgeons after they complete instructional courses that use animal models and cadaveric spines (10). Surgeons must have mastered the open techniques for lumbar interbody fusion cages before they attempt to perform endoscopic procedures.

Indications for laparoscopic lumbar interbody fusion with threaded lumbar interbody fusion implants (7, 8) include degenerative disc disease, degenerative lumbar instability, iaotrogenic lumbar instability (postlaminectomy, postfacetectomy or postdiscectomy), pseudarthrosis of posterior lumbar fusion, or Grade I isthmic or degenerative spondylolisthesis. When used to treat spondylolisthesis that is Grade II or greater, the anterior interbody fusion is followed by a posterior stabilization procedure using pedicle screws. Contraindications to laparoscopic interbody fusion include morbid obesity, extensive peritoneal adhesions (from prior laparotomies, peritonitis, or cancer), severe osteoporosis (cage subsidence), spinal ligamentous incompetence (Grade II or greater slip), a steep sacral inclination (interference with trajectory), pelvic deep venous thrombophlebitis, or aorto-iliac occlusive vascular disease.

Laparoscopy is best suited to access L5–S1 from a direct midline approach because the aorta and vena cava typically bifurcate rostral to the L5–S1 disc space, allowing easy exposure of the L5–S1 disc. Unless the bifurcation is high, it is much more difficult to expose L4–L5 endoscopically because the ileolumbar vessels and segmental vessels must be ligated and the aorta and vena cava retracted to expose the disc space. Levels rostral to L4–L5 are not approached by a midline anterior laparoscopic approach; they are best accessed by a lateral retroperitoneal approach.

Surgical Technique

We have previously reported the operative techniques used in the laparoscopic approach for lumbar interbody fusion (7, 8). The evening before surgery, patients drink magnesium citrate to clear their bowels. The patient is positioned supine on the operating room table and general endotracheal anesthesia is instituted. Normal lumbar lordosis is preserved by placing a pad or blanket under the lumbar spine. The operating room table is placed in a steep Trendelenburg, and gravity is used to retract the intestines rostrally. The entire abdomen, including both iliac crests and the suprapubic region, is prepared in a sterile fashion. Autograft cancellous bone is harvested from the iliac crest before and/or during the laparoscopic exposure of the ventral lumbar spine. The bone grafts are used to fill the hollow interbody cages.

A small incision is made above the umbilicus, and a Verees needle is inserted into the peritoneal cavity. Carbon dioxide is insufflated through the needle until a pressure of 10 to 15 mm Hg is achieved. A 10-mm portal is inserted through the incision. A high-resolution rigid endoscope is inserted through the portal, and the contents of the abdominal cavity are inspected. When the laparoscope is used, the transperitoneal approach is technically easier than the retroperitoneal approach (29). Throughout the procedure, we usually hold and manipulate the laparoscope using a voice-controlled robotic arm (*Fig. 37.12;* AESOP 2000, Computer Motion, Goleta, CA).

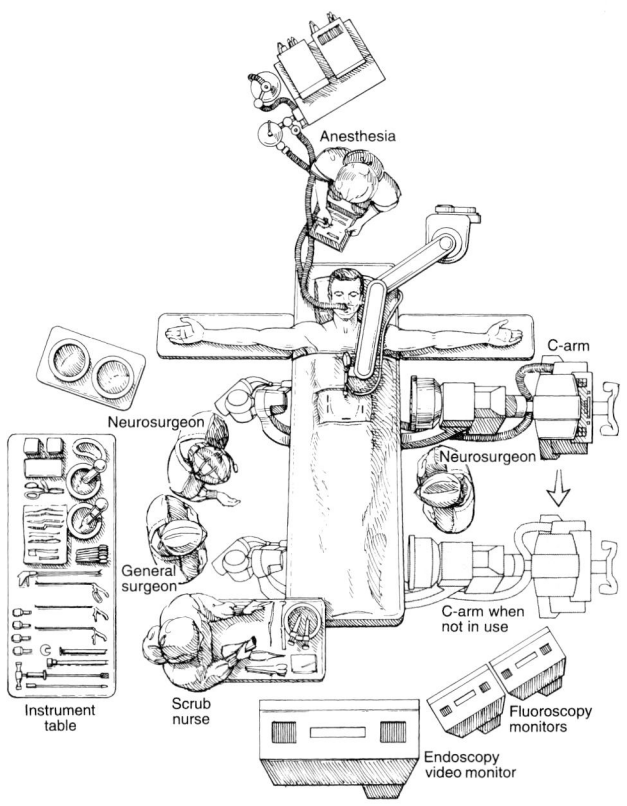

FIG. 37.12 Operating room setup for laparoscopic anterior lumbar interbody fusion. The movements of the laparoscope are performed by a voice-controlled robotic arm. Reprinted with permission from Barrow Neurological Institute.

The working portals are placed under direct visualization using the laparoscope to avoid injury to the abdominal organs. Typically, a 30°-angled endoscope is used during this portion of the procedure. The lateral working portals are usually 5 mm in diameter. The position of the suprapubic incision is precisely determined with fluoroscopy. The special 18-mm diameter portal placed through this incision is used for placing the interbody implants.

The bowel is mobilized out of the pelvis by gravity and by using a fan retractor. The sigmoid colon is retracted laterally with a suture passed through the ventral wall of the left abdomen: A Keith needle is placed through the anterior abdominal wall, through the sigmoid mesentery, and back through the abdominal wall. The suture is tied externally. Using sharp dissection, the posterior peritoneum is divided at the base of the sigmoid colon (*Fig. 37.13*).

The middle sacral artery and vein are identified, clipped, and divided (*Fig. 37.14*). The presacral autonomic plexus is mobilized laterally by blunt dissection. Damage to the autonomic plexus, which can lead to retrograde ejaculation (less than 5% incidence in men), is prevented by avoiding monopolar electrocauterization and by bluntly mobilizing the autonomic plexus laterally during the exposure.

After the appropriate disc space has been exposed, a suprapubic incision is made in a plane that allows the implant to be inserted parallel to the vertebral end-plates. An 18-mm diameter sealed trochar is placed through the suprapubic incision to allow the implant to be placed while maintaining pneumoperitoneum. During the procedure, the iliac vessels are protected with endoscopic vessel retractors.

Placement of the paired, threaded interbody implants (cadaveric cortical bone dowels or titanium cages) is the same as for an open procedure (*Fig. 37.15*). The paired cylindrical implants are inserted under fluoroscopic guidance into the distracted disc space. Pilot holes are cut, and the thread pattern is tapped into the vertebrae to anchor the implants. The cages are packed with autograft bone and securely inserted into the pilot holes (*Figs. 37.15* and *37.16*). The posterior peritoneum is closed with endoscopic suturing techniques. The pneumoperitoneum is then released, and the surgical field is meticulously visualized to ensure hemostasis. The portals are removed, and the fascia at the portal sites is closed with interrupted absorbable suture.

Clinical Results

Patients are mobilized postoperatively by wearing a lumbar elastic support brace for 6 weeks. Hospital stays are usually between 1 and 2 days. Several clinical centers perform the laparoscopic lumbar fusion

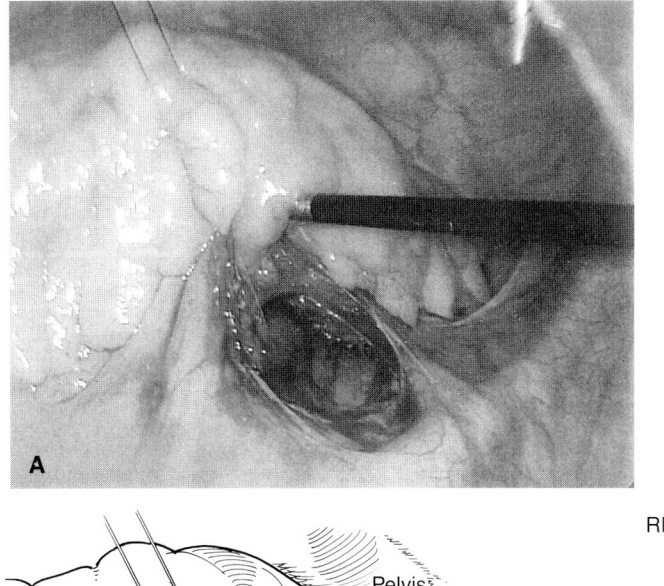
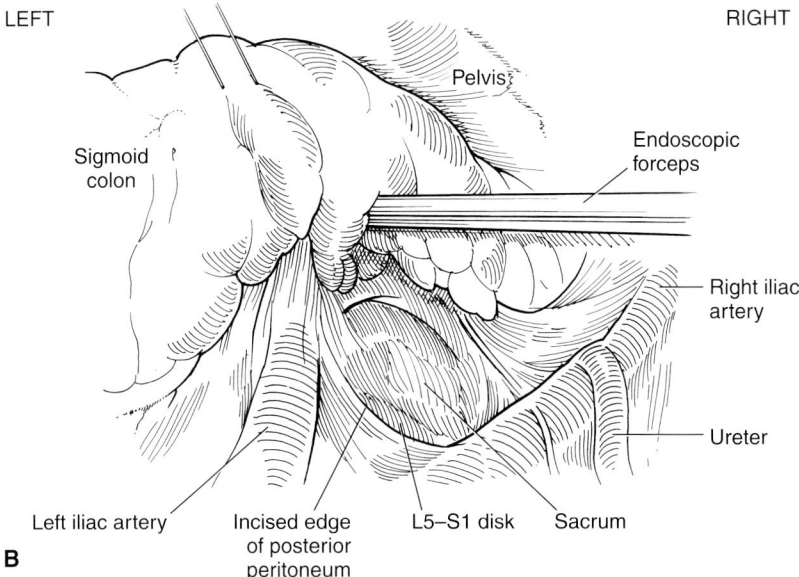

FIG. 37.13 (A) Intraoperative photograph and (B) illustration of the operative anatomy during a laparoscopic L5–S1 fusion. A suture has been placed in the sigmoid mesentery to retract the sigmoid colon from the surface of the spine. The suture was tied to the anterior abdominal wall. The posterior peritoneum was incised to provide access to the L5–S1 disc space. The common iliac arteries and the right ureter are visible (bottom = rostral, right = right. Subsequent intraoperative views have the same orientation). Reprinted with permission from Barrow Neurological Institute.

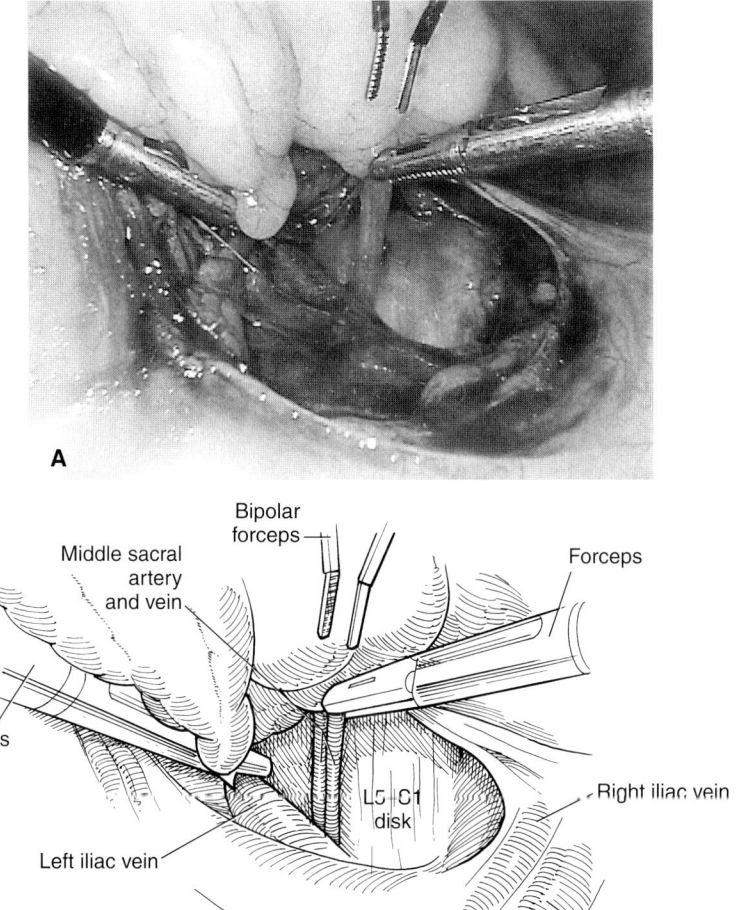

FIG. 37.14 (A) Intraoperative photograph and (B) illustration showing mobilization of the middle sacral vessels, which are held with a forceps. The vessels undergo bipolar cauterization. The left iliac vein was retracted laterally to expose the disc space. Reprinted with permission from Barrow Neurological Institute.

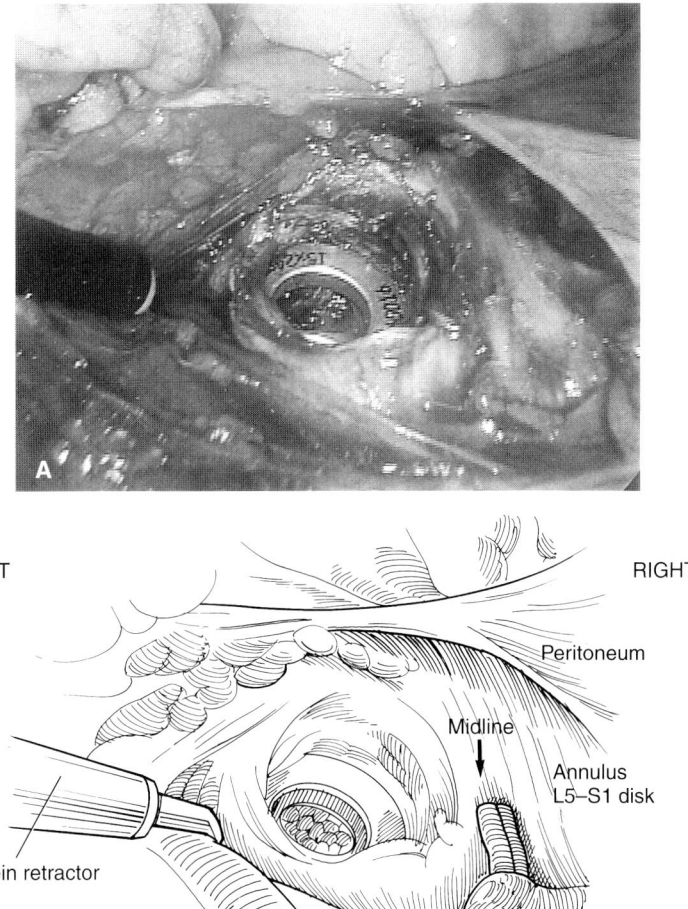

FIG. 37.15 (A) Intraoperative photograph and (B) illustration of a cage in its final position recessed beneath the surface of the L5–S1 disc. The cage was packed with cancellous bone. Two cages are inserted in the disc space using this technique. Reprinted with permission from Barrow Neurological Institute.

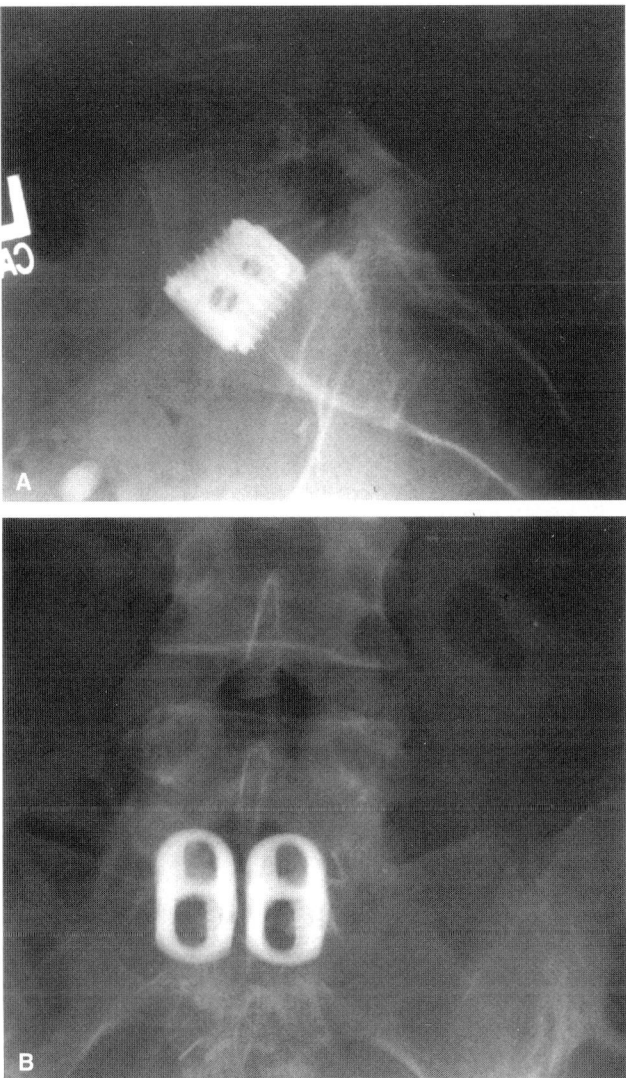

FIG. 37.16 Postoperative (A) lateral and (B) anteroposterior radiograph of L5–S1 threaded interbody fusion cages.

technique as an outpatient surgical procedure. Postoperatively, patients are restricted from repetitive bending, twisting, and heavy lifting. Fusion usually occurs within 3 months of the procedure. The fusion rate exceeds 95% for one-level anterior interbody cage constructs (31). The clinical outcome associated with this approach has been satisfactory in terms of improving patients' radicular pain, neurological deficits, back pain, and level of functioning (2, 3, 16, 22, 24, 31, 32). Our initial clinical experience with laparoscopic lumbar fusion has been very promising. It is a useful method that has significant potential advantages. We look forward to elucidating the long-term and large-scale results of these techniques.

REFERENCES

1. Ahn SS, Machleder HI, Concepcion B, et al: Thoracoscopic cervicodorsal sympathectomy: Preliminary results. **J Vasc Surg** 20:511–519, 1994.
2. Brantigan JW, Stefee AD: A carbon fiber implant to aid interbody lumbar fusion. Two-year clinical results in the first 26 patients. **Spine** 18:2106–2117, 1993.
3. Brodke DS, Dick JC, Kunz DN, et al: Posterior lumbar interbody fusion. A biomechanical comparison, including a new threaded cage. **Spine** 22:26–31, 1997.
4. Byrne J, Walsh TN, Hederman WP: Endoscopic transthoracic electrocautery of the sympathetic chain for palmar and axillary hyperhidrosis. **Br J Surg** 77:1046–1049, 1990.
5. Claes G, Drott C, Göthberg G: Thoracoscopy for autonomic disorders. **Ann Thorac Surg** 56:715–716, 1993.
6. Coltharp WH, Arnold JH, Alford WC Jr, et al: Videothoracoscopy: Improved technique and expanded indications. **Ann Thorac Surg** 53:776–779, 1992.
7. Detwiler PW, Porter RW, Dickman CA, et al: Lumbar spine interbody fusion with use of synthetic implants. **Oper Tech Neurosurg** 1:142–150, 1998.
8. Dickman CA: Internal fixation and fusion of the lumbar spine using threaded interbody cages. **BNI Quarterly** 13:4–25, 1997.
9. Dickman CA, Apfelbaum RI: Thoracoscopic microsurgical excision of a thoracic schwannoma. Case report. **J Neurosurg** 88:898–902, 1998.
10. Dickman CA, Karahalios DG: Thoracoscopic spinal surgery. **Clin Neurosurg** 43:392–422, 1996.
11. Dickman CA, Mican CA: Multilevel anterior thoracic discectomies and anterior interbody fusion using a microsurgical thoracoscopic approach. Case report. **J Neurosurg** 84:104–109, 1996.
12. Dickman CA, Rosenthal D, Karahalios DG, et al: Thoracic vertebrectomy and reconstruction using a microsurgical thoracoscopic approach. **Neurosurgery** 38:279–293, 1996.
13. Drott C, Göthberg G, Claes G: Endoscopic procedures of the upper-thoracic sympathetic chain. A review. **Arch Surg** 128:237–241, 1993.
14. Edmondson RA, Banerjee AK, Rennie JA: Endoscopic transthoracic sympathectomy in the treatment of hyperhidrosis. **Ann Surg** 215:289–293, 1992.
15. Friedel G, Linder A, Toomes H: Selective video-assisted thoracoscopic sympathectomy. **Thorac Cardiovasc Surg** 41:245–248, 1993.

16. Hacker RJ: Comparison of interbody fusion approaches for disabling low back pain. **Spine** 22:660–666, 1997.
17. Landreneau RJ, Mack MJ, Hazelrigg SR, et al: Video-assisted thoracic surgery: Basic technical concepts and intercostal approach strategies. **Ann Thorac Surg** 54:800–807, 1992.
18. Mack MJ, Aronoff RJ, Acuff TE, et al: Present role of thoracoscopy in the diagnosis and treatment of diseases of the chest. **Ann Thorac Surg** 54:403–409, 1992.
19. Mack MJ, Regan JJ, Bobechko WP, et al: Application of thoracoscopy for diseases of the spine. **Ann Thorac Surg** 56:736–738, 1993.
20. Malone PS, Cameron AEP, Rennie JA: The surgical treatment of upper limb hyperhidrosis. **Br J Dermatol** 115:81–84, 1986.
21. Malone PS, Duignan JP, Hederman WP: Transthoracic electrocoagulation (TTEC)—A new and simple approach to upper limb sympathectomy. **Ir Med J** 75:20–21, 1982.
22. McAfee PC, Regan JR, Zdeblick T, et al: The incidence of complications in endoscopic anterior thoracolumbar spinal reconstructive surgery. A prospective multicenter study comprising the first 100 consecutive cases. **Spine** 20:1624–1632, 1995.
23. Plas EG, Függer R, Herbst F, et al: Complications of endoscopic thoracic sympathectomy. **Surgery** 118:493–495, 1995.
24. Ray CD: Threaded fusion cages for lumbar interbody fusions. An economic comparison with 360° fusions. **Spine** 22:681–685, 1997.
25. Robertson DP, Simpson RK, Rose JE, et al: Video-assisted endoscopic thoracic ganglionectomy. **J Neurosurg** 79:238–240, 1993.
26. Rosenthal D, Dickman CA: Thoracoscopic microsurgical excision of herniated thoracic discs. **J Neurosurg** 89:224–235, 1998.
27. Rosenthal D, Rosenthal R, de Simone A: Removal of a protruded thoracic disc using microsurgical endoscopy. A new technique. **Spine** 19:1087–1091, 1994.
28. Rutherford, RB: Role of sympathectomy in the management of vascular disease, in Moore, WS (ed): *Vascular Surgery. A Comprehensive Review.* Philadelphia, W.B. Saunders, 1993, p 300–311.
29. Southerland SR, Remedios AM, McKerrell JG, et al: Laparoscopic approaches to the lumbar vertebrae. An anatomic study using a porcine model. **Spine** 20:1620–1623, 1995.
30. Weale FE: Upper thoracic sympathectomy by transthoracic electrocoagulation. **Br J Surg** 67:71–72, 1980.
31. Yuan HA, Kuslich SD, Dowdle JA Jr, et al: *Prospective Multi-Center Clinical Trial of the BAK™ Interbody Fusion System.* Minneapolis, Spine Tech, Inc., 1997.
32. Zucherman JF, Zdeblick TA, Bailey SA, et al: Instrumented laparoscopic spinal fusion. Preliminary results. **Spine** 20:2029–2035, 1995.

CHAPTER

38

Honored Guest Presentation: Contemporary Treatment of Skull Base Meningiomas

ANDREW J. KOKKINO, M.D., KHALED M. ABDEL AZIZ, M.D., AND JOHN M. TEW, JR., M.D.

The outcome of intracranial tumors is based on the clinical nature, biological characteristics, and the safety and efficacy of treatment. Meningiomas of the skull base are a unique category of lesions because most are benign and originate in anatomically challenging areas. The clinical behavior and biological character of most skull base meningiomas require that treatment be based on a multifactorial analysis of surgical options and adjuncts that offer the individual patient the most favorable quality of life.

BIOLOGICAL NATURE AND CLINICAL PRESENTATION

Cushing and Eisenhardt stated in 1938 that " . . . with a well taken case history, supplemented by thorough neurological and roentgenological studies, it should become possible in most cases before operation to determine not only the site, nature and status of the lesion but to form an estimate of its probable future course" (7).

The majority of meningiomas are benign, slow-growing tumors arising from arachnoidal cap cells. These cells arise predominantly from arachnoid villi at the dural venous sinuses and at sites of passage of cranial nerves at their foramina. Meningothelial cells functioning as the precursors of meningiomas are also present in the choroid plexus, the tela choroidea, and at the passage zones of spinal nerves. As expected, the origin of meningioma correlates with the sites of arachnoid cells.

The growth patterns of meningiomas reflect their possible clinical presentations. Slow growth in areas of the cranial vault or nonfunctional brain can support an expanding mass, leading to very large tumors that present with symptoms referable to mass effect, including headaches, lethargy, dizziness, transient memory problems, and focal neurological deficits. Growth of meningiomas abutting the cortical brain surface can cause seizures. Small tumors in functional areas of the brain or along cranial nerves can present with focal symptoms of anosmia, visual disturbance, diplopia, and paresis in the absence of substantial mass effect.

CLASSIFICATION OF SKULL BASE MENINGIOMAS

Classification of skull base meningiomas with convexity and parasagittal meningiomas must take into consideration the unique anatomic locations that can be affected. Histopathological classification does not correlate with intraoperative findings such as adhesion and infiltration of surrounding structures that can significantly affect surgical resectability. The significance of tumor aggressiveness is addressed by the inclusion of subcategories that are based on operative findings of invasiveness and infiltration. Therefore, the imaging characteristics, anatomy, histopathology, and invasive potential must be jointly considered to fully appreciate the biology and natural history of skull base meningiomas.

Pathology

Cushing coined the term "meningioma" to describe tumors that arise from the meninges (6). This term broadly described the primary meningeal neoplasms that had characteristic histological features and biological behavior. The traditional histopathological classification has undergone recategorization most recently in 1993 by the World Health Organization (Ref. 17; *Table 38.1*). This classification scheme attempts to correlate biological aggressiveness with histological appearance into three broad categories: classic, atypical, and malignant. Classic meningiomas have moderate cellularity and low mitotic activity. The invasion of bone, muscle, or dura is a characteristic behavior and not evidence of more aggressive biological behavior. Atypical meningiomas may have foci of necrosis, increased cellularity, and mitotic figures. Malignant meningiomas have characteristics of atypical meningiomas but also demonstrate brain invasion.

Proliferative Potential

Histological features do not independently determine the aggressiveness of skull base meningiomas. The growth rate and potential for recurrence can be assessed more accurately by the proliferative index, which is an objective measure of the biological nature of a meningioma. Proliferative indices include bromodeoxyuridine and MIB-1 (Ki-67) labeling. Recent studies have correlated the results of bromodeoxyuridine and MIB-1 proliferative indices and further demonstrated that elevation of these indices corresponded to more biologically aggressive

TABLE 38.1
New Classification Proposed by the World Health Organization for Tumors of the Meninges

Tumors of the meningothelial cells
  Meningioma (histological types)
    Meningothelial (syncytial)
    Transitional mixed
    Fibrous (fibroblastic)
    Psammomatous
    Angiomatous
    Microcystic
    Secretory
    Clear cell
    Choroid
    Lymphoplasmacyte-rich
    Metaplastic variants (xanthomatous, myxoid, osseous, chondroid)
  Atypical
  Malignant (anaplastic)
Tumors of uncertain origin
  Capillary hemangioblastoma
  Hemangiopericytoma
Mesenchymal, nonmeningothelial tumors
Primary melanocytic lesion

neoplasms (20). These authors reported their results with MIB-1 median staining indices (MIB-1 SI) in classic (3.4%), atypical (6.6%), and malignant (11.4%) meningiomas. An elevated MIB-1 SI has also been correlated to an increased incidence of recurrence (21). Meningiomas with an MIB-1 SI of 3% or more demonstrate a significantly higher tendency for recurrence, especially within the first 10 years of clinical follow-up. Additionally, a statistically significant correlation is recorded between the MIB-1 SI and recurrence in each Simpson grade. Conversely, no statistically significant relationship between the MIB-1 SI and cellularity could be established.

Several studies had addressed the prognostic significance of the MIB-1 SI. In a study of 425 meningioma patients who underwent gross total resection, an MIB-1 SI of 4.2% or more was strongly associated with decreased recurrence-free survival (26).

Anatomy

The skull base extends from the anterior aspect of the anterior fossa to the caudal aspect of the foramen magnum. Meningiomas grow at any point along the skull base, but certain foci of tumor growth are common (*Fig. 38.1*). The major anatomic categorization of these lesions is dis-

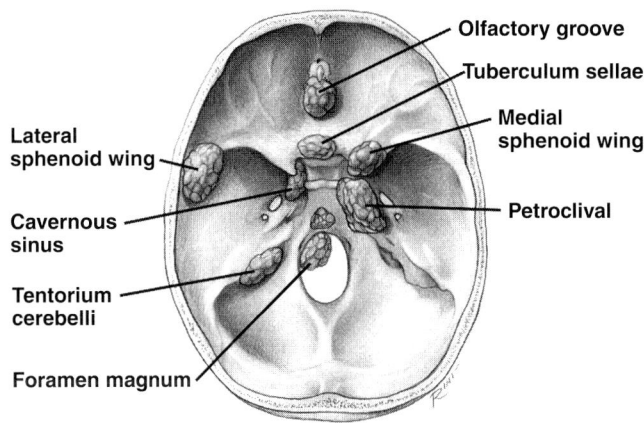

FIG. 38.1 The common sites of meningioma origin along the skull base reveal foci of predilection for tumor growth. Printed with permission from the Mayfield Clinic.

tinguished by the three cranial fossae. Meningiomas of the anterior fossa skull base include the olfactory groove, clinoidal, and tuberculum sellae meningiomas. Meningiomas of the middle fossa grow along the sphenoid wing, cavernous sinus, and petrous ridge. Meningiomas of the posterior fossa involve the clivus, petroclival region, and the foramen magnum. Occasionally, skull base meningiomas may expand to involve two, and possibly all three, fossae. At the craniocervical junction, foramen magnum meningiomas can expand beyond the posterior fossa into the spinal canal. Tumors may also arise from the tentorium cerebelli.

Imaging Characteristics

Neuroimaging of a skull base meningioma provides the surgeon with the most important information in the preoperative assessment of these lesions. The required preoperative information includes the presence of reactive bony changes (hyperostosis), brain distortion or edema, the integrity of the subarachnoid space immediately adjacent to the tumor, and invasion of the brain, cranial nerves, vessels, or cavernous sinus (*Fig. 38.2*). Cerebral angiography provides information regarding tumor vascularity; as well as carotid encasement, narrowing, or occlusion, it also provides the opportunity to perform preoperative balloon test occlusion or embolization if sacrifice of the internal carotid artery (ICA) is considered. Computed tomography with contrast enhancement reveals the majority of meningiomas and determines their extent. Bone

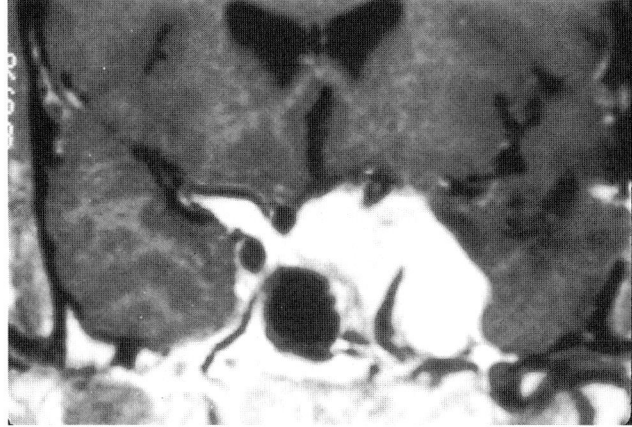

FIG. 38.2 Coronal MRI, T2-weighted image with gadolinium enhancement reveals a left holocavernous sinus meningioma encasing and narrowing the carotid, compressing the optic apparatus, filling the cavernous sinus, and extending across the sella to the contralateral medial sylvian fissure.

window settings are helpful in distinguishing hyperostosis or bone lysis. These images are particularly helpful in skull base surgery to identify the presence and integrity of bony landmarks that determine the particular approach required to reach a skull base meningioma. Magnetic resonance imaging (MRI) provides specific detail of the location and nature of skull base meningiomas. The relation of the meningioma to the cavernous sinus and the intracavernous ICA, as well as other arteries, can be delineated. Tumor vascularity and extracavernous ICA involvement or encasement can also be appreciated. Invasion of the pia-arachnoid membrane can be deduced when perifocal edema extends into the brain. Evaluation of the dural sinuses is important and can be achieved by magnetic resonance venography or contrast venography.

Cerebral edema is demonstrated on T2-weighted MRIs, and its presence in association with meningiomas is multifactorial. Its presence is more common with meningothelial or angioblastic variants (5). Peritumoral brain edema, as assessed on MRI, has demonstrated a statistically significant direct correlation to MIB-1 (15). This report demonstrated a rise in MIB-1 SI in order of increasing brain edema severity and a statistically significant direct relationship between size and brain edema. The significance of changes on T2-weighted MRIs has also been correlated with pial and brain invasion and, thus, more aggressive anaplastic variants (16).

DECISION ANALYSIS

Once the assessment of a skull base meningioma has been completed, a thorough communication of expectations, options, and expected results must occur. Patients deserve complete information to facilitate their decision process. Ultimately, the decision to pursue a treatment course relies on the patient's evaluation of risks, understanding of the natural history, and options.

Certain patient factors may greatly influence the morbidity of surgery. For an objective measure of a patient's anesthetic risk, a quick assessment is provided by using the Dripps-ASA scale (10). Patients are stratified according to the presence and severity of systemic disease, and the expected mortality for a period of 48 hours to 7 days postoperatively can be quoted (36). Comorbidities of increased age, heart disease, and respiratory disease must be carefully weighed in the decision process.

The imaging characteristics of the tumor should be reviewed with the patient to demonstrate the size, aggressiveness, location, surrounding structures, and their relation to anticipated postoperative deficits or complications. A review of the imaging characteristics provides the anatomic delineation needed to make the requisite decision of surgical accessibility and goals or the advisability of nonoperative approaches.

The decision to treat a skull base meningioma is not determined solely by the size of the lesion at the time of diagnosis. Rather, knowledge of the natural history of each particular lesion is critical when deciding the treatment algorithm, particularly in the elderly patient. Observation of serial imaging studies may be important in selecting a treatment option. A thorough outcome analysis should be presented to the patient as the final critical piece of data that must be understood to proceed with a treatment intervention for a skull base meningioma. An analysis of radiation results should include the expectation of tumor control, tumor shrinkage, treatment-related cranial neuropathies, and the risk of adverse effects induced by radiation. Similarly, a discussion of a surgical approach must include the expectations of the operation, in terms of tumor resection, operative risks, risks of recurrence in the absence of a complete resection, and the long-term anticipated outcome for subtotal versus complete resections.

Determination of the natural history of meningiomas, particularly skull base meningiomas, must be considered to improve the outcome analysis for the treatment of such lesions. If the growth rate, clinical course, and potential for malignant transformation are known, then accurate assessments are more confidently made regarding the indications for treatment. Recently, the natural history of asymptomatic meningiomas was documented for a group of 60 patients with incidental meningiomas (24). Of this group, only 19 were skull base meningiomas. The average clinical follow-up for 57 patients was 32 months, with an average radiological follow-up of 47 months. None of the patients demonstrated symptoms of an enlarging tumor during follow-up. Ten patients had radiographic evidence of (asymptomatic) growth. By measurement of the maximal diameter of the tumor, an average growth rate of 0.24 cm per year was recorded.

A recent effort to address this issue reported the natural history of 39 patients with skull base meningiomas (3). For a mean follow-up of 77 months, the investigators reported that 15 of 32 initially symptomatic patients developed worsening neurological deficits. None of the seven initially asymptomatic patients developed worsening deficits. Progression-free survival was 89%, 80%, 70%, and 54% at 2, 3, 5, and 7 years, respectively, whereas radiographic-free survival was 97%, 93%, 78%, and 78%, respectively. Symptoms worsened only in patients with a symptomatic presentation, with an incidence of 47%. Twelve patients eventually underwent treatment for progression. Three underwent surgery, whereas nine underwent radiation therapy. This report supports the indolent nature of skull base meningiomas. One may anticipate a significantly benign clinical course for many patients who present with minimal symptoms.

TREATMENT OPTIONS

The treatment options available to patients with skull base meningiomas have broadened steadily with advances in microsurgery, radiation, and chemotherapy and with an advanced understanding of the natural history of these lesions.

Observation

Several factors may support a course of observation in patients with skull base meningiomas. A review of the natural history, clinical presentation, patient age, and general medical condition determines the requirement for intervention. The growth rate of a particular meningioma can be established with serial MRIs at intervals of 6 to 12 months.

Chemotherapy

The majority of skull base meningiomas that require intervention can be controlled by surgical excision or radiotherapy. In cases of aggressive, recurrent, or unresectable meningeal tumors, several authors advocate the use of immunotherapy, chemotherapy, or hormonal therapy. In aggressive meningeal tumors, protocols have included combinations of ifosfamide/mesna, cisplatin/doxorubicin, and doxorubicin/dacarbazine (19, 34). In similar challenging cases, immunotherapy with interferon-alfa has been proposed (40). Its mechanism of action involves direct cytotoxic effect, activation of natural killer cells, modulation of antibody production, antiangiogenesis, and induction of major histocompatibility complex antigens on tumor cell surfaces (19).

The cytotoxic agent, hydroxyurea, has received growing attention in the treatment of unresectable or recurrent meningiomas. Preliminary reports indicate the stabilization of symptoms in most patients with benign meningiomas (28). Specifically, in 14 patients with benign meningiomas, 13 experienced stable clinical and radiographic responses (median duration 27 weeks, range 5–39 weeks), and 1 patient had a partial radiographic and clinical response maintained for 39 weeks. Longer evaluation of a larger treatment group is needed.

Radiation Therapy

Radiation therapy has been reported to be effective for incompletely resected meningiomas. Skull base meningiomas have a higher rate of incomplete resection than do convexity meningiomas (2, 12). Therefore, adjunct treatments play an important role when considering how to provide clinical stabilization and prevent tumor progression or recurrence.

The earliest attempts to irradiate meningiomas occurred with external beam radiotherapy for residual, recurrent, or histopathologically aggressive tumors (2, 12, 39). Methods designed to focus radiation delivery have improved in an effort to selectively maximize the dose to the tumor while limiting exposure to adjacent critical structures. This is particularly important when treating skull base meningiomas because of the proximity of these tumors to the optic nerves, cranial nerves, and brainstem. Stereotactic radiosurgery (SRS) and three-dimensional conformal radiotherapy have added precision and improved dosimetry for treatment of residual and primary meningiomas.

The goal of focused radiotherapy in skull base meningiomas is to prevent further growth and preserve neurological function. Immediate advantages of SRS include patient tolerance, low cost of treatment, and avoidance of the surgical morbidity and mortality.

Since the natural history of skull base meningiomas has documented the slow growth of many of these tumors, appropriate follow-up has been required to determine the safety and efficacy of SRS. Recently, Hakim et al. and Subach et al. presented their experience with linear accelerator-based radiosurgery and gamma knife radiosurgery for meningiomas, respectively (13, 35). Subach et al. focused on 62 patients with petroclival meningiomas who underwent SRS. Thirty-nine patients had previous surgery, and seven had previous fractionated radiation therapy. The neurological status of these patients was followed for a mean period of 37 months and demonstrated clinical improvement in 21%, stabilization in 66%, and worsening in 13%. Radiographic tumor volumes had decreased in 23%, stabilized in 68%, and increased in 8%. Hakim et al. reported on 127 patients with 155 meningiomas, of which 82 involved the skull base. For the entire group, 107 patients had prior treatment of their meningiomas. After a median follow-up of 22.9 months, 84% demonstrated freedom from progression, and 15.7% showed disease progression at a median of 19.6 months. Tumor control rates were similar for both studies. Hakim et al. reported tumor control rates for benign cranial base meningiomas at 1, 2, 3, 4, and 5 years as 100%, 92%, 92%, 92%, and 92%, respectively. Similar tumor control rates of 100% and 86.7% were reported by Subach et al. at 12 and 96 months, respectively, for all patients.

Complications from SRS can be divided into transient and permanent events. Hakim et al. reported a complication rate of 4.7% at 10.3 months for all meningioma patients. The types of complications seen in skull base patients included death, hearing loss, and monocular blindness. Subach et al. reported a rate of transient cranial neuropathies of 8%. Two of six patients experienced abducens palsies that resolved. Three patients (5%) developed permanent cranial nerve deficits after radiosurgery. From the same institution, Duma et al. reported a delayed complication rate of 11.7% (4 of 34) in patients who received SRS for cavernous sinus meningiomas (11). Two of these cranial nerve deficits resolved within 12 months.

Microsurgery

Surgical treatment of skull base meningiomas has evolved significantly in the past 15 years. The traditional approaches that gave access to a particular fossa have undergone modifications to provide enhanced access to the skull base through an expanded corridor to the dural base and blood supply. A fundamental principle has been an attempt to convert skull base meningiomas into convexity meningiomas (38). Specifically, we seek the ability to circumferentially expose and resect the dura that is involved with a basal meningioma. Certain structures along the skull base require particular attention during their exposure and subsequent tumor resection. Anatomic danger zones that limit complete resectability include the optic canal, cavernous sinus, medial sphenoid wing, and clivus.

Anterior Fossae

Olfactory groove and tuberculum sellae meningiomas (*Fig. 38.3A*) have been traditionally resected via a bifrontal craniotomy. Approaching this region via a frontotemporal craniotomy with an orbital osteotomy, in which the tumor favors a particular side, allows for drilling of involved bone along the anterior fossa and devascularization of tumor. This strategy is beneficial in the resection of optic nerve sheath meningiomas. Bone drilling includes an optic foraminotomy and exposure of the carotid cave after removal of the anterior clinoid process (*Fig. 38.3B*). A complete resection of bone and dural attachment of the tumor can be performed by this technique (*Fig. 38.3, C and D*). Tuberculum sellae meningiomas often require the removal of the tuberculum sellae to gain access to the basal dural attachment (*Fig. 38.3E*).

Middle Fossae

Before the development of skull base modifications, surgical approaches to meningiomas of the cavernous sinus and medial sphenoid wing (*Fig. 38.4A*) involved access through the middle fossa via either a subtemporal or frontotemporal craniotomy. These approaches allowed poor vascular exposure and control, leading to significant morbidity. Inadequate identification of the cranial nerves also led to a significant morbidity from cranial nerve deficits. Significant tumor often remained on the medial sphenoid wing and lateral wall of the cavernous sinus.

New operative approaches to the cavernous sinus begin with either a frontotemporal or subtemporal craniotomy. An orbitozygomatic osteotomy can be added for expanded exposure. Four basic variations of this osteotomy are proposed: frontal orbitozygomatic, temporal orbitozygomatic, total orbitozygomatic, and the zygomatic arch (38). Further dural exposure can be gained by performing an anterior clinoidectomy and expanding the superior orbital fissure, foramina of rotundum and ovale (*Fig. 38.4B*). Exposure is required to mobilize the lateral wall of the cavernous sinus and protect cranial nerves III, IV, V, and VI. The subsequent resection of tumor (*Fig. 38.4C*) from within the lateral wall of the cavernous sinus and extending along the medial sphenoid wing (*Fig. 38.4D*) along with resection of the involved dura can be performed.

Petroclival Region Including Posterior Fossae

The surgical approaches for petroclival and clival meningiomas are chosen with primary consideration given to the specific relationship of the tumor base and extent along the petroclival bony anatomy. The transverse sigmoid sinuses are carefully considered. This information

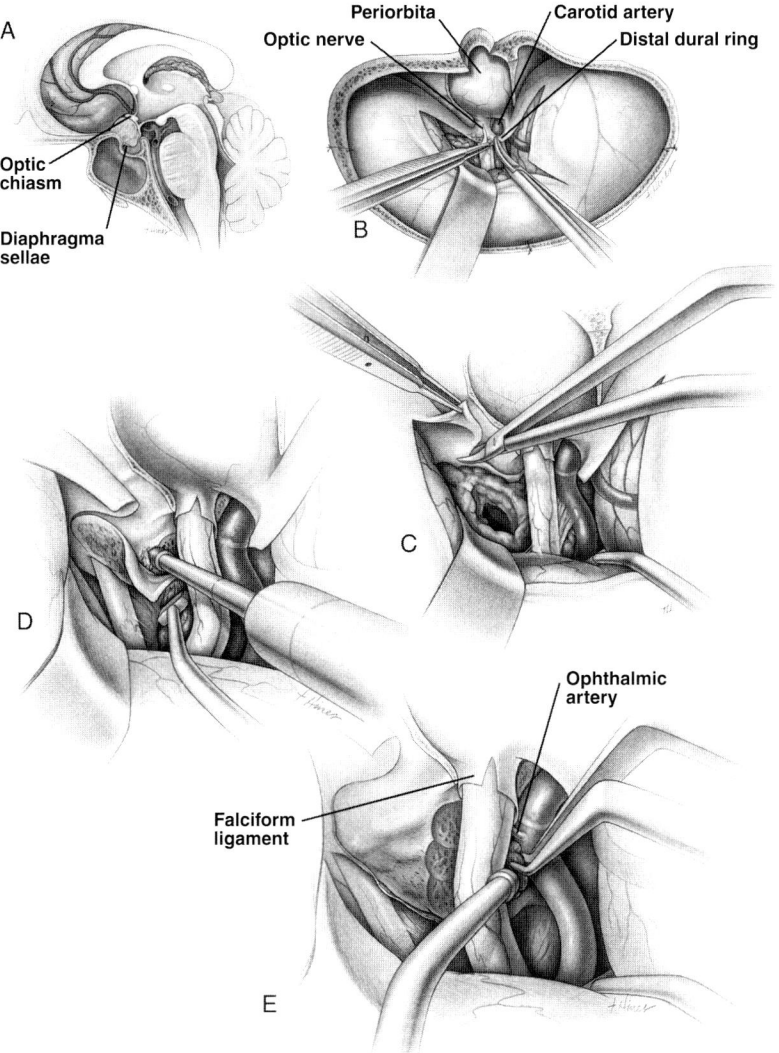

FIG. 38.3 Tuberculum sellae meningioma: operative technique. *A*, lateral schematic diagram demonstrates a tumor with mild posterior compression of the optic chiasm. *B*, an orbital osteotomy and optic foraminotomy are performed before opening the dura to allow subsequent safe retraction of the brain and optic nerve. *C*, dura infiltrated with tumor is excised to prevent recurrence. *D*, similarly, involved bone is drilled to minimize recurrence. *E*, after excision of the tumor and involved bone, final tumor remnants are removed along the falciform ligament near the ophthalmic artery. Reprinted with permission from Tew JM, van Loveren HR, Keller JT: *Atlas of Operative Microneurosurgery*, Philadelphia, W.B. Saunders, vol II, in press.

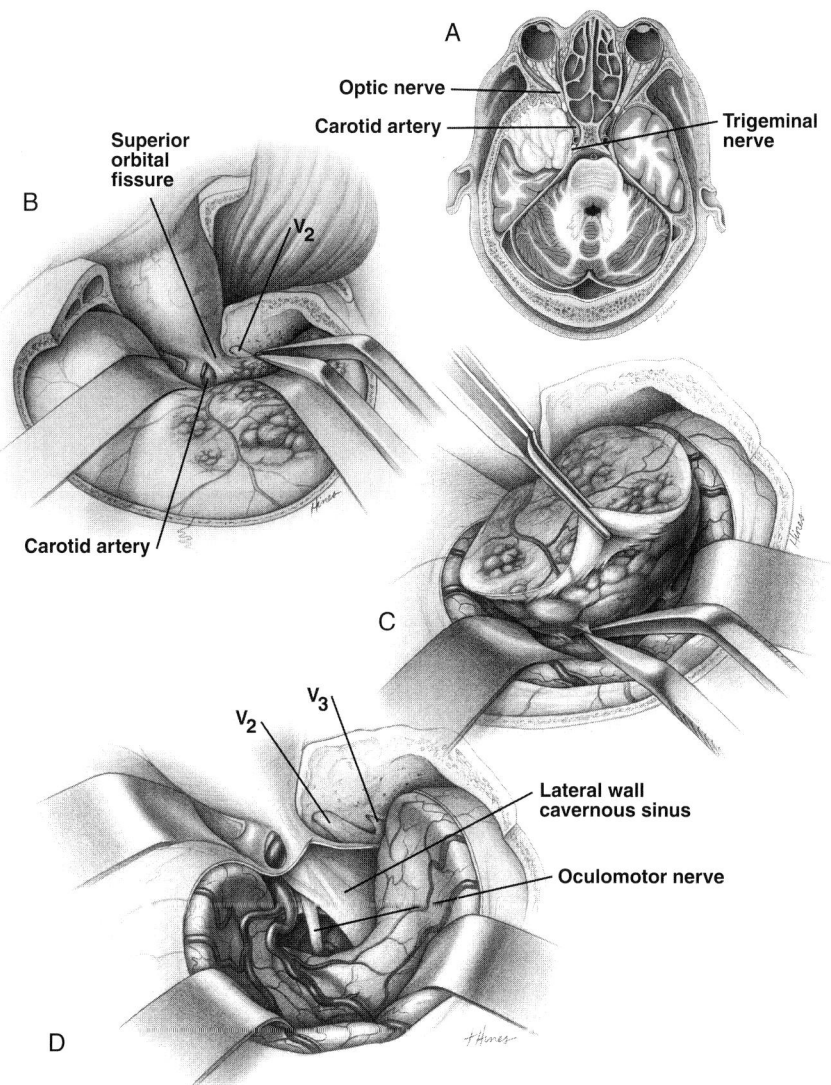

FIG. 38.4 Medial sphenoid wing meningioma: operative technique. *A,* axial schematic diagram demonstrates a right medial sphenoid wing meningioma. *B,* after a frontotemporal craniotomy, an orbital osteotomy, optic foraminotomy, anterior clinoidectomy, and drilling of the floor of the middle fossa are performed to expose the dural base of the tumor. *C,* the dura is circumferentially incised around the tumor. *D,* complete resection of the tumor is obtained, and inspection of the lateral wall of the cavernous sinus is explored for residual tumor. Reprinted with permission from Tew JM, van Loveren HR, Keller JT: *Atlas of Operative Microneurosurgery.* Philadelphia, W.B. Saunders, vol II, in press.

determines where a nondominant sinus is located and establishes the location of the vein of Labbe. Performance of a petrosectomy on the ipsilateral side of a dominant sinus requires verification of the patency of a sinus.

Petrosal approaches have proven most useful for surgical exposure of the petroclival region. Lateral skull base approaches to petroclival meningiomas have been listed under a plethora of names (*Table 38.2*). We designate transpetrosal approaches as either anterior or posterior petrosal approaches (23). Lesions above the internal auditory canal are exposed by using an anterior petrosal approach. The anterior petrosectomy provides a corridor to the posterior fossa between the internal carotid artery, trigeminal root, and the facial nerve (23). The anterior petrosectomy with a dural opening includes a transtentorial sectioning that provides adequate access to the upper clivus and exposure of the ventrolateral brainstem.

Tumors that extend below the internal auditory canal require a posterior petrosal approach. This approach exposes the area from the trigeminal nerve down to the upper border of the jugular tubercle. If a tumor extends into the area between the internal auditory canal or posterior aspect of the petrous surface (*Fig. 38.5A*), a posterior petrosectomy with a suboccipital-subtemporal craniotomy should be added to adequately expose the surface, including the anterior cerebellum and ventral brainstem. For larger tumors that require additional cerebellar

TABLE 38.2
Partial List of Names Given to Operations That Are Variations of Transpetrosal Approaches

Combined
Extended middle fossa
Infratemporal
Kawase's
Middle fossa transpetrosal
Presigmoid
Retroauricular-preauricular
Retrolabyrinthine
Subtemporal-suboccipital
Supratentoriual-infratentorial
Transcochlear
Translabyrinthine
Translabyrinthine-transtentorial
Transmastoid
Transpetrosal
Transpetrosal-transtentorial

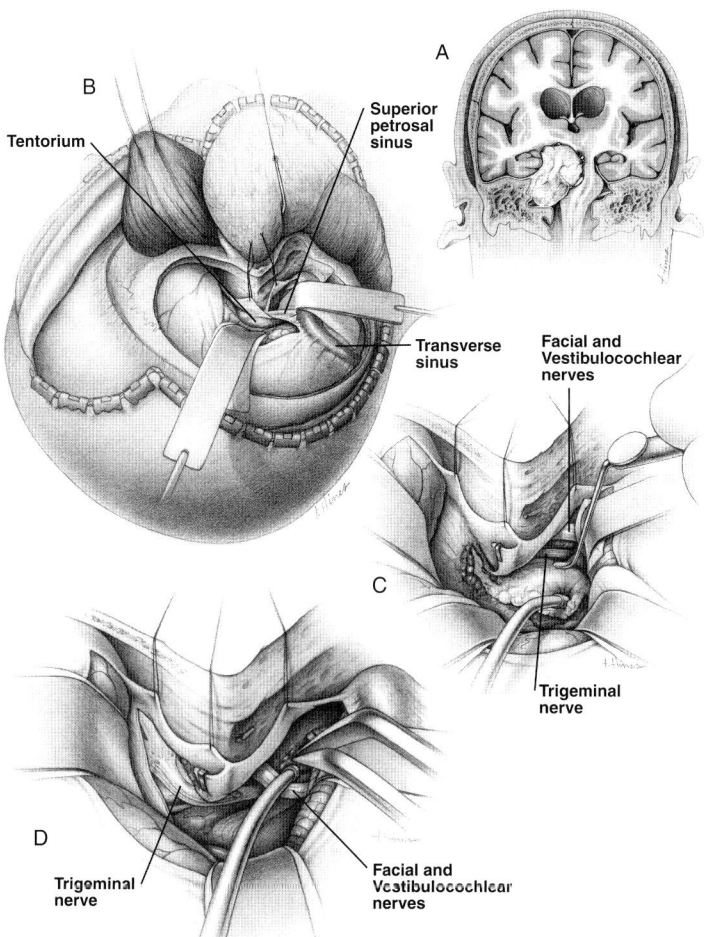

Fig. 38.5 Petroclival meningioma: coronal section and operative technique. *A*, coronal section reveals a large meningioma arising from the dural base of the clivus and the medial petrous ridge, causing compression and distortion of the brainstem and hydrocephalus. The inferior extent of the tumor is at the internal auditory meatus. *B*, after completion of a subtemporal-retrosigmoid craniotomy, a total petrosectomy is performed. The dura is incised, and the superior petrosal sinus is clipped to transect the tentorium. Careful attention is required to avoid injury to the trochlear nerve. *C*, the tumor is debulked, allowing decompression of the brainstem and relaxation of the affected cranial nerves. Excessive adherence of the capsule to the brainstem, basilar branches or perforators, or cranial nerves may necessitate a subtotal resection. *D*, the fifth, seventh, and eighth cranial nerves are seen after tumor resection. Medial tumor remnants are resected with concern toward excessive retraction against the brainstem. Reprinted with permission from Tew JM, van Loveren HR, Keller JT: *Atlas of Operative Microneurosurgery.* Philadelphia, W.B. Saunders, vol II, in press.

retraction, a retrosigmoid craniotomy and tentorial sectioning (*Fig. 38.5B*) are performed to provide anterolateral retraction of the sigmoid sinus and enhanced visualization of the lower brainstem (*Fig. 38.5, C and D*). When tumors extend to the dura of the medial clivus, additional exposure is obtained by resection of the labyrinth and mobilization of the facial nerve.

Tumors extending below the jugular tubercle (*Fig. 38.6A*) require exposure of the lower clivus to the foramen magnum, provided by the lateral suboccipital/transcondylar approaches. This exposure involves a retrosigmoid craniotomy that is placed laterally. Access to the ventrolateral brainstem is significantly hampered by the jugular tubercle if only a retrosigmoid craniotomy is performed. A modification of the retrosigmoid craniotomy to include a transcondylar exposure is preferred for meningiomas in this region (37). The patient is placed in the lateral oblique position, and a retrosigmoid craniotomy is performed. Depending on the location of the meningioma, the bony opening may be extended to include a posterior petrosectomy and/or a C1 laminectomy. The vertebral artery is identified at its dural entry point, and its medial retraction exposes the atlanto-occipital joint. Under microscopic magnification, a diamond drill is used to resect the posteromedial one-third of the occipital condyle and lateral mass of C1 to expose approximately 1 cm of the dura lateral to the dural entry point of the vertebral artery. An attempt is made to limit the condylar resection to the medial half of the joint (*Fig. 38.6B*). This limited resection preserves occipitocervical stability and avoids the need for subsequent fusion. The bony resection can be continued to skeletonize the jugular bulb to permit retraction. The dural incision extends from the inferomedial aspect of the dural entry point of the vertebral artery superiorly across the foramen magnum and suboccipital craniotomy. A small dural cuff can remain on the vertebral artery to facilitate dural closure (*Fig. 38.6C*). Using these techniques, we have been able to achieve gross total resections in nearly all patients. If occipital cervical instability is confirmed, instrumentation and fusion are performed as part of the same operative procedure (*Fig. 38.6D*).

For lesions of the inferior clivus, direct anterior transfacial/transbasal approaches may include the transoral, transmaxillary, transmandibular, and labiomandibuloglossotomy dissection. Transfacial approaches for intradural lesions provide a direct exposure of the lesion but are limited in lateral extension by the cranial nerves and carotid arteries. A watertight dural closure and reconstruction of the nasopharynx must be effective to prevent a cerebrospinal fluid leakage.

CONTEMPORARY TREATMENT OF SKULL BASE MENINGIOMAS 569

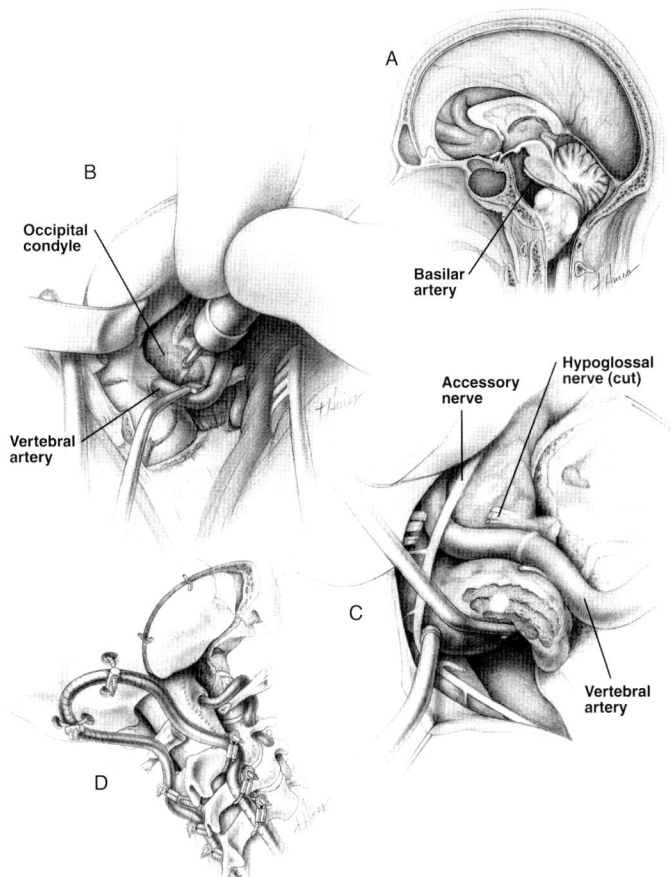

FIG. 38.6 Foramen magnum meningioma: sagittal section and operative technique. *A,* sagittal schematic diagram reveals a meningioma arising from the ventral foramen magnum with compression of the pontomedullary junction and displacement of the vertebrobasilar junction. *B,* after a lower lateral suboccipital craniotomy and C1 hemilaminectomy with partial mobilization of the vertebral artery, the medial aspect of the occipital condyle is resected. The partial condylectomy provides exposure to the ventral aspect of the lower skull base at the level of the foramen magnum, hypoglossal canal, and jugular tubercle. *C,* after the dura is incised, the tumor is mobilized without retracting on the medulla. If lower cranial neuropathies exist, sectioning of selected cranial nerve IX or X rootlets greatly assist in mobilizing the ventral tumor. Ultrasonic aspiration is often required to minimize tumor bulk without manipulation of the adjacent critical structures. *D,* occipitocervical instability may develop if more than half of a normal occipital condyle is resected. In such cases, occipitocervical fusion is performed, providing immediate stability. The dura is closed in a watertight fashion. Reprinted with permission from Tew JM, van Loveren HR, Keller JT: *Atlas of Operative Microneurosurgery.* Philadelphia, W.B. Saunders, vol II, in press.

OUTCOME ANALYSIS

Cavernous Sinus Meningiomas

Despite the technical advances in skull base approaches to cavernous sinus meningiomas, significant proportions of patients experience postoperative morbidity, partial resection, and the risk of recurrence after surgery. Analysis of our experience in 39 patients with cavernous sinus meningiomas revealed that two important factors affect the ability to achieve a total resection (25). First, the degree of ICA involvement as a result of invasion of the arterial wall was the primary determinant of total resectability (18, 25). Sacrifice of the ICA infiltrated by a meningioma carries a significant risk and has not been demonstrated to increase the long-term rate of cure. Second, tumor invasion of multiple fossae greatly decreases the ability to achieve a complete resection. In the face of these complicating factors, the surgical goal must be reassessed, and the strategy may dictate cytoreduction of extracavernous tumor and subsequent treatment of intracavernous tumor with adjunctive therapies. The incidence of total resection from five recent large series from skull base centers varied from 20.5 to 87.1% (8, 9, 25, 31, 33) (*Table 38.3*). These differences represent different surgical strategies regarding the need for complete resection. In our opinion, the treatment of holocavernous lesions should be limited to radiotherapy.

Clival and Petroclival Meningiomas

Experience with a suboccipital, retrosigmoid approach to petroclival meningiomas has been tarnished by significant morbidity and a high incidence of residual tumors. The development of skull base techniques has led to a renewed enthusiasm for more complete resection of meningiomas in this region. Improved exposure and more complete resection has been achieved. We must now wait to determine whether follow-up results will justify the aggressive attempts at total removal. A review of 11 large surgical series of petroclival meningiomas from established skull base centers reveals the continuing challenge of these tumors (1, 4, 14, 16, 22, 27, 29, 30, 32, 41) (*Table 38.4*). Total excision was achieved in 303 of 459 patients (66%), whereas new cranial neuropathies occurred in 12 to 83% of cases. Mortality has reached 0% in our experience, and the Karnofsky score has been either retained or improved in 91% of patients.

CONCLUSION

Several innovations have changed the approach to skull base meningiomas. First, improved diagnostic imaging clarifies issues regarding

TABLE 38.3
Review of Surgery for Cavernous Sinus Meningiomas

Reference	No. of Cases	Total Excision	Follow-up (mos)
Sepehrnia et al., 1991	36	50% (18/36)	Unclear
Sekhar et al., 1992	70	87% (61/70)	36
De Monte et al., 1994	41	76% (31/41)	36
De Jesus et al., 1996	119	61% (73/119)	36–60
O'Sullivan et al., 1997	39	20.5% (8/39)	24

the tumor's location, pathology, and vascularity. Second, understanding the significance of the biological potential of individual tumors by analyzing their proliferative potential not only guides initial and adjunct treatment but also provides information regarding the potential for recurrence and ultimate prognosis. Third, a better comprehension of the natural history of skull base meningiomas has been achieved, and these critical factors must be analyzed in the context of the individual patient's neurological presentation before developing a treatment plan.

The treatment of skull base meningiomas has evolved at an equally rapid pace. Observation is advocated in subsets of patients who are asymptomatic or mildly symptomatic. Patients with advanced risk factors or age considerations may be best observed or treated with radiotherapy. Microsurgeons have improved the techniques of accessing and resecting these tumors, but significant morbidity and recurrence rates still exist because of the difficulty in resecting the entire tumor, its dural base, and its blood supply. An increasing emphasis is being placed on the value of conformal and stereotactic radiotherapy to treat residual tumor, tumor recurrences, and aggressive pathological variants. Because of the low cranial nerve morbidity associated with radiating skull base meningiomas that abut and potentially invade critical structures, the tolerability of SRS, improved tumor control rates, and significant incidence of surgical morbidity, the initial treatment of these tumors with focused radiotherapy or SRS is being advocated and favored in several skull base centers. Because their natural history involves slow growth, an appropriate follow-up period of at least 10 years is required to verify the tumor control rates and long-term complication rates related to radiation therapy. We believe that current wisdom advocates the use of judicious microsurgery employing skull base techniques and focused radiotherapy. The operative survival and resection of these treacherous lesions has been greatly improved by this approach. The role of adjunctive chemotherapy is being evaluated but has proved to be of limited value, even in malignant lesions.

TABLE 38.4
Review of Surgery for Petroclival Meningiomas

Reference	No. of Cases	Total Excision	Postoperative Mortality	Major Morbidity	New CN Deficit	Recurrence
Mayberg and Simon, 1980	35	26% (9/35)	9%	34%	54%	20% (11 died)
Yasargil et al., 1980	20	35% (7/20)	10%	30%	50%	25%
Sekhar et al., 1987	30	70% (21/30)	0%	13%	20%	10%
Al-Mefty et al., 1988	13	85% (11/13)	0%	8%	31%	8%
Hakuba et al., 1988	13	85% (11/13)	0%	35%	31%	Unclear
Samii et al., 1988	24	71% (17/24)	0%	17%	46%	Unclear
Hakuba et al., 1988	24	71% (17/24)	8%	29%	83%	33%
Sekhar et al., 1990	41	78% (32/41)	2%	7%	12%	10%
Bricolo et al., 1929	33	79% (26/33)	9%	18%	76%	Unclear
Kawase et al., 1994	42	76% (32/42)	0%	12%	36%	7%
Sekhar et al., 1994	75	60% (45/75)	1%	16%	60%	3%

REFERENCES

1. Al-Mefty O, Fox JL, Smith RR: Petrosal approach for petroclival meningiomas. **Neurosurgery** 22:510–517, 1988.
2. Barbaro NM, Gutin PH, Wilson CB, Sheline GE, Boldrey EB, Wara WM: Radiation therapy in the treatment of partially resected meningiomas. **Neurosurgery** 20:525–528, 1987.
3. Bindal RK, Goodman JM, Kuzma BB, Kawasaki A: Long-term natural history of skull base (abstract). **Neurosurgery** 43:696, 1998.
4. Bricolo AB, Turazzi S, Talacchi A, Cristofori L: Microsurgical removal of petroclival meningiomas: A report of 33 patients. **Neurosurgery** 31:813–828, 1992.
5. Chen TC, Zee CS, Miller CA, et al: Magnetic resonance imaging and pathological correlates of meningiomas. **Neurosurgery** 31:1015–1022, 1992.
6. Cushing H: The meningiomas (dural endotheliomas): Their source and favoured seats of origin (Cavendish lecture). **Brain** 45:282–316, 1922.
7. Cushing H, Eisenhardt L (eds): Meningiomas: Their classification, regional behavior, life history, and surgical end results. Springfield, IL, Charles C Thomas, 1938.
8. De Jesus O, Sekhar LN, Parikh HK, Wright DC, Wagner DP: Long-term follow-up of patients with meningiomas involving the cavernous sinus: Recurrence, progression, and quality of life. **Neurosurgery** 39:915–920, 1996.
9. De Monte F, Smith H, Al-Mefty O: Outcome of aggressive removal of cavernous sinus meningiomas. **J Neurosurg** 81:245–251, 1994.
10. Dripps RD, Lamon A, Eckenhoff JE: The role of anesthesia in surgical mortality. **JAMA** 178:261–266, 1961.
11. Duma CM, Lunsford LD, Kondziolka D, Harsh GR IV, Flickinger JC: Stereotactic radiosurgery of cavernous sinus meningiomas as an addition or alternative to microsurgery. **Neurosurgery** 32:699–705, 1993.
12. Goldsmith BJ, Wara WM, Wilson CB, Larson DA: Postoperative irradiation for subtotally resected meningiomas: A retrospective analysis of 140 patients treated from 1967 to 1990. **J Neurosurg** 80:195–201, 1994.
13. Hakim R, Alexander E III, Loeffler JS, et al: Results of linear accelerator-based radiosurgery for intracranial meningiomas. **Neurosurgery** 42:446–454, 1998.
14. Hakuba A, Nishimura S, Jang BJ: A combined retroauricular and preauricular transpetrosal-transtentorial approach to clivus meningiomas. **Surg Neurol** 30:108–116, 1988.
15. Ide M, Jimbo M, Yamamoto M, Umebara Y, Hagiwara S, Kubo O: MIB-1 staining index and peritumoral brain edema of meningiomas. **Cancer** 78:133–143, 1996.
16. Kawase T, Shiobara R, Toya S: Middle fossa transpetrosal-transtentorial approaches for petroclival meningiomas. Selective pyramid resection and radicality. **Acta Neurochir (Wien)** 129:113–120, 1994.
17. Kleihues P, Burger PC, Scheithauer BW: *Histological Typing of Tumours of the Central Nervous System.* Berlin, Springer, 1993, pp 33–37.
18. Kotapka MJ, Kalia KK, Martinez AJ, Sekhar LN: Infiltration of the carotid artery by cavernous sinus infiltration. **J Neurosurg** 81:252–255, 1994.
19. Kyritsis AP: Chemotherapy for meningiomas. **J Neurooncol** 29:269–272, 1996.
20. Langford LA, Cooksley CS, DeMonte F: Comparison of MIB-1 (Ki-67) antigen and bromodeoxyuridine proliferation indices in meningiomas. **Hum Pathol** 24:350–354, 1996.
21. Matsuno A, Fujimaki T, Sasaki T, et al: Clinical and histopathological analysis of proliferative potentials of recurrent and non-recurrent meningiomas. **Acta Neuropathol (Berl)** 91:504–510, 1996.

22. Mayberg M, Symon L: Meningiomas of the clivus and apical petrous bone: Report of 35 cases. **J Neurosurg** 65:160–167, 1980.
23. Miller CG, van Loveren HR, Keller JT, Pensak M, El-Kalliny M, Tew JM Jr: Transpetrosal approach: Surgical anatomy and technique. **Neurosurgery** 33:461–469, 1993.
24. Olivero WC, Lister JR, Elwood PW: The natural history and growth rate of asymptomatic meningiomas: A review of 60 patients. **J Neurosurg** 83:222–224, 1995.
25. O'Sullivan MG, van Loveren HR, Tew JM: The surgical resectability of meningiomas of the cavernous sinus. **Neurosurgery** 40:238–247, 1997.
26. Perry A, Stafford SL, Scheithauser BW, Suman VJ, Lohse CM: The prognostic significance of MIB-1, p53, and DNA flow cytometry in completely resected primary meningiomas. **Cancer** 82:2262–2269, 1998.
27. Samii M, Ammirati M: The combined supratentorial presigmoid sinus avenue to the petroclival region: Surgical technique and clinical applications. **Acta Neurochir** 95:6–12, 1988.
28. Schrell UMH, Rittig MG, Andres M, et al: Hydroxyurea for treatment of unresectable and recurrent meningiomas: II. Decrease in the size of meningiomas in patients with hydroxyurea. **J Neurosurg** 86:840–844, 1997.
29. Sekhar LN, Janetta PJ: Petroclival and medial tentorial meningiomas, in Sekhar LN, Schramm VL Jr (eds): *Tumors of the Cranial Base: Diagnosis and Treatment.* New York, Futura Publishing Co., 1987, pp 623–640.
30. Sekhar LN, Janetta PJ, Burkhart LE, Janosky JE: Meningiomas involving the clivus: A six-year experience with 41 patients. **Neurosurgery** 27:764–781, 1990.
31. Sekhar LN, Ross DA, Sen CN: Cavernous sinus and sphenocavernous neoplasms: Anatomy and surgery, in Sekhar LN, Jancecka IP (eds): *Surgery of Cranial Base Tumors.* New York, Raven Press, 1992, pp 605–659.
32. Sekhar LN, Swamy NKS, Jaiswal U, Rubenstein E, Hirsch WE Jr, Wright DC: Surgical excision of meningiomas involving the clivus: Preoperative and intraoperative features as predictors of postoperative functional deterioration. **J Neurosurg** 81:860–868, 1994.
33. Sepehrnia A, Samii M, Tatagiba M: Management of intracavernous tumors: An 11-year experience. **Acta Neurochir Suppl (Wien)** 53:122–126, 1991.
34. Stewart DJ, Dahrouge S, Wee M, Aitken S, Hugenholtz H: Intra-arterial cisplatin plus intravenous doxorubicin for inoperable recurrent meningiomas. **J Neurooncol** 24:189–194, 1995.
35. Subach BR, Lunsford LD, Kondziolka D, Maitz AH, Flickinger JC: Management of petroclival meningiomas by stereotactic radiosurgery. **Neurosurgery** 42:437–445, 1998.
36. Vacanti CJ, Van Houten RJ, Hill RC: A statistical analysis of the relationship of physical status to postoperative morbidity in 68,388 cases. **Anesth Analg Curr Res** 49:564–566, 1970.
37. Van Loveren HR, Liu SS, Tew JM: Trancondylar approach. **Oper Techniques Otolaryngol Head Neck Surg** 7:151–158, 1996.
38. Van Loveren HR, Mahmood A, Liu SS: Innovations in cranial approaches and exposures: Anterolateral approaches, in Loftus CM (ed): *Clinical Neurosurgery.* Baltimore, Williams & Wilkins, 1996, pp. 44–52.
39. Wilson CB: Meningiomas: Genetics, malignancy, and the role of radiation in induction and treatment. **J Neurosurg** 81:666–675, 1994.
40. Wober-Bingal C, Wober C, Marosi C, Prayer D: Interferon-alpha-2b for meningioma (letter). **Lancet** 345:331, 1995.
41. Yasargil MG, Mortara RW, Curcic M: Meningiomas of basal posterior cranial fossa, in Krayenbuhl H (ed): *Advances and Technical Standard in Neurosurgery,* Wien, Springer-Verlag, 1980, vol 7, pp 3–115.

Author Index

A
Alleyne, Cargill H., Jr., 339–349
Andrews, Brian T., 196–201
Andrius, L. John, 12–21
Apfelbaum, Ronald I., 473–495
Apuzzo, Michael L. J., 44–66
Armonda, Rocco A., 237–256
Awad, Issam A., 363–387
Aziz, Khaled M. Abdel, 554–571

B
Barrow, Daniel L., 285–293, 392–406
Batjer, H. Hunt, 319–325
Beal, M. Flint, 12–21
Bentson, John, 295–316
Bogdanov, Mikhail, 12–21
Brown, Jeffrey A., 455–470
Burchiel, Kim J., 435–444
Butler, William E., 12–21

C
Carter, Bob S., 351–361
Cawley, C. Michael, 392–406
Chen, Joseph C. T., 44–66
Chestnut, Randall M., 185–187

D
Detwiler, Paul W., 526–552
Dickman, Curtis A., 526–552
Doberstein, Curt, 295–316

E
Endres, Matthias, 12–21

F
Fink, Klaus B., 12–21
Frank, Jeffrey I., 261–265
Friedlander, Robert M., 12–21
Friedman, William A., 1–11

G
Gopal, Harsha, 507–514

H
Hadley, Mark N., 153–166

Heilbrun, M. Peter, 89–100
Heilman, Carl B., 507–514
Holland, Martin, 216–226

K
Kalfas, Iain H., 70–87
Kaye, Andrew H., 499–505
Khan, Sohail Q., 12–21
Khanna, Rohit, 295–316
Kilburn, Michael P. B., 153–166
Kokkino, Andrew J., 554–571

L
Lee, Sunghoon, 363–387
Lewis, Adam I., 267–282
Li, Mingwei, 12–21
Link, Michael J., 326–334
Luerssen, Thomas G., 170–181

M
Marshall, Lawrence F., 105–112
Martin, Neil A., 295–316
Mayberg, Marc R., 231–235
McDonald, Jeffrey D., 89–100
Meagher, Richard J., 127–140
Moskowitz, Michael A., 12–21

N
Namura, Shobu, 12–21
Narayan, Raj K., 127–140

O
Ogilvy, Christopher S., 351–361
Ojemann, Robert G., 351–361
Ona, Victoria O., 12–21

P
Pitts, Lawrence H., 216–226
Porter, Randall W., 526–552
Povlishock, John T., 113–124
Putman, Christopher, 351–361

R
Rebeiz, Elie E., 507–514
Rosenwasser, Robert H., 237–256

S
Sagher, Oren, 446–453
Shucart, William A., 507–514
Spetzler, Robert F., 339–349

T
Taha, Jamal M., 410–429
Teo, Charles, 515–525
Tew, John M., Jr., 27–43, 267–282, 326–334, 410–429, 554–571
Tomsick, Thomas A., 326–334

V
Vishteh, A. Giancarlo, 339–349

W
Walters, Beverly C., 203–215
Wilberger, Jack E., 143–151

Y
Yuan, Junying, 12–21

Subject Index

A

Abernethy, John, 363–364
Ablation procedures, with stereotaxy, 64–65
Acetyl-Tyr-Val-Ala-Asp-chloromethylketone, for traumatic brain injury, 17–21, *18*
AcYVAD-cmk, 17–21, *18*
Adenomas, endoscopic surgery for, 507–514
Airway management, in head injury, 131–132
  pediatric, 172–173, 175
American Association for the Surgery of Trauma (AAST), 224
American Association of Neurological Surgeons/Congress of Neurological Surgeons (AANS/CNS)
  Carotid Endarterectomy Task Force, 231, 235
  Cerebrovascular Section, 235
  legislative initiative of, 220
  Neuroendovascular Task Force, 235
American College of Surgeons, Committee on Trauma (ASCOT), 217–218, 218*t*
Amitriptyline, for facial pain, 452*t*, 468
Anesthesia
  endotracheal, 526–530
  for percutaneous treatment of trigeminal neuralgia, 468, 493
  risk assessment, 559
  for thoracoscopy, 526–530
Anesthesia dolorosa, with trigeminal neuralgia treatment, 448*t*, 468–469, 473, 490, 493, 495
Anesthetic, local, for facial pain, 453
Aneurysm(s), intracranial. *See also* Pseudoaneurysms
  basilar tip, 517
  cavernous
    asymptomatic, therapeutic carotid artery occlusion for, 327, 366, 366*t*
    symptomatic, therapeutic carotid artery occlusion for, 327, 340, 366, 366*t*

  therapeutic carotid artery occlusion for, 366, 366*t*, 394–395, *395*, 401–402
  treatment of, historical perspective on, 364, 392–394
  cluster headache with, 428
  collateral or retrograde blood flow to, after therapeutic carotid artery occlusion, *395*, 402, 406
  contralateral to side of therapeutic carotid artery occlusion, 373, 402, 406
  de novo formation of, after therapeutic carotid artery occlusion, 330–332, 333*t*, 342, *345*, 371–373, *372*, 375, 402–403
  endoscopic-assisted microneurosurgery for, 515–525, *523–524*
  extracranial-intracranial bypass surgery for, 406. *See also* Extracranial-intracranial bypass surgery
  literature on, 357–359, 358*t*
  giant, treatment of, historical perspective on, 364
  high cervical, management of, 398
  with intracranial arteriovenous malformations, 267–269
    management of, 271–272, *272*, 296
    ruptured, management of, 274–277, *276*
  large/giant supraclinoid, management of, 395–397, *396–397*, 401–402
  petrous segment, management of, 398
  rupture, after therapeutic carotid artery occlusion, 371–373, 375, 402–403
  trapping procedure for, 406
  treatment of, historical perspective on, 364
  untreated, rupture, after therapeutic carotid artery occlusion, 371–373, 375, 402–403
Angiography. *See also* Magnetic resonance angiography
  in cerebrovascular disease, 238
  of skull base meningioma, 557

Angioplasty, in acute stroke, 255–256
Anterior commissure-posterior commissure line, 50
Anterior fossa, meningiomas of, 557
  operative technique for, 563, *564*
Anterior inferior cerebellar artery, trigeminal nerve compression by, 474, 483
Anticoagulation
  in percutaneous treatment of trigeminal neuralgia, 469–470
  with therapeutic carotid artery occlusion, 334, 371, 384, 386, 405–406
    benefits of, 369
    contraindications to, 367, 368*t*
Anticonvulsant(s), for facial pain, 437, 439–440, 449–450, 451*t*, 462–463, 478
Antidepressant(s), for facial pain, 441–442, 449–451, 452*t*, 468
Apoptosis, traumatic brain injury and, 12–23, 116
Arteriovenous malformations, intracranial. *See also* Venous malformations, intracranial
  aneurysms associated with, 267–269
    management of, 271–272, *272*, 296
    ruptured, management of, 274–277, *276*
  angioarchitecture, and risk of hemorrhage, 267
  arterial supply to, 298
  cavernous, treatment of, 268–269, 277, *277–279*
  cerebral perfusion pressure compromise with, 303
  cluster headache with, 428
  embolization, 268–273, *270–271*, 295–315, 321
    anatomic and physiologic effects of, 295–296
    applications of, 295–296
    complications of, 296–300
    as cure, 296, *297*, 300–301, *302*
    delayed refilling or recanalization after, 300–301, *302*
    draining vein occlusion with, 298, *299*
    to facilitate hemostasis and nidus dissection, 307–313, *309*, 310*t*–311*t*, *312*

for feeding artery embolization, 301–302
feeding artery perforation with, 297
hemodynamic complications of, prevention of, 303–307
hemorrhagic complications of, 298, *299*
historical perspective on, 295
incomplete nidus occlusion with, 298–300
indications for, 300, 305*t*
ischemic complications of, 297
limitations of, 296–300
mortality with, 298
neurologic complications of, 297
palliative partial, 315–316
partial, and risk of future hemorrhage, 316
perfusion pressure breakthrough after, prevention of, 303–307
as preoperative adjunct, 295–296, 300–301, 307–313, *309*, 310*t*–311*t*, *312*
reflux of embolic material in, 297–298
restoration of normal cerebral autoregulation after, 303–307, *306*
rupture after, 298, *299*
state of the art, 296
for stepwise preoperative flow reduction, 303–307, *307*
before stereotactic radiosurgery, 272–273, 280, 313–315
technical advances in, 295–296
feeding arteries
  deep/inaccessible, embolization, 302–303, *304*
  embolization, 301–302
  perforation, with embolization, 297
giant, management of, 281
global hemispheric, management of, 273
grade, and treatment modality, 268
grading system for, 286
hemorrhage with
  partial embolization and, 316
  risk factors for, 267–268
inoperable, 273, 291
large
  management of, 303–313
  surgical reduction, preoperative embolization and, 307–313, 310*t*

surgical resection, preoperative embolization and, 307–313, 311t
location, and risk of hemorrhage, 267
microsurgery for, 267–268, 273–279
  advantages and disadvantages of, 285
  arguments against, 324
  arguments for, 323–324
  cost-effectiveness of, 287–288, 289t
  efficacy of, 287, 288t
  minor unreported complications of, 291
  neurosurgeon's experience and, 290, 292
  outcomes with, 286–287, 288t
  patient preference and, 288–290
  quality-adjusted life years gained with, 288, 289t–290t
  and radiosurgery, comparison of, 274, 275, 285–293
  risk assessment for, 290–291
mixed venous and cavernous, 279
morbidity and mortality with, 268–269
natural history of, 319–320
postoperative residual, stereotactic radiosurgery for, 280
prognostic factors for, 286
radiosurgery for, 267–268
  advantages and disadvantages of, 285
  embolization before, 272–273, 280, 313–315
  image-guided technique, 99, 100
  and microsurgery, comparison of, 274, 275, 285–293
  neurosurgeon's experience and, 292
  outcomes with, 286–287
  patient preference and, 288–290
  risks of, 292–293
recurrence of, 268
resection
  with embolization, 307–313, 309, 310t–311t, 312
  risk-benefit analysis for, 285–286
  without embolization, 313, 314
ruptured, management of, 274
size
  and hemodynamic complications, 305
  and management, 286, 305
  and risk of hemorrhage, 267

treatment of
  case selection and, 322–323
  controversy about, 267
  to eliminate risk for recurrent hemorrhage, 267–268
  goal of, 268, 319–320
  historical perspective on, 364
  by observation, 269, 321
  options for, 268–269, 321
  outcome analysis, 281
  principles of, 320–321
  rationale for, 319–320
  strategies for, 321–322
  successful, requirements for, 322
Astrolabe, 46
Atelectasis, postoperative, 535, 541
Atlases, stereotactic, 33, 50, 50–51
  MRI-based, 59
Augmentative procedures, stereotaxy for, 64–65
Autoregulation, in head-injured patients, 144

B
Baclofen, for facial pain, 449–450, 451t
Bailes, Julian, 234
Balloon compression
  anesthetic for, 468, 493
  hemorrhagic complications of, 470
  for multiple division pain, 467
  selective injury with, 466–467
  for trigeminal neuralgia, 413, 416t, 417–418, 419t, 457–460, 466–468, 470, 493–494
    advantages and disadvantages of, 418, 419t
    trigeminal motor weakness after, 416t, 417
Barbiturates
  adjunctive, in therapeutic carotid artery occlusion, 346
  in head injury, pediatric, 175–176, 178
  in management of traumatic brain injury, 186, 186t
N-Benzyloxycarbonyl-Val-Ala-Asp-fluoromethylketone, for traumatic brain injury, 17–21, 18
Birley, J.L., 393
Blood pressure, in head injury. See Hypotension

Brain
  function
    equipotential school of, 47
    heterogenous nature of, 47–48
    localized, 47–48
  injury. See Head injury; Traumatic brain injury
  structures, variability in location of, 51
Brain Attack Coalition, Acute Stroke Toolbox, 234–235
Bromodeoxyuridine index, 555–556
Brown, Russell, 56, 90
Brown-Roberts-Wells (BRW) apparatus, 56–58, *58,* 61, 90
Burr hole(s), by general surgeons, 130
Burr-hole mounted devices, for stereotaxy, 51, *52*
Business plans, 38–39

C

Calcium, neuronal, after traumatic brain injury, 116
  neuroprotection targeted at, 119, 121*t*
Capsaicin, for facial pain, 453
Carbamazepine, for facial pain, 437, 439, 449–450, 451*t*, 462–463, 478
Cardiac tamponade, 135
Carotid artery
  puncture, with percutaneous treatment of trigeminal neuralgia, 470, 491
  rupture
    management of, 364, 366*t*, 366–367
    risk factors for, 367
    traumatic, 367
  therapeutic occlusion. See Therapeutic carotid artery occlusion
Carotid cavernous fistulae, management of, 327–328, 340, 397–398
Carotid endarterectomy
  frequency of, 231, *232*
  neurosurgeons' role in, 231–232, *233*
Carotid stent, *247–248*
Caspase(s), 12
  in acute and chronic neurological disorders, 20
  in traumatic brain injury, 12–23
Caspase-1, 12–23
Caspase inhibitors
  therapeutic window for, 17
  for traumatic brain injury, 17–21, *18*

Causalgia, thoracoscopic sympathectomy for, 530
Cavernous sinus, meningiomas of
  operative outcomes with, 570, 571*t*
  operative technique for, 563, *565*
Celestial navigation, *46,* 46–47
Cell death
  speed of, trigger event and, 20
  in traumatic brain injury, 12–23
Central nervous system, injury. See Neurotrauma
Central sulcus, localization of, 48
Central venous catheterization, with therapeutic carotid artery occlusion, 382–384
Cerebral blood flow, measurement of
  with HMPAO SPECT, 251–253, 328–330, 355, 360, 377–378, *379,* 404
  qualitative methods, 328, 353, 404. See also Single photon emission computed tomography (SPECT)
  quantitative methods, 254, 328, 353, 404. See also Xenon computed tomography (CT)
  in stroke, 254
  before therapeutic carotid artery occlusion, 341–343, 353–355, 360, 375–378
Cerebral edema
  in head injury, 145
  with meningioma, 558
Cerebral ischemia. See also Stroke, ischemic
  early acute
    computed tomography of, 241
    magnetic resonance imaging of, 241
  hemodynamic, after therapeutic carotid artery occlusion, 351, 353, 367–368, *370*
  thromboembolic, after therapeutic carotid artery occlusion, 351, 353, 368–369, *369*
Cerebral perfusion pressure
  in management of traumatic brain injury, 186–188, 188*t*
  normal, in children, 174–175
Cerebral perfusion pressure therapy, with head injury, 145, 147, *147,* 186–188, 188*t*
  pediatric contraindication to, 174–175

Cerebral vasospasm, with subarachnoid hemorrhage, 274, *276*, 277
Cerebrospinal fluid, drainage, with pediatric head injury, 175–176
Cerebrovascular disease
  computed tomography in, 238–241, *239*
  diagnostic studies for, 238–254
  digital subtraction angiography in, 238
  emergency services related to, 234
  incidence of, 231
  magnetic resonance imaging in, 238, 241–250, *244*
    apparent diffusion coefficient maps, 245–247
    diffusion-weighted imaging, *244*, 245–250, *249*
    magnetic resonance spectroscopy of, 251, *252*
  management of, guidelines for, 235
  outcomes of, assessment instruments, 235
  research on, neurosurgeons' role in, 232–234
  single photon emission computed tomography in, 250–254, *253*
  treatment of, neurosurgeons' role in, 232
Cervical spine
  C1–2 transarticular screw fixation, spinal imaging for, 74–75, 81–82, *83*
  lateral mass plate fixation, spinal imaging for, 83–84
Chemotherapy, for skull base meningiomas, 560–561, 571
Children
  head injury in
    airway management with, 172–173, 175
    barbiturates in, 175–176, 178
    cerebral perfusion pressure in, 174–175
    cerebrospinal fluid drainage in, 175–176
    fluid resuscitation in, 172–173, 178
    hyperventilation for, 175, 178
    hypotension with, 174–175
    integration and design of therapies for, 176–178
    intracranial pressure in, measurement and management of, 173–178
    mild or minor, 179
    osmotic therapies for, 175–176
    prehospital management in, 172–173
    severe, 170–178
    ventriculostomy for, 178
  neurological injuries in, current management strategies for, 170–184
  spinal cord injury in, 179–181
    anatomic properties and, 180–181
    management of, 181
    mechanisms of, 180
    patterns of, 180
    pharmacological therapy for, 181
    without radiographic abnormality (SCIWORA), 180–181
  traumatic brain injury in, 170–178
  standard therapies for, 171–172, 176
Chordoma, endoscopic-assisted microsurgery for, 519, *520*
Chronometers, 46–47
Cingulotomy, 469
Clival meningiomas, 563–568, 570
Clonazepam, for facial pain, 451*t*
Cluster headache
  with intracranial pathology, 428
  nervus intermedius-superficial petrosal-sphenopalatine system in, 426
  surgery of, 426–429, 427*t*
  pathogenesis of, 425–426
  treatment of, 426*t*, 426–429, 427*t*
    innovative approaches, 428
  trigeminovascular system in, 426
  surgery of, 426*t*, 426–428
Columbus, Christopher, 45–46
Common carotid artery, stenosis, *248*
Compasses, 45, *46*
Computed tomography (CT)
  and brain shift monitoring, 92
  in cerebrovascular disease, 238–241, *239*
  development of, 56, *57*
  of disc herniation, 539, *539*
  of head injury
    in hypotensive patients, 137, *138*
    pediatric, 173, 176, 178–179
  of skull base meningioma, 557
  of spinal cord injury, 157, *157*

stereotaxy with, 29, 33–34, 56, 63–64, 89–90
  instrumentation for, 56–58, *58*
  in trigeminal neuralgia, 436–438
Computer, stereotactic technique with, 31
Contralateral endoscopic method, 516
Cooper, Astley, 363–364, 393
Core curriculum, in neurosurgical critical care, 199, 200*t*
  and certification, 201
Cornea
  anesthesia, after trigeminal neuralgia treatment, 414*t*–416*t*, 417
  damage, with trigeminal neuralgia treatment, 412*t*, 414*t*–416*t*, 417, 456, 473, 490, 493, 495
Cortical stimulation, with awake craniotomy, 96–97, *98*
Costotransversectomy, versus thoracoscopic discectomy, 541
Cranial injuries, as domain of neurosurgeon, 153–155, 216–226
Cranial nerve(s)
  V (trigeminal), compression of, 499. *See also* Trigeminal *entries*
  VII (facial)
    compression of, 475–476, 480, 499. *See also* Hemifacial spasm
    palsy, after trigeminal neuralgia treatment, 412*t*, 414*t*–416*t*, 417
  IX (glossopharyngeal). *See also* Glossopharyngeal neuralgia; Vagoglossopharyngeal neuralgia
    transient paresis, after vagoglossopharyngeal neuralgia treatment, 424
  X (vagus). *See also* Vagoglossopharyngeal neuralgia
    transient paresis, after vagoglossopharyngeal neuralgia treatment, 424
  hyperactive dysfunction of, 473–474, 476, 502
Cranial neuralgias, 442–443, 443*t*. *See also* Trigeminal neuralgia
Craniofacial pain, 435–445. *See also* Trigeminal neuralgia
Craniometric localization, 48–49
Craniopharyngioma, endoscopic-assisted microsurgery for, 518–519

Craniospinal traction, 154–155, 157–158
Craniotomy, neurosurgeon's role in, 191
Critical care
  competency in, 189, 192–193
  neurosurgical
    core curriculum in, 199, 200*t*
    credentialing in, 201
  for neurotrauma, models of, 185–194
  special qualifications in, 197
  for traumatic brain injury, neurosurgeon's role in, 187–191
    as team leader, 189–190
    as team member, 190
    as technical consultant, 190–191
Critical care neurologist, 198
CRW frame, 61, *61*
Cushing, Harvey, 364
Cushing's disease, endoscopic surgery in, 513–514

D
Dandy, Walter, 327, 364, 393–394, 474, 481, 499
Database
  for neurosurgical research
    characteristics of, 204–211
    and confidentiality, 210–211
    data collection for, 205, 212–215
    data entry for, 205
    design of, 211, 214
    device-specific, 204
    disease-oriented, 204
    funding for, 211–212
    goal(s) for, 212
    hardware and software requirements for, 205–210
    information storage in, 210
    maintenance of, 211
    organization of, 204–205
    population-oriented, 204
    and privacy, 210–211
    procedure-specific, 204
    successful, characteristics of, 212
    therapy-specific, 204
  on neurotrauma, 203–215
    actuarial outcome variables for, 213–214
    clinical outcome variables for, 213–214
    clinical variables for, 213

cost-effectiveness variables for, 213–214
data collection for, 212–215
demographic variables for, 213
functional outcome variables for, 213–214
injury variables for, 213
on-line data collection for, 205, *208–209*
outcome variables for, 213–214
quality of life variables for, 213–214
treatment variables for, 213
for trauma assessment, 205, *206–207*
Dead reckoning, 44–45, *46*, 48–49, 63
Decompression
cerebral, in head injury
by general surgeons, 130
timing of, 137–139
neurovascular, 455–457, 473–498, 503–505
spinal
in spinal cord injury, 155–159, 165–166
in thoracoscopic discectomy, 535–541
Deep brain stimulation, for trigeminal neuropathic pain, 464, 468–469
Demyelination, and trigeminal neuralgia, 455, 458, 477–478, 481
Depression, and facial pain, 441–442, 451
Desipramine, for facial pain, 452t
Diagnostic imaging, for stroke, 237–256
Diagnostic peritoneal lavage (DPL), for hypotensive head-injured patients, 137, *138*
Diffuse axonal injury, pathophysiology of, 113–115
Digital subtraction angiography, in cerebrovascular disease, 238
Discectomy, thoracoscopic, 526, 530, 535–541
bleeding with, 537, 539, *540*, 541
clinical results of, 541
versus costotransversectomy, 541
operative time of, 541
patient positioning for, *536*, 536–537
technique of, 536–539, *538*, *540*
Disc herniation
clinical manifestations of, 535
computed tomography of, 539, *539*
thoracoscopic discectomy for, 535–541

DNA fragmentation, in traumatic brain injury, 14–16, *15,* 20
Doppler ultrasound
carotid, in pre-procedural evaluation for therapeutic carotid artery occlusion, 382
transcranial
in cerebrovascular disease, 238
with clinical balloon test occlusion of ICA, 356, 385
predictive value, for ischemic risk, 376
Dorsal root entry zone surgery, for cluster headache, 428
Doxepin, for facial pain, 452t
Dripps-ASA scale, 559
Dysesthesia, after trigeminal neuralgia treatment, 412t, 413–417, 414t–416t, 423, 459–460, 468, 473
Dysphagia, after vagoglossopharyngeal neuralgia treatment, 424

E
Electrical stimulation
for navigation, 54–55
for trigeminal neuropathic pain, 463–465, 468–469
Electroencephalography (EEG), 95
with clinical balloon test occlusion of ICA, 356
Electrophysiological localization, 54–56, *55*
Emergency rooms, specialty coverage in, 127–130
Endoscopic-assisted microneurosurgery, 515–525
aim of, 515
benefits of, 515, 521–525
objective, 515–516, 521
subjective, 521
complications of, 517–518
contralateral, 516
definition of, 515, 521
ipsilateral, 516
materials and methods of, 515–517
for neurovascular procedures, 515–525, *523–524*
patient pathologies in, 518t
questionnaire for assessing efficacy of, 517, 518t
results of, 517–519

safety rules for, 521
as teaching aid, 521
transsphenoidal, 517
transventricular, 516–517
for tumors, 515–525, *520, 522*
Endoscopic-guided surgery, 521
Endoscopic pituitary surgery, 507–514
 sphenoidotomy approach for, 507*t*, 507–514
  anatomical considerations in, 508
  complications of, 514
  hospital stay after, 513*t*, 513–514
  instrumentation for, 508–509
  patient positioning for, 509
  results of, 513–514
  surgeon positioning for, 509
  technique of, 508–513, *510–512*
 sublabial transseptal approach for, 507
Endoscopic spine surgery, 526–553. *See also specific procedures*
 Barrow Neurological Institute experience with, 526, 529*t*
 comparison of approaches in, 526, 527*t*
 laparoscopic, 526, 527*t*, 543–552
 thoracoscopic, 526–543, 527*t*
Endoscopic surgery. *See also specific procedures*
 pure, 519–521
Endoscopy, applications of, 519–521
Endotracheal anesthesia, for thoracoscopy, 526–530
Ependymoma, endoscopic-assisted microsurgery for, *522*
Ephapse, in trigeminal neuralgia, 477
Epileptiform neuralgia, 446
European Cooperative Acute Stroke Study (ECASS), 261, 263
European Cooperative Acute Stroke Study II (ECASS II), 263
Excitatory amino acids, elevation, after traumatic brain injury, 115–117
 neuroprotection targeted at, 118, 120*t*
Extracranial injury, and hypotension with head injury, 134–135
Extracranial-intracranial bypass surgery. *See also* Therapeutic carotid artery occlusion, revascularization for
 algorithm for, 358*t*, 360–361
 for aneurysm treatment, 379, 394–395, *395, 397*
 complications of, 358*t*, 359
 literature on, 357–359, 358*t*
 goal of, 351
 high-flow, 405
 ischemic risk with, 380
 low-flow, 404–405
 morbidity and mortality with, 358*t*, 359, 380
 patient selection for, 405
 selective, 326, 328, 341–343, 351–352, 381, *382*
  for borderline-risk (at-risk) patients, 360, 380, 405
  risk-benefit analysis for, 357*t*–358*t*, 359, 405
  versus universal (prophylactic), 339–340, 346–347, 348*t*, 352–353, 405
 thromboembolic risk with, 369, 380
 universal (prophylactic), 332–334, 343–346, 351, 378–381, 405
  arguments against, 381
  delayed occlusion after, 333–334
  for high-risk group, 360–361, 385, 405
  morbidity and mortality with, 332–333, 358*t*, 359
  results with, 333
  risk-benefit analysis for, 357*t*–358*t*, 359, 405
  versus selective, 339–340, 346–347, 348*t*, 352–353, 405

F
Facial nerve, compression of, 475–476, 480, 499. *See also* Hemifacial spasm
Facial pain. *See also* Trigeminal neuralgia
 anticonvulsants for, 437, 439–440, 449–450, 451*t*, 462–463
 antidepressants for, 441–442, 449–451, 452*t*, 468
 atypical, 441–442, 448*t*, 469
 characteristics of, 441*t*
 conditions associated with, 441–442
 treatment of, 410
 capsaicin for, 453
 clinical diagnosis of, 436–443
 constant, 449
 as continuum of diagnosis, 443–444, *444*

depression and, 441–442, 451
diagnostic clues in, 447, 448t
differential diagnosis of, 435–436,
    436t, 447, 447t–448t
as discrete diagnosis, 443, 443–444
dysesthetic, treatment of, 410
local anesthetics for, 453
with malignancy, 448t, 450, 452
medical management of
    contemporary, 446–454
    general principles of, 447–449, 450
    history of, 446–447
    medications used in, 449–452
    pain characteristics and, 448–449, 450
neuralgic, treatment of, 410
neuroleptics for, 451–452
neuropathic, treatment of, 410
nociceptive, 448–449, 452
opioids for, 448, 452–453
paroxysmal, 446, 448–449
pathogenesis of, 447, 447t
patient's history of, 436
physical examination in, 436
postoperative, neuroma and, 423
posttraumatic, neuroma and, 423
practical considerations in, 435–445
psychogenic, 441, 452
salicylates for, 453
surgical intervention for, 444
treatment of
    effectiveness, 410
    failure, 410
    guidelines for, 410
    individualization, 410
    medical, 410
    surgical, 410
Ferrier, David, 48
Fluid restriction
    in head-injured patients, 135, 145
    in traumatic brain injury, 185
Fluid resuscitation
    in head injury, 135–136, 145
        pediatric, 172–173, 178
    in spinal cord injury, 162–163, 164t
        pediatric, 181
Fluoroscopy
    and brain shift monitoring, 92
    intraoperative, 71
Fluphenazine, for facial pain, 452
Foramen magnum, meningiomas of, 557,
    568, 569

Foramen of Monro-posterior commissure
    line, 50
Frankel, Viktor, 5–7, 9
Free radical production, in traumatic
    brain injury, 13, 19, 19, 21
Friedman, Bill, 90
Functional imaging
    in diagnosis, 96
    image-guided surgery and, 94–97, 98
    stereotactic combination with
        anatomic imaging, 96
Funding
    for database maintenance, 211–212
    for trauma research, 220t, 220–221,
        225–226

G
Gabapentin, for facial pain, 437, 440,
    449–450, 462–463
Gamma knife, 90
Gamma knife radiosurgery, 60
    for meningiomas, 561–562
    for trigeminal neuralgia, 461–462, 494
Ganglioneurofibroma, endoscopic
    surgery for, 528
Gardner, William J., 477, 500
Gasserian ganglion
    decompression of, 501
    electrical stimulation of, 464
    in trigeminal neuralgia, 458–459, 464,
        501
Gastric dilatation, with spinal cord in-
    jury, in children, 181
Gene therapy, for head injury, 150
Geniculate neuralgia, 442
Gildenberg, Phil, 91
Glasgow Coma Score, assessment of,
    131
Global Positioning System, 47
Globus pallidum, localization of, 33, 34
Glossopharyngeal neuralgia, 442, 448t,
    465, 476, 499, 502–503
    bilateral, 425
    treatment of, 425
    treatment of
        hemodynamic instability with,
            424–425
        perioperative management of,
            424–425
Glutamate, release, after traumatic
    brain injury, 115–117

Glycerol rhizotomy (rhyzolysis)
  for multiple division pain, 467
  selective injury with, 466–467
  for trigeminal neuralgia, 413, 415t, 417–418, 419t, 460–461, 466–467, 491–494
    advantages and disadvantages of, 418, 419t
    repeat, 418, 421
G_{M1} ganglioside, for spinal cord injury, 161–162
  mechanism of action, 161t
Gunther, John, 5–6

H
Habenular calcification, as landmark, 50
Haller, Albrecht von, 47
Halo rings, 157–158
Harbaugh, Bob, 235
Head injury. *See also* Traumatic brain injury
  airway management in, 131–132
    pediatric, 172–173, 175
  autoregulation in, 144
  basic therapy for, 176–178, 177t
  brain versus body dilemma in, 136–137
  cerebral perfusion pressure therapy in, 145, 147, *147*
    contraindication in children, 174–175
  cerebrospinal fluid drainage for, pediatric, 175–176
  chemical paralysis in, 132–133
  in children
    integration and design of therapies for, 176–178
    mild or minor, 179
    prehospital management of, 172–173
    severe, 170–178
  computed tomography of, 137, *138*
    pediatric, 173, 176, 178–179
  cost of, 105, 108–110, 109t–110t
  epidemiology of, 105–112
  escalated therapy for, 176–178, 177t
  extracranial injury with, 134–135
  fluid resuscitation in, 135–136, 145
    pediatric, 172–173, 178
  gene therapy for, 150
  genetic response to, 144, 150, *150*
  heterogeneity of, 144–145
  hyperventilation for, 133–134, 145
    pediatric, 175, 178
  hypotension with, 131, 134–137, 143–144
    causes and effects of, 134–135
    diagnostic algorithm for, 137, *138*
    pediatric, 174–175
    as predictor of mortality, 135
  incidence of, 143, *144*
    in Sand Diego County, 105–110, 107t
  intensive therapy for, 176–178, 177t
  intracranial pressure with, 132–136, 145, *146*
    pediatric, 173–178
  literature on, 216–217, 217t
  medical therapies for, levels of, 176–178, 177t
  mild or minor, pediatric, 179
  mortality from, 135, 143, *144,* 216
  multimodality cerebral monitoring in, 148
  neurological examination in
    initial, 130–131
    postresuscitation, 131
    procedures complicating, 131–133
  neuroprotection in, *149,* 149–150
  neurosurgeon availability for treatment of, 127–130
  osmotic therapies for, pediatric, 175–176
  oxygenation with, management of, 147–148, *148*
  prevention of
    helmets in, 221
    neurosurgeons' role in, 216–217, 217t
  secondary injury with, 143–145
    biochemical substrates of, 144, 149–150
  sedation in, 132–133
    pediatric, 175–176, 178
  severe
    guidelines for management of, 145–147
    pediatric, 170–178
    treatment of, clinical trials in, 222
    triage and acute management of, 127–142
  surgery for, timing of, 137–139
  targeted therapy for, 147–148, *147–148*
  treatment of

SUBJECT INDEX 587

algorithm for, 146, *146*
contemporary paradigms for,
  143–152
guidelines for, 223–224
in millennium, 151
protocols for, 223–224
strategies, 145
Health Professions' Education Partnership, 220
Hearing loss, after trigeminal neuralgia treatment, 412*t*, 414*t*–416*t*, 417–418
Helmets, in trauma prevention, 221
Hematomas
  decompression for, 137–139
  extra-axial, 137
  subdural, 139
Hemifacial spasm, 474
  neurovascular decompression for, 473, 475–476, 500, 503–505
  pathophysiology of, 476–481
  unilateral symptoms of, 502–503
  vascular compression in, 474–476, 480, 499, 502–503
Hemodynamic support, with therapeutic carotid artery occlusion, 371
Heparin therapy, with therapeutic carotid artery occlusion, 384
Heros, Roberto, 234
High thoracic epidural block, for neuralgia, 465
Hormonal therapy, for skull base meningiomas, 560–561
Horsley, Victor, 326, 393, 474
Horsley-Clarke stereotactic frame, 28, *28*, 49, 52, *53*
Hunter, John, 392
Hydroxyl radical detection, in traumatic brain injury, 14
Hydroxyurea, for meningioma, 561
Hyperactive cranial nerve dysfunction, 473–474, 476, 502
Hypercarbia, in head-injured patients, 131–132
Hyperhidrosis
  axillary, 530
  debilitating effects of, 530
  medical treatment of, 530
  mimicking conditions, 530
  open procedures for, 530–531
  palmar, 530

plantar, 530
thoracoscopic sympathectomy for, 530–535
Hyperpathia, 468
Hypertension, after therapeutic carotid artery occlusion, 402
Hypertonic solutions, for head-injured patients, 136
Hyperventilation
  in management of traumatic brain injury, 185–187, 186*t*, 188*t*
  prophylactic, for head injury, 133–134
  negative effects of, 133–134, 145
  optimized, 134
  pediatric, 175, 178
Hypotension
  with head injury, 131, 134–137, 143–144
  brain versus body dilemma in, 136–137
  causes and effects of, 134–135
  diagnostic algorithm for, 137, *138*
  extracranial injury and, 134–135
  fluid resuscitation and, 135–136, 145
  pediatric, 174–175
  as predictor of mortality, 135
  hypovolemic, in traumatic brain injury, 185
  with spinal cord injury, 163
Hypothermia, for head-injured patient, 222
Hypoxia
  definition of, 131
  with head injury, 131–132, 144
  with spinal cord injury, 161

I

Image guided surgery, 34–37. *See also* Spinal navigation, image-guided
  and brain shift monitoring, 91–92
  components of, 34
  and conformal radiation delivery, *99*, 99–100
  evaluation of, 36–37
  frame-based, 90
  frameless, 90
  and functional imaging, 94–97, *98*
  future of, 89–100
  historical perspective on, 89–91
  history of, 28–31

and operating room robotics, 92–93, *93–94*
reference points for, 96
and stimulation for functional disorders, 97–98
Imaging, intraoperative, in spinal surgery, 70–71, 78–80
Imipramine, for facial pain, 452*t*
Immobilization, for spinal cord injury, 155, 157–159, 165–166
pediatric, 181
Immunotherapy, for skull base meningiomas, 560–561
Impedance measurements, 54–55
Industry, and technical innovation, 40–43
Infants, neurological injuries in, current management strategies for, 170–184
Infrasellar tumors, 517
Intensive care unit
competing interests in, 197–198
neurosurgical care in, 196
and patient outcome, 196–197
patient management in, models of, 197
Intensivists
neurosurgical procedures performed by, 198
in neurotrauma care, 224
Interbody fusion, of lumbar spine, laparoscopic, 543–552
benefits of, 545
clinical results of, 547–552
contraindications to, 545
indications for, 545
versus open approach, 545
patient positioning for, 545
technique of, 545–547, *548–551*
voice-controlled robotic arm for, 546, *546*
Intercostal neuralgia, 541
Interferon, alpha, for meningioma, 561
Interleukin-1β, in traumatized brain
mature, 14, *16,* 16–17
quantification of, 14
Interleukin-1β converting enzyme, in traumatic brain injury, 12–23
Internal carotid artery
dissection, therapeutic carotid artery occlusion for, 340

meningioma and, 557, 570
neoplasms involving
benign, 340, 400
malignant, 340–341, 399–400
management of, 340–341, 399–400
occlusion, thrombolytic therapy for, *243*
therapeutic occlusion. *See* Therapeutic carotid artery occlusion
Intracranial carotid to carotid bypass, for cerebral revascularization, 380
Intracranial hemorrhage, after intravenous recombinant tissue plasminogen activator, 262–263
Intracranial pressure (ICP)
with head injury
chemical paralysis and sedation and, 132
fluid resuscitation and, 135–136
hyperventilation and, 133–134
monitoring of, 145, 173–174
pediatric, measurement and management of, 173–178
surgery and, 137–139
treatment algorithm for management of, *146*
monitoring, in management of traumatic brain injury, 185–186, 186*t,* 188*t*
monitor insertion for, neurosurgeon's role in, 191
normal, in children, 173–174
Intubation, of head-injured patients, 131–132
Ipsilateral endoscopic method, 516
Ischemia, with spinal cord injury, 161–166

J
Jannetta, Peter, 473–474, 481–484, 483*t*–485*t,* 499, 501, 503
Jugular saturation monitoring, 133–134, 148

K
Kaufman, Bruce, 234
Kelly, Patrick, 90
Keratitis, with trigeminal neuralgia treatment, 473, 490
Kushner, Harold, 4–6
Kyphosis, endoscopic surgery for, 526

L

Lamotrigine, for trigeminal neuralgia, 463
Laparoscopic interbody fusion of lumbar spine, 543–552
  benefits of, 545
  clinical results of, 547–552
  contraindications to, 545
  indications for, 545
  versus open approach, 545
  patient positioning for, 545
  technique of, 545–547, *548–551*
  voice-controlled robotic arm for, 546, *546*
Laparoscopy, for spine surgery, 526, 527*t*, 543–552
Legislation, and neurotrauma prevention, 219*t*, 219–221, 225
Leksell, Lars, 52, 60, *60*, 90
Leksell G-frame, 60, *61*
Leksell stereotactic frame, 33, *34*, 52, *53*, 60, *61*
Lidocaine, for facial pain, 453
Life, meaning of, 1–11
Linear accelerator, 90
Local anesthetics, for facial pain, 453
Localization
  of brain function, 47–48
  craniometric, 48–49
  electrophysiological, 54–56, *55*
  stereotactic, 33–37, *35–36*, 49–63
Localizing the point, 44. *See also* Navigation
Lodestones, 45
Long bone fractures, and hypotension with head injury, 134–135
Lumbar spine, endoscopic procedures for, 526, 527*t*, 543–552
Lumbar spine interbody fusion, laparoscopic, 526, 543–552
  benefits of, 545
  clinical results of, 547–552
  contraindications to, 545
  indications for, 545
  versus open approach, 545
  patient positioning for, 545
  technique of, 545–547, *548–551*
  voice-controlled robotic arm for, 546, *546*
Lumbosacral spine, pedicle screw placement, spinal imaging for, 71, 75, *76*, 76–81, *77*

Lund method, for management of traumatic brain injury, 187, 188*t*
Lunsford, Dade, 90

M

M17Z, in traumatic brain injury, 12–23, *18*
Macroadenoma, endoscopic surgery for, 513
Magnet(s), 45
Magnetic neurosurgery, 93
Magnetic resonance angiography (MRA)
  in pre-procedural evaluation for therapeutic carotid artery occlusion, 382
  of vertebral artery stenosis, *250*
Magnetic resonance imaging (MRI)
  and brain shift monitoring, 92
  in cerebrovascular disease, 238, 241–250, *244*
    diffusion-weighted imaging, *244*, 245–250, *249*
    perfusion techniques, 241–245
  diffusion scanning, 95–96
  functional, 94–95
  image distortion with, 58
  of meningiomas, 558, *558*
  operating room, 39–40, *40*
  of spinal cord injury, *154*
    without radiographic abnormality, 181
  stereotaxy with, 29–30, 33–34, 58–59, *59*, 63–64, 89–90
  in transient ischemic attacks, diffusion-weighted imaging, 247
  in trigeminal neuralgia, 436–438
  versatility of, 58
Magnetic resonance spectroscopy, of cerebrovascular disease, 251, *252*
Magnetic source imaging (MSI), 94–95
Magnetoencephalography (MEG), 95
Maimonides, Moses, 10–11
Mannitol, in management of traumatic brain injury, 185–186, 186*t*
Matas, R., 326, 393
Matas test, 326, 393, 403–404
Mayfield ACCISS system, 34–35, *35*
McGill pain questionnaire, 468
Mechanical arms, as surgical localizers, 34–35, *35–36*
Mechanical coupled point stereotaxy,

60–61, 60–62. *See also* Stereotaxy, frames
Medial sphenoid wing, meningioma of, 563, *565*
Medial thalamotomy, 469
Meningiomas
  anatomical considerations in, 556–557
  anterior fossa, 557
    operative technique for, 563, *564*
  atypical, 555
  biological nature of, 554–555, 571
  carotid artery preservation with, 340
  cavernous sinus
    operative outcomes with, 570, 571*t*
    operative technique for, 563, *565*
    treatment of, 327
  cerebral edema with, 558
  chemotherapy for, 560–561, 571
  classic, 555
  classification of, 555
    World Health Organization, 555, 556*t*
  clinical presentation of, 554–555
  clival, 563–568, 570
  cluster headache with, 428
  decision analysis in, 559–560
  definition of, 555
  foci of growth, 556–557, *557*
  foramen magnum, 557, 568, *569*
  growth patterns of, 554–555
  hormonal therapy for, 560–561
  imaging characteristics of, 557–558, *558*
  immunotherapy for, 560–561
  malignant, 555
  microsurgery for, 562–571, *564–565*, 566*t*, *567, 569*
    endoscopic-assisted, 519
  middle fossa, 557
    operative technique for, 563, *565*
  natural history of, 559–560, 571
  observation of, 560, 571
  olfactory groove, 563
  optic nerve sheath, 563
  pathology of, 555
  petroclival
    operative outcomes with, 570, 572*t*
    operative technique for, 563–568, *567*
  posterior fossa, 557
    operative technique for, 563–568, 566*t*, *567, 569*
  preoperative assessment of, 557
  proliferative potential of, 555–556
  radiation therapy for, 561–562
  skull base, contemporary treatment of, 554–574
  stereotactic radiosurgery for, 561–562, 571
  tentorium cerebelli, 557
  transfacial approaches to, 568
  transpetrosal approaches to, 563–568, 566*t*
  tuberculum sellae, 563, *564*
Methohexitol, 468
Methylprednisolone (Sygen), for spinal cord injury, 161
  mechanism of action, 161*t*
  pediatric, 181
Mexiletine, for facial pain, 453
MIB-1 (Ki-67) index, 555–556
Microadenoma, endoscopic surgery for, 513
Microelectrode recording, 33, 54–56, *55*
Microsurgery, 41, *42*
  endoscopic, pituitary, 507–514
  endoscopic-assisted, for tumors and neurovascular procedures, 515–525
  for intracranial arteriovenous malformations, 267–268, 273–279
    advantages and disadvantages of, 285
    arguments against, 324
    arguments for, 323–324
    cost-effectiveness of, 287–288, 289*t*
    efficacy of, 287, 288*t*
    minor unreported complications of, 291
    neurosurgeon's experience and, 290, 292
    outcomes with, 286–287, 288*t*
    patient preference and, 288–290
    quality-adjusted life years gained with, 288, 289*t*–290*t*
    and radiosurgery, comparison of, 274, *275*, 285–293
    risk assessment for, 290–291
  for skull base meningiomas, 562–571, *564–565*, 566*t*, *567, 569*
Microvascular decompression
  failure of, 478–479, 488, 503–505
  for hemifacial spasm, 473, 475–476, 500, 503–505

for trigeminal neuralgia, 455–457, 473–498
 advantages and disadvantages of, 418, 419*t*
 age factors and, 494–495
 author's experience with, 484–488, 486*t*–488*t*
 comparison with alternative procedures, 488–494
 complications of, 412*t*, 413, 417–418, 483, 484*t*, 485, 487*t*
 effectiveness, 411–413, 412*t*
 Jannetta's series on, 481–484, 483*t*–485*t*, 501, 503
 long-term follow-up of, 487–488
 morbidity and mortality after, 412*t*, 417–418
 as procedure of choice, 494–495, 500
 repeat, 420–421
 results of, 481–488, 485*t*, 487*t*–489*t*, 503–505, 504*t*
 risks of, 495
 for vagoglossopharyngeal neuralgia, 420*t*, 423–425
Microvasculature, diffuse damage to, in traumatic brain injury, 113, 115
Middle cerebral artery (MCA)
 hyperdense, computed tomography of, 238–241
 occlusion
  angiography of, *240, 242, 246*
  computed tomography of, 238–241
 stroke, endovascular therapy in, 255–256
Middle fossa, meningiomas of, 557
 operative technique for, 563, *565*
Middle fossa technique, for trigeminal neuralgia, 473–474
Monoamine oxidase inhibitors, for facial pain, 452*t*
Moore's Law, 65
Motor cortex stimulation
 complications of, 464–465
 for trigeminal neuropathic pain, 463–465, 468–469
Multidisciplinary teams, for technical innovation, 37–38
Multimodality cerebral monitoring, in head-injured patients, 148

Multiple sclerosis, trigeminal neuralgia with, 421–422, 478, 481
Myelopathy, 535, 539, 541–542

N
Nasal septum, 508, *511*
National Institutes of Neurological Disorders and Stroke (NINDS), recombinant tissue plasminogen activator trial, 261–265
 inclusion and exclusion criteria, 261–262, 262*t*, 264–265
Nattrass, F. J., 326, 393
Navigation
 celestial, *46*, 46–47
 comparison with geographical, 44–48
 computed tomography in, 56–58, *58*
 craniometric, 48–49
 dead reckoning, 44–45, *46*, 48–49, 63
 electrophysiological, 54–56, *55*
 evolving principles of, 44–69
 history of, 44–47
 primordial, 44–45
 stereotactic, 49–63
 voice-activated computer, 31
Neoplasm(s)
 with carotid artery involvement
  benign, 340, 400
  malignant, 340–341, 399–400
  management of, 340–341, 399–400
 head and neck, management of, 364–366, 366*t*, 370–371
 skull base, management of, 364–366, 366*t*, 370–371, 399
 spinal column, surgery for, spinal imaging for, 84–85, *86*
Nerve block, for trigeminal neuropathic pain, 440–441
Nerve of Kuntz, accessory, 533
Nervus intermedius-superficial petrosal-sphenopalatine system, in cluster headache, 426
 surgery of, 426–429, 427*t*
Neuralgia
 cranial, 442–443, 443*t*
 epileptiform, 446
 geniculate, 442
 glossopharyngeal, 442, 448*t*, 465, 476, 499, 502–503
 intercostal, 541
 occipital, 442

postherpetic, 442, 448t, 450, 452–453
Raeder's paratrigeminal, 442–443
sphenopalatine, 442–443
trigeminal. *See* Trigeminal neuralgia
Neural injury. *See also* Head injury;
  Spinal cord injury; Traumatic
  brain injury
 pathophysiology of, 113–124
Neuroexcitation, in traumatic brain injury, 113–117
Neurointensivist, 192
Neuroleptics, for facial pain, 451–452
Neurological examination, in head injury, 130–133
 initial, 130–131
 postresuscitation, 131
 procedures complicating, 131–133
Neurological injuries, in children and infants, current management strategies for, 170–184
Neuromuscular blockade, in head injury, 132–133
Neuron(s), intracellular calcium, after traumatic brain injury, 116
Neuron-specific enolase promoter, in traumatic brain injury, 12–23, *18*
Neuron theory, 48
Neuropathic pain, 448–449
 antidepressants for, 450–451, 468
 constant, 449
 paroxysmal, 446, 448–449
 percutaneous treatment of, 469
 trigeminal, 435, 440t, 440–441, 448t, 450, 463–465
Neuroprotection
 clinical trials of, 149, *149*, 222
 in head injury, 149–150
 preclinical trials of, 223
Neuroscience, advances in, and stereotaxy, 64–65
Neurosurgeons
 availability of, 127–130
 neurotrauma as domain of, 153–155, 216–226
 in triage and management
  of head injury, 127–130
  of spinal cord injury, 153–155, 166
Neurosurgery, in traumatic brain injury management, 189–193, 194t
Neurotrauma
 critical care for, models of, 185–194

as neurosurgeon's domain, 153–155, 216–226
 outcomes with, national database of, 203–215
 pathophysiology of, 113–124
 pediatric, 170–184
 prevention of, 224–225
  legislation and, 219t, 219–221, 225
  neurosurgeons' role in, 216–219
 regionalization of care for, 193–194
 treatment of
  clinical trials in, 203
  education and information dissemination on, 225
  evidence-based, 203–204
  literature review on, 203
  research on, 203
Neurotrauma research
 funding for, 220t, 220–221, 225–226
 neurosurgeons' role in, 221–223
Neurotraumatologists, neurosurgical, 193
Neurovascular decompression
 failure of, 478–479, 488, 503–505
 for hemifacial spasm, 473, 475–476, 500, 503–505
 historical perspectives on, 474–476
 for trigeminal neuralgia, 455–457, 473–498
  age factors and, 494–495
  author's experience with, 484–488, 486t–488t
  comparison with alternative procedures, 488–494
  complications of, 483, 484t, 485, 487t
  Jannetta's series on, 481–484, 483t–485t, 501, 503
  long-term follow-up of, 487–488
  as procedure of choice, 494–495, 500
  results of, 481–488, 485t, 487t–489t, 503–505, 504t
  risks of, 495
Neurovascular procedures, endoscopic-assisted, 515–525, *523–524*
Nimodipine
 for severe head injury, 222
 for traumatic subarachnoid hemorrhage, 222
Nociceptive pain, 448–449, 452
Nortriptyline, for facial pain, 452t

O

Oath of Maimonides, 10–11
Observation, of skull base meningiomas, 560, 571
Occipital neuralgia, 442
Ocular pneumoplethysmography, for measurement of cerebral blood flow, 376
Olfactory groove, meningiomas of, 563
Operating Arm System, 35, *36*
Opioids, for facial pain, 448, 452–453
Optical tracking system, 34–36
Optic nerve sheath, meningiomas of, 563
Orofacial pain, 436
Osmotic therapies, for head injury, pediatric, 175–176
Oxygenation, with head injury, management of, 147–148, *148*
Oxygen free radicals, damage due to, after traumatic brain injury, 117–118
  neuroprotection targeted at, 119, 121*t*

P

Pain
  constant, 449
  facial. *See also* Trigeminal neuralgia
    paroxysmal, 446, 448–449
    practical considerations in, 435–445
    neuropathic, 448–449
    nociceptive, 448–449, 452
    paroxysmal, 446, 448–449
    psychogenic, 441, 452
Paralysis, chemical, in head injury, 132–133
Paré, Ambroise, 392
Parkinson's disease, ablative pallidal and thalamic lesions for, image-guided surgery and, 97–98
Paroxysmal pain, facial, 446, 448–449
Pedicle screw placement, lumbosacral, spinal imaging for, 71, 75, *76*, 76–81, *77*
Pelorus stereotactic system, *30*, 30–31
Pelvic fractures, and hypotension in head-injured patient, 134–135
Percutaneous stereotactic radiofrequency rhizotomy
  for trigeminal neuralgia
    advantages and disadvantages of, 418, 419*t*

corneal anesthesia after, 414*t*, 417
    effectiveness, 411–413, 414*t*
    trigeminal motor weakness after, 414*t*, 417
  for vagoglossopharyngeal neuralgia, 423–424
Percutaneous treatment, of trigeminal neuralgia. *See* Percutaneous stereotactic radiofrequency rhizotomy; Trigeminal neuralgia, percutaneous treatment of
Peripheral neurectomy, for trigeminal neuralgia, 418, 419*t*
Peroxynitrite formation, and cell death, 20–21
Petroclival region, meningiomas of
  operative outcomes with, 570, 572*t*
  operative technique for, 563–568, *567*
Petrosal approaches, to meningiomas, 563–568, 566*t*
Petrosectomy, 566–568
Phenelzine, for facial pain, 452*t*
Phenytoin (Dilantin), for facial pain, 437, 449, 451*t*, 463, 478
Phrenology, 47
Pilz, C., 364, 393
Pineal gland, center of, as landmark, 50
Pituitary surgery, endoscopic, 507–514
  sphenoidotomy approach for, 507*t*, 507–514
    anatomical considerations in, 508
    complications of, 514
    hospital stay after, 513*t*, 513–514
    instrumentation for, 508–509
    patient positioning for, 509
    results of, 513–514
    surgeon positioning for, 509
    technique of, 508–513, *510–512*
  sublabial transseptal approach for, 507
Pituitary tumors, cluster headache with, 428
Pneumoencephalography, 49
Positron emission tomography (PET)
  with clinical balloon test occlusion of ICA, 356, 404
  stereotactic technique with, 30
Posterior commissure-pontomedullary line, 50
Posterior fossa
  ependymoma of, endoscopic surgery for, *522*

meningiomas of, 557
  operative technique for, 563–568, 566t, 567, 569
Posterior fossa technique, for trigeminal neuralgia, 474
Postherpetic neuralgia, 442, 448t, 450, 452–453
Potassium bromide, for facial pain, 449
Primordial navigation, 44–45
PROACT study, 255–256
Proliferative indices, 555–556
Propofol
  for facial pain procedures, 468
  for head-injured patients, 133
  vasopressors with, 133
Pro-urokinase, recombinant, in acute MCA stroke, 255–256
Pseudoaneurysms
  carotid, traumatic, 398, 398
  intracranial, traumatic, 398, 399
Psychogenic pain, 441, 452
Psychogenic pain disorder, 441

Q
Quadrant, 46

R
Radiation therapy
  fractionated
    image-guided delivery techniques, 99, 99–100
    for intracranial arteriovenous malformations, 268
    for meningiomas, 561–562
Radiculopathy, 535, 541–542
Radio frequency generators, 42–43
Radiosurgery, 60
  for arteriovenous malformations, image-guided technique, 99, 100
  for cluster headache, 428
  conformal, image-guided technique, 99, 99–100
  for intracranial arteriovenous malformations, 267–268
    advantages and disadvantages of, 285
    embolization before, 272–273, 280, 313–315
    image-guided technique, 99, 100
    and microsurgery, comparison of, 274, 275, 285–293

neurosurgeon's experience and, 292
outcomes with, 286–287
patient preference and, 288–290
risks of, 292–293
stereotactic, 267–268, 272–274, 275, 279–281, 285–293, 562
  for meningiomas, 561–562, 571
stereotactic
  complications of, 562
  embolization before, 272–273
  for intracranial arteriovenous malformations, 267–268, 279–281
  for meningiomas, 561–562, 571
  and microsurgery, comparison of, 274, 275, 285–293
  for trigeminal neuralgia, 413, 414t, 417–418, 419t, 461–462, 488–491, 491t, 494
Raeder's paratrigeminal neuralgia, 442–443
Raynaud's disease, thoracoscopic sympathectomy for, 530
Reactive oxygen species (ROS), in traumatic brain injury, 13, 20–21
Reflex sympathetic dystrophy, thoracoscopic sympathectomy for, 533–534
Remote surgery, 64
Research, on trauma, funding for, 220t, 220–221, 225–226
Revascularization, cerebral. See also Extracranial-intracranial bypass surgery
  in acute stroke, 255–256
  bonnet bypass for, 343, 345
  high-flow, 343
  intracranial carotid to carotid bypass for, 380
  long-term graft occlusion rate with, 346
  low-flow, 343
  morbidity and mortality with, 346, 347t
  neurological complications of, 346, 347t
  recommendations for, 347–349
  selective, 341–343
  universal, 343–346, 344
Rhizotomy
  open
    contraindications to, 425

SUBJECT INDEX

for vagoglossopharyngeal neuralgia, 423–424
for vagoglossopharyngeal syncope, 425
for trigeminal neuralgia, advantages and disadvantages of, 418, 419*t*
for vagoglossopharyngeal neuralgia, 420*t*, 423
Ringer's solution, 136
Roberts, David, 90
Roberts, Theodore, 56, 90
Robotics
  in laparoscopic interbody fusion of lumbar spine, 546, *546*
  stereotaxy with, 64
Rostrum of sphenoid sinus, 508, *511*

S

Salicylates, for facial pain, 453
Schorstein, J., 364, 394
SCIWORA, 180–181
Scoliosis, endoscopic surgery for, 526
Seatbelts, in trauma prevention, 221
Secondary injury
  with head injury, 143–145
    biochemical substrates of, 144, 149–150
  with spinal cord injury, 160–166
Sedation, in head injury, 132–133
  pediatric, 175–176, 178
Selective injury, for trigeminal neuralgia, 466–467, 470
Sella, endoscopic sphenoidotomy approach to, 507*t*, 508, 511–513, *512*
Selman, Warren, 234
Sextant, 46, *46*
Shank, Chuck, 9, *10*
Shingles, and neuralgia, 442
Shock, with spinal cord injury, 161
Siegrist, A., 393
Single-lung ventilation, for thoracoscopy, 526–529, 537
Single photon emission computed tomography (SPECT)
  in cerebrovascular disease, 250–254, *253*
  for measurement of cerebral blood flow, 355, 360, 377–378, *379*
  stereotactic technique with, 30
  in stroke, 253
  Tc-99m hexamethylpropylene amineoxime (HMPAO), for measurement of cerebral blood flow, 251–253, 328–330, 355, 360, 377–378, *379*, 385, 404
Sinuses
  endoscopic approach through, 507–514, 517
  meningioma of, 563, *565*, 570, *571*
Skull base, anatomy of, 556–557
Skull base meningiomas
  anatomical considerations in, 556–557
  cerebral edema with, 558
  chemotherapy for, 560–561, 571
  contemporary treatment of, 554–574
  decision analysis in, 559–560
  foci of growth, 556–557, *557*
  hormonal therapy for, 560–561
  imaging characteristics of, 557–558, *558*
  immunotherapy for, 560–561
  microsurgery for, 562–571, *564-565*, 566*t*, *567*, *569*
  natural history of, 559–560, 571
  observation of, 560, 571
  preoperative assessment of, 557
  radiation therapy for, 561–562
  stereotactic radiosurgery for, 561–562, 571
Skull features, and navigation, 48
SMART program, in cerebrovascular disease, 234
Somatosensory evoked potentials, monitoring, in therapeutic carotid artery occlusion, 346
Sphenoidotomy approach, for endoscopic pituitary surgery, 507*t*, 507–514
  anatomical considerations in, 508
  complications of, 514
  hospital stay after, 513*t*, 513–514
  instrumentation for, 508–509
  patient positioning for, 509
  results of, 513–514
  surgeon positioning for, 509
  technique of, 508–513, *510–512*
Sphenoid sinus
  endoscopic approach through, 507–514, 517
  meningioma of, 563, *565*
  ostium, 508–509, *510*
  rostrum of, 508, *511*
  septations, 508, 511–512

Sphenopalatine neuralgia, 442–443
Spiegel-Wycis stereotactic frame, 28, *29*, 49, 52, *53*
Spinal column
  anatomy of, contour map of, 74
  neoplasms, surgery for, spinal imaging for, 84–85, *86*
  three-dimensional anatomy of, 70–71
Spinal cord compression, 155, *158*
Spinal cord deformities, endoscopic surgery for, 526
Spinal cord injury
  aggressive medical intervention in, 162–166
    studies in support of, 164t
  and blood flow, 162, *163–164*
  cellular and subcellular events with, 160–161
  in children, 179–181
    anatomic properties and, 180–181
    management of, 181
    mechanisms of, 180
    patterns of, 180
    without radiographic abnormality (SCIWORA), 180–181
  computed tomography of, 157, *157*
  cost of, 105, 110–112
  detection of, 155, 157–159, 165–166
  epidemiology of, 105–112
  fracture and fracture dislocations, *154*, 155–159, *156–158*
  immobilization for, 155, 157–159, 165–166
    pediatric, 181
  incidence of, in Sand Diego County, 105–108, 108t
  ischemia with, 161–166
  literature on, 216–217, 217t
  pharmacological therapy for, 161–162, 165–166
    mechanism of action, 161t
    pediatric, 181
  prevention of, neurosurgeons' role in, 216–217, 217t
  reduction/realignment for, 155–159, *160*, 165–166
  resuscitation/perfusion for, 162–163, 164t
    pediatric, 181
  secondary injury with, 160–166
  surgical intervention for, 155–159, *160*, 165–166
    studies in support of, 159t
  treatment of
    algorithm for, *165*
    contemporary paradigms in, 153–169
    history of, 155–158
    optimal, 163–166
  triage and management of
    hallmarks of, 155–159
    role of neurosurgeon in, 153–155, 166
Spinal cord tumors, endoscopic surgery for, 526, *528*
Spinal navigation, image-guided
  applications of, 70–72, 76–85
  benefits of, 87
  drill guide for, *73*
  frame of reference for, 73–74
  image planes for, 75
  rationale for, 70–71
  registration process for, 73–75
  segmental registration for, 80
  technique for, *72*, 72–76
  views for, 75, *76*
  wand for, *73*, 74
Spinal surgery
  anterior, image-guided technology for, 74, 76–81, 84, *85*
  endoscopic, 526–553. *See also specific procedures*
    Barrow Neurological Institute experience with, 526, 529t
    comparison of approaches in, 526, 527t
    laparoscopic, 526, 527t, 543–552
    thoracoscopic, 526–543
  posterior, image-guided technology for, 73, 81–82
  stereotactic, applications of, 70–72
Status trigeminus, diagnosis of, 411
Stellate ganglion, 532
Stellate ganglion block, for neuralgia, 465
Stereoencephalotome, 28, *29*
Stereoencephalotomy, 50, *50*
Stereotactic radiosurgery (SRS). *See* Radiosurgery
Stereotaxy, 49–63
  ablation procedures with, 64–65

SUBJECT INDEX

acceptance of techniques, factors controlling, 65–66
atlases for, 33, *50,* 50–51, 59
augmentative procedures with, 64–65
burr-hole mounted devices for, 51, *52*
with computed tomography, 29, 33–34, 56–58, *58,* 63–64
computer-directed, 31
frameless, 31, 33–37, *62,* 62–63
  components of, 34
  for endoscopic pituitary surgery, 508–509, 512
  evaluation of, 36–37
  operative microscope in, 41, *42*
  three-dimensional localizers for, 34–36, *35-36*
frames
  applications of, 30, 33
  arc-centered, 52, *53*
  current, 60–61, *61*
  development of, 28–31, 49, 52–54, *60*
  Horsley-Clarke, 28, *28,* 49, 52, *53*
  image problems with, 30, 54
  indications for, 61
  Leksell, 33, *34,* 52, *53,* 60, *61*
  rectilinear, 52, *53*
  simplified, *30,* 30–31
  Spiegel-Wycis, 28, *29,* 49, 52, *53*
future directions in, 63–66
heterogeneity of brain function and, 47
history of, 28–31, 33, 49–54
instrumentation for, 28–31, 51–54
  CT-optimized, 56–58, *58*
  with magnetic resonance imaging, 29–30, 33–34, 58–59, *59,* 63–64
  mechanical coupled point, *60–61,* 60–62
neuroscience advances and, 64–65
positron emission tomography, 30
real-time problem with, 63–64
robotic, 64
state of art, 60–63
volumetric, 62–63
x-ray, 49–50
Steroids, in management of traumatic brain injury, 186*t,* 187
Stroke
  acute, treatment of, time goals for, 264, 264*t*
  acute ischemic
    diagnostic imaging for, 237
    endovascular therapy in, 254–256
    thrombolysis in, 254–256, 261
    treatment of, 237
  after therapeutic carotid artery occlusion
    rates for, 357*t*–358*t,* 359
    risk for, 352
  borderzone (watershed), after therapeutic carotid artery occlusion, 370, *370*
  diagnostic imaging for, 237–256
  hemorrhagic
    after intravenous recombinant tissue plasminogen activator, 262–263
    emergency triage for, 263–264
  incidence of, 231
  ischemic. *See also* Cerebral ischemia
    after therapeutic carotid artery occlusion, 370
    single photon emission computed tomography in, 253
Stroke Team
  development of, 234
  members of, 234
Subarachnoid hemorrhage
  after therapeutic carotid artery occlusion, 327, 330–332, 333*t,* 342, 371–372, *372,* 375, 402
  cerebral vasospasm with, 274, *276,* 277
  traumatic, outcome predictors, 222
Sublabial transseptal approach, for endoscopic pituitary surgery, 507
Superior cerebellar artery, trigeminal nerve compression by, *475, 482,* 483, 501, 501*t,* 503
Superior nasal turbinate, 508
Suprasellar tumors, 517
Surgical navigation. *See* Navigation
Sweating, excessive. *See* Hyperhidrosis
Sygen. *See* Methylprednisolone
Sylvian fissure, localization of, 48
Sympathectomy, thoracoscopic, 526, 530–535
  anesthesia for, 529–530
  clinical results of, 533–535
  complications of, 531, 531*t,* 533
  conversion to open procedure, 532
  for hyperhidrosis, 530–535
  indications for, 530

palmar skin temperature monitoring with, 533
patient positioning for, 531–532
for reflex sympathetic dystrophy, 533–534
in situ chain transection with, 534, *535*
technique of, 531–533, *532, 534-535*

T

Talairach apparatus, 54
Targeted therapy, for head injury, 147–148, *147–148*
Taylor-Haughton line, 48
Team building, for technical innovation, 37–38
Technical innovations
　determining effectiveness of, 33–37
　history of, 28–31
　improving patient care with, 33
　integration in everyday practice, 27–43
　　model for, 31–43, *32*
　multidisciplinary teams for, 37–38
　principles for, 32–43
　relationship with industry in, 40–43
　　commitments in, 41–43
　　development of, 40–41
　relationship with institution in, 38–40
Tension pneumothorax, 135
Tentorium cerebelli, meningiomas of, 557
Therapeutic carotid artery occlusion
　adjunctive studies with, 354–356, 357*t*, 384–385, 404
　adjunctive therapy with, 346, 365, 385–386
　for aneurysm, 364, 366, 366*t*, 394–396, *395–396*, 401–402
　in carotid artery rupture (blowout), 364, 366*t*, 366–367
　central venous catheterization with, 382–384
　cerebral blood flow measurement before, 328–330, 341–343, 353–355, 360, 375–378, 384–385, 404
　clinical balloon test occlusion before, 331, 341–343, 353, 360, 373–375, 384, 404
　　additional adjunctive studies with, 356
　　complications of, 342–343, 356–357, 357*t*

　　with HMPAO SPECT, 253, 328–330, 355, 360, 385
　　with hypotensive challenge, 354–355, 360, 374, *374*, 384–385
　　protocol for, 328–329, *329*
　　reliability of, 332
　　safety of, 331–332, 342–343
　　University of Cincinnati procedure, 328–331
　　with xenon-enhanced CT, 253, 328, 341–343, 355–356, 385, 405
　clip/clamp ligation technique, 364, 373–375
　and collateral circulation, 392–393
　complications of, 331, 367–373, 375, 401–403
　　long-term (delayed), 330–332, 332*t*
　　prevention/reduction of, 403–406
　　rate for, 353
　contraindications to, 342–343
　　absolute, 367, 368*t*, 403
　　relative, 367, 368*t*, 403
　cost-effectiveness of, 330–331
　delayed infarcts after, 331–332, 332*t*
　delayed management paradigm for, 386
　device embolization in, prevention of, *400*, 406
　endovascular balloon technique, 365
　　complications of, 375
　　long-term follow-up of, 375
　　outcomes with, 375
　follow-up, 373, 386
　gradual, 326–327, 341, 364–365, 374–375, 401
　hemodynamic support after, 382–386, 405–406
　hemorrhagic complications of, delayed, 330, 371–373, 372*f*, 375
　high-risk patient and, 385
　historical perspective on, 326–328, 339, 341, 363–365, 392–394
　hypertension after, 402
　and inadequate hemodynamic support, 367, 368*t*
　indications for, 327, 340–341, 365–367, 366*t*, 394–400
　　vascular, 394–398
　ischemic complications of
　　delayed (late), 352, 369–370, 375, 386, 402–403

hemodynamic, 334, 351, 353,
    367–368, *370*, 386
  prevention/reduction of, 403–406
  risk of, 352, 401
  thromboembolic, 334, 351, 353,
    368–369, *369*, 375, 386, 401,
    405–406
low-risk patient and, 386
in management of neoplasms,
    340–341, 364–366, 366*t*, 399–400
  ischemic complications of, 370–371,
    401
moderate-risk patient and, 385–386
neurologic sequelae
  patients at risk for, identification of,
    353–357, 385–386
  risk of, 352
noninvasive surveillance after, 373,
    386
outcomes with, 331
periprocedural management of, 369,
    371
post-procedural care with, 385–386
practical management protocol for,
    381–386, *383*
pre-procedural evaluation for,
    375–378, *379*, 381–382, 403–404
provocative testing before, 373–375,
    384–386
quality of life after, 330
revascularization for. *See also* Extracranial-intracranial bypass surgery
  bonnet bypass for, 343, *345*
  high-flow, 343
  long-term graft occlusion rate with,
    346
  low-flow, 343
  morbidity and mortality with, 346,
    347*t*
  neurological complications of, 346,
    347*t*
  recommendations for, 347–349
  selective, 341–343
  universal, 343–346, *344*
risk assessment for, 341–343, 385–386
risk management with, 381–384, *383*
stroke rates with, 357*t*–358*t*, 359
subclinical ischemia after, 370, *371*
Thermal rhizotomy
  carotid artery puncture with, 470

for multiple division pain, 467
selective injury with, 466–467
trigeminal nerve-evoked potential
    guidance for, 457
for trigeminal neuralgia, 455–457,
    466–467, 470, 488–491
Think First, 218–219
  For Kids, 218
  For Teens, 218–219
Thoracic spine
  endoscopic procedures for, 526–543,
    527*t*
  pedicle screw fixation, spinal imaging
    for, *80*, 80–81
Thoracolumbar spine, anterior surgery,
    spinal imaging for, 84, *85*
Thoracoscopic discectomy, 526, 530,
    535–541
  bleeding with, 537, 539, *540*
    mean blood loss, 541
  clinical results of, 541
  versus costotransversectomy, 541
  operative time, mean, of, 541
  patient positioning for, *536*, 536–537
  technique of, 536–539, *538, 540*
Thoracoscopic sympathectomy, 526,
    530–535
  anesthesia for, 529–530
  clinical results of, 533–535
  complications of, 531, 531*t*, 533
  conversion to open procedure, 532
  for hyperhidrosis, 530–535
  indications for, 530
  palmar skin temperature monitoring
    with, 533
  patient positioning for, 531–532
  for reflex sympathetic dystrophy,
    533–534
  in situ chain transection with, 534, *535*
  technique of, 531–533, *532, 534–535*
Thoracoscopic vertebrectomy, 526,
    541–543
  clinical results of, 542–543
  complications of, 543
  technique of, 541–542, *542–544*
  versus thoracotomy, 543
Thoracoscopy, 526–543, 527*t*
  anesthesia for, 526–530
  applications of, 526
  Barrow Neurological Institute experience with, 526, 529*t*

versus thoracotomy, 535–536, 541, 543
Thoracotomy, thoracoscopy versus, 535–536, 541, 543
Three-dimensional localizers, 34–36, *35–36*
Thrombolytic therapy. *See also specific thrombolytic agent*
  in acute stroke, 255, 261
  candidates for, evaluation of, 238
  eligibility for, physician accuracy in determination of, 241
  outcomes, angiography of, *240, 243*
Tic douloureux. *See* Trigeminal neuralgia
Tissue plasminogen activator, recombinant, intravenous, 261–265
Tocainide, for facial pain, 453
Todd, Edwin M., *60*, 60–61
Todd-Wells stereotactic frame, 61
Transfacial approaches, to meningiomas, 568
Transient ischemic attacks (TIA), diffusion-weighted magnetic resonance imaging in, 247
Transpetrosal approaches, to meningiomas, 563–568, 566t
Transsphenoidal endoscopic method, 517
Transtentorial herniation, 137–139
Transventricular endoscopic method, 516–517
Trauma. *See also* Head injury; Spinal cord injury; Traumatic brain injury
  prevention of, legislation and, 219t, 219–221, 225
Trauma systems
  neurosurgeon availability for, 127–130
  organization of, 225
  pediatric, 172–173
Traumatic brain injury (TBI). *See also* Head injury
  basic therapy for, 176–178, 177t
  brain metabolism after, neuroprotection targeted at, 118, 119t
  caspase inhibitors for damage mediation, 17–21, *18*
  in children, 170–178
  cholinergic suppression after, neuroprotection targeted at, 118, 119t
  critical care for, 187–193
  diffuse, 113–114. *See also* Diffuse axonal injury
  DNA fragmentation in, 14–16, *15*, 20
  escalated therapy for, 176–178, 177t
  focal, 113
  free radical production in, 13, 19, *19*, 21
  hydroxyl radical detection in, 14
  intensive therapy for, 176–178, 177t
  interleukin-1β converting enzyme in, 12–23
  interleukin-1β in
    mature, 14, *16*, 16–17
    quantification of, 14
  management of
    cardiovascular system in, 189
    critical care and, 187–191
    neurosurgery's role in, 189–193, 194t
    outcomes with, 188
    pulmonary system in, 189
    variability of, 185–187, 188t
  medical therapies for, levels of, 176–178, 177t
  microvascular damage in, 113, 115
  neuroexcitation due to, 113–117
  neuroprotection targeted at, 118, 120t
  neuroprotection in, clinical trials, 118–122, 119t-122t
  oxygen free radical-induced damage after, 117–118
  neuroprotection targeted at, 119, 121t
  pathophysiology of, 113–124
  reactive oxygen species in, 13, 20–21
  regionalization of care for, 193–194
  standard therapies for, 171–172
    application to children, 171–172, 176
  therapeutic intervention in
    future directions for, 122–124
    ongoing clinical trials, 119, 122, 122t
Triangulated emitters, as surgical localizers, 34–36
Tricyclic antidepressants, for facial pain, 441–442, 450–451, 452t
Trigeminal memalgia, 450
Trigeminal motor weakness, after trigeminal neuralgia treatment, 412t, 414t–416t, 417
Trigeminal nerve-evoked potentials (TNEPs), 457
Trigeminal neuralgia, 435–440
  abnormal intraneuronal circuits in, 478–479

anticonvulsants for, 437, 439, 449–450, 462–463, 478
associated with multiple sclerosis, 421–422
atypical, 435, 439t, 439–440
  diagnosis of, 411
balloon compression for, 413, 457–460, 466–468, 470, 493–494
  advantages and disadvantages of, 418, 419t
  trigeminal motor weakness after, 416t, 417
clinical features of, 437, 437t, 478
as continuum of diagnosis, 443–444, 444
demyelination and, 455, 458, 477–478, 481
diagnosis, 410
diagnostic clues in, 448t
as discrete diagnosis, 443, 443–444
electrical stimulation for, 463–465, 468–469
etiology of, 455
glycerol rhizotomy for
  advantages and disadvantages of, 418, 419t
  repeat, 418, 421
glycerol rhyzolysis for, 413, 415t, 417–418, 419t, 460–461, 466–467, 491–494
idiopathic, 435, 437
imaging studies in, 436–438
intermittent symptoms of, 502
medical treatment of, 446–454, 462–463
microvascular decompression for. See Microvascular decompression
middle fossa technique for, 473–474
with multiple sclerosis, 478, 481
nerve impulse at false synapse in, 477
neuropathic, 423
neurophysiological theory of, 477–478
neurovascular decompression for, 455–457, 473–498
  age factors and, 494–495
  author's experience with, 484–488, 486t–488t
  comparison with alternative procedures, 488–494
  complications of, 483, 484t, 485, 487t

  failure of, 478–479, 488, 503–505
  Jannetta's series on, 481–484, 483t–485t, 501, 503
  long-term follow-up of, 487–488
  as procedure of choice, 494–495, 500
  results of, 481–488, 485t, 487t–489t, 503–505, 504t
  risks of, 495
pathophysiology of, 476–481
percutaneous stereotactic radiofrequency rhizotomy for
  advantages and disadvantages of, 418, 419t
  corneal anesthesia after, 414t, 417
  effectiveness, 411–413, 414t
  trigeminal motor weakness after, 414t, 417
percutaneous treatment of, 455–472, 488–494, 492t
  advances in, 455–465
  adverse effects of, 414t, 417, 468–470, 473, 490–491, 493, 495
  anesthetic for, 468, 493
  anticoagulation in, 469–470
  and carotid artery puncture, 470, 491
  mass lesions and, 470
  medical issues in, 469–470
  for multiple division pain, 467
  problems with, 465–469
  selective injury with, 466–467, 470
peripheral neurectomy for, 418, 419t
posttraumatic, 435
radiosurgery for, 413, 414t, 417 418, 419t, 461–462, 488–491, 491t, 494
recurrent
  with analgesia, 421
  in other trigeminal divisions, 420
  treatment of, 420–421
rhizotomy for, advantages and disadvantages of, 418, 419t
secondary, 435, 438t, 438–439
surgery for, 411, 444, 473–498
  advantages and disadvantages of, 418, 419t
  results of, 418, 419t
symptomatic, 435
with tumor, 422–423
thermal rhizotomy for, 455–457, 466–467, 470, 488–491
treatment of, 411–420

dysesthesia after, 412t, 413–417,
    414t–416t, 423, 459–460, 468, 473
  unilateral symptoms of, 502–503
  vascular compression in, 473–498
    aging and, 479
    contradictions in, 501–505
    debate over, 499–500
    duration of, 479
    minimalists' view of, 501–502
    negative explorations for, 480–481,
      482
    pulsatile, 480, 500–501
    root entry zone, 479–480, 501
    theory of, 499–506
    type of, 479, 487, 488t
    vascular elongation and, 479
    vessels involved in, 475, 479, 483,
      501, 501t
Trigeminal neuropathic pain, 435–436,
    440–441, 448t
  characteristics of, 440, 440t
  motor cortex stimulation for, 463–465,
    468–469
  treatment of, 440–441, 450, 463–465
Trigeminal nucleotomy-tractotomy
  percutaneous, 423, 425
  ultrasonic, for cluster headache, 428
Trigeminovascular system, in cluster
    headache, 426
  surgery of, 426t, 426–428
Trotter, W., 393
Trousseau, Armand, 446
Tuberculum sellae, meningiomas of, 563,
    564
Tumor(s)
  with carotid artery involvement
    benign, 340, 400
    malignant, 340–341, 399–400
    management of, 340–341, 399–400
  endoscopic-assisted microneurosurgery
    for, 515–525, 520, 522
  head and neck, management of,
    364–366, 366t, 370–371
  infrasellar, 517
  pituitary
    cluster headache with, 428
    endoscopic surgery for, 507–514
  skull base. See also Meningiomas
    contemporary treatment of, 554–574
    management of, 364–366, 366t,
      370–371, 399

  spinal
    endoscopic surgery for, 526, 528
    surgery for, spinal imaging for,
      84–85, 86
  suprasellar, 517
  symptomatic trigeminal neuralgia
    with, 422–423
  therapeutic carotid artery occlusion
    for, 340–341, 364–366, 366t,
    399–400
    ischemic complications of, 370–371,
      401
TUNEL immunohistochemistry, 14
Tuner, George Gray, 393

U
Ultrasound (US)
  abdominal, in hypotension with head
    injury, 137, 138
  and brain shift monitoring, 92
  intraoperative, 71
Urokinase
  endovascular, in acute stroke, 255
  for ruptured intracranial AVMs, 277

V
Vagoglossopharyngeal neuralgia, treat-
    ment of, 420t, 423–425
Vagoglossopharyngeal syncope, open rhi-
    zotomy for, 425
Valproic acid, for facial pain, 451t
Vascular compression. See also Neu-
    rovascular decompression
  asymptomatic, 502
  definition of, 500–501
  in hemifacial spasm, 474–476, 480,
    499, 502–503
  lack of effect on other cranial nerves,
    502
  in trigeminal neuralgia, 473–498
    aging and, 479
    contradictions in, 501–505
    debate over, 499–500
    duration of, 479
    and intermittent symptoms, 502
    minimalists' view of, 501–502
    negative explorations for, 480–481,
      482
    pulsatile, 480, 500–501
    root entry zone, 479–480, 501
    theory of, 499–506

type of, 479, 487, 488t
and unilateral symptoms, 502–503
vascular elongation and, 479
vessels involved in, *475,* 479, 483, 501, 501t
Venous malformations, intracranial, treatment of, 268–269, 279
Ventilation, in head injury. *See* Airway management
Ventricular system, as landmark, 49–50
Ventriculography, 49
Ventriculostomy, in pediatric head injury, 178
Vertebral artery, intracranial, stenosis, magnetic resonance angiography of, *249–251*
Vertebral column, 155
fractures and fracture dislocations of, *154,* 155–159, *156–158*
pediatric injuries of, 179–181
Vertebral reconstruction, 542, *544*
Vertebrectomy, thoracoscopic, 526, 541–543
clinical results of, 542–543
complications of, 543
technique of, 541–542, *542–544*
versus thoracotomy, 543

Virtual reality, 31
Vocal cord paralysis, after vagoglossopharyngeal neuralgia treatment, 424
Voice-activated computer navigation, 31
Voice-controlled robotic arm, for laparoscopy, 546, *546*
Vomer, 508

W
Watanabe, Eli, 90
Wells, Trent H., Jr., 56–57, *60,* 61, 90
Wepler, Johann J., 363
Willis, Thomas, 47
Winston, Ken, 90

X
Xenon computed tomography (CT), for measurement of cerebral blood flow, 250, 254, 328, 341–343, 355–356, 376–377, 385, 405
disadvantages of, 253, 377
flow activation with, 377
in stroke, 254
X-ray, in stereotactic technique, 49–50

Z
zVAD-fmk, 17–21, *18*